ORTHOPEDIC RADIOLOGY

A Practical Approach

Second Edition

ORTHOPEDIC RADIOLOGY

A Practical Approach

Second Edition

Adam Greenspan, M.D.

Professor of Radiology and Orthopedic Surgery
University of California,
Davis School of Medicine
Chief, Musculoskeletal Radiology
UCD Medical Center
Sacramento, California

Forewords by
Michael W. Chapman, M.D.
and
Harold G. Jacobson, M.D.

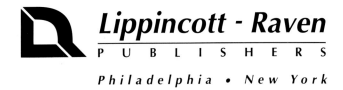

Lippincott - Raven
P U B L I S H E R S

Philadelphia • New York

Distributed in the USA and Canada by:
Lippincott-Raven Publishers, 227 East Washington Square,
Philadelphia, Pennsylvania 19106 USA

Distributed in Japan by:
Nankodo Company Ltd., 42-6, Hongo 3-Chome, Bunkyo-Ku
Tokyo 113, Japan

Printed in Singapore by Imago Productions (FE) Pte Ltd.

Library of Congress Cataloging-in-Publication Data
Greenspan, Adam.
Orthopedic radiology: a practical approach/Adam
Greenspan; foreword by Michael W. Chapman and
Harold G. Jacobson.—2nd ed.
p.   cm.
Includes bibliographical references and index.
ISBN 1-56375-023-6 (hard cover)
1. Radiography in orthopedics.   I. Title.
[DNLM: 1. Bone and Bones–radiography   WE
200 G815o]
RD734.5.R33G74   1992
617.3–-dc20
                                        92-1440

British Library Cataloguing-in-Publication Data.
A catalogue record for this book is available from the British Library.

Editor: Elizabeth Greenspan
Illustration Director: Laura Pardi Duprey
Illustrators: Laura Pardi Duprey (1st edition)
            Patricia Gast
Art Director: Jill Ruscoll, Kathryn Greenslade
Design Supervisor and Cover Design: Jeffrey S. Brown
Production Coordinator: Judy Ray
Editorial Assistant: Alison Marek

Acknowledgments

I would like to express appreciation to my colleagues from the Departments of Radiology and Orthopedic Surgery, University of California at Davis, for their invaluable comments that were extremely helpful in revising the older edition of this book.

I am also indebted to many friends from Gower Medical Publishing who helped me in the tedious work on this text. In particular, I am grateful to Elizabeth Greenspan, the editor and project manager, who, through her editorial skills and endurance in dealing with many technical difficulties, led this project to the happy ending. I would also like to express my thanks to the illustration director Laura Pardi Duprey and the illustrator Patricia Gast for the exceptional quality line drawings and schematics, to Daniel Benevento for the expert and high quality photographic work, and to Art Directors Kathryn Greenslade and Jill Ruscoll and designer Jeff Brown for the beautiful design. Finally, special thanks to Valerie Anderson and Carol Harris for their invaluable secretarial assistance. Without the cooperation and collective effort of these individuals this work would have never been accomplished.

To my wife Barbara, whose love and devotion made it all possible.

Preface

During the preparation of the first edition of *Orthopedic Radiology*, MRI was just evolving as a new modality with promise in musculoskeletal imaging, but was not yet in wide use. Since publication of the volume, MRI has proven to be an excellent noninvasive means of effectively evaluating many musculoskeletal abnormalities. Its high resolution and superb tissue contrast can delineate muscles, tendons, ligaments, menisci, cartilage, and bone marrow, and allow accurate assessment of these structures. The rapid and wide acceptance of MRI as an indispensable part of the diagnostic armamentarium of skeletal radiologists prompted the need to revise the book to include this modality. Sections on traumatic conditions of shoulder girdle, knee and spine, as well as the imaging of musculoskeletal tumors have received the preponderance of the added MR images, but this new modality is now represented in virtually every chapter.

There are also other changes. Two new chapters have been added: one on the use of the different radiologic imaging techniques in the evaluation of musculoskeletal disorders, and the other on bone formation and growth, which also clarifies the processes at work in several musculoskeletal abnormalities, particularly the skeletal dysplasias. The trauma section has updated text and new diagrams, especially in the chapters dealing with the shoulder and hand.

This section also features the addition of circular diagrams whose role is to give a quick visual reference to the spectrum of radiologic imaging techniques for evaluating injury in the various regions of the axial and appendicular skeleton.

The text of the arthritides section has been augmented with some important clinical information on hyperuricemia, rheumatoid factors, antinuclear antibodies, and the general examination of synovial fluid. In addition, new sections have been included on polymyositis and dermatomyositis, mixed connective tissue disease, vasculitis, calcium hydroxyapatite crystal deposition disease, hemochromatosis arthropathy, alkaptonuria, amyloid arthropathy, multicentric reticulohis-tiocytosis, hemophilic arthropathy, and arthritis associated with AIDS. Moreover, the section on musculoskeletal tumors now contains brief but pertinent information on the histopathologic findings in each entity to give the reader a more meaningful view of these abnormalities. Finally, the section on congenital and developmental anomalies has been updated to reflect the newest concepts concerning many of these disorders, particularly the sclerosing dysplasias for which a new classification has been developed. The references have been brought up to date, and instead of being grouped at the end of the book, they now appear at the end of each chapter for the reader's convenience.

These additions and changes, it is hoped, strengthen the overall usefulness of this volume to its primary audience—medical students and residents in radiology and orthopedics—and reinforce its purpose as stated in the Preface to the first edition: to facilitate the complex process of diagnostic investigation in a broad range of orthopedic disorders:

- by providing a basic understanding of the currently available imaging modalities,
- by helping in the choice of the most effective radiologic techniques with a view to minimizing the cost of examination and the exposure of patients to radiation, and
- by emphasizing the need for providing the orthopedic surgeon with the information required to choose the right therapy.

Although its aim is to teach, *Orthopedic Radiology* is also meant to serve as a quick and convenient reference for physicians interested in bone and joint disorders and those customarily employing radiologic studies in their everyday practice.

Adam Greenspan, M.D.
Sacramento, California

Forewords

The first edition of *Orthopedic Radiology* by Adam Greenspan was published just about the time that MRI began to make inroads as a new and important modality for use in studying the skeletal system. Because of the timing, only a handful of MRI illustrations were included in his book. The second edition, however, has been revised to include numerous illustrations and in-depth discussions relating to the use of this virtually indispensable modality.

It is of interest to note that MRI's development and the publication of the second edition of this book are consonant with the acceptance of skeletal radiology as a major discipline in the practice of medicine. MRI has rapidly become widely accepted in skeletal imaging as a method for graphically delineating both the normal and pathologic states of the various structures considered to be a part of the musculoskeletal system. This new modality has provided skeletal radiologists and orthopedic clinicians with an invaluable tool in their daily missions. Such structures as the various muscles, tendons, and ligaments, as well as other areas of the MS system, are now delineated by the radiologist with an incredible degree of accuracy. At the same time, skeletal radiology with MRI has furnished vital information concerning newly described tissue structures in the various organ systems. In addition to MRI, CT, plain film radiography, and scintigraphy play fundamental roles in the care of patients by the orthopedic clinician. This new edition of *Orthopedic Radiology* includes sections that discuss all of the various new imaging techniques used in MS disorders.

The chapters on trauma, particularly those sections dealing with the shoulder and hand, have been totally updated. The addition of circular diagrams provides a quick reference for considering and utilizing relevant techniques in evaluating skeletal trauma.

The material on the arthritides has been enlarged and modified. The section dealing with various crystal deposition disorders (e.g., calcium pyrophosphate deposition disease) is presented in a particularly pragmatic manner. Other related connective tissue abnormalities (e.g., scleroderma, dermatomyositis, polymyositis) are also included. Up-to-date material on such important entities as hemachromatosis, alkaptonuria, and amyloid arthropathy has been added. A section that deals with AIDS represents a timely addition to an extremely important field.

Also of significance is the expansion of a section on MS neoplasms, which contains concise descriptions of imaging features and other pertinent data. Included are fundamentally important pathologic findings presented in a correlative fashion.

Dr. Greenspan lists three basic goals of this new edition:
1. Providing the orthopedic clinician with an understanding of the currently available imaging;
2. Aiding all concerned with the choice of the most effective radiologic techniques, including plain films;
3. Aiding the orthopedic clinician in determinations regarding therapy for an individual patient.

Dr. Greenspan has carried out these goals admirably. His timely, important work adds positively to current literature on skeletal imaging.

In his preface for the new edition, Dr. Greenspan states that "these additions and changes, it is hoped, strengthen the work and insure its continued availability to its primary audience—medical students and residents in radiology and orthopedic surgery." Here I must demur. Dr. Greenspan is too modest to appreciate the quality and importance of his work or how helpful such a text is in providing information to experienced radiologists and orthopedic clinicians, as well as to medical students and residents. This book will help everyone.

The exciting world of skeletal radiology is comprised of clinical data, laboratory results, and relevant imaging, combined with information provided by the skilled and experienced skeletal pathologist, all acting in unison. Such close collaboration serves to establish this discipline of MS disorders as one of the most stimulating to which medical students and residents are exposed. In-depth studies of the musculoskeletal system may reach levels of complexity that are difficult to absorb. However, collaborative efforts must be encouraged and the concepts of cooperation must continue to grow. In this connection, Dr. Greenspan has added materially in the second edition of his work. The various imaging techniques and their results play a fundamental role in studying the musculoskeletal system. They are utilized constantly in conjunction with the histologic patterns in a multitude of areas in the musculoskeletal system.

The experienced skeletal radiologist and the skeletal pathologist must learn to work as a single functioning unit. Dr. Greenspan has added to this concept notably and he deserves heartfelt congratulations for a task well done.

Harold G. Jacobson, M.D.
Distinguished University Professor
Emeritus Professor and Chairman of Radiology
Albert Einstein College of Medicine and
 Montefiore Medical Center
Bronx, New York

Orthopedic Radiology: A Practical Approach was written with the student of musculoskeletal radiology in mind. It is aimed primarily at medical students and residents in radiology, orthopedics, and other specialties dealing with the musculoskeletal system. Dr. Greenspan's goals are to provide a basic understanding of imaging modalities, to help the clinician choose imaging modalities in a logical sequence, which is most effective from both a diagnostic and cost viewpoint, and to help provide the clinician with the information necessary to choose the appropriate treatment. Dr. Greenspan achieves his goals well, using over 1,400 superb x-ray film reproductions, diagrams, and tables.

Since Dr. Greenspan wrote the first edition in 1988, amazing advances have been made in the imaging of the musculoskeletal system, most notably in the technology and understanding of MRI as well as significant improvements in other imaging methods. In this second edition Dr. Greenspan provides us the current state of the art in this rapidly evolving field.

As I perused the text to prepare this foreward, I was enticed to continue reading by the superb reproductions of x-ray films with associated line drawings and the accompanying algorithms. As a result, I read the text from cover to cover. The text sharpened my understanding of the radiographic characteristics of many bone disorders, helped me to better understand the methodologies for obtaining special views, and increased the sophistication of my knowledge on selected disorders.

Chapter One, on the role of the orthopedic radiologist, establishes a logical stepwise sequence for the utilization of radiologic techniques, which is useful to any physician confronted with a musculoskeletal disorder. I commend this chapter not only to students of orthopedic radiology but to all primary care and specialty physicians and surgeons who encounter musculoskeletal disorders in their practice. The physician who follows Dr. Greenspan's approach to diagnostic imaging will better utilize both routine and specialized techniques. This will result in less exposure of patients to radiation and will substantially control the cost of imaging—an extremely important contribution in this era of rising medical costs and overutilization of diagnostic modalities.

Two new chapters on basic principles have been added to the second edition. The chapter on imaging techniques will help the reader understand better the advantages and disadvantages of the various imaging techniques. Keeping in mind the reader of this book, Dr. Greenspan does not explain the complex physics of MRI in great detail but provides excellent guidelines for the clinical use of this modality. The other new chapter is on bone formation and growth. The development of bone is basic to understanding the pathophysiology of bone dysplasias, growth disorders, and a host of skeletal disorders related to remodeling of bone.

Advances in genetics are increasing our knowledge about the pathophysiology of congenital and inherited disorders. A thorough knowledge of these processes is essential to understanding the pathology of the musculoskeletal system.

Chapter Four, on the radiologic evaluation of trauma, is beautifully presented and delineates a solid basis for fracture description, which provides a common ground of understanding and terminology useful to both the radiologist and the orthopedist. The standard it sets is helpful to us all and will enhance our communication and documentation of musculoskeletal disorders. I commend to the reader the excellent illustrations on positioning for radiographic views in the trauma chapters.

Each section begins with a chapter on the basic principles of radiologic evaluation, followed by chapters discussing specific disorders. The section-opening chapters are useful to all readers, but I strongly recommend that students and residents new to the field read each of them first. For example, Chapter Fifteen on the radiologic evaluation of tumors includes a wonderful series of charts, drawings, and x-ray film reproductions on how to approach bone lesions. These clear illustrations, such a Figure 15.29 on the distribution of tumors in vertebrae and Figure 15.46 on the differential diagnosis of primary soft tissue tumors versus primary bone tumors, offer quick guidelines to tumor recognition and easily remembered hints to diagnosis. Practitioners who are having difficulty establishing the differential diagnosis of an unusual bone lesion will find the points on differential diagnosis in these introductory chapters extremely useful.

The presentations of various entities in subsequent chapters in each section are very well illustrated and provide the clinician with an excellent guide to radiographic diagnosis on the majority of commonly encountered disorders. Moreover, a strong feature of this text is the "practical points to remember" at the end of each chapter, which student and practitioner alike will find helpful.

In summary, I believe *Orthopedic Radiology* will be an essential resource for medical students, residents, and fellows concerned with imaging of the musculoskeletal system. This text, especially the chapters on basic principles and the presentations on positioning, will also be a useful reference source for radiology technicians, paramedical personnel, and all physicians who need to have knowledge of imaging of the musculoskeletal system.

Michael W. Chapman, M.D.
Professor and Chairman
Department of Orthopaedic Surgery
University of Califormia
Davis School of Medicine
Sacramento, California

Table of Contents

Part IV Tumors and Tumor-Like Lesions

Part V Infections

Part VI Metabolic and Endocrine Disorders

Part VII Congenital and Developmental Anomalies

28 Scoliosis and Anomalies With General Affect on the Skeleton

PART I

Introduction to Orthopedic Radiology

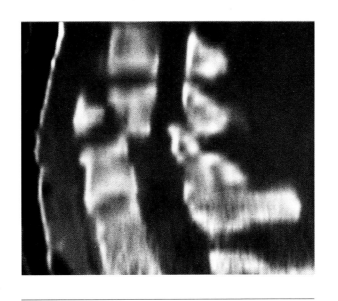

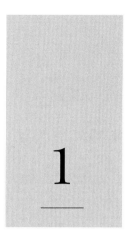

The Role of the
Orthopedic Radiologist

SPECTACULAR PROGRESS HAS BEEN MADE, and continues to be made, in the field of radiology. The introduction of new imaging modalities—computed tomography (CT) and its tridimensional (3-D) variant, digital subtraction radiography and its variant, digital subtraction angiography (DSA), radionuclide angiography and perfusion scintigraphy, magnetic resonance imaging (MRI), positron emission tomography (PET), single photon emission computerized tomography (SPECT), among others—has expanded the armamentarium of the radiologist, facilitating the sometimes difficult process of diagnosis. Yet these new technological developments have also brought with them some disadvantages. They have contributed to a dramatic rise in the cost of medical care and have often led clinicians, trying to keep up with new imaging modalities, to order too many, and frequently unnecessary, radiologic examinations.

This situation has served to emphasize the crucial importance of the role of the orthopedic radiologist and the place of conventional radiography. The radiologist must not only comply with prerequisites for various examinations but also—and more important—screen them to choose only those procedures that will lead to the correct diagnosis and evaluation of a given disorder. To this end, the radiologist should bear in mind the following objectives in the performance of his or her role:

1. To *diagnose an unknown disorder* preferably by using standard projections, along with the special views and techniques obtainable in conventional radiography before employing the more sophisticated modalities now available.
2. To perform examinations in the *proper sequence* and to know what should be done *next* in radiologic investigation.

3. To demonstrate the determining *radiologic features of a known disorder*, and the *distribution* of a lesion in the skeleton and its *location* in the bone, as well as to monitor the *progress of therapy* and possible *complications.*
4. To be aware of what *specific information* is important to the orthopedic surgeon.
5. To recognize the *limits of noninvasive radiologic investigation* and to know when to *proceed with invasive techniques.*
6. To recognize lesions that require biopsy and those that do not ("don't touch" lesions).
7. To assume occasionally a more active role in therapeutic management, such as performing an embolization procedure or delivering chemotherapeutic material by means of selective catheterization.

The radiologic diagnosis of many bone and joint disorders cannot be made solely on the basis of particular, recognizable radiographic patterns. Clinical data—the patient's age, sex, symptoms, history, and laboratory findings—are also important to the radiologist in correctly interpreting a radiograph. Occasionally, clinical information is so typical of a certain disorder that it alone may suffice as the basis for diagnosis. Pain that is characteristically most severe at night and is promptly relieved by salicylates, for example, is so highly suggestive of osteoid osteoma that often the radiologist's only task is finding the lesion. However, in many cases clinical data do not suffice and may even be misleading.

When presented with a patient, the etiology of whose complaint is *unknown* (Fig. 1.1) or *suspected* on the basis of clinical data (Fig. 1.2), the radiologist should avoid, as a point of departure in the examination, the more technologically sophisticated imaging modalities in favor of making a diagnosis, whenever possible, on the basis of simple conventional films. This approach is essential not only to maintain cost effectiveness but to decrease the amount of radiation to which a patient is exposed. Proceeding first with conventional technique also has a firm basis in the chemistry and physiology of bone. The calcium apatite crystal, one of the mineral constituents of bone, is an intrinsic contrast agent, which gives skeletal radiology a great advantage over other radiologic subspecialties and makes information on bone production and destruction readily available through conventional radiography. Simple observation of changes in the shape or density of normal bone, for example, in the vertebrae, can be a deciding factor in arriving at a specific diagnosis (Figs. 1.3, 1.4).

To aid the radiologist in the analysis of radiographic patterns and signs, some of which may be pathognomonic and others nonspecific, a number of options within the confines of conventional radiography are available. Certain *ways of positioning the patient* when radiographs are obtained afford the radiologist the opportunity to evaluate otherwise hidden anatomic sites and more suitably demonstrate a particular abnormality. The frog-lateral projection of the hip, for example, is better than the anteroposterior view for imaging the

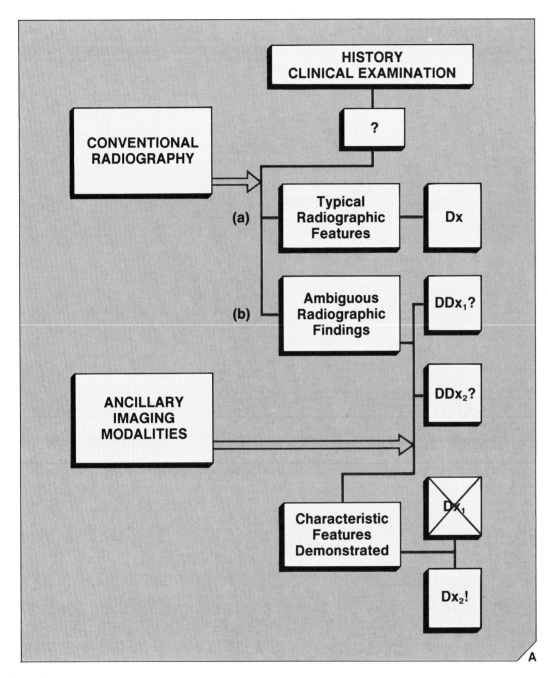

Figure 1.1 (A,B) The patient's history and the results of the clinical examination, supplied to the radiologist by the referring physician, are not sufficient to form a diagnosis (?). On the basis of conventional radiographic studies, (a) the diagnosis is established (Dx), or (b) the studies may suggest the differential possibilities (DDx). In the latter case, ancillary imaging techniques, such as tomography, arthrography, scintigraphy, computed tomography, or magnetic resonance imaging, among others, are called upon to confirm or exclude one of the options.

signs of suspected osteonecrosis of the femoral head by more readily demonstrating the crescent sign, the early radiographic feature of this condition (see Fig. 4.51B). The frog-lateral view is also extremely helpful in early diagnosis of slipped femoral capital epiphysis (see Fig. 27.30B). Likewise, the application of *special techniques* can help to identify a lesion that is difficult to detect on routine radiographs. Fractures of such complex structures as the elbow, wrist, ankle, and foot are not always demonstrated on the standard projections. Because of the overlap of bones on the lateral view of the elbow, for example, detecting a nondisplaced or minimally displaced fracture

of the radial head occasionally requires a special 45°-angle view (called the radial head-capitellum view) that projects the radial head free of adjacent structures, making an otherwise obscure lesion evident (see Fig. 5.49). Stress radiographic views are similarly useful, particularly in evaluating tears of various ligaments of the knee and ankle joints (see Figs. 4.3, 8.56, 9.9, 9.10).

An accurate diagnosis, then, depends on the radiologist's acute observations and careful analysis, in light of clinical information, of the radiographic findings regarding the size, shape, configuration, and density of a lesion, its location within the bone, and its distribu-

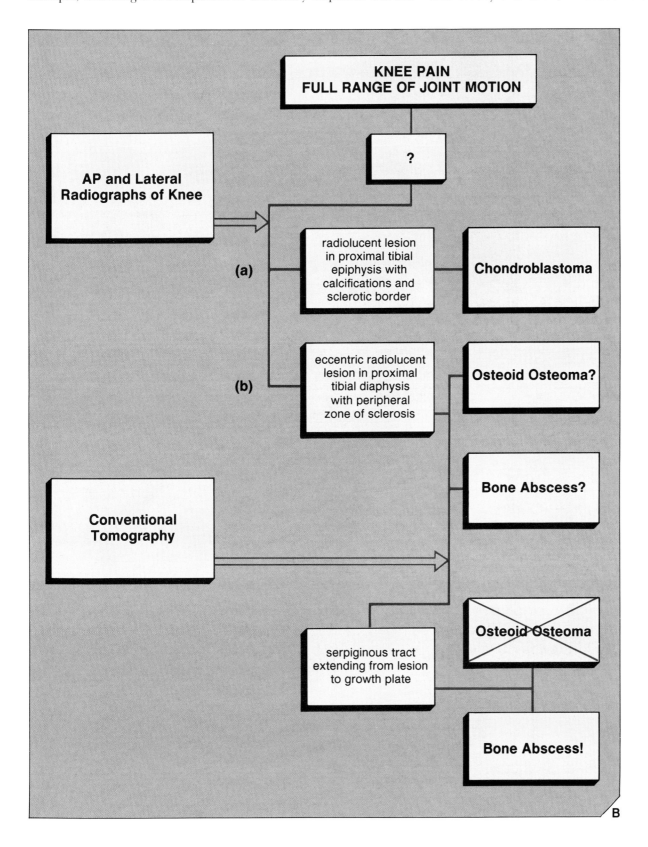

tion in the skeletal system. Until the conventional approach with its range of options fails to provide the radiographic findings necessary for correct diagnosis and precise evaluation of an abnormality, the radiologist need not turn to more costly procedures.

Knowing the *proper sequence* of procedures in radiologic investigation depends, to a great extent, on the pertinent clinical information provided by the referring physician. The choice of modality or modalities for imaging a lesion or investigating a pathologic process is dictated by the clinical presentation as well as by the equipment available, physician expertise, cost, and individual patient restrictions. Knowing *where to begin* and *what to do next*, as rudimentary as it may sound, is of paramount importance in reaching a precise diag-

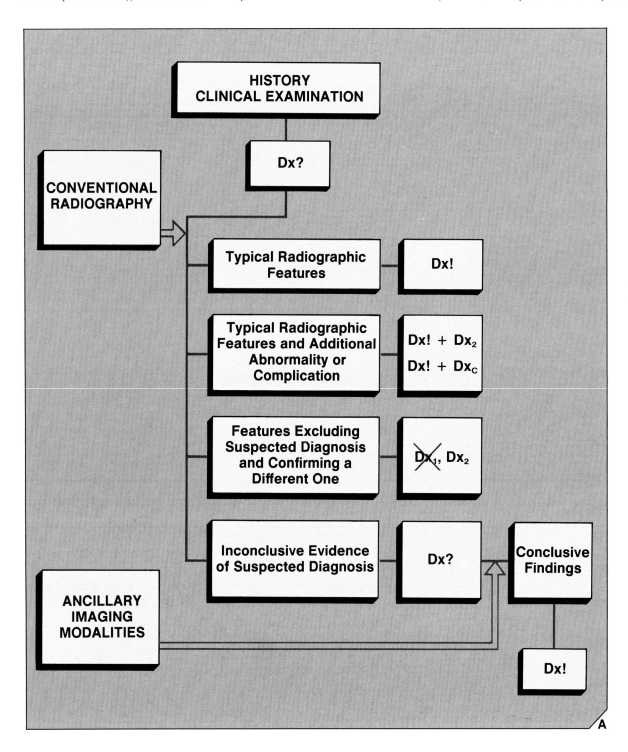

Figure 1.2 (A,B) From the information supplied by the referring physician, the radiologist may suspect the diagnosis (Dx?) and proceed with conventional radiographic studies. The results of the examination may confirm the suspected diagnosis (Dx!), reveal an additional abnormality (Dx! + Dx$_2$) or an unsuspected complication (Dx! + Dx$_c$), or exclude the suspected diagnosis and confirm a different one (~~Dx~~$_1$, Dx$_2$). The studies may also show inconclusive evidence of the original suspected diagnosis, in which case ancillary imaging modalities, such as scintigraphy, conventional tomography, computed tomography, or magnetic resonance imaging, among others, are employed (see Fig. 1.5).

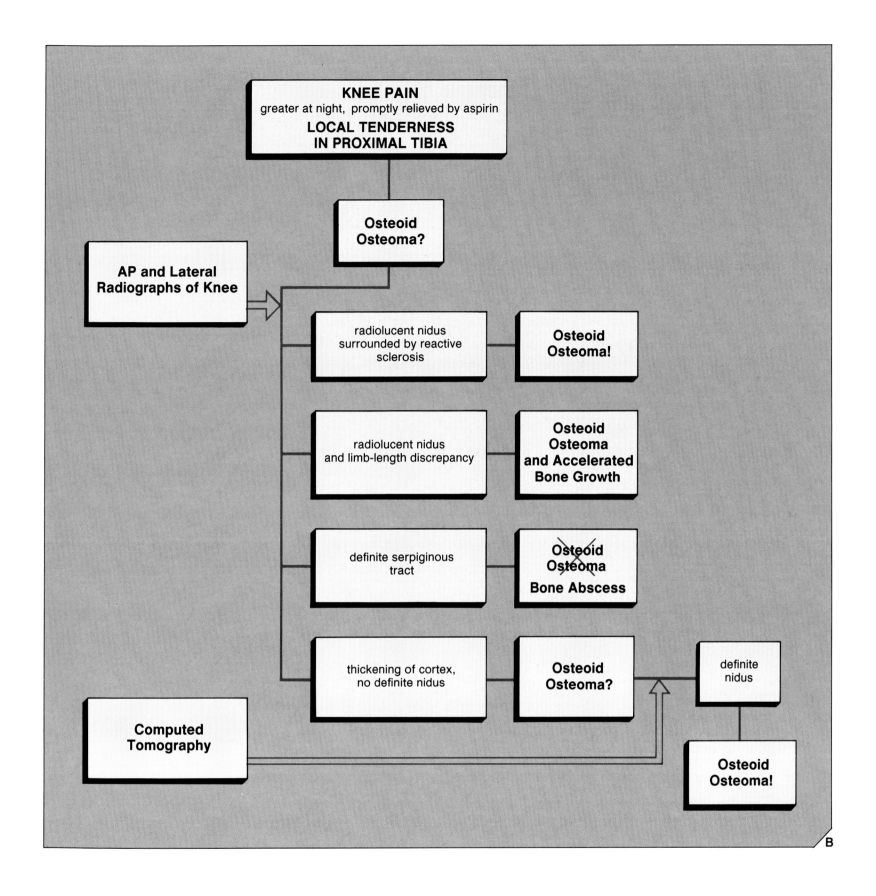

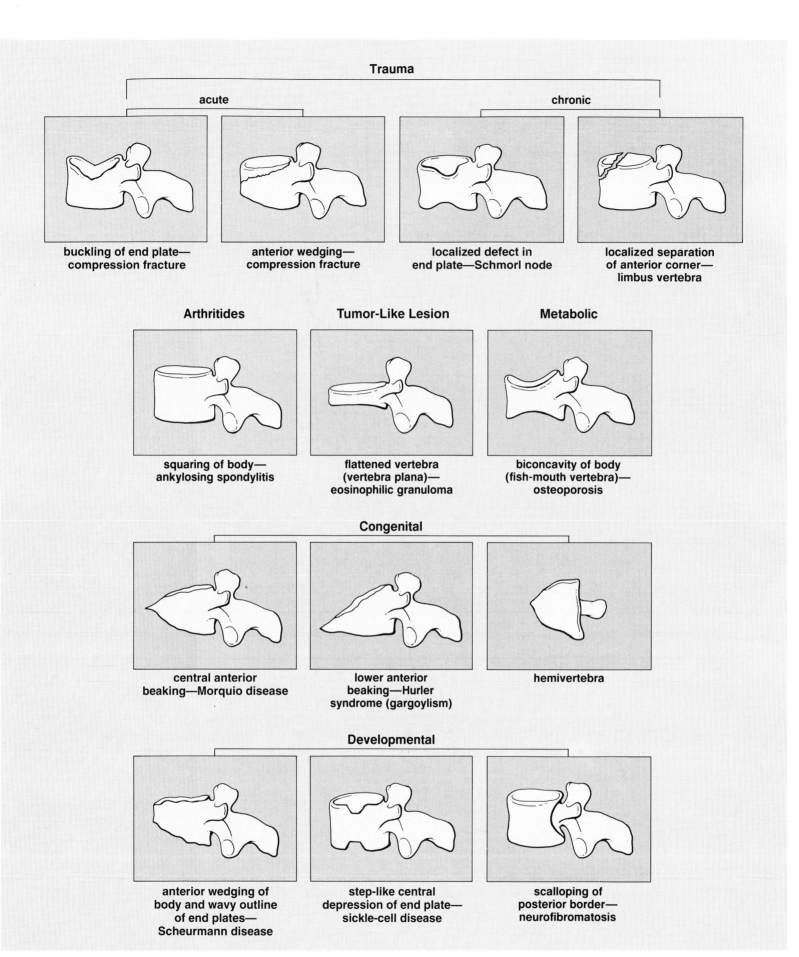

Figure 1.3 Observation of changes in the shape and contour of a vertebral body on conventional radiographs may disclose critical information leading to a correct diagnosis.

nosis by the shortest possible route with the least expense and detriment to the patient. Redundant studies should be avoided. For example, if a patient presents with arthritis, and the clinician is interested in demonstrating the distribution of "silent" sites of the disorder, the radiologist should not begin by obtaining radiographs of every joint—a so-called joint survey. It is instead more sensible to perform a scintigraphy and, afterward, to order films of only those areas showing increased uptake of radiopharmaceutical. A simple radionuclide bone scan rather than a broad-ranging bone survey is likewise a reasonable starting point in investigating other possible sites of involvement when a lesion is detected in a single bone and is

suspected of representing part of a multifocal or systemic disorder, such as polyostotic fibrous dysplasia or metastatic disease. Similarly, if a patient is suspected of having osteoid osteoma around the hip joint, and standard radiography has not demonstrated the nidus, a radionuclide bone scan should be performed next to determine the site of the lesion. This should be followed by conventional tomography and CT scan for more precise localization of a nidus in the bone. On the other hand, if the routine examination demonstrates the nidus, scintigraphy and conventional tomography can be omitted from the sequence of examination. At this point only CT scan is required to determine the lesion's exact location in the bone and to

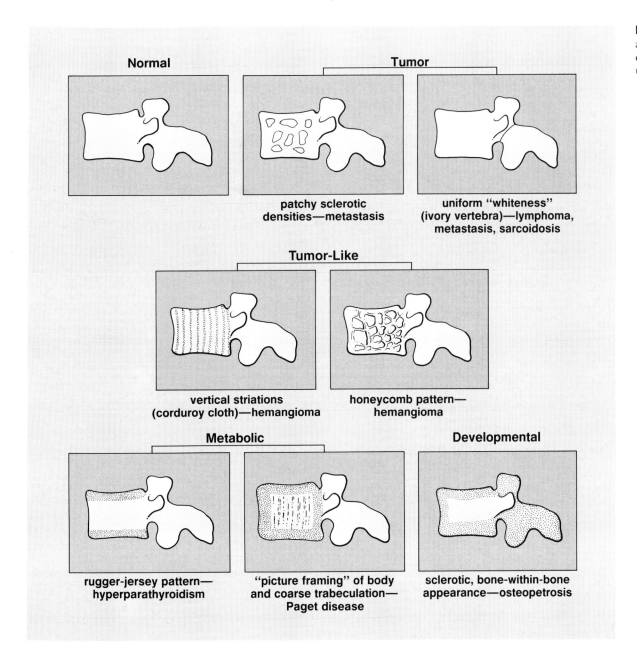

Figure 1.4 Changes in the density and texture of a vertebral body on conventional radiographs may offer useful data for arriving at a diagnosis.

obtain specific measurements of the nidus (Fig. 1.5; see also Fig. 16.9). If osteonecrosis (AVN) of the femoral head is suspected and the plain radiographs are normal, MRI should be ordered as the next diagnostic procedure, since it is a more sensitive modality than conventional tomography, CT, or even scintigraphy. The text that follows presents many similar situations in which the proper sequence of imaging modalities may dramatically shorten the diagnostic investigation.

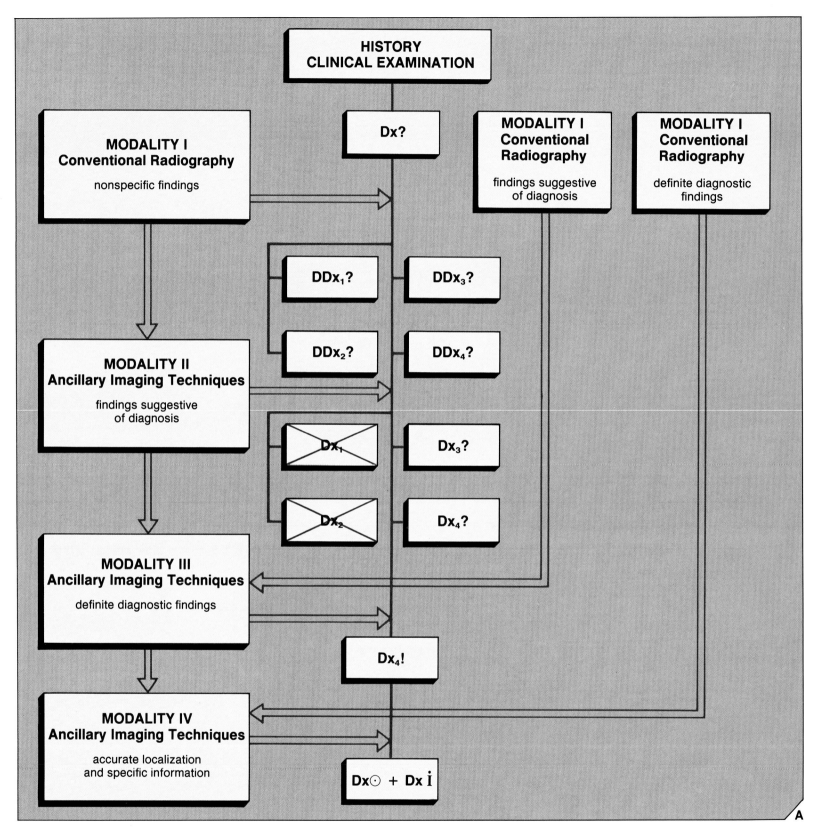

Figure 1.5 (A,B) A diagnosis is suspected (Dx?) on the basis of a patient's history and the results of the clinical examination. The radiologist suggests the proper sequence of imaging modalities, eliminating various disorders in the process and narrowing the differential possibilities to arrive at one correct diagnosis.

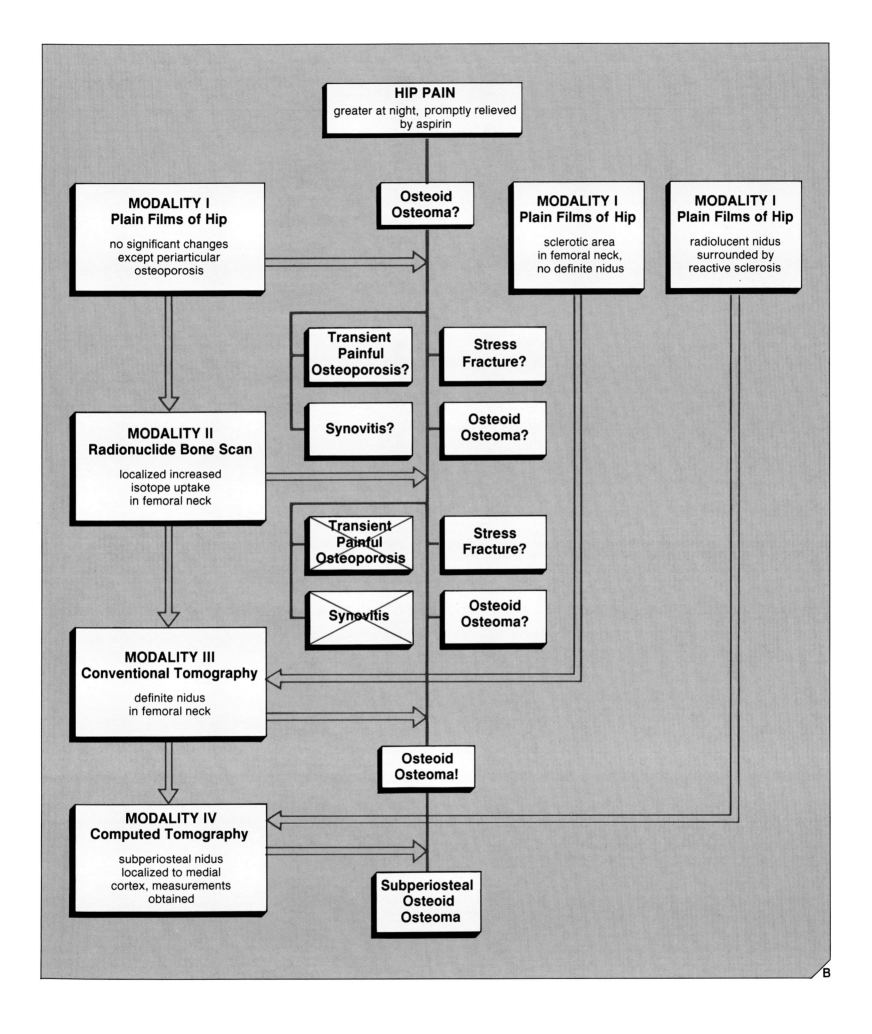

HIP PAIN
greater at night, promptly relieved by aspirin

Osteoid Osteoma?

MODALITY I
Plain Films of Hip
no significant changes except periarticular osteoporosis

MODALITY I
Plain Films of Hip
sclerotic area in femoral neck, no definite nidus

MODALITY I
Plain Films of Hip
radiolucent nidus surrounded by reactive sclerosis

Transient Painful Osteoporosis?

Stress Fracture?

Synovitis?

Osteoid Osteoma?

MODALITY II
Radionuclide Bone Scan
localized increased isotope uptake in femoral neck

Transient Painful Osteoporosis

Stress Fracture?

Synovitis

Osteoid Osteoma?

MODALITY III
Conventional Tomography
definite nidus in femoral neck

Osteoid Osteoma!

MODALITY IV
Computed Tomography
subperiosteal nidus localized to medial cortex, measurements obtained

Subperiosteal Osteoid Osteoma

B

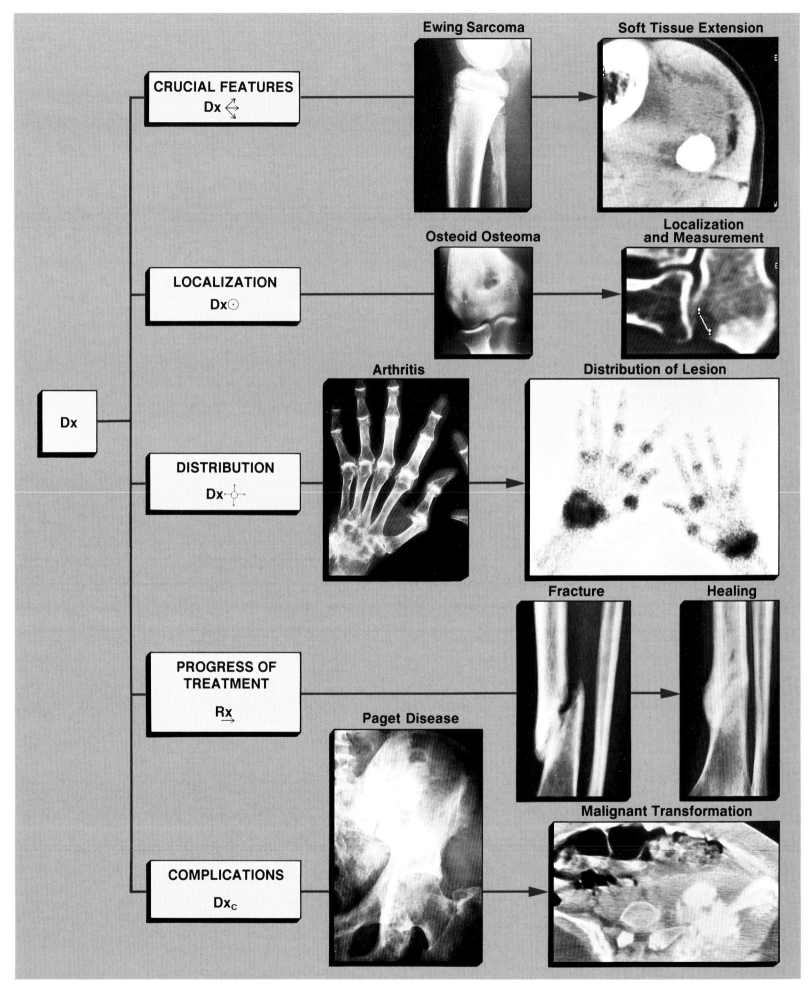

Figure 1.6 The diagnosis is known (Dx). The clinician is interested in demonstrating: (1) the crucial features of the lesion (Dx ⇄)—its character, extent, stage, and other pertinent data; (2) the location of the lesion in the bone (Dx ⊙); (3) the distribution of the lesion in the skeleton (Dx-⟡-); (4) the progress of treatment (Rx); and (5) the emergence of any complications (Dx_c).

Reaching a correct diagnosis does not end the process of radiologic investigation, since the course of treatment often depends on the *identification of distinguishing features of a particular disorder* (Fig. 1.6). For example, the diagnosis of Ewing sarcoma by plain-film radiography is only the beginning of a radiologic workup of the patient. The *crucial features* of this tumor must be identified, such as intraosseous and soft tissue extension (by CT or MRI) and the vascularity of the lesion (by arteriography). Similarly, a diagnosis of osteosarcoma must be followed by determination of the exact extent of the lesion in the bone and the status of bone marrow in the vicinity of the tumor. This can be accomplished by precise measurement of bone marrow density using Hounsfield numbers during CT examination (see Fig. 15.10) or by using MR images with or without contrast enhancement. Diagnosing Paget disease may be an important achievement in the investigation of an unknown disorder, but even more important is the further search for an answer to a crucial question: Is there any sign of malignant transformation (see Fig. 24.16)? *Localization* of a lesion in the skeleton or in a particular bone can frequently be more important than diagnosis itself. The best example of this is, again, the precise localization of the nidus of osteoid osteoma, since incomplete resection of this lesion invariably results in recurrence. Determining the *distribution of a lesion* in the skeleton is helpful in planning the treatment of various arthritides and the management of a patient with metastatic disease. Scintigraphy is an invaluable technique in this respect.

Many of the most important questions put to the radiologist by the orthopedic surgeon concern monitoring the *progress of treatment* and the appearance of possible *complications*. At the stage when the

diagnosis is already established, the fate of the lesion, and consequently the patient, must be established. Comparison of earlier radiographic examinations with present findings plays a crucial role at this stage, since it may disclose the dynamics of specific conditions (see Figs. 15.23, 27.22). Likewise, in monitoring the progress of healing fractures, study of the diagnostic sequence of radiographs complemented by tomography should decide questionable cases. Ancillary imaging techniques such as scintigraphy, CT, and MRI play an essential role in evaluating one of the most serious complications of benign tumors and tumor-like lesions—malignant transformation as may occur in enchondroma, osteochondroma, fibrous dysplasia, or Paget disease (see Figs. 16.46, 18.54, 24.16).

Providing the orthopedic surgeon with *specific information* is also an important function of the radiologist at the time when a diagnosis is being established. If, for example, osteochondritis dissecans is diagnosed, the decision on the choice of therapy requires information on the status of the articular cartilage covering the lesion. This information is obtainable by contrast arthrography, alone or combined with CT, or by MRI (see Figs. 8.43, 8.44). If the cartilage is intact, conservative treatment should be contemplated; if it is damaged, surgical intervention is the more likely course of treatment. Similarly, in contributing to the plan of treatment of anterior dislocation in the shoulder joint, the radiologist should be aware of the importance to the surgeon of information about the status of the cartilaginous labrum of the glenoid (see Fig. 5.16) and the possible presence of osteochondral bodies in the joint (see Fig. 5.72); these features must be confirmed or excluded by arthrography combined with tomography (arthrotomography), CT (computed arthrotomography), or MRI (Fig. 1.7).

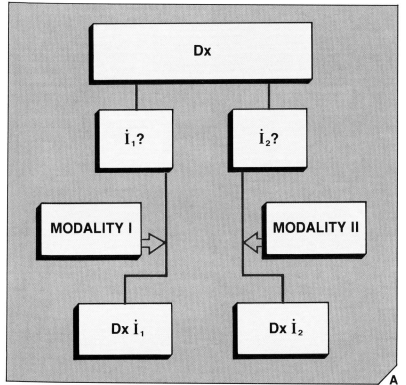
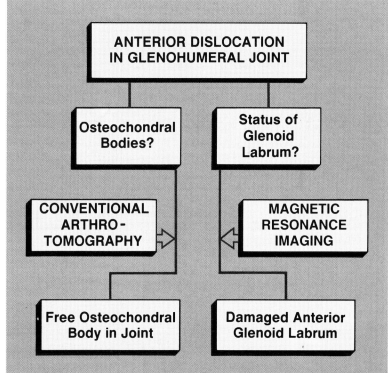

Figure 1.7 (A,B) The diagnosis is known (Dx). The radiologist should be aware of the specific information (i)—for example, regarding the features (i_1?) or extent (i_2?) of a lesion—that is required by the orthopedic surgeon in planning treatment. The information may also concern the distribution of a lesion and its localization, the progress of treatment, or the emergence of complications. Application of the best radiologic modality for demonstrating the required information is one of the radiologist's primary functions. The modalities may vary depending on the specific information needed.

References

Deutsch AL, Mink JH: Magnetic resonance imaging of musculoskeletal injuries. *Radiol Clin North Am* 27:983, 1989.

Elkin M: Issues in radiology related to new technologies. *Radiology* 143:1, 1982.

Margulis AR: Introduction to the algorithmic approach to radiology. In: Eisenberg RL, Amberg JR: *Critical Diagnostic Pathways in Radiology.* Philadelphia, Lippincott, 1981.

Nelson SW: Some important diagnostic and technical fundamentals in the radiology of trauma, with particular emphasis on skeletal trauma. *Radiol Clin North Am* 4:241, 1966.

Pitt MJ, Speer DP: Radiologic reporting of skeletal trauma. *Radiol Clin North Am* 28:247, 1990.

Renner RR, Mauler GG, Ambrose JL: The radiologist, the orthopaedist, the lawyer and the fracture. *Semin Roentgenol* 13:7, 1978.

Sartoris DJ: Musculoskeletal imaging: An evolving subspecialty. *Am J Roentgenol* 148:1186, 1987.

Straub WH: Current diagnostic imaging methods: Relative strengths and limitations. In: *Manual of Diagnostic Imaging: A Clinician's Guide to Clinical Problem Solving.* Boston, Little Brown, 1984.

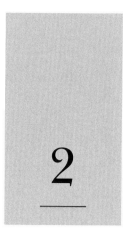

2

Imaging Techniques in Orthopedics

CHOICE OF IMAGING MODALITY

IN THIS CHAPTER, THE PRINCIPLES and limitations of current imaging modalities are described. Understanding the basis of the imaging modalities available to diagnose many commonly encountered disorders of the bones and joints is of utmost importance. It may help determine the most effective radiologic technique, minimizing the cost of examination as well as the exposure of patients to radiation. To this end, it is important to choose the modality appropriate for specific types of orthopedic abnormalities and, when using conventional techniques (namely plain radiography), to be familiar with the views and the techniques that best demonstrate the abnormality. It is important to re-emphasize that plain-film radiography remains the most effective means of demonstrating a bone and joint abnormality.

Use of radiologic techniques differs in evaluating the presence, type, and extent of various bone, joint, and soft-tissue abnormalities. Therefore, both the radiologist and orthopedic surgeon must know the indications for use of each technique, the limitations of a particular modality, and the appropriate imaging approaches for abnormalities at specific sites. The question "What modality should I use for this particular problem?" is frequently asked by radiologists and orthopedic surgeons alike and, although there are numerous algorithms available to evaluate various problems at different anatomic sites, the answer cannot always be clearly stated. The choice of techniques for imaging bone and soft-tissue abnormalities is dictated not only by clinical presentation but by equipment availability, expertise, and cost. Restrictions may also be imposed by the needs of individual patients. For example, allergy to ionic or nonionic iodinated contrast agents may preclude the use of arthrography; the presence of a pacemaker would preclude the use of magnetic resonance imaging (MRI); physiologic states, such as pregnancy, preclude the use of ionized radiation, favoring, for instance, sonography. Time and cost consideration should discourage redundant studies.

No matter what ancillary technique is used, plain film should be available for comparison. Most of the time, the choice of imaging technique is dictated by the type of suspected abnormality. For instance, if osteonecrosis is suspected after obtaining plain radiographs, the next examination should be MRI, which detects necrotic changes in bone long before plain films, tomography, computed tomography (CT), or scintigraphy becomes positive. In evaluation of internal derangement

of the knee, plain films should be obtained first and, if the abnormality is not obvious, should again be followed by MRI, since this modality provides exquisite contrast resolution of the bone marrow, articular cartilage, ligaments, menisci, and soft tissues. Arthrography and MRI are currently the most effective procedures for evaluation of rotator cuff abnormalities, particularly when detecting a partial or complete tear. Although ultrasonography can also detect a rotator cuff tear, its low sensitivity (68%) and low specificity (75% to 84%) make it a less definitive diagnostic procedure. In evaluating a painful wrist, conventional radiographs and trispiral tomography should precede use of more sophisticated techniques, such as arthrotomography or CT-arthrography. MRI is less desirable, since its sensitivity and specificity in detecting abnormalities of triangular fibrocartilage and various intercarpal ligaments is lower than that of CT-arthrotomography, particularly if a three-compartment injection is used. However, if carpal tunnel syndrome is suspected, MRI is preferred because it provides a high-contrast difference among muscles, tendons, ligaments, and nerves. Similarly, if osteonecrosis of carpal bones is suspected and the plain films are normal, MRI would be the method of choice to demonstrate this abnormality. In evaluation of fractures and fracture healing of carpal bones, trispiral tomography is still the procedure of choice—preferred over CT or MRI—because of the high degree of spatial resolution. In evaluation of bone tumors, plain-film radiography and tomography are still the gold standard for diagnostic purposes. However, to evaluate the intraosseous and soft-tissue extension of tumor, they should be followed by either CT scan or MRI, the latter modality being more accurate. To evaluate the results of radiotherapy and chemotherapy of malignant tumors, dynamic MRI using Gd-DTPA as a contrast enhancement is far superior to scintigraphy, CT, or even plain MRI.

IMAGING TECHNIQUES
Plain Film Radiography

The most frequently used modality for the evaluation of bone and joint disorders, and particularly traumatic conditions, is plain-film radiography. The radiologist should obtain at least two views of the bone involved, at 90° angles to each other, with each view including two adjacent joints. This decreases the risk of missing an associated fracture, subluxation, and/or dislocation at a site remote from the apparent primary injury. In children, it is frequently necessary to obtain a radiograph of the normal unaffected limb for comparison. Usually the standard films comprise the anteroposterior and lateral views; occasionally oblique and special views are necessary, particularly in evaluating complex structures, such as the elbow, wrist, ankle, and pelvis. A weight-bearing view may be of value for a dynamic evaluation of the joint space under the weight of the body. Special projections, such as those described in the following chapters, may at times be required to demonstrate an abnormality of the bone or joint to further advantage (see Figs. 4.2, 9.21, 9.22, 9.23, 10.10, etc.).

Magnification Radiography

Magnification radiography is occasionally used to enhance bony details not well appreciated on the standard radiographic projections and to maximize the diagnostic information obtainable from a radiographic image. This technique involves a small focal-spot radiographic tube, a special screen-film system, and increased object-to-film distance, resulting in a geometric enlargement that yields magnified images of the bones and joints with greater sharpness and greater bony detail. This technique is particularly effective in demonstrating early changes in some arthritides (see Fig. 11.7) as well as in various metabolic disorders (see Fig. 21.10B). Occasionally, it may be useful in demonstrating subtle fracture lines otherwise not seen on routine projections.

Stress Views

Stress views are important in evaluating ligamentous tears and joint stability. In the hand, abduction-stress film of the thumb may be obtained when gamekeeper's thumb, resulting from disruption of the ulnar collateral ligament of the first metacarpophalangeal joint, is suspected. In the lower extremity, the stress views of the knee and ankle joints are frequently obtained. Evaluation of knee instability due to ligament injuries may require use of this technique in cases of a suspected tear of the medial collateral ligament (see Fig. 8.16), and less frequently in evaluating an insufficiency of the anterior and posterior cruciate ligaments (see Fig. 8.17). Evaluation of ankle ligaments also requires stress radiography. Inversion (adduction) and anterior-draw stress films are the most frequently obtained stress views (see Figs. 9.9, 9.10).

Scanogram

The scanogram is the most widely used method for limb-length measurement. This technique requires a slit-beam diaphragm with a $\frac{1}{16}$-inch opening attached to the radiographic tube and a long film cassette. The radiographic tube moves in the long axis of the radiographic table. During exposure, the tube traverses the whole length of the film, scanning the entire extremity. This technique allows the x-ray beam to intersect the bone ends perpendicularly; therefore, comparative limb lengths can be measured. When a motorized radiographic tube is not available, a modified technique may be used with three separate exposures over the hip joints, knees, and ankles. In this technique, an opaque tape measure is placed longitudinally down the center of the radiographic table.

Fluoroscopy and Video Taping

Fluoroscopy is a fundamental diagnostic tool for many radiologic procedures including arthrography, tenography, bursography, arteriography, and percutaneous bone or soft tissue biopsy. Fluoroscopy combined with videotaping is useful in evaluating the kinematics of joints. Because of the high dose of radiation, however, it is only occasionally used, such as in evaluating the movement of various joints, or to detect transient subluxation (i.e., carpal instability). Occasionally, it is used after fractures in follow-up examination of the healing process to evaluate the solidity of the bony union. Fluoroscopy is still used in conjunction with myelography, where it is important to observe the movement of the contrast column in the subarachnoid space; in arthrography, to check proper placement of the needle and to monitor the flow of contrast medium; and intraoperatively, to assess reduction of a fracture or placement of hardware.

Digital Radiography

In digital radiography, a video processor and a digital disk are added to a fluoroscopy-imaging complex to provide on-line viewing of subtraction images. This technique is most widely used in evaluation of the vascular system, but it may also be used in conjunction with arthrography to evaluate various joints. Employment of high-performance video cameras with low noise characteristics allows single video frames of precontrast and postcontrast images to be used

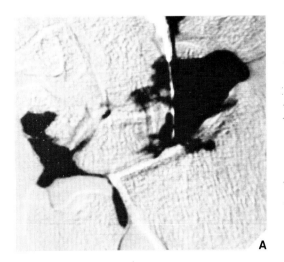
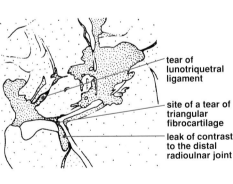

tear of
lunotriquetral
ligament

site of a tear of
triangular
fibrocartilage

leak of contrast
to the distal
radioulnar joint

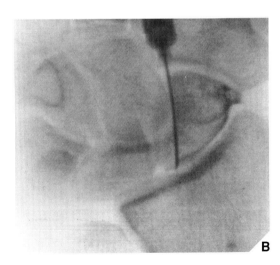

Figure 2.1 Digital subtraction arthrogram demonstrates tears of the lunotriquetral ligament and the triangular fibrocartilage complex. (A) This image was obtained by subtracting the digitally acquired preinjection image (B) from postinjection film. (Courtesy Dr. BJ Manaster, Salt Lake City, Utah)

for subtraction. Spatial resolution can be maximized using a combination of geometric magnification, electric magnification, and a small anode-target distance. The subtraction technique removes surrounding anatomic structures and thus isolates the opacified vessel or joint, making it more conspicuous.

Nonvascular digital radiography may be used to evaluate various bone abnormalities and, in conjunction with contrast injection, a procedure called digital subtraction arthrography (Fig. 2.1), to evaluate subtle abnormalities of the joints, such as tears of the triangular fibrocartilage or intercarpal ligaments in the wrist, or to evaluate the stability of prosthesis replacement. Digital radiography offers the potential advantages of improved image quality, contrast sensitivity, and exposure latitude, and provides efficient storage, retrieval, and transmission of radiographic image data. Digital images may be displayed on the film or on a video monitor. A significant advantage of image digitization is the ability to produce data with low noise and a wide dynamic range suitable for window-level analysis in a manner comparable to that employed in a CT scanner.

Digital subtraction angiography

Digital subtraction angiography (DSA), the most frequently used variant of digital radiography, can be employed in the evaluation of trauma, bone and soft-tissue tumors, and in general evaluation of the vascular system. In trauma to the extremity, DSA is effectively used to evaluate arterial occlusion, pseudoaneurysms, arteriovenous fistulas, and transection of the arteries. Some advantages of DSA over conventional film techniques are that its images can be studied rapidly and multiple repeated projections can be obtained. Bone subtraction is useful in clearly delineating the vascular structures. In evaluation of bone and soft-tissue tumors, DSA is an effective tool for mapping tumor vascularity.

Tomography

Tomography is a body section radiography that permits more accurate visualization of lesions too small to be noted on conventional radiographs or demonstrates anatomic detail obscured by overlying structures. It employs continuous motion of the radiographic tube and film cassette in opposite directions throughout exposure, with the fulcrum of the motion located in the plane of interest. By blurring structures above and below the area being examined, the object to be studied is sharply outlined on a single plane of focus. The focal plane may vary in thickness according to the distance the x-ray tube travels: the longer the distance (or arc) traveled by the tube, the thinner the section in focus. Newly developed tomographic units can localize the image more precisely and have aided greatly in the ability to detect lesions as small as approximately 1 mm.

The simplest tomographic movement is linear with the radiographic tube and film cassette moving on a straight line in opposite directions. This linear movement has little application in the study of bones because it creates streaks that often interfere with radiological interpretation. Resolution of the plane of focus is much clearer when there is more uniform blurring of undesired structures. This requires a multidirectional movement, such as in zonography or in circular tomography, in which the radiographic tube makes one circular motion at a preset angle of inclination. More complex multidirectional hypocycloidal or trispiral movements increase the distance the tube moves and create a varying angle of projection of the x-ray beam during the exposure. These complex movements are more advantageous because they produce even greater blurring and yield the sharpest images. Trispiral tomography is an important radiographic technique in the diagnosis and management of a variety of bone and joint problems. It continues to be a basic tool for examining patients who have sustained trauma to the skeletal system. Its advantages over conventional radiographs include the visualization of subtle fractures (see Fig. 4.4). It is not only helpful in delineating the fracture line and demonstrating its extent but also in evaluating the healing process (see Fig. 4.49B), posttraumatic complications (see Figs. 4.45, 4.51), and bone grafts in the treatment of nonunions. It is also invaluable in evaluating various tumor and tumor-like lesions (for instance, to

demonstrate a nidus of osteoid osteoma or to delineate calcific matrix in enchondroma or chondrosarcoma). Small cystic and sclerotic lesions and subtle erosions can also be better demonstrated. As a rule, the tomograms should be interpreted together with a plain radiograph for comparison.

Computed Tomography (CT)

CT is a radiologic modality containing an x-ray source, detectors, and a computer data-processing system. The essential components of a CT system include a circular scanning gantry, which houses the x-ray tube and image sensors, a table for the patient, an x-ray generator, and a computerized data processing unit. The patient lies on the table and is placed inside the gantry. The x-ray tube is rotated 360° around the patient while the computer collects the data and formulates an axial image, or "slice." Each cross-sectional slice represents a thickness between 0.3 cm to 1.5 cm of body tissue.

The newest CT scanners use a rotating fan of x-ray beams, a fixed ring of detectors, and a predetector collimator. A highly collimated x-ray beam is transmitted through the area being imaged. The tissues absorb the x-ray beam to various degrees depending on the atomic number and density of the specific tissue. The remaining, unabsorbed (unattenuated) beam passes through the tissues and is detected and processed by the computer. The CT computer software converts the x-ray beam attenuations of the tissue into a CT number (Hounsfield units) by comparing it with the attenuation of water. The attenuation of water is designated as 0 (zero) H, the attenuation of air is designated as -1000 H, and the attenuation of normal cortical bone is +1000 H. Routinely, axial sections are obtained; however, computer reconstruction (reformation) in multiple planes may be obtained if desired.

CT is indispensable in the evaluation of many traumatic conditions and various bone and soft tissue tumors because of its cross-sectional imaging capability. In trauma, CT is extremely useful to define the presence and extent of fracture or dislocation; to evaluate various intra-articular abnormalities such as damage to the articular cartilage or the presence of noncalcified and calcified osteocartilaginous bodies; and to evaluate adjacent soft tissues. CT is of particular importance in the detection of small bony fragments displaced into the joints following trauma; in the detection of small displaced fragments of the fractured vertebral body; and in the assessment of concomitant injury to the cord or thecal sac. The advantage of CT over conventional radiography is its ability to provide excellent contrast resolution, accurately measure the tissue attenuation coefficient, and obtain direct transaxial images (see Figs. 10.23C, 10.29B, 10.31B, 10.51C). A further advantage is its ability—through data obtained from thin, contiguous sections—to image the bone in the coronal, sagittal, and oblique planes, using reformation technique. This multiplanar reconstruction is particularly helpful in evaluating vertebral alignment (Fig. 2.2), demonstrating horizontally oriented fractures of the vertebral body, or evaluating complex fractures of the pelvis or calcaneus, abnormalities of the sacrum and sacroiliac joints, and sternum and sternoclavicular joints, as well as the temporomandibular joints and wrist. Modern CT scanners employ collimated fan beams directed only at the tissue layer under investigation. The newest advances in sophisticated software enable three dimensional reconstruction, which is helpful in analyzing regions with complex anatomy, such as the face, pelvis, vertebral column, foot, ankle, and wrist (Fig. 2.3). New computer systems now permit the creation of plastic models of the area of interest based on three-dimensional images. These models facilitate operative planning and allow rehearsal surgery of complex reconstructive procedures.

CT plays a significant role in the evaluation of bone and soft-tissue tumors, owing to its superior contrast resolution and its ability to accurately measure the tissue attenuation coefficient (see Fig. 2.4). Although CT by itself is rarely helpful in making a specific diagnosis, it can precisely evaluate the extent of the bone lesion and may demonstrate a break through the cortex and the involvement of surrounding soft tissues. Moreover, CT is very helpful in delineating a tumor in bones having complex anatomic structures, such as the

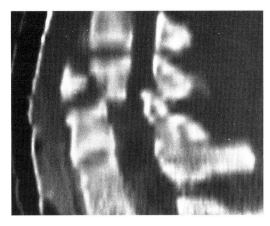
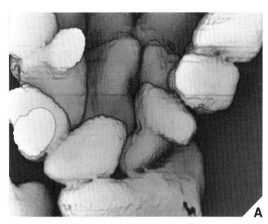

Figure 2.2 Sagittal CT reformation image demonstrates the flexion tear-drop fracture of C-5. It also effectively shows malalignment of the vertebral body and narrowing of the spinal canal. (Reproduced with permission from Greenspan A, 1992)

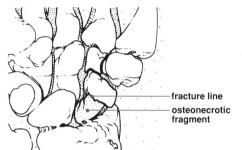

fracture line

osteonecrotic fragment

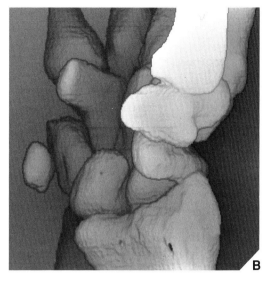

Figure 2.3 Anteroposterior (A) and oblique (B) 3-D CT reformation of the wrist demonstrates a fracture through the waist of the scaphoid bone, complicated by osteonecrosis of the proximal fragment.

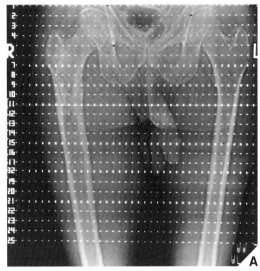

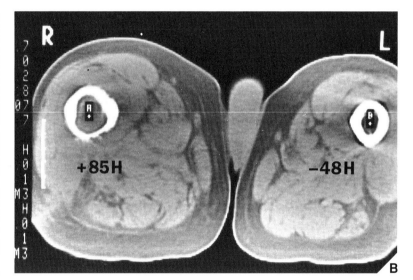

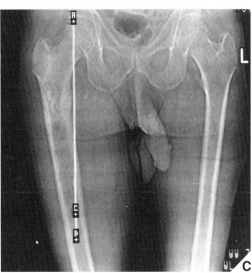

Figure 2.4 CT evaluation of intraosseous extension of chondrosarcoma is an important part of the radiologic work-up of a patient if limb salvage is contemplated. (A) Several contiguous axial sections, preferably 1 cm in thickness, of both affected and nonaffected limbs are obtained. (B) Hounsfield values of the bone marrow are measured to determine the distal extent of tumor in the medullary cavity. A value of +85 indicates the presence of tumor; a value of –48 is normal for fatty marrow. (C) The linear measurement is obtained from the proximal articular end of the bone *A* to the point located 5 cm distally to the tumor margin *B*. Point *C* corresponds to the most distal axial section that still shows tumor in the marrow. (Reproduced with permission from Greenspan A, 1989)

scapula, pelvis, and sacrum, which may be difficult to image fully with conventional radiographic techniques or even conventional tomography. CT examination is crucial to determine the extent and spread of a tumor in the bone if limb salvage is contemplated, so that a safe margin of resection can be planned (Fig. 2.4). It can effectively demonstrate the intraosseous extension of a tumor and its extraosseous involvement of soft tissues such as muscles and neurovascular bundles. It is also useful for monitoring the results of treatment, evaluating for recurrence of resected tumor, and demonstrating the effect of nonsurgical treatment such as radiation therapy and chemotherapy.

Occasionally iodinated contrast agents may be used intravenously to enhance the CT images. Contrast medium directly alters image contrast by increasing the x-ray attenuation, thus displaying increased brightness in the CT images. It can aid in identifying a suspected soft tissue mass when initial CTs are unremarkable, or it can assess the vascularity of the soft tissue or bone tumor.

CT has a crucial role in bone mineral analysis. The ability of CT to measure the attenuation coefficients of each pixel provides a basis for accurate quantitative bone mineral analysis in cancellous and cortical bone. The evaluation of bone mass measurement provides valuable insight into improving the evaluation and treatment of osteoporosis and other metabolic bone disorders.

CT is also a very important modality for successful aspiration or biopsy of bone or soft tissue lesions, since it provides visible guidance for precise placement of the instrument within the lesion (Fig. 2.5).

Some disadvantages of CT include the so-called average volume effect, which results from lack of homogeneity in the composition of the small volume of tissue. In particular, the measurement of Hounsfield units results in average values for the different components of the tissue. This partial volume effect becomes particularly important when normal and pathologic processes interface within a section under investigation. The other disadvantage of CT is poor tissue characterization. Despite the ability of CT to discriminate among some differences in density, a simple analysis of attenuation values does not permit precise histologic characterization. Moreover, any movement of the patient will produce artifacts that degrade the image quality. Similarly, an area that contains metal (for instance, prosthesis or various rods and screws) will produce significant artifacts. Finally, the radiation dose may occasionally be high, particularly when contiguous and overlapping sections are obtained during examination.

Arthrography

Arthrography is introduction of a contrast agent ("positive" contrast—iodide solution, "negative" contrast—air, or a combination of both) into the joint space. Despite the evolution of newer diagnostic imaging modalities, such as CT and MRI, arthrography has retained its importance in daily radiologic practice. The growing popularity of arthrography has been partially due to advances in its techniques and interpretation. The fact that it is not a technically difficult procedure and is much simpler to interpret than ultrasound, CT, or MRI makes it very desirable for evaluating various articulations. Although virtually every joint can be injected with contrast, the examination, at the present time, is most frequently performed in the shoulder, wrist, ankle, and elbow. It is important to obtain preliminary films prior to any arthrographic procedure, since contrast may obscure some joint abnormalities (i.e., osteochondral body) that can be easily detected on plain-film radiography. Arthrography is particularly effective in demonstrating rotator cuff tear (Fig. 2.6; see also Figs. 5.33B,C, 15.34) and adhesive capsulitis in the shoulder (see Fig. 5.36), and

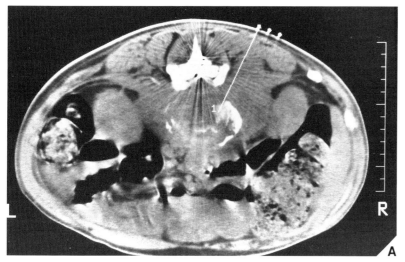

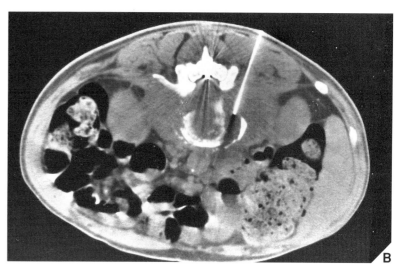

Figure 2.5 Aspiration biopsy of an infected disk is performed under CT guidance. (A) Measurement is obtained from the skin surface to the area of interest (intervertebral disk). (B) The needle is advanced under CT guidance and placed at the site of the destructive lesion.

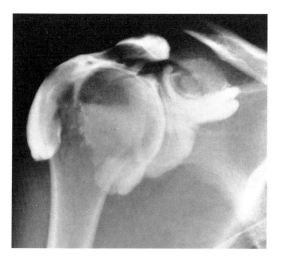

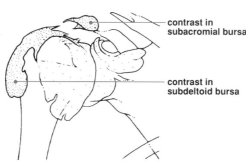

contrast in subacromial bursa

contrast in subdeltoid bursa

Figure 2.6 Shoulder arthrogram. After injection of contrast into the glenohumeral joint there is filling of subacromial-subdeltoid bursae complex, indicating rotator cuff tear.

osteochondritis dissecans, osteochondral bodies, and subtle abnormalities of the articular cartilage in the elbow joint (see Fig. 5.72). In the wrist, it is still the best procedure for evaluating triangular fibrocartilage complex abnormalities (see Figs. 6.7B,C, 6.20). Recent introduction of the three-compartment injection technique and the combination of arthrographic wrist examination with digital subtraction arthrography and postarthrographic CT examination have made this modality almost the procedure of choice when evaluating a painful wrist.

Although arthrography of the knee has been almost completely replaced by MRI, it still may be used to demonstrate injuries to the soft-tissue structures, such as the joint capsule, menisci, and various ligaments (see Fig. 8.51). It also provides important information on the status of the articular cartilage, particularly when subtle chondral or osteochondral fracture is suspected, or when the presence or absence of osteochondral bodies (i.e., in osteochondritis dissecans) must be confirmed (see Fig. 8.43).

In the examination of any of the joints, arthrography can be combined with tomography (so-called arthrotomography), with CT (CT-arthrography), or with digitization of image (digital subtraction arthrography), thus providing additional information (Fig. 2.7).

There are relatively few absolute contraindications to arthrography. Even hypersensitivity to iodine is a relative contraindication since, in this case, a single contrast study using only air can be performed.

Tenography and Bursography

Occasionally, in order to evaluate the integrity of a tendon, contrast material is injected into the tendon sheath. This procedure is known as a tenogram (see Figs. 9.12, 9.59). Since introduction of newer diagnostic modalities, such as CT and MRI, this procedure is seldom performed; it has relatively limited clinical application, being used mainly to evaluate traumatic or inflammatory conditions of the tendons (such as peroneus longus and brevis, tibialis anterior and posterior, and flexor digitorum longus) of the lower extremity, and in the upper extremity to outline the synovial sheaths within the carpal tunnel.

Bursography involves the injection of contrast agent into various bursae. This procedure in general has been abandoned, and only occasionally is subacromial-subdeltoid bursae complex directly injected with contrast agent to demonstrate partial tears of the rotator cuff.

Angiography

The use of contrast material injected directly into selective branches of both the arterial and venous circulation has aided greatly in assessing the involvement of the circulatory system in various conditions and has provided a precise method for defining local pathology. With arteriography, a contrast agent is injected into the arteries and films are made, usually in rapid sequence. With venography, contrast material is injected into the veins. Both procedures are frequently used in evaluation of trauma, particularly if concomitant injury to the vascular system is suspected (see Fig. 4.10).

In evaluation of tumors, arteriography is used mainly to map out bone lesions, demonstrate the vascularity of the lesion, and assess the extent of disease. It is also used to demonstrate the vascular supply of a tumor and to locate vessels suitable for preoperative intra-arterial chemotherapy. It is very useful in demonstrating the area suitable for open biopsy, since the most vascular parts of a tumor contain the most aggressive component of the lesion. Occasionally, arteriography can be used to demonstrate abnormal tumor vessels, corroborating findings with plain-film radiography and tomography (see Fig. 15.13). Arteriography is often extremely helpful in planning for limb-salvage procedures, since it demonstrates the regional vascular anatomy and thus permits a plan to be drawn up for the resectioning. It is also sometimes used to outline the major vessels prior to resection of a benign tumor (see Fig. 15.14). It can also be combined with an interventional procedure, such as embolization of hypervascular tumors, prior to further treatment (see Fig. 15.15).

Myelography

During this procedure, water-soluble contrast agents are injected into the subarachnoid space, mixing freely with the cerebrospinal fluid to produce a column of opacified fluid with a higher specific gravity than the nonopacified fluid. Tilting the patient will allow the opacified fluid to run up or down the thecal sac under the influence of gravity (see Figs. 10.17, 10.44). The puncture usually is done in the lumbar area at the L2-3 or L3-4 levels. For examination of the cervical segment, a C1-2 puncture is performed (see Fig. 10.17A). Myelographic examination has been almost completely replaced by high-resolution CT and high-quality MRI.

Diskography

Diskography is an injection of contrast material into the nucleus pulposus. Although this is a controversial procedure that has been abandoned by many investigators, under tightly restricted indications and immaculate technique a diskogram can yield valuable information. Diskography is a valuable aid to determine the source of a patient's low back pain. It is not purely an imaging technique, since the symptoms produced during the test (pain during the injection) are considered to have even greater diagnostic value than the obtained radiographs. It should always be combined with CT examination (so-called CT-diskogram) (see Figs. 10.45, 10.73B,C). According to the official position statement on diskography by the Executive Committee of the North American Spine Society in 1988, this procedure "is indicated in the evaluation of patients with unremitting spinal pain, with or without extremity pain, of greater than four months duration, when the pain has been unresponsive to all appropriate methods of conservative therapy." According to the same statement, before a diskogram is performed, the patient should have undergone investigation with other modalities (such as CT, MRI, and myelography) and the surgical correction of the patient's problem should be anticipated.

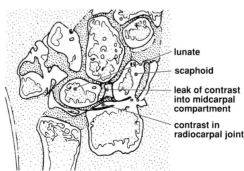

Figure 2.7 Coronal CT arthrogram of the wrist demonstrates a subtle leak of contrast from the radiocarpal joint through a tear in the scapholunate ligament, a finding not detected on routine arthrographic examination of the wrist.

lunate

scaphoid

leak of contrast into midcarpal compartment

contrast in radiocarpal joint

Ultrasonography

Over the past several years, ultrasound has made an enormous impact in the field of radiology; however, it is only rarely used in skeletal radiology. It has several inherent advantages: It is relatively inexpensive, allows comparisons with the opposite, normal side, uses no ionizing radiation, and can be performed at bedside or in the operating room. It is a noninvasive modality, relying upon the interaction of propagated sound waves with tissue interfaces in the body. Whenever the directed pulsing of sound waves encounters an interface between tissues of different acoustic impedance, reflection or refraction occurs. The sound waves reflected back to the ultrasound transducer are recorded and converted into images.

Various types of ultrasound scanning are available. Most modern ultrasound equipment displays dynamic information in "real time" similar to information that is provided by fluoroscopy. With real-time sonography, the images may be obtained in any scan plane by simply moving the transducer. Thus, imaging may include transverse or longitudinal images and any obliquity can also be produced. Modern probe technology has extended to some degree the use of ultrasound in orthopedic radiology (Fig. 2.8). Higher frequency transducers of 7.5 MHz and 10 MHz have excellent spatial resolution and are ideal for imaging the appendicular skeleton.

Applications of ultrasound in orthopedics include the evaluation of infants with suspected congenital hip dislocations, evaluation of the rotator cuff, injuries to various tendons (for instance, the Achilles tendon), and, occasionally, soft tissue tumors (such as hemangioma). Ultrasound has recently been applied to certain areas in rheumatic disorders, in particular to detect intra-articular and periarticular fluid collection, and to the differentiation of popliteal fossa masses (e.g., aneurysm versus Baker cyst versus hypertrophied synovium).

More recent ultrasound techniques such as Doppler ultrasound or colorflow imaging, which expresses motion from moving red blood cells in color, have found limited applications in orthopedic radiology. This modality is used mainly to detect arterial narrowing and venous thrombosis. However, there have been a limited number of reports regarding the use of this technology in detecting tumor vascularity within soft tissue masses.

Scintigraphy (Radionuclide Bone Scan)

Scintigraphy is a modality that detects the distribution in the body of a radioactive agent injected into the vascular system. Following an intravenous injection of radiopharmaceutical agent, the patient is placed under a scintillation camera, which detects the distribution of radioactivity in the body by measuring the interaction of gamma rays emitted from the body with sodium iodide crystals in the head of the camera. The photoscans are obtained in multiple projections and may include either the entire body or selected parts.

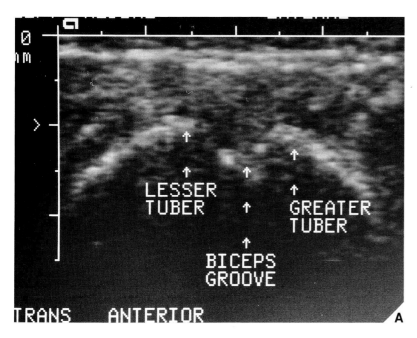

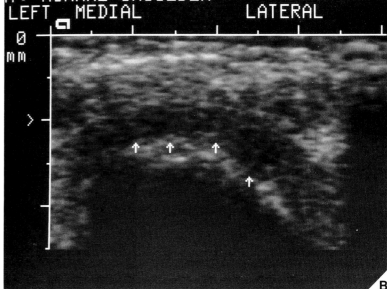

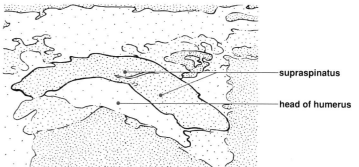

Figure 2.8 Ultrasonography of the shoulder. (A) The bony landmarks (lesser and greater tuberosities, bicipital tendon groove) and (B) tendinous structures (supraspinatus) are well outlined.

One major advantage of skeletal scintigraphy over all other imaging techniques is its ability to image the entire skeleton at once (Fig. 2.9). Bone scan may confirm the presence of the disease, demonstrate the distribution of the lesion, and help evaluate the pathologic process. Indications for skeletal scintigraphy include traumatic conditions, tumors (primary and metastatic), various arthritides, infections, and metabolic bone disease. The detected abnormality may consist of either decreased uptake of bone-seeking radiopharmaceutical (for instance, in the early stage of osteonecrosis) or increased uptake (such as in the case of fracture, neoplasm, a focus of osteomyelitis, etc.). Some structures under normal conditions may show increased activity (such as sacroiliac joints or normal growth plates).

Scintigraphy is a very sensitive imaging modality; however, it is not very specific, and it is impossible to distinguish various processes that can cause increased uptake. Occasionally, however, the bone scan may yield very specific information and even suggest diagnosis, for instance, in multiple myeloma or osteoid osteoma. In the search for myeloma, scintigraphy can distinguish between similar looking bony metastases since in most myeloma cases no significant increase in the uptake of the radiopharmaceutical agent occurs, while in skeletal metastasis invariably the uptake of the tracer is significantly elevated. In the case of osteoid osteoma, the typical bone scan demonstrates the so-called double density sign—greater increased uptake in the center, related to the nidus of the lesion, and lesser increased uptake at the periphery, related to the reactive sclerosis surrounding the nidus (Fig. 2.10).

Radionuclide bone scan is an indicator of mineral turnover. Because there is usually an enhanced deposition of bone-seeking radiopharmaceuticals in areas of bone undergoing change and repair, bone scan is useful in localizing tumors and tumor-like lesions in the skeleton. This is particularly helpful in such conditions as fibrous dysplasia, eosinophilic granuloma, or metastatic cancer, where more than one lesion is encountered, and some may represent a "silent" site of disorder. It also plays an important role in localizing small lesions, such as osteoid osteoma, which may not always be seen on plain-film studies. In most instances radionuclide bone scan cannot distinguish benign lesions from malignant tumors, since increased blood flow with consequently increased isotope deposition and osteoblastic activity will take place in both conditions. However, it occasionally makes the differentiation in a benign lesion (such as a bone island) that does not absorb the radioactive isotope (see Fig. 15.21).

In traumatic conditions, scintigraphy is extremely helpful in the early diagnosis of stress fractures. These fractures may not be seen on conventional radiographs or even on tomographic studies. It also has value in diagnosing fractures of the scaphoid or the femoral neck in elderly patients when routine radiographic examinations appear normal.

In metabolic bone disorders, bone scintigraphy is helpful, for instance, in establishing the extent of skeletal involvement in Paget disease (see Fig. 21.12) and assessing response to treatment. Although it is of no value for patients with generalized osteoporosis, it may occasionally be helpful in differentiating osteoporosis from osteomalacia and multiple vertebral fractures resulting from osteoporosis from those occurring in metastatic carcinoma.

Skeletal scintigraphy is frequently used in evaluation of infections. In particular, technetium-99m MDP and indium-111 are highly sensitive in detecting early and occult osteomyelitis. In chronic osteomyelitis, imaging with Gallium-67 citrate is more accurate in detecting the response or lack of response to treatment than ^{99m}Tc-phosphate bone imaging. For detecting recurrent active infection in patients with chronic osteomyelitis, ^{111}In appears to be the radiopharmaceutical of choice. The three-phase technique using technetium phosphate tracers can be effectively employed to distinguish between soft tissue infection (cellulitis) and osseous infection (osteomyelitis).

In neoplastic conditions, the detection of skeletal metastasis is probably the most common indication for skeletal scintigraphy. It also is used frequently to determine the extent of a lesion or the presence of so-called skipped lesions or intraosseous metastases. It

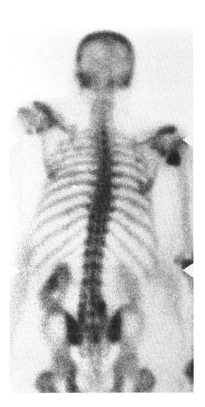 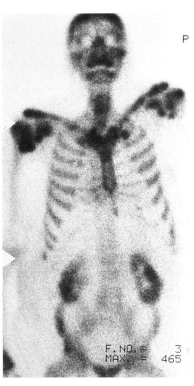 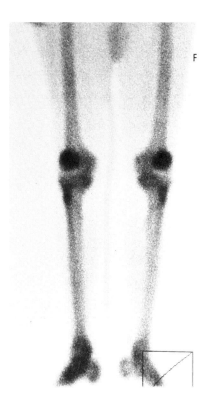

Figure 2.9 Radionuclide bone scan obtained in a patient with renal disease and secondary hyperparathyroidism demonstrates several abnormalities: left hydronephrosis secondary to urinary obstruction, resorptive changes of the distal ends of both clavicles, and periarticular soft tissue calcifications around both shoulders.

is not, however, the method of choice to determine the extent of the lesion in bone. It is important to stress that scintigraphy alone cannot diagnose the type of tumor; however, it may be useful to detect and localize some primary tumors as well as multifocal lesions (such as multicentric osteosarcoma).

Technetium-99m MDP scans are used primarily to determine whether a lesion is monostotic or polyostotic. Such a study is therefore essential in staging a bone tumor. It is important to remember that, although the degree of abnormal uptake may be related to the aggressiveness of the lesion, this does not correlate well with histologic grade. Gallium-67 may show uptake in a soft-tissue sarcoma and may help to differentiate a sarcoma from a benign soft-tissue lesion.

Although a bone scan may be useful in demonstrating the extent of the primary malignant tumor in bone, it is not as accurate as CT or MRI. It may be useful in the detection of a local recurrence of the tumor and occasionally indicates the response or lack of response to treatment (in the case of radiotherapy or chemotherapy).

In the evaluation of arthritides, a bone scan is extremely helpful in

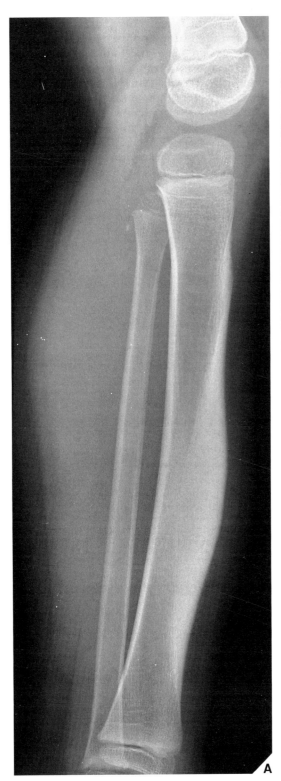

A

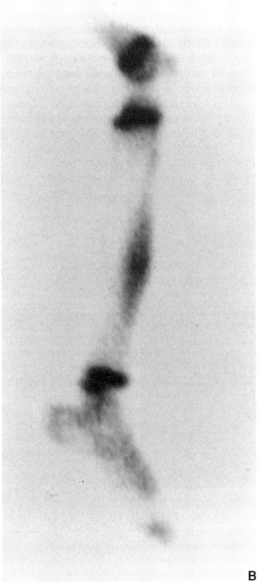

B

Figure 2.10 A four-year-old girl had symptoms suggesting a diagnosis of osteoid osteoma; however, a plain radiograph (A) failed to demonstrate the nidus. Scintigraphic examination (B) demonstrates a characteristic "double density" sign: More increased uptake in the center is related to the nidus of osteoid osteoma, while less increased uptake at the periphery denotes reactive sclerosis.

muscle and b) signal higher than muscle but lower than subcutaneous fat (bright). *High signal intensity* may be subdivided into a) signal equal to normal subcutaneous fat (bright) and b) signal higher than subcutaneous fat (extremely bright). High signal intensity of fat planes and differences in signal intensity of various structures allow separation of the different tissue components including muscles, tendons, ligaments, vessels, nerves, hyalin cartilage, fibrocartilage, cortical bone, and trabecular bone (Fig. 2.12). For instance: fat and yellow (fatty) bone marrow display high signal intensity on T1- and intermediate signal on T2-weighted images; hematoma display relatively high signal intensity. Cortical bone, air, ligaments, tendons, and fibrocartilage display low signal intensity on T1- and T2-weighted images; muscle, nerves, and hyaline cartilage display intermediate signal intensity on T1- and T2-weighted images. Red (hematopoietic) marrow displays low signal on T1- and low-to-intermediate signal on T2-weighted images. Fluid displays intermediate signal on T1- and high signal on T2-weighting. Most tumors display low to intermediate signal intensity on T1-weighted images and high signal intensity on T2-weighted images. Lipomas display high signal intensity on T1- and intermediate signal on T2-weighted images.

Occasionally MR images may be enhanced by intravenous injection of gadopentate dimeglumine (Gd-DTPA), known as gadolinium. The mechanism by which gadolinium produces enhancement in MRI is fundamentally different from the mechanism of contrast enhancement in CT. Unlike iodine in CT, gadolinium itself produces no MRI signal. Instead it acts by shortening the T1- and T2-relaxation times of tissues into which it extravasates, resulting in an increase in signal intensity on T1-weighted (short TR/TE) imaging sequences.

Although MRI has many advantages, disadvantages exist as well. These include the typical contraindications of scanning patients with cardiac pacemakers, cerebral aneurysm clips, and claustrophobia. The presence of metallic objects, such as ferromagnetic surgical clips, causes focal loss of signal with or without distortion of image. Metallic objects create "holes" in the image, but ferromagnetic objects cause more distortion. Another disadvantage is that MRI still lacks high resolution in evaluation of osseous anatomy and fractures compared to CT and conventional tomography. Similar to CT, an average volume effect may be observed in MR images, causing occasional pitfalls in the interpretation.

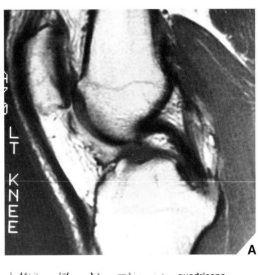
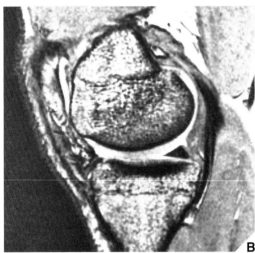

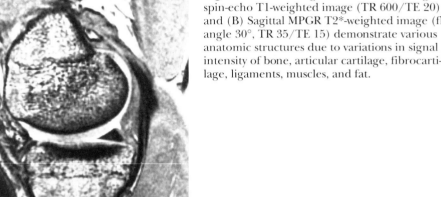

Figure 2.12 MR image of the knee. (A) Sagittal spin-echo T1-weighted image (TR 600/TE 20) and (B) Sagittal MPGR T2*-weighted image (flip angle 30°, TR 35/TE 15) demonstrate various anatomic structures due to variations in signal intensity of bone, articular cartilage, fibrocartilage, ligaments, muscles, and fat.

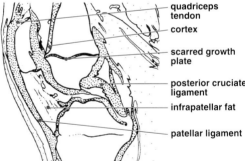
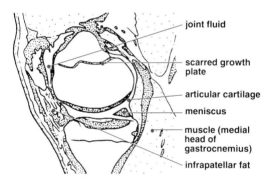

References

Aisen AN, Martel W, Braunstein EM, McMillin KI, Phillips WA, Kling TF: MRI and CT evaluation of primary bone and soft tissue tumors. *Am J Radiol* 146:749, 1986.

Al Sheikh W, Sfakianakis GN, Mnaymneh W, et al: Subacute and chronic bone infections: Diagnosis using In-111, Ga-67, and Tc-99m MDP bone scintigraphy and radiography. *Radiology* 155:501, 1985.

Baker LL, Goodman SB, Perkash I, Lane B, Enzmann DR: Benign versus pathologic compression fractures of vertebral bodies: Assessment with conventional spin-echo, chemical-shift, and STIR MR imaging. *Radiology* 174:495, 1990.

Ballinger PW: *Merrill's Atlas of Radiographic Positions and Radiologic Procedures vol 1*, ed 3. St. Louis, Mosby, 1986.

Beck RN: Radionuclide Imaging principles. In: Taveras JM, Ferrucci JT (eds): *Radiology — Diagnosis, Imaging, Intervention vol 1*. Philadelphia, Lippincott, 1990, ch 19.

Berman L, Klenerman L: Ultrasound screening for hip abnormalities: Preliminary findings in 1001 neonates. *Br Med J* 293:719, 1986.

Borders J, Kerr E, Sartoris DJ, et al: Quantitative dual-energy radiographic absorptiometry of the lumbar spine: In vivo comparison with dual-photon absorptiometry. *Radiology* 170:129, 1989.

Brandt TD, Cardone BW, Grant TH, Post M, Weiss CA: Rotator cuff sonography: A reassessment. *Radiology* 173:323, 1989.

Brower AC: *Arthritis in Black and White*. Philadelphia, Saunders, 1988.

Burk DL, Mears DC, Kennedy WH, Cooperstein LA, Herbert DL: Three-dimensional computed tomography of acetabular fractures. *Radiology* 155:183, 1985.

Colhoun EN, Johnson SR, Fairclough JA: Bone scanning for hip fracture in patients with osteoarthritis: Brief report. *J Bone Joint Surg (Br)* 69:848, 1987.

Dalinka MK, Boorstein JM, Zlatkin MB: Computed tomography of musculoskeletal trauma. *Radiol Clin North Am* 27:933, 1989.

Derchi LE, Balconi G, DeFlaviis L, Oliva A, Rosso F: Sonographic appearance of hemangiomas of skeletal muscle. *J Ultrasound Med* 8:263, 1989.

Dewhirst MW, Sostman HD, Leopold KA, et al: Soft-tissue sarcomas: MR imaging and MR spectroscopy for prognosis and therapy monitoring.*Radiology* 174:847, 1990.

Erlemann R, Reiser MF, Peters PE, et al: Musculoskeletal neoplasms: Static and dynamic Gd-DTPA-enhanced MR imaging. *Radiology* 171:767, 1989.

Erlemann R, Sciuk J, Bosse A, et al: Response of osteosarcoma and Ewing sarcoma to preoperative chemotherapy: Assessment with dynamic and static MR imaging and skeletal scintigraphy. *Radiology* 175:791, 1990.

Erlemann R, Vasallo P, Bongartz G, et al: Musculoskeletal neoplasms: Fast low-angle shot MR imaging with and without Gd-DTPA. *Radiology* 176:489, 1990.

Errico TJ: The role of diskography in the 1980s. *Radiology* 162:285, 1989.

Ferrucci JT: Imaging algorithms for radiologic diagnosis. In: Taveras JM, Ferrucci JT (eds): *Radiology—Diagnosis, Imaging, Intervention vol I*. Philadelphia, Lippincott, 1990, ch 36.

Flannigan B, Kursunoglu-Brahme S, Snyder S, Karzel R, Del Pizzo W, Resnick D: MR Arthrography of the shoulder: Comparison with conventional MR imaging. *Am J Roentgenol* 155: 829, 1990.

Foley WD, Wilson CR: Digital orthopedic radiography: Vascular and non-vascular In: Galasko CSB, Isherwood I (eds): *Imaging Techniques in Orthopedics*. London, Springer-Verlag, 1989, pp 145-158.

Fornage BD: Achilles tendon: US examination. *Radiology* 159:759, 1986.

Freiberger RH, Pavlov H: Knee arthrography. *Radiology* 166:489, 1988.

Fuchs AW: Cervical vertebrae (part I). *Radiogr Clin Photogr* 16:2, 1940.

Genant HK, Boyd DP: Quantitative bone mineral analysis using dual-energy computed tomography. *Invest Radiol* 12:545, 1977.

Genant HK, Cann CE, Chafetz NI, Helms CA: Advances in computed tomography of the musculo-skeletal system. *Radiol Clin North Am* 19:645: 1981.

Genant HK, Resnick D: Magnification radiography. In: Resnick D (ed): *Bone and Joint Imaging*. Philadelphia, Saunders, 1989, pp 85-92.

Goodman PC, Jeffrey RB Jr, Brant-Zawadzki M: Digital subtraction angiography in extremity trauma. *Radiology* 153:61, 1984.

Greenfield GB: *Radiology of Bone Diseases*, ed 5. Philadelphia, Lippincott, 1990, p 12.

Greenspan A: Tumors of cartilage origin. *Orthop Clin North Am* 20:347, 1989.

Greenspan A: Imaging modalities in orthopedics. In: Chapman MW (ed): *Operative Orthopedics*, ed 2. Philadelphia, Lippincott, 1992.

Greenspan A, Norman A: The radial head-capitellum view: Useful technique in elbow trauma. *Am J Roetgenol* 138:1186, 1982.

Gundry CR, Schils JP, Resnick D, Sartoris DJ: Arthrography of the post-traumatic knee, shoulder, and wrist. Current status and future trends. *Radiol Clin North Am* 27:957, 1989.

Haacke EM, Tkach JA: Fast MR imaging: Techniques and clinical applications. *Am J Roentgenol* 155:951, 1990.

Ho C, Sartoris, DJ, Resnick D: Conventional tomography in musculoskeletal trauma. *Radiol Clin North Am* 27:929, 1989.

Hodler J, Fretz CJ, Terrier F, Gerber C: Rotator cuff tears: Correlation of sonographic and surgical findings. *Radiology* 169:791, 1988.

Jones MM, Moore WH, Brewer EJ, Sonnemaker RE, Long SE: Radionuclide bone/joint imaging in children with rheumatic complaints. *Skeletal Radiol* 17:1, 1988.

Kaplan PA, Matamaros A Jr, Anderson JC: Sonography of the muscoloskeletal system. *Am J Roengenol* 155:237, 1990.

King JB, Turnbull TJ: An early method of confirming scaphoid fracture. *J Bone Joint Surg (Br)* 63:287, 1981.

Levinsohn EM, Palmer AK, Coren AB, Zinberg E: Wrist arthrography: The value of the three compartment injection technique. *Skeletal Radiol* 16:539, 1987.

Magid D, Fishman EK: Imaging of musculoskeletal trauma in three dimensions. *Radiol Clin North Am* 27:945, 1989.

McAfee JG: Update on radiopharmaceuticals for medical imaging. *Radiology* 171:593, 1989.

McAfee JG, Samin A: Indium-111 labeled leukocytes: A review of problems in image interpretation. *Radiology* 155:221, 1985.

Merchant AC, Mercer RL, Jacobson RH, Cool CR: Roentgenographic analysis of patello-femoral congruence. *J Bone Joint Surg* 56A:1391, 1974.

Murray IPC, Dixon J: The role of single photon emission computed tomography in bone scintigraphy. *Skeletal Radiol* 18:493, 1989.

Negendank WG, Crowley MG, Ryan JR, Keller NA, Evelhoch JL: Bone and soft-tissue lesions: Diagnosis with combined H-1 MR imaging and P-31 MR spectroscopy. *Radiology* 173:181, 1990.

Pugh DG, Winkler TN: Scanography of leg-length measurement: An easy satisfactory method. *Radiology* 87:130, 1966.

Reinus WR, Hardy DC, Totty WG, Gilula LA: Arthrographic evaluation of the carpal triangular fibrocartilage complex. *J Hand Surg* 12A:495, 1987.

Reuther G, Mutschler W: Detection of local recurrent disease in musculoskeletal tumors: Magnetic resonance imaging versus computed tomography. *Skeletal Radiology* 19:85, 1990.

Rosenberg ZS, Cheung Y: Diagnostic imaging of the ankle and foot. In: Jahss MH (ed): *Disorders of the Foot and Ankle*, ed 2. Philadelphia, Saunders, 1991, pp 109-154.

Sartoris DJ, Resnick D: Current and innovative methods for noninvasive bone densitometry. *Radiol Clinics North Am* 28:257, 1990

Sartoris DJ, Sommer FG: Digital film processing: Applications to the musculo-skeletal system. *Skeletal Radiol* 11:274, 1984.

Schmalbrock P, Beltran J: Principles of magnetic resonance imaging. In: Beltran J: *MRI Musculoskeletal System*. Philadelphia, Lippincott, 1990.

Shapiro R: Current status of lumbar diskography (letter). *Radiology* 159:815, 1986.

Soble MG, Kaye AD, Guay RC: Rotator cuff tear: Clinical experience with sonographic detection. *Radiology* 173:319, 1989.

Sostman HD, Charles HC, Rockwell S, et al: Soft-tissue sarcomas: Detection of metabolic heterogeneity with P-31 MR spectroscopy. *Radiology* 176:837, 1990.

Sundaram M, McLeod RA: MR imaging of tumor and tumorlike lesions of bones and soft tissues. *Am J Roentgenol* 155:817, 1990.

Suzuki S, Awaya G, Wakita S, Maekawa M, Ikeda T: Diagnosis by ultrasound of congenital dislocation of the hip joint. *Clin Orthop* 217:171, 1987.

Vanharanta H, Guyer RD, Ohnmeiss DD, et al: Disc deterioration in low-back syndromes. A prospective, multi-center CT/discography study. *Spine* 13:1349, 1988.

Zucherman J, Derby R, Hsu K, et al: Normal magnetic resonance imaging with abnormal discography. *Spine* 13:1355, 1988

3

Bone Formation and Growth

THE SKELETON IS MADE UP of cortical and cancellous bone, which are highly specialized forms of connective tissue. Each type of bony tissue has the same basic histologic structure, but the cortical component has a solid, compact architecture interrupted only by narrow canals containing blood vessels (haversian system), while the cancellous component consists of trabeculae separated by fatty or hematopoietic marrow. Bone is rigid calcified material and grows by the addition of new tissue to existing surfaces. The removal of unwanted bone, called *simultaneous remodeling*, is also a necessary component of skeletal growth, as Sissons pointed out. Unlike most tissues, bone grows only by apposition on the surface of an already existing substrate, such as bone or calcified cartilage. Cartilage, however, grows by interstitial cellular proliferation and matrix formation.

Normal bone is formed through a combination of two processes: *endochondral ossification* and *intramembranous ossification*. In general, the spongiosa develops by endochondral ossification and the cortex by intramembranous ossification. Once formed, living bone is never metabolically at rest. Beginning in the fetal period, it constantly remodels and reappropriates its minerals along lines of mechanical stress. This process continues throughout life, accelerating during infancy and adolescence. The factors controlling bone formation and resorption are still not well understood, but one fact is clear: Bone formation and bone resorption are exquisitely balanced, coupled processes that result in net bone formation equaling net bone resorption.

Most of the skeleton is formed by endochondral ossification (Fig. 3.1), a highly organized process that transforms cartilage to bone and contributes mainly to increasing bone length. Endochondral ossification is responsible for the formation of all tubular and flat bones, vertebrae, the base of the skull, the ethmoid, and the medial and lateral ends of the clavicle. For example, at about seven weeks of embryonic life, cartilage cells (chondroblasts and chondrocytes) produce a hyaline cartilage model of the long tubular bones

from the condensed mesenchymal aggregate. At about the ninth week, peripheral capillaries penetrate the model, inducing the formation of osteoblasts. Osseous tissue is then deposited on the spicules of calcified cartilage matrix that remain after osteoclastic resorption, thereby transforming the primary spongiosa into secondary spongiosa.

As this process moves rapidly toward the epiphyseal ends of the cartilage model, a loose network of bony trabeculae containing cores of calcified cartilage is left behind, creating a well defined line of advance. This line represents the growth plate (physis) (Fig. 3.2) and the adjacent metaphysis to which the secondary spongiosa moves as it is formed. The many trabeculae of the secondary spongiosa that are resorbed soon after being formed become the marrow cavity, while other trabeculae enlarge and thicken through the apposition of new bone, although these too eventually undergo resorption and remodeling. Others extend toward the shaft and become incorporated into the developing cortex of the bone, which is formed by intramembranous ossification. Endochondral bone formation is not normally observed after growth plate closure.

In intramembranous ossification, bone is formed directly without an intervening cartilaginous stage (Fig. 3.3). Initially, condensed mesenchymal cells differentiate into osteoprogenitor cells, which then differentiate into fibroblasts that produce collagen and fibrous connective tissues, and osteoblasts, which produce osteoid. Beginning at approximately the ninth week of fetal life, the fibrous membrane produced by the fibroblasts forms a periosteal collar and is replaced with osteoid by the action of the osteoblasts. Bones formed by this process include the frontal, parietal, and temporal bones and their squamae; bones of the upper face as well as the tympanic parts of the temporal bone; and the vomer and the medial pterygoid.

Intramembranous ossification also contributes to the appositional formation of periosteal bone around the shafts of the tubular bones,

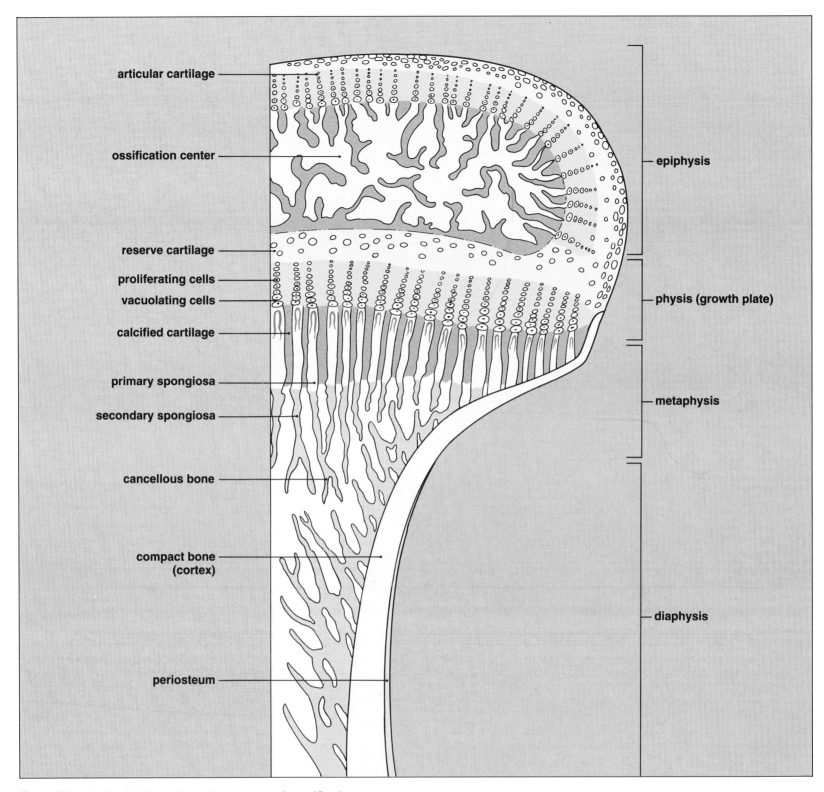

Figure 3.1 Endochondral bone formation occurs at the ossification center, growth plate, and metaphysis. (Modified from Dr. P. Rubin, 1964)

thus forming the cortex of the long and flat bones. This type of bone formation increases bone width. In addition to the periosteal envelope on the outer surface of bone, intramembranous ossification is active in the endosteal envelope covering the inner surface of the cortex and in the haversian envelope at the internal surface of all intracortical canals. These three envelopes are sites of potent cellular activity involving both resorption and formation of bone throughout life.

It is interesting to note that the mandible and middle portions of the clavicle are formed by a process that shares features of both endochondral and intramembranous ossification. These bones are preformed in cartilage in embryonic life, but they do not undergo endochondral ossification in the conventional manner. Instead, the cartilage model simply serves as a surface for the deposition of bone by connective tissues. Eventually, the cartilage is resorbed and the bones become fully ossified.

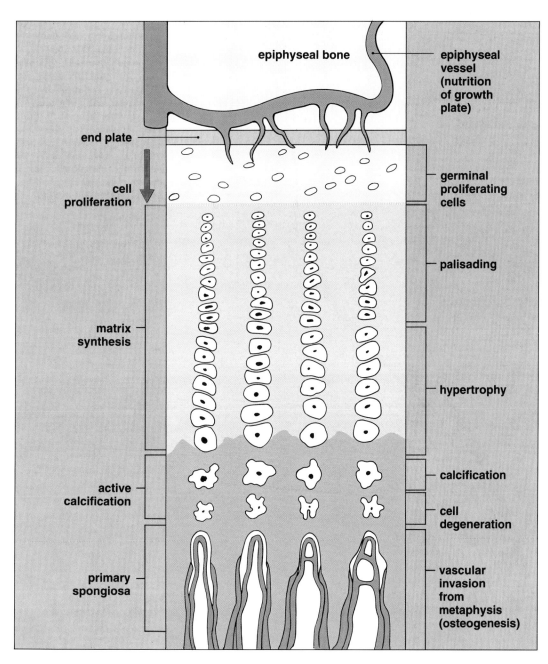

Figure 3.2 Growth plate during active bone growth. At the top of the diagram the epiphyseal vessels are supplying nutrition to the germinal proliferating cells. Further down the cells begin to palisade into vertical columns, and as they approach the metaphysis, the cells undergo hypertrophy and the matrix calcifies. The calcified matrix is then invaded by blood vessels and the primary spongiosa forms. (Adapted from Bullough PG, Vigorita VJ, 1984)

PART II

Trauma

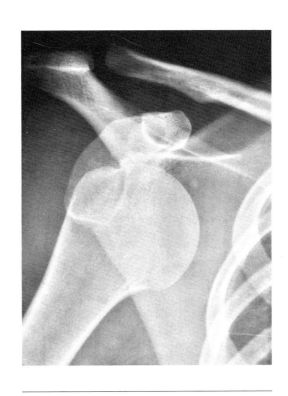

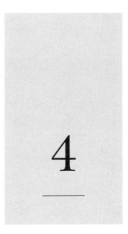

4

Radiologic Evaluation of Trauma

RADIOLOGIC IMAGING MODALITIES

The radiologic modalities most often used in analyzing injury to the skeletal system are:

1. Conventional radiography, including routine views (specific for various body parts), special views, and stress views
2. Digital radiography, including digital subtraction angiography (DSA)
3. Fluoroscopy, alone or combined with videotaping
4. Tomography (particularly trispiral tomography)
5. Computed tomography (CT)
6. Arthrography, tenography, and bursography
7. Myelography and diskography
8. Angiography (arteriography and venography)
9. Scintigraphy (radionuclide bone scan)
10. Magnetic resonance imaging (MRI).

In most instances, radiographs obtained in two orthogonal projections—usually the anteroposterior and lateral—at 90° to each other are sufficient (Fig. 4.1). Occasionally, oblique and special views are necessary, particularly in evaluating fractures of complex structures such as the pelvis, elbow, wrist, and ankle (Fig. 4.2).

Certain special modalities are used more often in evaluating different types of injuries in specific anatomic locations. Fluoroscopy and videotaping are useful in evaluating the kinematics of joints. Stress views are important in evaluating ligamentous tears and joint stability (Fig. 4.3). Tomography (zono- or trispiral) is useful in con-

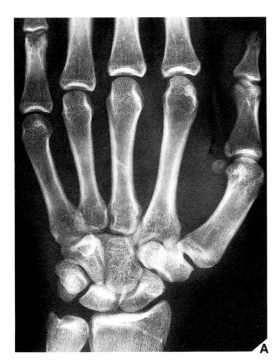
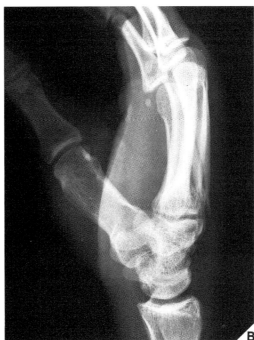
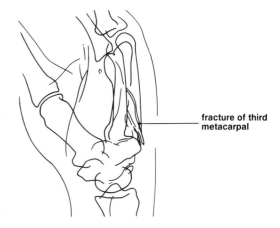

Figure 4.1 (A) Dorsovolar (posteroanterior) view of the hand does not demonstrate a fracture. (B) The lateral view reveals a fracture of the third metacarpal bone.

fracture of third metacarpal

firming the presence of a fracture (Fig. 4.4), delineating the extent of a fracture line, and assessing the position of the fragments. It is also valuable in monitoring the progress of healing.

Computed tomography (CT) is essential in the evaluation of complex fractures, particularly in the spinal and pelvic regions (Fig. 4.5). The advantages of CT over conventional radiography are its ability to provide three-dimensional imaging, excellent contrast resolution, and accurate measurement of the tissue attenuation coefficient. The use of sagittal, coronal, and multiplanar reformation provides an added advantage over other imaging modalities.

Radionuclide bone scan can detect occult fractures or fractures too subtle to be seen on conventional radiographs or tomograms

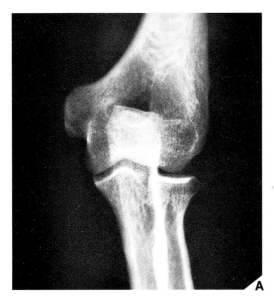 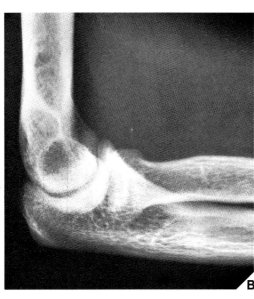 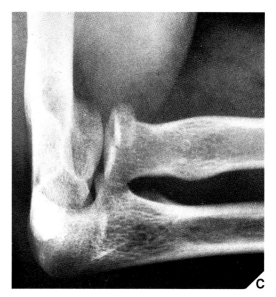

Figure 4.2 A patient presented with elbow pain after a fall. Anteroposterior (A) and lateral (B) views are normal; however, the radial head and coronoid process are not well demonstrated because of bony overlap. A special 45°-angle view of the elbow (C) is used to project the radial head ventrad, free of the overlap of other bones. A short, intra-articular fracture of the radial head is now clearly visible.

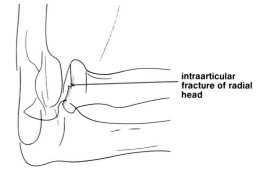

intraarticular fracture of radial head

Figure 4.3 In most ankle injuries, if a ligamentous tear is suspected, conventional films should be supplemented by stress views. The standard anteroposterior radiograph of this ankle (A) is not remarkable. The same view after application of adduction (inversion) stress (B) shows widening of the lateral compartment of the tibiotalar (ankle) joint, indicating a tear of the lateral collateral ligament.

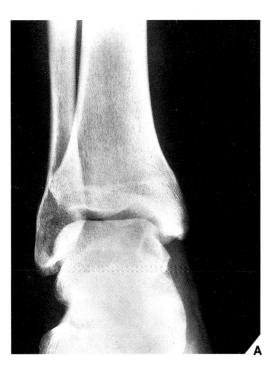 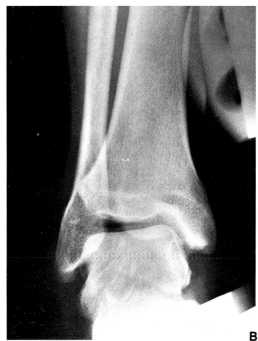

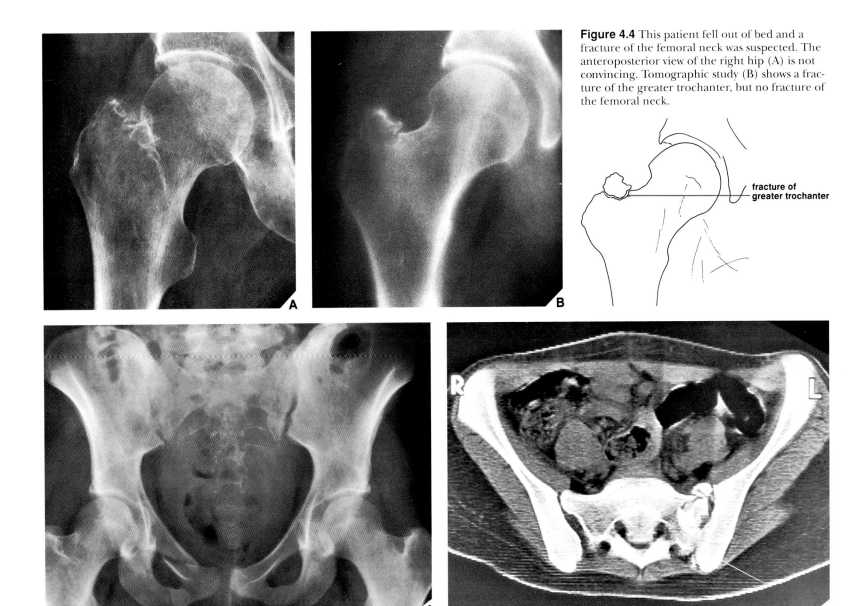

Figure 4.4 This patient fell out of bed and a fracture of the femoral neck was suspected. The anteroposterior view of the right hip (A) is not convincing. Tomographic study (B) shows a fracture of the greater trochanter, but no fracture of the femoral neck.

fracture of greater trochanter

Figure 4.5 (A) Standard anteroposterior view of the pelvis shows obvious fractures of the right obturator ring. (B) CT section demonstrates an unsuspected fracture of the sacrum and disruption of the left sacroiliac joint.

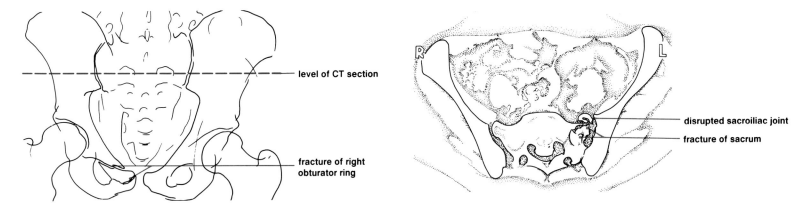

level of CT section

fracture of right obturator ring

disrupted sacroiliac joint

fracture of sacrum

(Fig. 4.6). Scintigraphy occasionally aids in making a differential diagnosis of old-versus-recent fractures and in detecting such complications as early-stage osteonecrosis. However, bone scans seldom provide new information about the status of fracture healing and, in particular, static bone scans fail to separate normally healing fractures from delayed–healing fractures or those that result in nonunion. Also, a bone scan cannot indicate the point at which clinical union is established. Scintigraphy is, however, helpful in distinguishing noninfected fractures from infected ones. With osteomyelitis, scanning, using gallium citrate (^{67}Ga) and indium labeled white blood cells (^{111}In), demonstrates a significant increase in the uptake of the tracer. Since ^{67}Ga is also actively taken up at the site of a normally healing fracture, but significantly less than that encountered with ^{99m}Tc (technetium) scanning agents, the combination of ^{67}Ga and ^{99m}Tc MDP has been suggested, using the ratio of uptake of ^{67}Ga to ^{99m}Tc to determine whether or not the fracture is infected. The ratio of ^{67}Ga to ^{99m}Tc MDP should be higher in infected fractures than in noninfected fractures. It is very difficult to

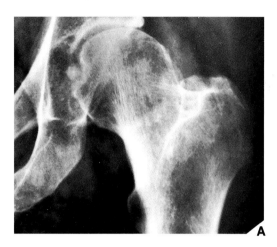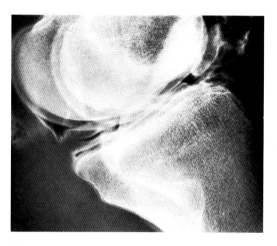

Figure 4.6 (A) Anteroposterior view of the left hip reveals a band of increased density, suggesting a fracture of the femoral neck. (B) A bone scan performed after administration of 15 mCi (555 MBq) of technetium-99m-labeled methylene diphosphonate shows increased uptake of isotope in the region of the femoral neck, confirming the fracture.

Figure 4.7 In this patient double-contrast arthrography of the knee shows a horizontal cleavage tear in the medial meniscus.

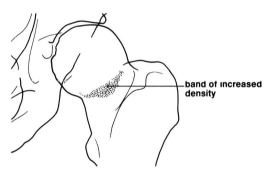

band of increased density

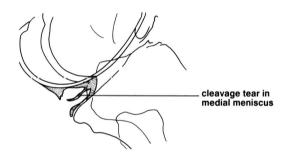

cleavage tear in medial meniscus

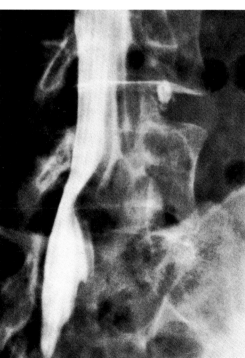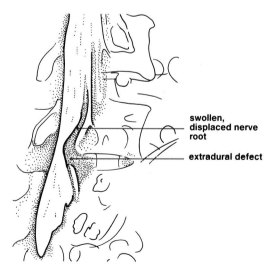

swollen, displaced nerve root

extradural defect

Figure 4.8 A patient strained his back by lifting a heavy object. Oblique view of the lower lumbosacral spine after injection of metrizamide contrast into the subarachnoid space shows an extradural pressure defect on the thecal sac at the L5-S1 intervertebral space characteristic of disk herniation. Note the markedly swollen, displaced nerve root.

differentiate pseudoarthrosis from infection at the fracture site. Standard ^{99m}Tc and ^{67}Ga bone scans are not helpful, since both may be positive for both conditions. In these instances, ^{111}In white-blood-cell scanning combined with ^{99m}Tc MDP scanning appears to be the best method for determining if a fractured or traumatized bone is infected.

Arthrography is still used in the evaluation of injuries to articular cartilage, menisci, joint capsules, and ligaments (Fig. 4.7). Although virtually every joint can be injected with contrast, the examination is most frequently performed in the knee, shoulder, ankle, and elbow articulations. Tenograms help evaluate injuries to the tendons. Myelography, either alone or in conjunction with CT scan, is used to evaluate certain traumatic conditions of the spine (Fig. 4.8). If a disk abnormality is suspected and a myelographic study is not diagnostic, diskography may yield information required for further patient management (Fig. 4.9). Angiography is indicated if concomitant injury to the vascular system is suspected (Fig. 4.10). Digital subtraction angiography (DSA) is preferred because subtraction of the overlying bones results in clear delineation of vascular structures.

Magnetic resonance imaging (MRI) plays a leading role in the evaluation of trauma to bone and soft tissue. MRI evaluation of trauma to the knee, particularly abnormalities of the menisci and ligaments, has a high negative predictive value. MRI can be used to screen patients before surgery so unnecessary arthroscopies are

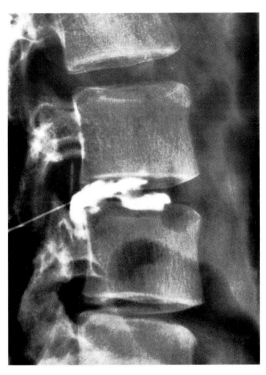

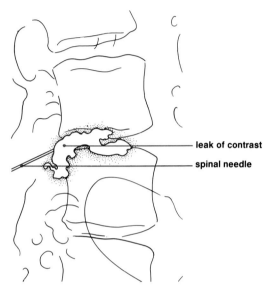

Figure 4.9 A spinal needle was placed in the center of the nucleus pulposus and a few milliliters of metrizamide were injected. The leak of contrast into the extradural space indicates a rupture of the annulus fibrosus and posterior disk herniation.

leak of contrast

spinal needle

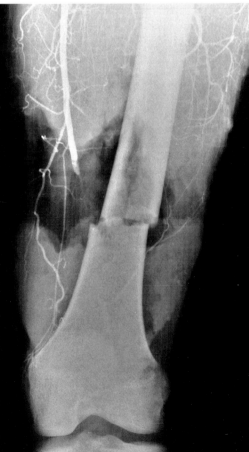

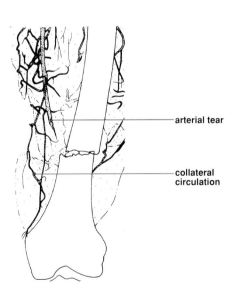

Figure 4.10 In this patient, a femoral arteriogram was performed to rule out damage to vascular structures by a fractured femur. Transverse fracture resulted in transsection of the superficial femoral artery.

arterial tear

collateral circulation

avoided. Subtle abnormalities of various structures and posttraumatic joint effusion can be well visualized (Fig. 4.11). Similarly, the medial and lateral collateral ligaments, anterior and posterior cruciate ligaments, and tendons around the knee joint can be well visualized (see Figs. 8.14, 8.15) and abnormalities of these structures diagnosed with high accuracy. Also difficult to detect are some types of meniscal injuries, such as bucket-handle tears, tears of the free edge, and peripheral detachments. In the shoulder, impingement syndrome and complete and incomplete rotator cuff tears may be effectively diagnosed most of the time (Fig. 4.12). Traumatic lesions of the tendons (such as biceps tendon rupture), traumatic joint effusions, and hematomas are easily diagnosed with MRI. Much more

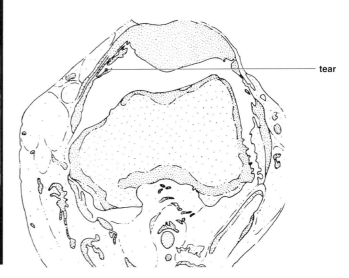

Figure 4.11 A 64-year-old man sustained injury to the left knee. Axial MRI (MPGR flip angle 30°, TR500/TE15) demonstrates a partial tear of the medial retinaculum. Posttraumatic knee effusion shows high signal intensity. Note marked thinning of patellar articular cartilage due to osteoarthritis.

tear

Figure 4.12 A 60-year-old man presented with right shoulder pain. Oblique coronal MRI (SE TR 2000/TE80) demonstrates complete rotator cuff tear. The supraspinatus muscle is retracted medially and no tendon tissue is present in the subacromial space. Joint fluid shows high signal intensity. (From Beltran J, 1990)

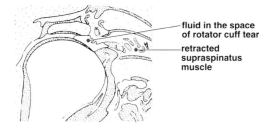

fluid in the space of rotator cuff tear

retracted supraspinatus muscle

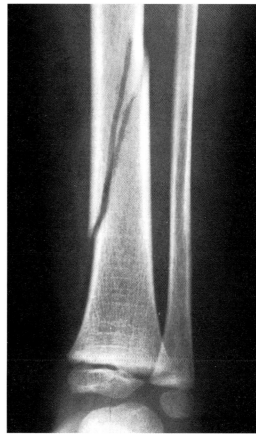

Figure 4.13 A complete fracture. The continuity of the bone is disrupted and there is a narrow gap between the bony fragments.

difficult to diagnose is a tear of the cartilaginous labrum. The changes of osteonecrosis at various sites, particularly in its early stage, may be detected by MRI when other modalities, such as plain-film radiography, tomography, and even radionuclide bone scan, may be normal. Imaging of the ankle and foot, using MRI, has been used in diagnosing tendon ruptures and posttraumatic osteonecrosis of the talus. In the wrist and hand, MRI has been successfully used in early diagnosis of posttraumatic osteonecrosis of the scaphoid. MRI is still not the technique of choice in evaluation of abnormalities of the triangular fibrocartilage complex, where arthrography is preferred, particularly in conjunction with digital imaging and CT. The greatest use of MRI is for evaluating trauma of the spine, the spinal cord, the thecal sac, and nerve roots, as well as disk herniation (see Fig. 10.74). MRI is also useful in evaluation of spinal ligament injury. Demonstration of the relationship of vertebral fragments to the spinal cord with direct sagittal imaging is extremely helpful, particularly to evaluate injury in the cervical and thoracic area.

FRACTURES AND DISLOCATIONS

Fractures and dislocations are among the most common traumatic conditions encountered by radiologists. By definition, a *fracture* is a complete disruption in the continuity of a bone (Fig. 4.13). If only some of the bony trabeculae are completely severed while others are bent or remain intact, the fracture is incomplete (Fig. 4.14). A *dislocation* is a complete disruption of a joint; articular surfaces are no longer in contact (Fig. 4.15). A *subluxation*, on the other hand, is a minor disruption of a joint where some articular contact remains (Fig. 4.16). Proper radiologic evaluation of these conditions contributes greatly to successful treatment by the orthopedic surgeon.

In dealing with trauma, the radiologist has two tasks:

1. Diagnosing and evaluating the type of fracture or dislocation
2. Monitoring the results of treatment and looking for possible complications.

Diagnosis

The important radiographic principle in diagnosing skeletal trauma is to obtain at least two views of the bone involved, with each view including two joints adjacent to the injured bone (Fig. 4.17). In so doing, the radiologist eliminates the risk of missing an associated fracture, subluxation, and/or dislocation at a site remote from the apparent primary injury. In children it is frequently necessary to obtain a radiograph of the normal, unaffected limb for comparison.

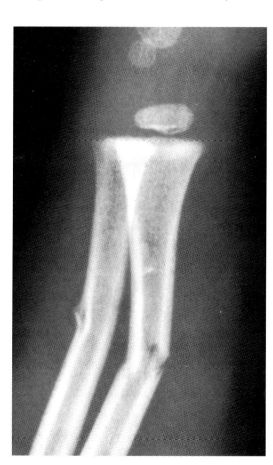

Figure 4.14 An incomplete (greenstick) fracture. The ulna is bent and there is a fracture line extending only through the posterior cortex. In the radial fracture some trabeculae remain intact.

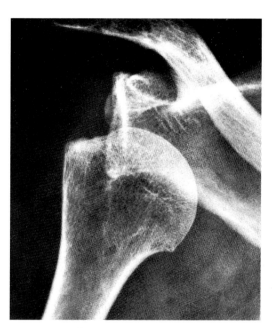

Figure 4.15 A typical anterior dislocation of the shoulder joint. The articular surface of the humerus loses contact with the articular surface of the glenoid.

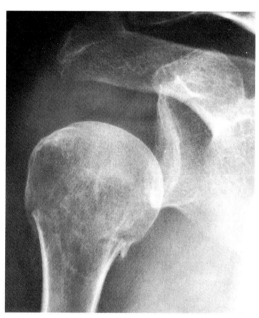

Figure 4.16 Subluxation of the shoulder joint. There is malalignment of the head of the humerus and the glenoid fossa, but some articular contact remains. Note the associated fracture of the surgical neck of the humerus.

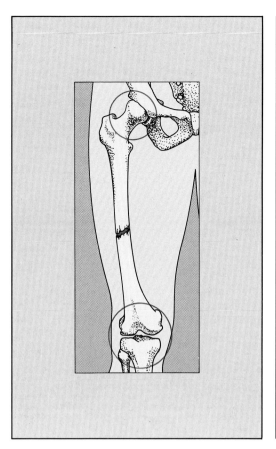

SITE AND EXTENT OF FRACTURE

junction of
middle and distal
thirds of femur

supracondylar

intra-articular

Figure 4.17 The radiograph of a suspected fracture of the femoral shaft should include the hip and knee articulations.

Figure 4.18 Factors in the radiographic evaluation of a fracture: the anatomic site and extent.

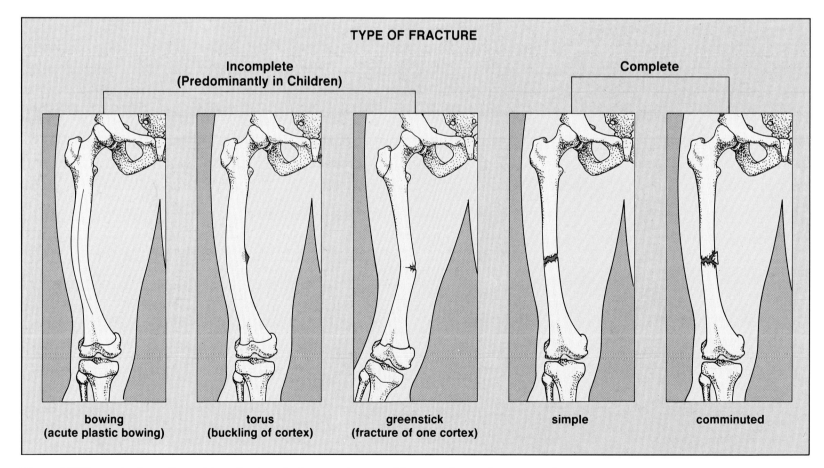

TYPE OF FRACTURE

**Incomplete
(Predominantly in Children)**

Complete

bowing
(acute plastic bowing)

torus
(buckling of cortex)

greenstick
(fracture of one cortex)

simple

comminuted

Figure 4.19 Factors in the radiographic evaluation of a fracture: the type of fracture—incomplete or complete.

Radiographic Evaluation of Fractures

The complete radiographic evaluation of fractures should include the following elements: (1) the anatomic *site* and *extent* of a fracture (Fig. 4.18); (2) the *type* of fracture, whether it is incomplete, as seen predominantly in children, or complete (Fig. 4.19); (3) the *alignment* of the fragments with regard to displacement, angulation, rotation, fore-shortening, or distraction (Fig. 4.20); (4) the *direction* of the fracture line in relation to the longitudinal axis of the bone (Fig. 4.21); (5) the presence of *special features* such as impaction, depression, or compression (Fig. 4.22); (6) the presence of *associated abnormalities* such as fracture with concomitant dislocation or diastasis (Fig. 4.23); and (7) *special types* of fractures that may occur as the result of abnormal stress

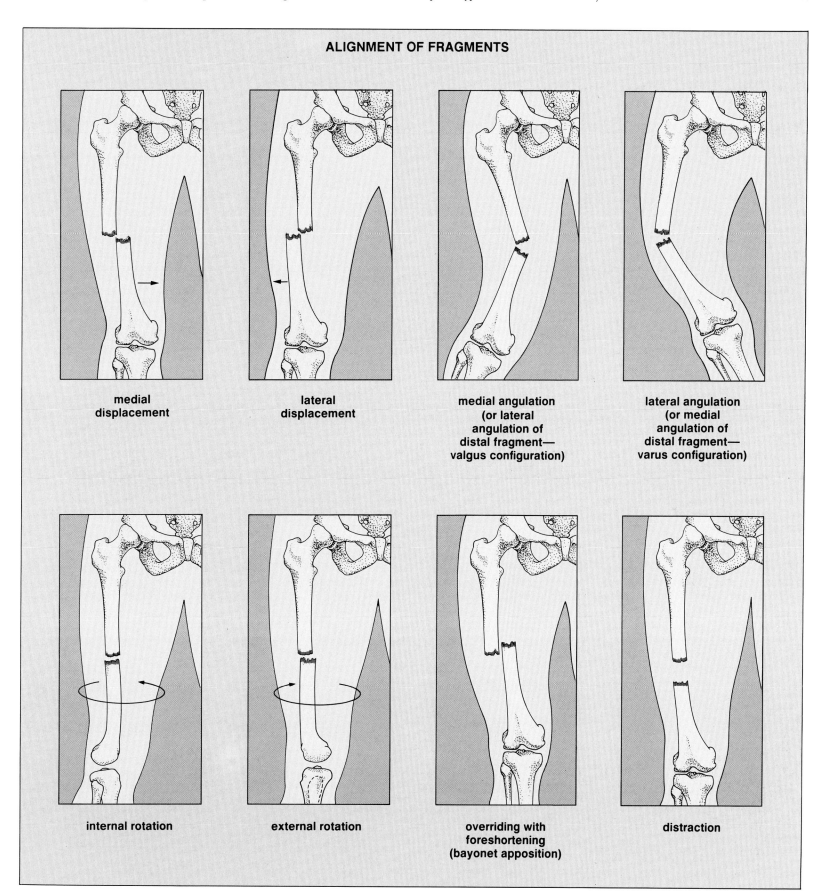

Figure 4.20 Factors in the radiographic evaluation of a fracture: the alignment of the fragments.

or secondary to pathologic processes in the bone (Fig. 4.24). The distinction between an *open* (or *compound*) fracture—one in which the fractured bone communicates with the outside environment through an open wound—and a *closed* (or *simple*) fracture—one which does not produce an open wound in the skin—should preferably be made by clinical rather than radiographic examination.

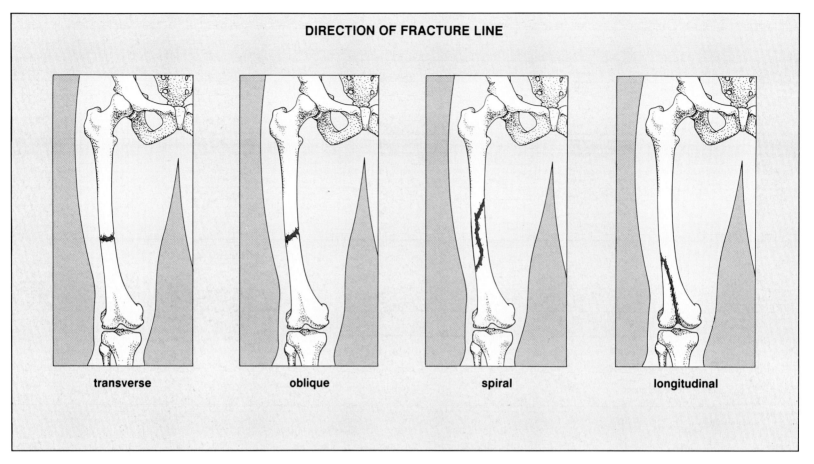

Figure 4.21 Factors in the radiographic evaluation of a fracture: the direction of the fracture line.

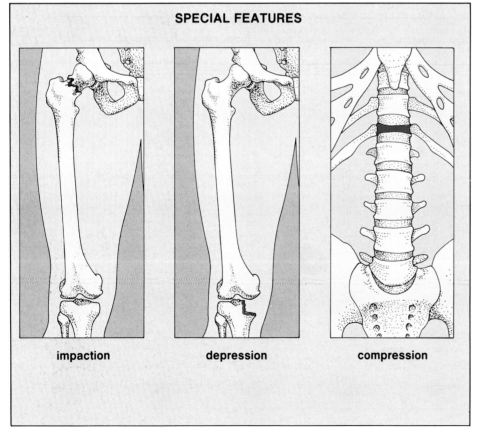

Figure 4.22 Factors in the radiographic evaluation of a fracture: special features.

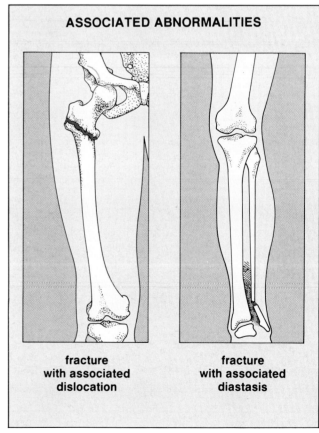

Figure 4.23 Factors in the radiographic evaluation of a fracture: associated abnormalities.

In children the radiographic evaluation of fractures, particularly of the ends of tubular bones, should also take into consideration the involvement of the growth plate (physis). Localization of the fracture line has implications with respect to the mechanism of injury and possible complications. A useful classification of injuries affecting the physis, metaphysis, epiphysis, or all of these structures has been proposed by Salter and Harris (types I-V) and has been expanded by Rang (type VI) and Ogden (types VII-IX) to include four additional types of fractures (Fig. 4.25). Although the injuries described by Rang and Ogden do not directly involve the growth plate, the sequelae of such trauma affect the physis in the same way as the direct injuries described by Salter and Harris. In type VI, which involves only the peripheral region of the growth plate, the injury may not always be associated with a fracture. It may result from a localized contusion, trauma-induced infection, or severe burn. Type VII injury consists of a purely transepiphyseal fracture,

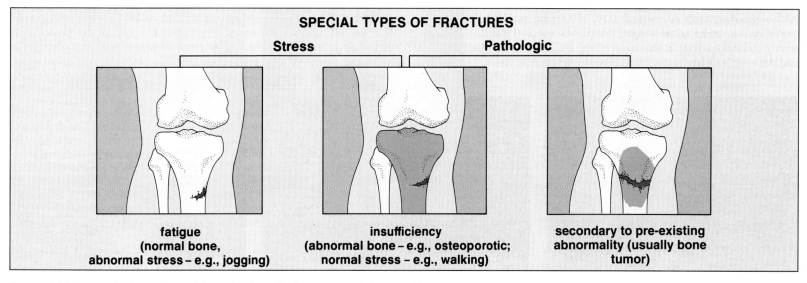

Figure 4.24 Factors in the radiographic evaluation of a fracture: special types of fractures.

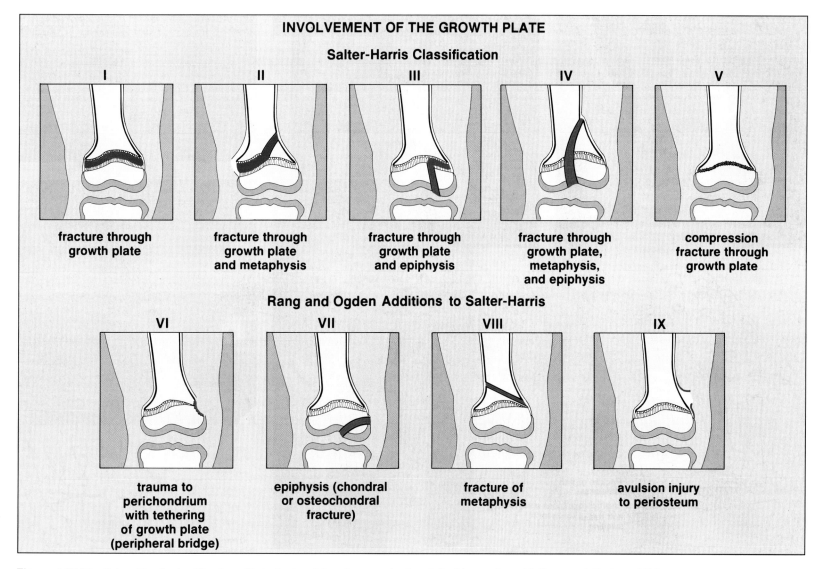

Figure 4.25 The Salter-Harris classification of injuries involving the growth plate (physis) together with Rang and Ogden additions.

PERIOSTEAL AND ENDOSTEAL REACTION The fracture line may not be visible, but the periosteal or endosteal response may be the first radiographic sign of a fracture (Fig. 4.29).

JOINT EFFUSION This finding, which results in the radiographic appearance of the fat-pad sign, is particularly useful in diagnosing elbow injuries. The posterior (dorsal) fat pad lies deep in the olecranon fossa and is not visible in the lateral projection. The anterior (ventral) fat pad occupies the shallower anterior coronoid and radial fossae and is usually seen as a flat radiolucent strip ventrad to the anterior cortex of the humerus. Distention of the articular capsule by synovial or hemorrhagic fluid causes the posterior fat pad to become visible and also displaces the anterior fat pad—yielding the *fat-pad sign* (Fig. 4.30). When there is a history of elbow trauma and the fat-pad sign is positive, there is usually an associated fracture and every effort should be made to demonstrate it. Even if the fracture line is not demonstrated on multiple films, the patient should be treated for fracture.

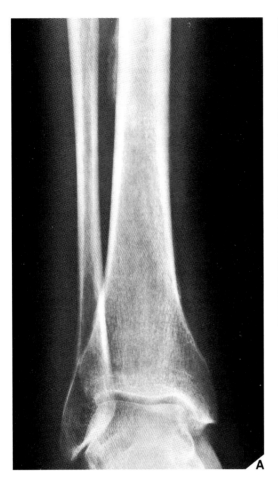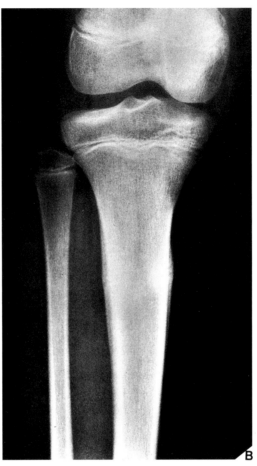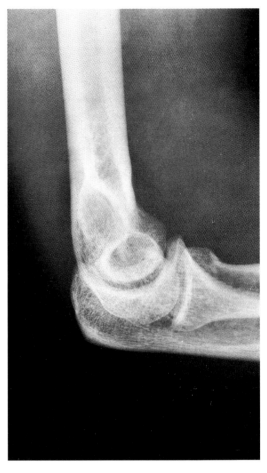

Figure 4.29 (A) A 49-year-old woman sustained an injury to the lower leg. Plain anteroposterior view shows periosteal new bone at the lateral cortex of the distal third of the tibia and on the medial aspect just above the malleolus. This indirect sign of a fracture represents an early stage of external callus formation. The actual hairline spiral fracture line is barely discernible.

(B) Example of periosteal callus formation at the medial and lateral cortices of the proximal tibial diaphysis. A transverse band of increased density, visible in the medullary portion of the bone, represents endosteal callus. The fracture line is practically invisible. These features are commonly seen in a stress fracture.

Figure 4.30 Lateral view of the elbow shows a positive fat-pad sign. The anterior fat pad is markedly elevated and the posterior fat pad is clearly visible in this patient. There is a subtle, nondisplaced fracture of the radial head.

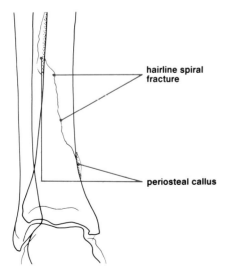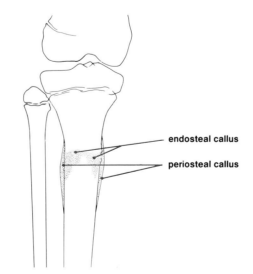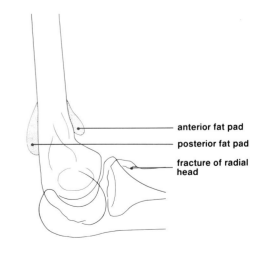

DOUBLE CORTICAL LINE Thi[...]
fracture. The actual fractur[...]
ble contour of the cortex re[...]

BUCKLING OF THE CORTEX [...]
the only sign of a tubular b[...]
finding is identified at time[...]
frontal projection.

IRREGULAR METAPHYSEAL C[...]
small avulsion fractures of [...]
to the bone caused by a rap[...]
insertion. As a result, smal[...]
the metaphysis. These *corne*[...]
children who sustain skelet[...]
particularly if battered chil[...]
syndrome" or PITS (paren[...]
(Fig. 4.35).

Radiographic Evaluation [...]
Dislocations are more obvi[...]
graphs, and consequently [...]
such a characteristic appea[...]
rior view) that this single e[...]
the same principle of obta[...]

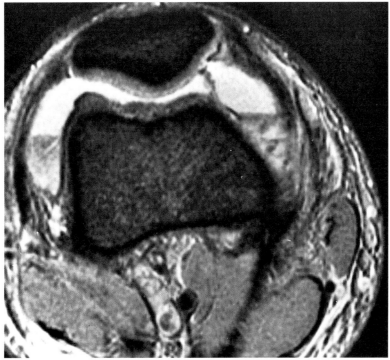

INTRACAPSULAR FAT-FLUID LEVEL If a fracture involves the articular end of a bone (particularly a long bone like the tibia, humerus, or femur), blood and bone-marrow fat enter the joint (lipohemarthrosis) and produce a characteristic layering of these two substances on the radiograph—the fat-blood interface, or *FBI sign* (Fig. 4.31) An MRI study can also demonstrate this phenomenon (Fig. 4.32). When the fracture line cannot be demonstrated, diagnosis should be made on the strength of this sign alone.

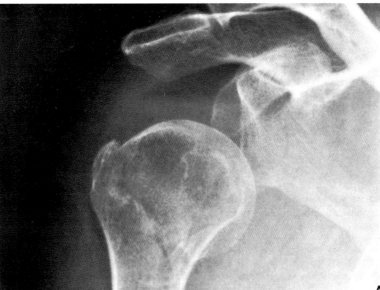
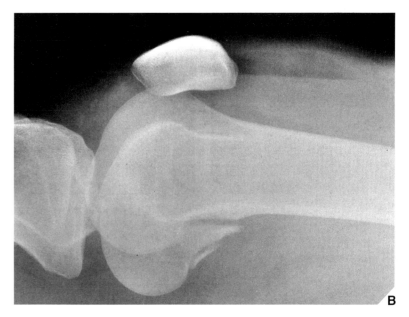

Figure 4.31 (A) Erect anteroposterior view of the shoulder demonstrates the fat-fluid level in the joint—an example of the FBI sign. The fracture line extends from the humeral neck cephalad to the humeral head. To demonstrate the FBI sign, the cassette should be positioned perpendicular to the expected fat-fluid level with the central ray directed horizontally. For example, in the shoulder, an upright radiograph (patient standing or sitting) should be obtained. In the knee (B), the patient should be supine and a cross-table lateral view should be taken.

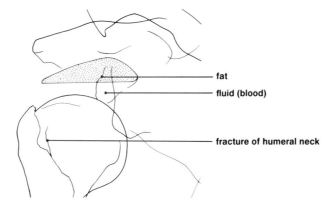

fat

fluid (blood)

fracture of humeral neck

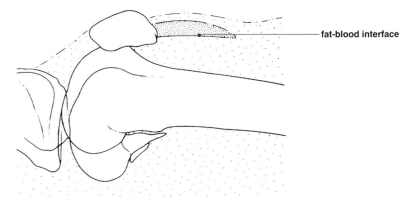

fat-blood interface

Figure 4.32 Axial MR image of the knee (MPGR flip angle 25°, TR 500/TE15) with patient in supine position demonstrates FBI sign secondary to differential layering of fat (high signal intensity) and blood (intermediate signal intensity). Note inhomogeneous appearance of blood due to partial clotting.

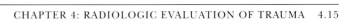

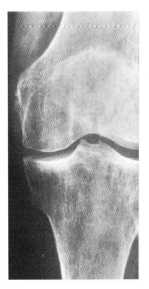

Figure 4.33 (A) On the a[...]
is not apparent, but a dep[...]
condyle projects proximal[...]
ment, producing a double[...]
ence of a subtle fracture o[...]

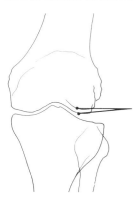

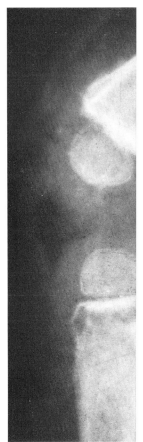

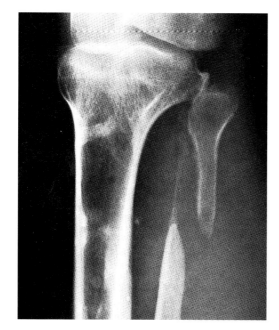

Figure 4.41 Nonunion of a fracture of the proximal fibula. Note the gap between the fragments, the complete lack of callus formation, and the rounding of the fragment edges.

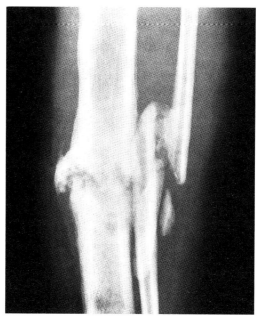

Figure 4.42 In hypertrophic nonunion, seen here in the shafts of the tibia and fibula, there is flaring of the bone ends, marked sclerosis, and periosteal response, but no evidence of endosteal callus formation. The gap between the bony fragments persists.

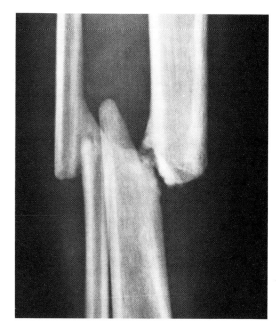

Figure 4.43 In atrophic nonunion, seen here at the junction of the middle and distal thirds of the tibia, there is a gap between the fragments, rounding of the edges, and an almost complete lack of bone reaction. Note the malunited fracture of the fibula.

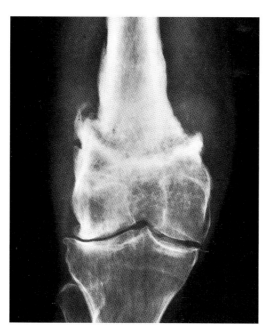

Figure 4.44 Nonunion of the fractured distal shaft of the femur with evidence of old, inactive osteomyelitis shows irregular thickening of the cortex, reactive sclerosis of the medullary portion of the bone, and well organized periosteal reaction.

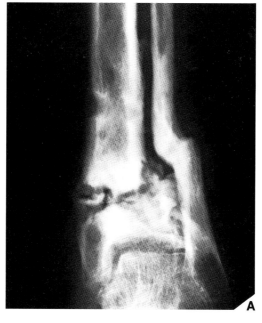

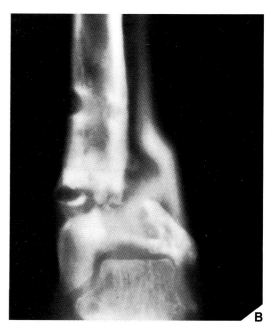

Figure 4.45 (A) Plain film of a nonunited fracture in the distal shaft of the tibia with associated active osteomyelitis shows thickening of the cortex, sclerosis of the cancellous bone, a gap

between the bony fragments, and several sequestra. (B) Tomographic examination provides a better demonstration of the multiple sequestra, the cardinal sign of active infection.

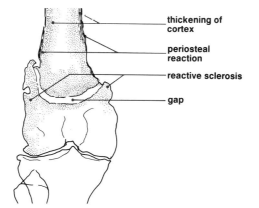

thickening of cortex

periosteal reaction

reactive sclerosis

gap

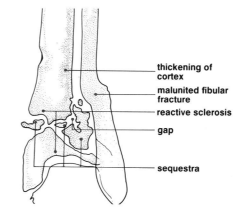

thickening of cortex

malunited fibular fracture

reactive sclerosis

gap

sequestra

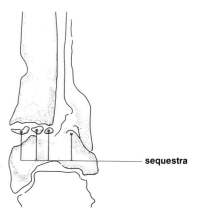

sequestra

age and the fracture site. *Nonunion*, on the other hand, applies to a fracture that simply fails to unite (Fig. 4.41). A *pseudoarthrosis* is a variant of nonunion where there is formation of a false joint cavity with a synovial-like capsule and even synovial fluid at the fracture site; however, some physicians refer to any fracture that fails to heal within eight months as a pseudoarthrosis and use the term as a synonym for nonunion. Radiographically, nonunion is characterized by rounded edges; smoothness and sclerosis (eburnation) of the fragment ends, which are separated by a gap; and motion between the fragments (demonstrated under fluoroscopy or on consecutive stress films).

To provide adequate evaluation of healing failure, the radiologist needs to distinguish between the three types of nonunion: reactive, nonreactive, and infected.

REACTIVE (HYPERTROPHIC AND OLIGOTROPHIC) NONUNION Radiographically, this type is characterized by exuberant bone reaction and resultant flaring and sclerosis of bone ends—the elephant-foot or horse-hoof type (Fig. 4.42). The sclerotic areas do not represent dead bone but the apposition of well vascularized new bone. Radionuclide bone scan shows a marked increase of isotope uptake at the fracture site. This type of nonunited fracture is usually treated by intramedullary nailing or compression plating.

NONREACTIVE (ATROPHIC) NONUNION With this type of nonunion the radiograph shows an absence of bone reaction at the fragment ends, and the blood supply is generally very scanty (Fig. 4.43). Bone scan shows either minimal or no isotope uptake. In addition to stable internal fixation, such fractures often require extensive decortication and bone grafting.

INFECTED NONUNION Radiographic presentation of infected nonunion depends on the infection's activity. Old, *inactive* osteomyelitis shows irregular thickening of the cortex, well organized periosteal reaction, and reactive sclerosis of cancellous bone (Fig. 4.44), whereas the *active* form shows soft tissue swelling, destruction of the cortex and cancellous bone associated with periosteal new bone formation, and sequestration (Fig. 4.45). Treatment of infected nonunion depends on the stage of osteomyelitis. Decortication and bone grafting combined with compression plating are used if

nonunion is accompanied by inactive osteomyelitis. Treatment of active osteomyelitis involves sequestrectomy usually followed by bone grafting and intramedullary stabilization. Different procedures are individually tailored, depending on the anatomic site and various general and local factors.

Other Complications of Fractures and Dislocations

In addition to the possible complications associated with the process of fracture healing, the radiologist may encounter complications that are not related to that process. Radiographic evidence of the presence of such complications may not show up on immediate follow-up examination, since they may occur weeks, months, or even years after the trauma and sometimes in a location distant from the original site of injury. Consequently, in dealing with patients presenting with a history of fracture or dislocation, the radiologist should direct his or her investigation to areas where these associated complications may occur and should be aware of their radiologic characteristics and appearance.

DISUSE OSTEOPOROSIS Mild or moderate osteoporosis, which can be generally defined as a decrease in bone mass, frequently occurs following a fracture or dislocation as a result of disuse of the extremity due to pain and immobilization in the plaster cast. Other terms often used to describe this condition are demineralization, deossification, bone atrophy, and osteopenia. The latter term is generally accepted as the best description of the nature of this complication. Radiographically, it is identified by radiolucent areas of decreased bone density secondary to thinning of the cortex and atrophy of the bony trabeculae. It may accompany united as well as nonunited fractures (Fig. 4.46).

REFLEX SYMPATHETIC DYSTROPHY SYNDROME (RSDS) Known also as posttraumatic painful osteoporosis or Sudeck atrophy, this severe form of osteoporosis may occur subsequent to a fracture or even a milder form of injury. It has also been reported as resulting from neurologic or vascular abnormalities unrelated to trauma. Clinically, the patient presents with a painful, tender extremity with hyperesthesia, diffuse soft tissue swelling, joint stiffness, vasomotor instability, and dystrophic skin changes. On the radiograph it is characterized by soft tissue swelling and severe, patchy osteoporosis,

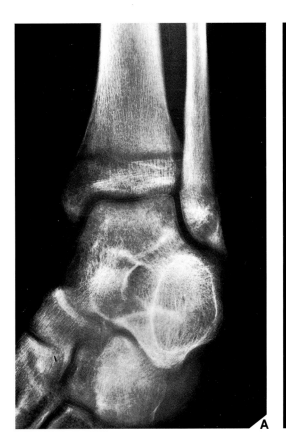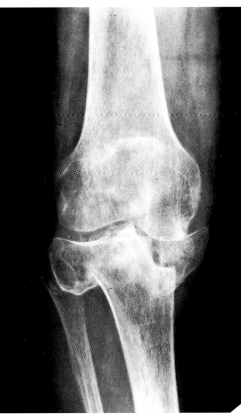

Figure 4.46 (A) Oblique view of the ankle shows a completely united fracture of the distal fibula. Disuse juxta-articular osteoporosis is evident from the thinning of the cortices associated with decreased bone density. (B) Anteroposterior view of the knee shows a nonunited fracture of the tibial plateau, with a moderate degree of disuse osteoporosis.

which progresses rapidly (Fig. 4.47). Technetium bone scan characteristically shows increased uptake in the affected areas, particularly around the joints.

VOLKMANN ISCHEMIC CONTRACTURE Developing usually after supracondylar fracture of the humerus, Volkmann contracture is caused by ischemia of the muscles followed by fibrosis. Clinically, it is characterized as the "five P's" syndrome—pulselessness, pain, pallor, paresthesia, and paralysis. Radiographic examination usually reveals flexion-contracture in the wrist and in the interphalangeal joints of the fingers and hyperextension (or, rarely, flexion) of the metacarpophalangeal joints associated with soft tissue atrophy (Fig. 4.48).

POSTTRAUMATIC MYOSITIS OSSIFICANS Occasionally after a fracture, dislocation, or even minor trauma to the soft tissues, an enlarging, painful mass develops at the site of injury. The characteristic feature of this lesion is the clearly recognizable pattern of its evolution, which correlates well with the lapse of time following the trauma. Thus, by the third to fourth week calcifications and ossifications in the mass begin to develop (Fig. 4.49A), and at six to eight weeks the periphery of the mass shows definite, well organized cortical bone

(Fig. 4.49B). The important radiographic hallmark of this complication is the presence of the so-called "zonal phenomenon." On the radiograph this phenomenon is characterized by a radiolucent area in the center of the lesion, indicating the formation of immature bone, and by a dense zone of mature ossification at the periphery. In addition, a thin radiolucent cleft separates the ossific mass from the adjacent cortex (Fig. 4.49C). These important features help differentiate this condition from juxtacortical osteosarcoma, which may at times appear very similar. It must be stressed, however, that occasionally the focus of myositis ossificans may adhere and fuse with the cortex, mimicking parosteal osteosarcoma on plain radiographs. In these cases, CT may provide additional information, such as the presence of the zonal phenomenon characteristic of myositis ossificans (Fig. 4.50).

OSTEONECROSIS (ISCHEMIC OR AVASCULAR NECROSIS) Osteonecrosis, the cellular death of bone tissue, occurs following fracture or dislocation when the bone is deprived of a sufficient supply of arterial blood. However, it is important to recognize that this condition may also develop as a result of factors unrelated to mechanical trauma. Among the reported causes of osteonecrosis are the following:

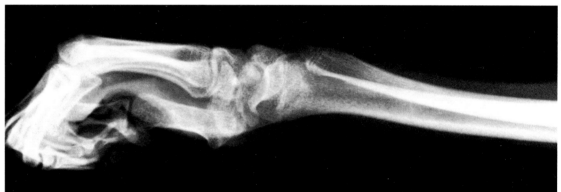

Figure 4.48 Having sustained a supracondylar fracture of the humerus, which united, a 23-year-old man presented with complaints typical of Volkmann ischemic contracture. Lateral view of the distal forearm including the wrist and hand shows flexion-contracture in the metacarpophalangeal and the interphalangeal joints, together with a marked degree of soft tissue atrophy.

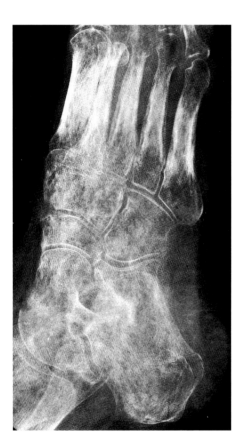

Figure 4.47 A 35-year-old man sustained fractures of the tibia and fibula, which eventually healed. Subsequently, however, he complained of weakness, stiffness, and pain in his foot. Radiographic examination showed changes typical of Sudeck atrophy in the foot: rapidly progressive, patchy osteoporosis associated with marked soft tissue swelling.

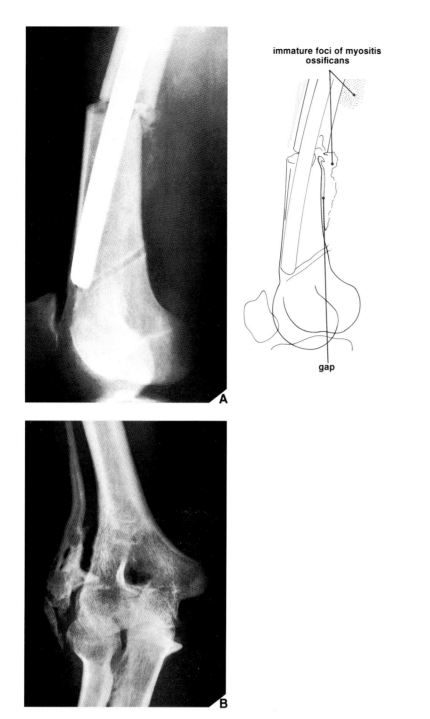

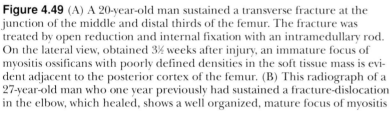

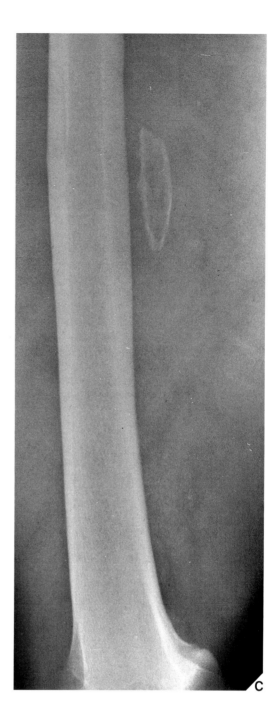

Figure 4.49 (A) A 20-year-old man sustained a transverse fracture at the junction of the middle and distal thirds of the femur. The fracture was treated by open reduction and internal fixation with an intramedullary rod. On the lateral view, obtained 3½ weeks after injury, an immature focus of myositis ossificans with poorly defined densities in the soft tissue mass is evident adjacent to the posterior cortex of the femur. (B) This radiograph of a 27-year-old man who one year previously had sustained a fracture-dislocation in the elbow, which healed, shows a well organized, mature focus of myositis ossificans. Note the well developed cortex at the periphery of the osseous mass and the radiolucent gap separating the lesion from the cortex of the humerus. (C) A 16-year-old boy presented with a history of trauma six weeks before this radiographic examination. The lateral view of the right femur demonstrates a lesion that exhibits features of the zonal phenomenon characteristic of juxtacortical myositis ossificans. Note the cleft separating the ossific mass from the posterior cortex.

1. Embolization of arteries. This may occur in a variety of conditions. It is seen, for example, in certain hemoglobinopathies, such as sickle-cell disease, where arteries are occluded by abnormal red blood cells; in decompression states of dysbaric conditions, such as caisson disease, where embolization by nitrogen bubbles occurs; or in chronic alcoholism and pancreatitis, when fat particles embolize arteries.
2. Vasculitis. Inflammation of the blood vessels may lead to interruption of the supply of arterial blood to the bone, as seen in collagen disorders such as systemic lupus erythematosus.
3. Abnormal accumulation of cells. In Gaucher disease, which is characterized by the abnormal accumulation of lipid-containing histiocytes in the bone marrow, or following steroid therapy, which can lead to an increase of fat cells, sinusoidal blood flow may be compromised, resulting in deprivation of blood supply to the bone.
4. Radiation exposure. Exposure to radiation may result in damage to the vascularity of bone.
5. Idiopathic. Often no definite etiology can be established, as in the case of spontaneous osteonecrosis that predominantly affects the medial femoral condyle; or in the case of certain osteochondroses such as Legg-Calvé-Perthes disease involving the femoral head, or Freiberg disease affecting the head of the second metatarsal.

Following trauma, osteonecrosis occurs most commonly in the femoral head, the carpal scaphoid, and the humeral head because of the precarious supply of blood to these bones.

Osteonecrosis of the femoral head is a frequent complication following intracapsular fracture of the femoral neck (60% to 75%), dislocation in the hip joint (25%), and slipped capital femoral epiphysis (15% to 40%). In its very early stages, radiographs may appear completely normal; radionuclide bone scan, however, may show increased isotope uptake at the site of the lesion—a very valuable indication of abnormality. The earliest radiographic sign of this complication is the presence of a radiolucent crescent, which may be seen as early as four weeks after the initial injury. This phenomenon, as Norman and Bullough have pointed out, is secondary to the subchondral structural collapse of the necrotic segment and is visible as a narrow radiolucent line parallel to the articular surface of the bone. Radiographically, the sign is most easily demonstrated on the frog-lateral view of the hip, but tomography provides the best modality for imaging the features of the complication itself (Fig. 4.51). Because the necrotic process does not affect the articular cartilage, the width of the joint space (that is, the radiographic joint space: the width of the articular cartilage of adjoining bones plus the actual joint cavity) is preserved. Preservation of the joint space helps to differentiate this condition from osteoarthritis. In its later stage osteonecrosis can be readily identified on the anteroposterior view of the hip by a flattening of the articular surface and the dense appearance of the femoral head (Fig. 4.52). The density is secondary to compression of bony trabeculae following microfracture of the nonviable bone, calcification of detritic marrow, and repair of the necrotic area by deposition of new bone—so-called

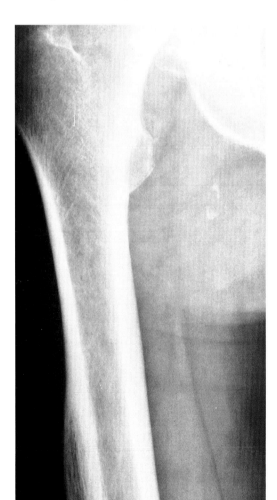

A

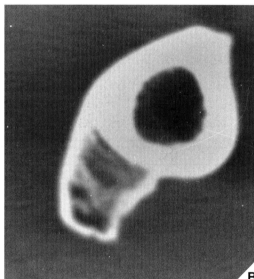

B

Figure 4.50 A 52-year-old man sustained injury to the lateral aspect of the left thigh six months previously. He was concerned about a hard mass he had palpated. (A) Plain film shows an ossific mass adherent to the lateral cortex of the left femur. (B) CT scan demonstrates the classic zonal phenomenon of myositis ossificans. Note radiolucent center surrounded by mature cortex.

creeping substitution. Tomographic examination frequently helps to delineate the details of this condition.

A significant breakthrough in identifying osteonecrosis in patients who had normal bone scans and conventional radiographs was achieved with MRI. Currently, this modality is considered the most sensitive and specific for the diagnosis and evaluation of osteonecrosis. In particular, several reports have established the diagnostic sensitivity of MRI in the early stages of osteonecrosis, when radiographic changes are not yet apparent or are nonspecific. MRI is indispensable in the accurate staging of osteonecrosis, since it reflects the size of the lesion and roughly the stage of the disease. Mitchell and colleagues have described a classification system of osteonecrosis based on alterations in the central region of MR signal intensity in the osteonecrotic focus. In early stages (class A or fat-like), there is preservation of a normal fat signal, except at the sclerotic reactive margin surrounding the lesion, that manifests as a central region of high signal intensity on short SE TR/TE images

(T1-weighted), and intermediate signal intensity on long TR/TE images (T2-weighted). Later, when there is sufficient inflammation or vascular engorgement, or if subacute hemorrhage is present (class B or blood-like), a high signal intensity is noted on short and long TR/TE images. This signal is similar to that of a subacute hemorrhage. If there is enough inflammation, hyperemia, and fibrosis present to replace the fat content of the femoral head (class C or fluid-like), a low intensity signal with short TR/TE and high intensity signal with long TR/TE is seen. Finally, in advanced stages, where fibrosis and sclerosis predominate (class D or fibrous-like), low signal intensity is present on both short and long TR/TE images (Fig. 4.53). MRI findings correlate well with histologic changes. The central region of high signal intensity corresponds to necrosis of bone and marrow. The low signal of the peripheral band corresponds to the sclerotic margin of reactive tissue at the interface between necrotic and viable bone. As Seiler and coworkers have pointed out, MRI evaluation of osteonecrosis of the femoral head has several

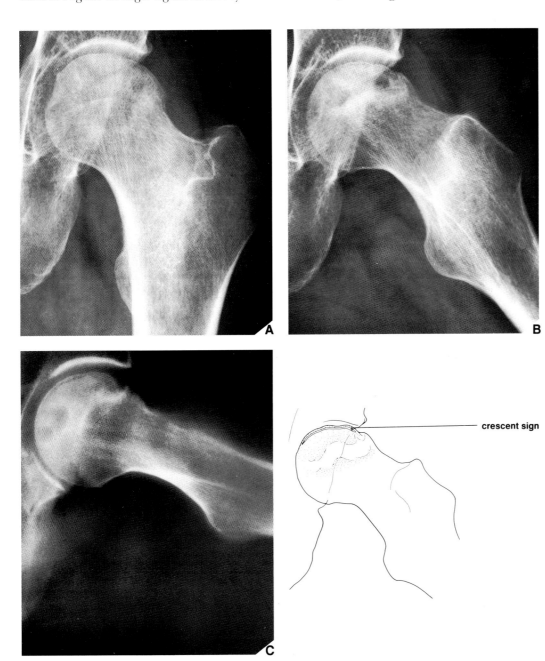

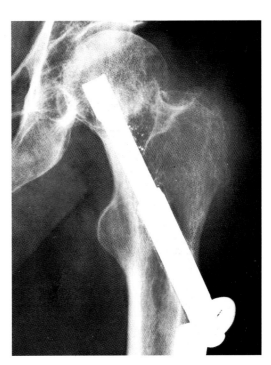

Figure 4.52 A 56-year-old woman sustained an intracapsular fracture of left femoral neck, which healed after surgical treatment by open reduction and internal fixation. The anteroposterior view shows a Smith-Peterson nail inserted into the femoral neck and head. The fracture line is obliterated. The dense appearance of the femoral head indicates the development of osteonecrosis.

Figure 4.51 (A) A 41-year-old man presented with a history of traumatic dislocation in the left hip joint. On frontal projection the increased density of the femoral head suggests osteonecrosis, but a definite diagnosis cannot be made. (B) The frog-lateral view demonstrates a thin radiolucent line parallel to the articular surface of the femoral head. This represents the crescent sign, a radiographic hallmark of osteonecrosis. (C) Tomographic examination confirms the features typical of osteonecrosis: the crescent sign, the dense femoral head, and the preservation of the joint space indicating intact articular cartilage.

advantages: It is noninvasive, does not require ionizing radiation, provides multiplanar images, reflects physiologic changes in the bone marrow, provides excellent resolution of surrounding soft tissues, and makes it possible to simultaneously evaluate the contralateral femoral head.

Osteonecrosis of the carpal scaphoid is a complication commonly seen in 10% to 15% of cases of carpal scaphoid fracture, increasing in incidence to 30% to 40% if there is nonunion. Necrosis generally involves the proximal bone fragment, but the distal fragment, although rarely, may also be affected. Evidence of this complication most frequently becomes apparent about four to six months after injury, when radiographic examination shows increased bone density. Although it is most often diagnosed on plain-film radiographs, tomographic study (Fig. 4.54) or MRI is indicated when conventional radiographic findings are equivocal.

Osteonecrosis may also develop in the humeral head following a fracture of the humeral neck (Fig. 4.55), but this complication is infrequently seen.

INJURY TO MAJOR BLOOD VESSELS   A relatively infrequent complication of a fracture or dislocation, injury to the major blood vessels occurs when bone fragments lacerate or completely transect an artery or a vein, resulting in bleeding, the formation of hematoma, arteriovenous fistula, or a pseudoaneurysm (Fig. 4.56). In order to demonstrate this abnormality, angiography is the procedure of choice. This technique is invaluable in visualizing the site of laceration, ascertaining the exact extent of vascular damage, and assessing the status of collateral circulation. It may also be combined with an interventional procedure, such as embolization to control hemorrhage.

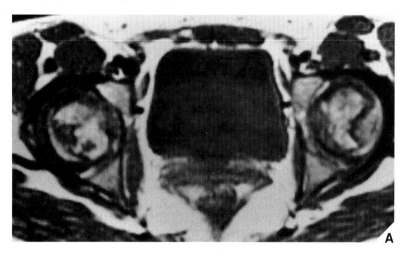

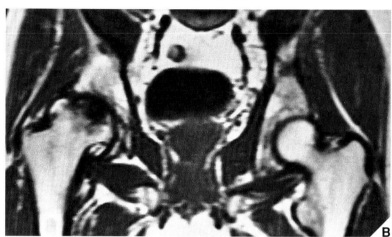

Figure 4.53 (A) Axial T1-weighted MR image of the pelvis (SE, TR 600/TE 20) shows early stage (class A) osteonecrosis of the left femoral head and a more advanced stage (class C) of the right. Note that in the central areas of necrosis of the left femoral head the high signal intensity is preserved, but it is surrounded by a rim of low signal intensity, representing reactive sclerosis . More advanced stage osteonecrosis of the right femoral head is imaged as areas of low signal density. (B) Coronal T1-weighted MR image of the right proximal femur (SE, TR 600/TE 20) demonstrates advanced (class D) osteonecrosis of the right femoral head. The necrotic focus displays low signal intensity. The identical low signal was present on T2-weighted images.

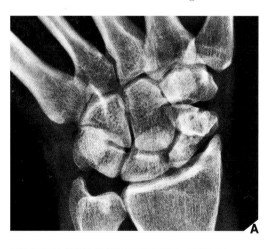

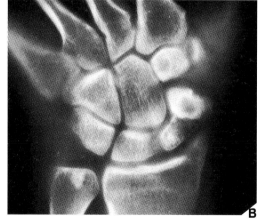

Figure 4.54 (A) Plain film of the wrist on the dorsovolar projection demonstrates a fracture of the carpal scaphoid; it is unclear, however, whether the fracture is complicated by osteonecrosis. (B) Trispiral tomogram clearly shows nonunion and the presence of osteonecrosis of the distal fragment, together with cystic degeneration. Note also the posttraumatic cyst in the trapezoid bone. The dense spot in the articular end of the ulna represents a bone island.

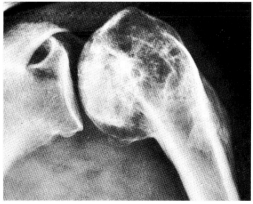

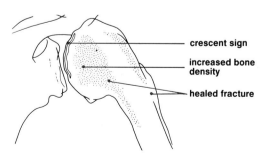

Figure 4.55 Six months after sustaining a fracture of the left humeral neck, which united, a 62-year-old man developed osteonecrosis of the humeral head, evident on the radiograph from the increased bone density and the collapse of the subchondral segment.

GROWTH DISTURBANCE A common complication of Salter-Harris type IV and V fractures involving the physis, growth disturbance may result from injury to the growth plate by the formation of an osseous bridge between the epiphysis and metaphysis. As a result of this tethering of the growth plate, localized cessation of bone growth occurs. If the entire physis in a single long bone stops growing, a limb length discrepancy will result (Fig. 4.57A). If only one growth plate at the articulations of parallel bones (the radius and ulna or the tibia and fibula) is damaged and ceases to grow, the uninjured bone continues to grow at the normal rate, leading to overgrowth and consequent joint deformity (Fig. 4.57B).

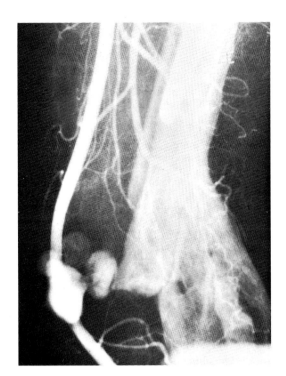

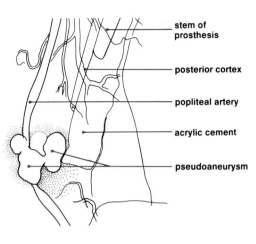

stem of prosthesis

posterior cortex

popliteal artery

acrylic cement

pseudoaneurysm

Figure 4.56 A 30-year-old woman with Gaucher disease and a total hip replacement as a result of osteonecrosis of the femoral head sustained a transverse fracture of the left femoral shaft through the acrylic cement just distal to the stem of the prosthesis. A femoral arteriogram revealed a pseudoaneurysm of the popliteal artery resulting from injury to the vessel by the fractured bone fragment and the acrylic cement. (Reprinted with permission of the author and the publisher from Baker ND, 1981)

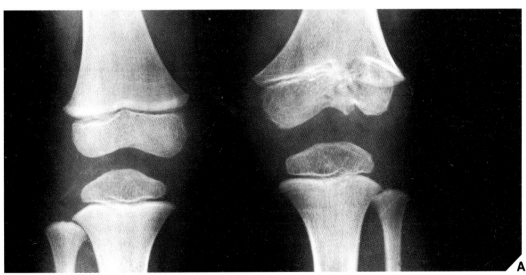

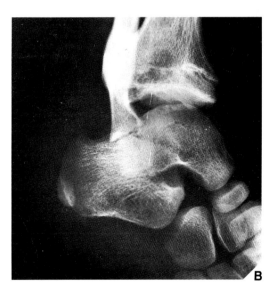

Figure 4.57 (A) A 3-year-old boy sustained a fracture of the left distal femur that extended through the growth plate. As a result, the bone at this end prematurely ceased to grow. The anteroposterior view of both knees shows a discrepancy in the length of the femora associated with deformity of the distal epiphysis of the left femur secondary to tethering of the growth plate.

(B) A 5-year-old girl sustained a Salter-Harris type V fracture of the distal tibia. On the lateral view a joint deformity is evident as a result of the fusion of the physis of the tibia and overgrowth of the distal fibula. Note also the posttraumatic synostosis of these two bones.

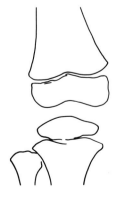

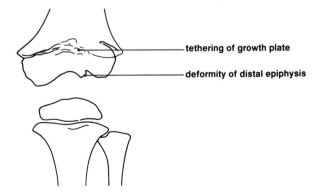

tethering of growth plate

deformity of distal epiphysis

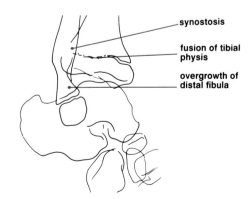

synostosis

fusion of tibial physis

overgrowth of distal fibula

POSTTRAUMATIC ARTHRITIS If a fracture line extends into the joint, the articular surface may become irregular. Such incongruity in the articular surfaces results in abnormal stresses that lead to precocious degenerative changes recognized on the radiograph by narrowing of the joint space, subchondral sclerosis, and formation of marginal osteophytes (Fig. 4.58). A similar complication may also be seen following a dislocation (Fig. 4.59).

INJURY TO SOFT TISSUES

Under normal physiologic circumstances, soft tissues such as muscles, tendons, ligaments, articular menisci, and intervertebral discs are only faintly outlined or not visible at all on plain-film radiographs. As a result, only rarely—as in such traumatic conditions as myositis ossificans or certain tears of ligaments and tendons—does conventional radiography suffice to demonstrate trauma to the soft tissues (Fig. 4.60). Adequate evaluation of injury to these structures and of the progress of treatment, consequently, requires supplemental studies, which may include stress radiography, arthrography, tenography, bursography, myelography, CT, and MRI.

MRI, in particular, is considered to be the best imaging modality for evaluating traumatic soft tissue injuries. Differences in signal intensity enable abnormalities of the various structures (muscles, tendons, ligaments, fascias, vessels, and nerves) to be effectively demonstrated. Posttraumatic tenosynovitis, joint effusion, and soft tissue hematomas are also well seen on MR images. Tears of various ligaments and tendons can be accurately diagnosed; for instance, when evaluating tendon injuries, MRI provides information regarding the location of the tear (whether it is within the tendon, at the tendon insertion, or at the musculotendinous interface), the size of the gap between both tendon ends, the size of the hematoma at the rupture site, and the presence of any inflammatory component (Fig. 4.61).

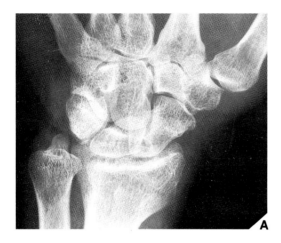

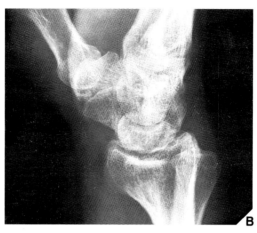

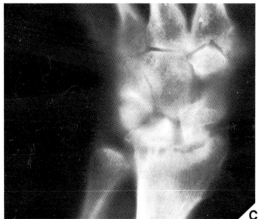

Figure 4.58 Dorsovolar (A) and lateral (B) views of the wrist of a 57-year-old man who had sustained an intra-articular fracture of the distal radius demonstrate residual deformity of this bone and narrowing of the radiocarpal articulation. Trispiral tomogram (C) shows, in addition, the multiple subchondral degenerative cysts often seen in posttraumatic arthritis.

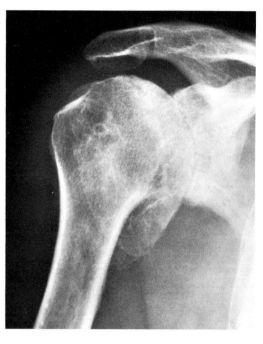

Figure 4.59 The anteroposterior view of the right shoulder of a 78-year-old man who presented with a history of several previous dislocations in that joint demonstrates the advanced degenerative changes resulting from repeated trauma to the articular surfaces of the humeral head and glenoid.

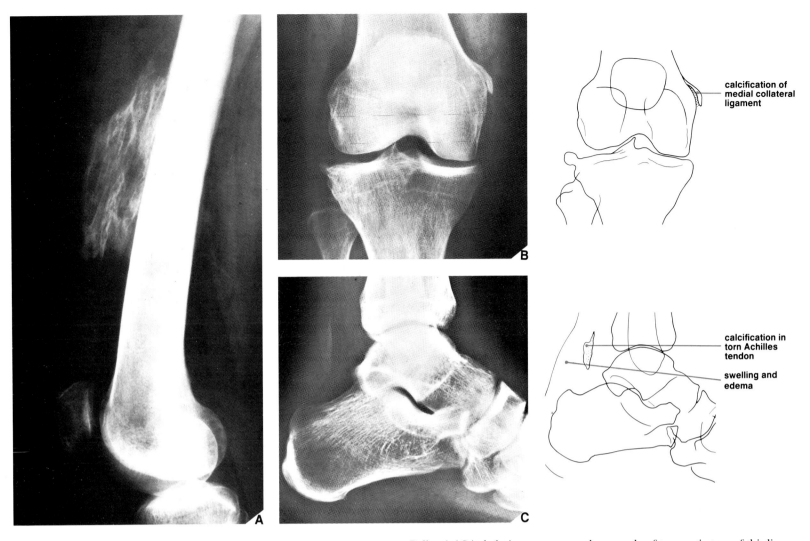

Figure 4.60 (A) A common complication of trauma to the muscular structures, myositis ossificans is characterized by the formation of bone in the injured muscle. This condition is apparent on the plain-film radiograph. (B) Calcification of the medial collateral ligament of the knee, known as Pellegrini-Stieda lesion, represents the sequela of traumatic tear of this ligament. (C) In certain instances the tear of a tendon may be diagnosed on the plain-film radiograph. The lateral view of the ankle shows the typical appearance of a torn Archilles tendon.

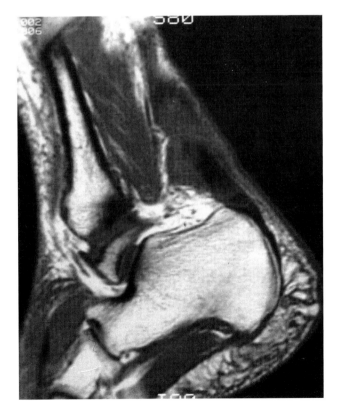

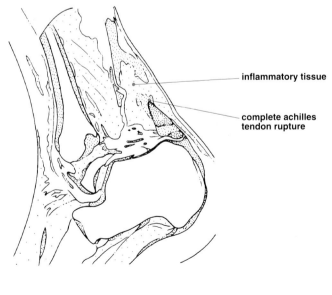

Figure 4.61 Sagittal MRI section of the ankle (SE TR2000/ TE20) shows discontinuity of the Achilles tendon near its insertion to the calcaneus. An inflammatory mass is seen at the rupture site. (From Beltran J, 1990)

PRACTICAL POINTS TO REMEMBER

[1] When dealing with suspected fractures and dislocations, obtain radiographs in at least two projections at 90° to each other.

[2] To eliminate the risk of missing an associated injury, include the adjacent joints on the film.

[3] When a fracture is suspected, look for subtle associated abnormalities such as:
  • soft tissue swelling
  • obliteration or displacement of fat stripes
  • periosteal and endosteal reaction
  • joint effusion
  • intracapsular fat-fluid level
  • double cortical line
  • buckling of the cortex
  • irregular metaphyseal corners.

[4] When reporting a fracture, describe:
  • the site and extent
  • the type
  • the direction of the fracture line
  • the alignment of the fragments
  • the presence of impaction, depression, or compression
  • the presence of associated abnormalities
  • whether the fracture is a special type
  • whether the growth plate is involved (in which case the Salter-Harris classification, together with Rang and Ogden additions, provides a useful method of precise evaluation of the injury).

[5] When a fracture fails to heal, distinguish between the three types of nonunion:
  • reactive (hypertrophic and oligotrophic)
  • nonreactive (atrophic)
  • infected.

[6] In patients presenting with a history of skeletal trauma, be aware of such possible complications as:
  • disuse osteoporosis (mild or moderate)
  • reflex sympathetic dystrophy syndrome
  • Volkmann ischemic contracture
  • posttraumatic myositis ossificans (the hallmarks of which are the clearly defined pattern of its evolution, the radiographic presence of the zonal phenomenon, and a radiolucent cleft)
  • osteonecrosis (the earliest signs may be demonstrated by MRI or later may manifest as an increased uptake of isotope on scintigraphy; the radiographic hallmark is the radiolucent crescent signs)
  • injury to vessels
  • growth disturbance
  • posttraumatic arthritis.

[7] When dealing with injury to soft tissues, consider using supplemental imaging modalities, including:
  • stress radiography
  • arthrography
  • tenography and bursography
  • myelography
  • computed tomography
  • magnetic resonance imaging.

References

Arger PH, Oberkircher PE, Miller WT: Lipohemarthrosis *Am J Roentgenol* 121:97, 1974.

Baker ND: Pseudoaneurysm—a complication of fracture through cement after total hip replacement *Orthop Rev* 10:110, 1981.

Bassett LW, Grover JS, Seeger LL: Magnetic resonance imaging of knee trauma. *Skeletal Radiol* 19:401, 1990.

Beltran J: *MRI: Musculoskeletal System.* Philadelphia, Lippincott, 1990.

Bohrer SP: The fat pad sign following elbow trauma. Its usefulness and reliability in suspecting "invisible" fractures. *Clin Radiol* 21:90, 1970.

Brody AS, Strong M, Babikian G, Sweet DE, Seidel FG, Kuhn JP: Avascular necrosis: Early MR imaging and histologic findings in a canine model. *Am J Roentegenol* 157:341, 1991.

Caffey J: *Pediatric X-Ray Diagnosis*, vol 2, ed 2. Chicago, Year Book Medical Publishers, 1973.

Coleman BG, Kressel HY, Dalinka MK, et al: Radiographically negative avascular necrosis: detection with MR imaging *Radiology* 168:525, 1988.

Conolly JF, Whittaker D, Williams E: Femoral and tibial fractures combined with injuries to the femoral or popliteal artery. *J Bone Joint Surg* 53A:56, 1971.

Deutsch AL, Mink JH: Magnetic resonance imaging of musculoskeletal injuries. *Radiol Clin North Am* 27:983, 1989.

Eisenberg RL: *Atlas of Signs in Radiology.* Philadelphia, Lippincott, 1984.

Genant HK, Kozin F, Bekerman C, McCarty DJ, Sims J: The reflect sympathetic dystrophy syndrome. *Radiology* 117:21, 1975.

Haughton VM: MR imaging of the spine. *Radiology* 166:297, 1988.

Hendrix RW, Rogers, LF: Diagnostic imaging of fracture complications. *Radiol Clin North Am* 27:1023, 1989.

Hermann LG, Reineke HG, Caldwell JA: Post-traumatic painful osteoporosis; a clinical and roentgenological entity. *Am J Roentgenol* 47:353, 1942.

Holt G, Helms CA, Steinbach L, Neumann C, Munk PL, Genant HK: Magnetic resonance imaging of the shoulder: Rationale and current applications. *Skeletal Radiol* 19:5, 1990.

Jones DA: Volkmann's ischemia. *Surg Clin North Am* 41:1099, 1970.

Jones G: Radiological appearance of disuse osteoporosis. *Clin Radiol* 20:345, 1969.

Kuhlman JE, Fishman EK, Magid D, et al: Fracture nonunion: CT assessment with multiplanar reconstruction. *Radiology* 167:483, 1988.

MacEwan DW: Changes due to trauma in the fat plane overlying the pronator quadratus muscle. A radiologic sign. *Radiology* 82:879, 1964.

Mazet R Jr, Hohl M: Fractures of the carpal navicular. *J Bone Joint Surg* 45A:82, 1963.

McDougall IR, Rieser RP: Scintigraphic techniques in musculoskeletal trauma. *Radiol Clin North Am* 27:1003, 1989.

Mitchell DG, Rao VM, Dalinka MK, et al: Femoral head avascular necrosis: correlation of MR imaging, radiographic staging, radionuclide imaging, and clinical findings. *Radiology* 162:709, 1987.

Müller ME, Allgower M, Schneider R, Willenegger H: *Manual of Internal Fixation. Techniques Recommended by the AO Group*, ed 2. Berlin, Springer-Verlag, 1979.

Nelson SW: Some important diagnostic and technical fundamentals in the radiology of trauma, with particular emphasis on skeletal trauma. *Radiol Clin North Am* 4:241, 1966.

Norell HG: Roentgenologic visualization of the extracapsular fat, its importance in the diagnosis of traumatic injuries to the elbow. *Acta Radiol* 42:205, 1954.

Norman A, Bullough P: The radiolucent crescent line—an early diagnostic sign of avascular necrosis of the femoral head. *Bull Hosp J Dis Orthop Inst* 24:99, 1963.

Norman A, Dorfman HD: Juxtacortical circumscribed myositis ossificans: Evolution and radiographic features. *Radiology* 96:301, 1970.

Ogden JA: Skeletal growth mechanism injury patterns. *J Pediatr Orthop* 2:371, 1982.

Rang M: *The Growth Plate and Its Disorders.* Baltimore, Williams & Wilkins, 1969.

Richardson ML, Kilcoyne RF, Mayo KA, Lamont JG, Hastrup W: Radiographic evaluation of modern orthopedic fixation devices. *RadioGraphics* 7:685, 1987.

Rockwood CA Jr, Green DP: *Fractures in Adults*, vol 1. Philadelphia, Lippincott, 1984.

Rockwood CA Jr, Wilkins KE, King RE: *Fractures in Children*, vol 3. Philadelphia, Lippincott, 1984.

Rogers LF: *Radiology of Skeletal Trauma.* New York, Churchill Livingstone, 1982.

Salter RB: *Textbook of Disorders and Injuries of the Musculoskeletal System.* Baltimore, Williams & Wilkins, 1970.

Salter RB, Harris WR: Injuries involving the epiphyseal plate *J Bone Joint Surg* 45A:587, 1963.

Seiler JG III, Christie MJ, Homra L: Correlation of the findings of magnetic resonance imaging with those of bone biopsy in patients who have stage I or II ischemic necrosis of the femoral head. *J Bone Joint Surg* 71A:28, 1989.

Stoller DW, Genant HK: The hip. In: Stoller DW (ed.): *Magnetic Resonance Imaging in Orthopaedics and Rheumatology.* Philadelphia, Lippincott, 1989.

Terry DW Jr, Ramin JE: The navicular fat stripe: A useful roentgen feature for evaluating wrist trauma. *Am J Roentgenol* 124:25, 1975.

Weissman BNW, Sledge CB: *Orthopedic Radiology* (Chapter 1: General Principles). Philadelphia, Saunders, 1986.

Wenzel WW: The FBI sign. *Rocky Mount Med J* 69:71, 1972.

ating suspected abnormalities of the fibrocartilaginous glenoid labrum (Fig 5.16). The effectiveness of this combination lies in the fact that the injected air outlines the anterior and posterior labrum for better demonstration of subtle traumatic changes on CT images. For this study the patient is placed supine in the CT scanner with the arm of the affected side in the neutral position to allow the air to rise and enhance the outline of the anterior labrum; to evaluate the posterior labrum, the arm is externally rotated (or the patient is positioned prone) to force the air to move posteriorly.

Recent studies have shown the considerable advantage of MRI in the examination of the shoulder. This modality is particularly effective in demonstrating traumatic abnormalities of the soft tissues, such as impingement syndrome, partial and complete rotator cuff tears, biceps tendon rupture, glenoid labrum tears, and demonstration of the traumatic joint effusion. However, the shoulder presents unique difficulties for imaging. Because of space limi-

tations in the magnet, the shoulder cannot be positioned in the center of the magnetic field. This necessitates lateral shift for image centering and scanning a region where the signal-to-noise ratio is relatively low. These problems have been overcome by combining high-resolution scanning with the use of special surface coils. Because the bones and muscles of the shoulder girdle are oriented along multiple nonorthogonal axes, scanning in oblique planes is more effective.

The patient should be positioned in the magnet supine with the arms along the thorax and the affected arm externally rotated. The scanning planes include oblique coronal (along the long axis of the belly of the supraspinatus muscle), oblique sagittal (perpendicular to the course of supraspinatus muscle), and axial (Fig. 5.17). The first two planes are ideal for evaluating all of the structures of the rotator cuff; the axial plane is ideal for evaluating the glenoid labrum, bicipital groove, biceps tendon, and subscapularis tendon.

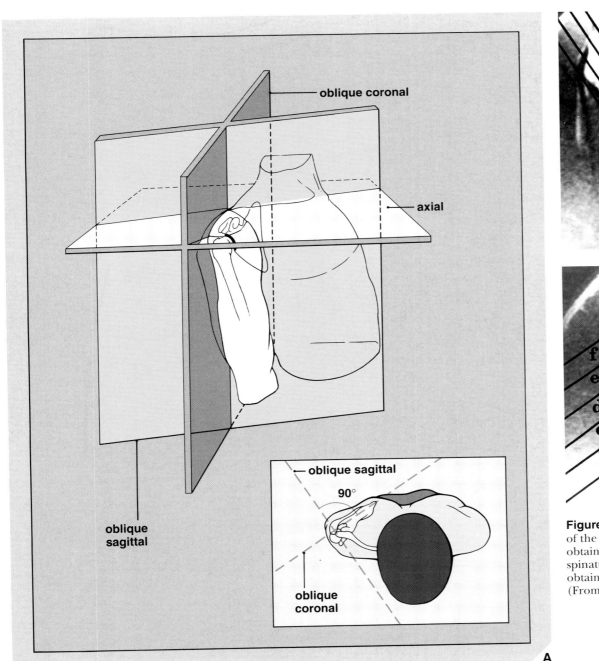

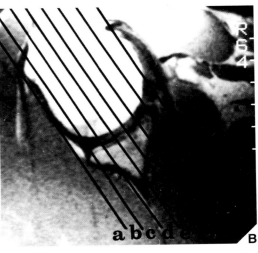

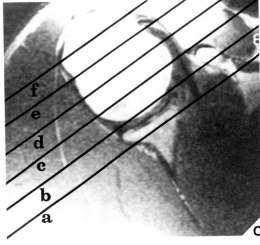

Figure 5.17 (A) Standard planes of MRI sections of the shoulder. (B) Oblique coronal sections are obtained parallel to the long axis of the supraspinatus muscle. (C) Oblique sagittal sections are obtained perpendicular to the coronal sections. (From Beltran J, 1990)

Figure 5.18 Standard and Special Radiographic Projections for Evaluating Injury to the Shoulder Girdle

PROJECTION	DEMONSTRATION	PROJECTION	DEMONSTRATION
Anteroposterior		*Axillary*	Relationship of humeral head and glenoid fossa
Arm in neutral position	Fractures of: Humeral head and neck Clavicle Scapula Anterior dislocation Bankart lesion		Anterior and posterior dislocations Compression fractures secondary to anterior and posterior dislocations Fractures of: Proximal humerus Scapula
Erect	Fat–blood interface (FBI sign)		
Arm in internal rotation	Hill–Sacks lesion	*West Point*	Same structures and conditions as axillary projection Anteroinferior rim of glenoid
Arm in external rotation	Compression fracture of humeral head (through line impaction) secondary to posterior dislocation	*Lateral Transthoracic*	Relationship of humeral head and glenoid fossa Fractures of proximal humerus
40°posterior oblique (Grashey)	Glenohumeral joint space Glenoid in profile Posterior dislocation	*Tanget (Humeral Head)*	Bicipital groove
15° cephalad tilt of radiographic tube	Acromioclavicular joint Acromioclavicular separation Fracture of clavicle	*Trans-Scapular (Y)*	Relationship of humeral head and glenoid fossa Fractures of: Proximal humerus Body of scapula Coracoid process Acromion
Stress	Occult acromioclavicular subluxation Acromioclavicular separation		

Figure 5.19 Ancillary Imaging Techniques for Evaluating Injury to the Shoulder Girdle

TECHNIQUE	DEMONSTRATION	TECHNIQUE	DEMONSTRATION
Tomography	Position of fragments and extension of fracture line in complex fractures Healing process: Nonunion Secondary infection	*Ultrasonography*	Rotator cuff tear
		Arthrography **Single- or double-contrast**	Complete rotator cuff tear Partial rotator cuff tear Abnormalities of articular cartilage and joint capsule* Synovial abnormalities* Adhesive capsulitis Osteochondral bodies in joint* Abnormalities of bicipital tendon* Intra-articular portion of bicipital tendon*† Inferior surface of rotator cuff*†
Computed Tomography	Relationship of humeral head and glenoid fossa Multiple fragments in complex fractures (particularly of scapula) Intra-articular displacement of bony fragments in fractures		
Magnetic Resonance Imaging	Impingement syndrome Partial and complete rotator cuff tear Biceps tendon rupture Glenoid labrum tears Traumatic joint effusion	**Double-contrast combined with CT**	All of the above in addition to: Abnormalities of cartilaginous glenoid labrum Osteochondral bodies in joint Subtle synovial abnormalties

*These conditions are usually best demonstrated using double-contrast arthrography.
†These features are best demonstrated on erect films.

Appropriate pulse sequences are critical in displaying normal anatomy and traumatic abnormalities. T1-weighted pulse sequences sufficiently demonstrate the structural anatomy (see Figs. 5.4, 5.5). Proton density and T2-weighted pulse sequences provide the information necessary to evaluate pathology of rotator cuff, joint space and bones (see Figs. 5.31, 5.35).

For a summary of the foregoing discussion in tabular form, see Figures 5.18, 5.19, and 5.20.

Injury to the Shoulder Girdle
Fractures About the Shoulder

FRACTURES OF THE PROXIMAL HUMERUS Fractures of the upper humerus involving the head, the neck, and the proximal shaft usually result either from a direct blow to the humerus or—as is more often seen in elderly patients—from a fall on the outstretched arm. Nondisplaced fractures are the most common, representing about 85% of all such proximal humeral injuries.

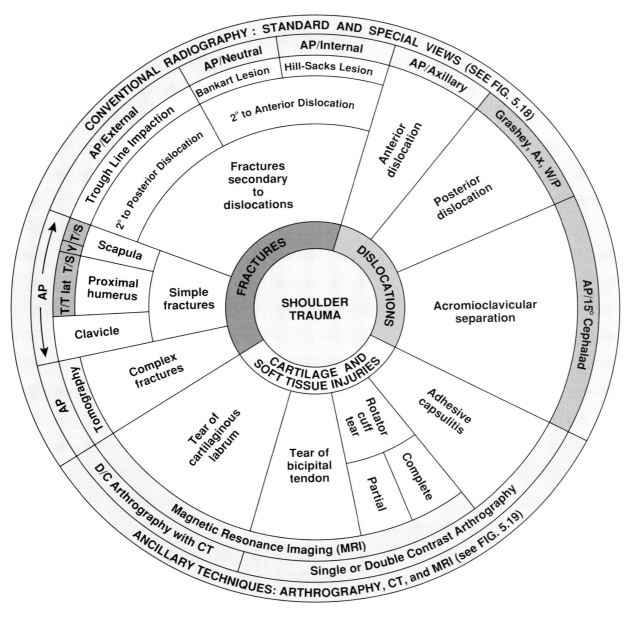

SPECTRUM OF RADIOLOGIC IMAGING TECHNIQUES FOR EVALUATING INJURY TO THE SHOULDER GIRDLE*

*The radiographic projections or radiologic techniques indicated throughout the diagram are only those that are the most effective in demonstrating the respective traumatic conditions.

Figure 5.20 Spectrum of radiologic imaging techniques for evaluating injury to the shoulder girdle.

The anteroposterior projection is usually sufficient to demonstrate the abnormality, but the transthoracic lateral or the transscapular (or Y) projection may be required to provide a fuller evaluation, particularly of the degree of displacement or angulation of the bony fragments (Fig. 5.21). In cases of comminution, conventional tomography may also need to be employed to assess the degree of displacement of the various fragments. The erect anteroposterior radiograph may demonstrate the presence of fat and blood within the joint capsule (the FBI sign of lipohemarthrosis; see Fig. 4.31), indicating intra-articular extension of the fracture.

Traditional classifications of trauma to the proximal humerus, according to the level of the fracture or the mechanism of injury, have been inadequate to identify the various types of displaced fractures. The four-segment classification described by Neer in 1970 was complex and difficult to follow. He later modified this classification and simplified divisions to various groups. Classification of a displacement pattern depends on two main factors: the number of displaced segments and the key segment displaced. Fractures of the proximal humerus occur between one or all of four major segments: the articular segment (at the level of the anatomic neck), the greater tuberosity, the lesser tuberosity, and the humeral shaft (at the level of the surgical neck). One-part fracture occurs when there is minimal or no displacement between the segments. In the two-part fractures, only one segment is displaced. In the three-part fractures, two segments are displaced, one tuberosity remaining in continuity with the humeral head. In the four-part fractures, three segments are displaced, including both tuberosities. Two-part, three-part, and four-part fractures may or may not be associated with dislocation, either anterior or posterior. The involvement of the articular surface is classified separately into two groups: the anterior fracture-dislocation, termed by Neer "head splitting," and posterior fracture-dislocation termed "impression" (Fig. 5.22).

One-part fracture may involve any or all of the anatomic segments of the proximal humerus. There is no or minimal (less than 1 cm) displacement and no or minimal (less than 45°) angulation; the fragments are being held together by the rotator cuff, the joint capsule, and the intact periosteum.

Two-part fracture indicates that only one segment is displaced in relation to the three that remain undisplaced. It may involve either anatomic neck, surgical neck, greater tuberosity, or lesser tuberosity. The two-part fracture involving the anatomic neck of the humerus with displacement of the articular end may be associated with tear of the rotator cuff, and complications such as malunion or osteonecrosis may later develop. In two-part fractures involving the surgical neck of the humerus with displacement or angulation of the shaft, three types may be seen: impacted, unimpacted, and comminuted. These fractures may be associated with either anterior or posterior dislocation. With anterior dislocation, the fracture invariably involves the greater tuberosity; with posterior dislocation, the lesser tuberosity.

Three-part fracture may involve either greater tuberosity or lesser tuberosity and may be associated with anterior or posterior dislocation. Two segments are displaced in relation to two other segments that are not displaced.

Four-part fracture involves both the greater and lesser tuberosity in addition to the fracture of the surgical neck, and four major segments are displaced. This may be associated with anterior or posterior dislocation. The four-part fracture is usually associated with impairment of the blood supply to the humeral head, and osteonecrosis of the humeral head is a frequent complication.

FRACTURES OF THE CLAVICLE   A common injury—in infancy during delivery, in adolescence due to a direct blow or fall, and in adulthood as the result of a motor vehicle accident—fracture of the clavicle can be divided into three types according to the anatomic segment involved. The most common site of injury is the middle third of the clavicle, representing 80% of all clavicular fractures. Fractures of the distal (lateral) third (15%) and the proximal (medial) third (5%) are less commonly seen. If displacement is present, the proximal fragment is usually elevated and the distal fragment is displaced medially and caudally. The anteroposterior projection of the shoulder usually allows sufficient evaluation of any type of clavicular fracture (Fig. 5.23), but the same projection obtained with 15° cephalad angulation of the radiographic tube

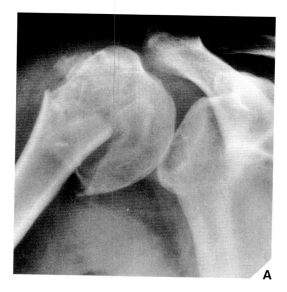

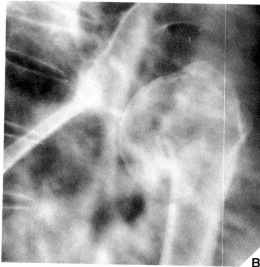

Figure 5.21 A 60-year-old man fell on a staircase and injured his right arm. (A) Anteroposterior view of the shoulder demonstrates a comminuted fracture through the surgical neck of the humerus. The greater tuberosity is fractured as well, but not significantly displaced. To better assess the degree of displacement of the various fragments, the transthoracic lateral view (B) was obtained. It demonstrates slight anterior angulation of the humeral head, which in addition is inferiorly subluxed—a finding not well appreciated on the anteroposterior projection.

A

B

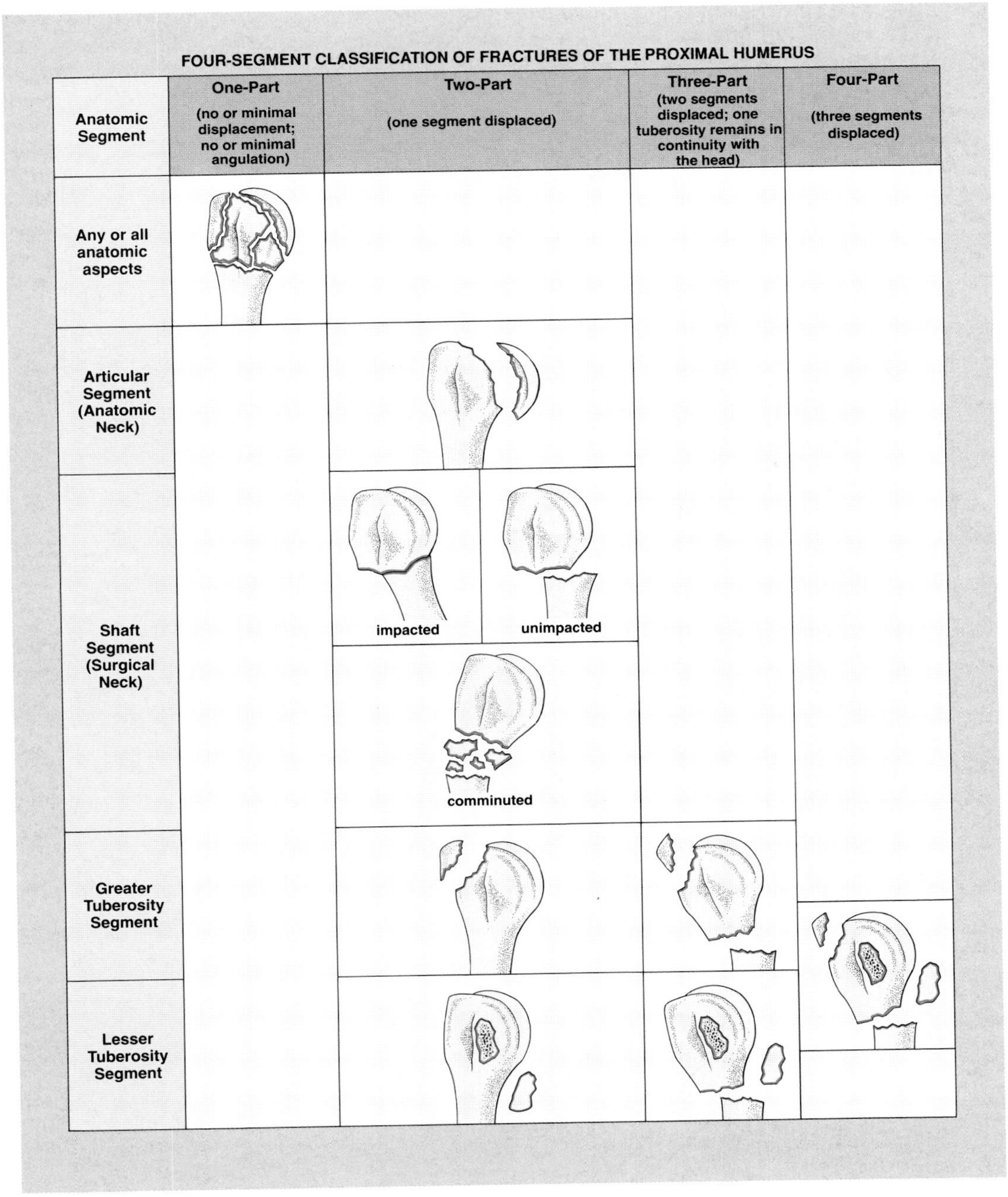

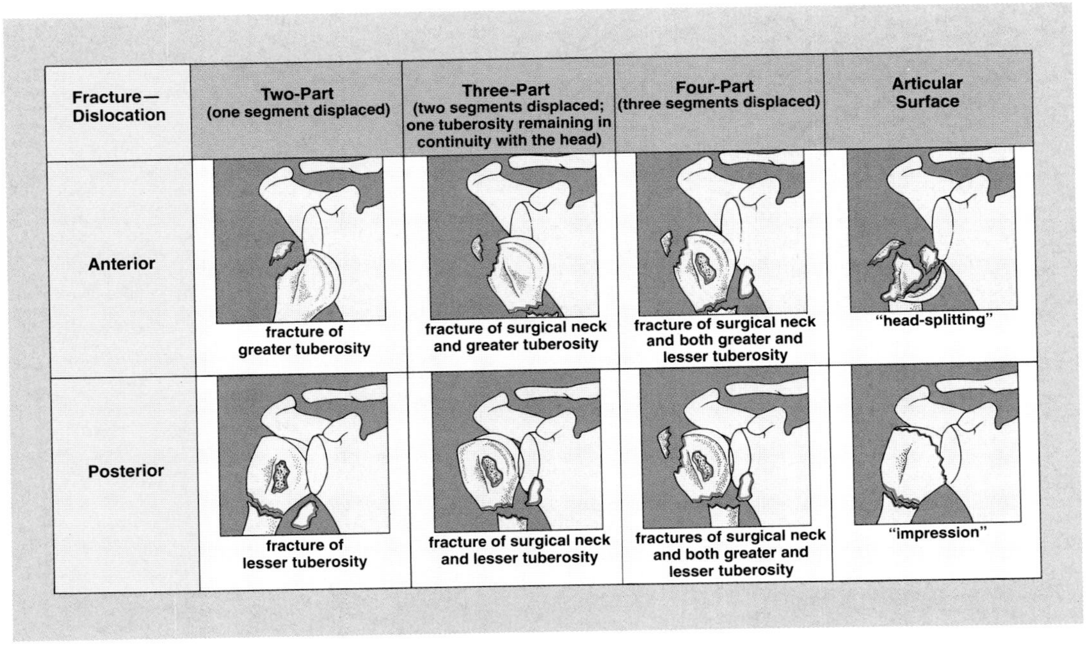

Figure 5.22 Fractures of the proximal humerus based on the presence or absence of displacement of the four major fragments that may result from fracture. (Modified from Neer CS II, 1975)

FOUR-SEGMENT CLASSIFICATION OF FRACTURES OF THE PROXIMAL HUMERUS

Anatomic Segment	One-Part (no or minimal displacement; no or minimal angulation)	Two-Part (one segment displaced)	Three-Part (two segments displaced; one tuberosity remains in continuity with the head)	Four-Part (three segments displaced)
Any or all anatomic aspects				
Articular Segment (Anatomic Neck)				
Shaft Segment (Surgical Neck)		impacted unimpacted comminuted		
Greater Tuberosity Segment				
Lesser Tuberosity Segment				

Fracture—Dislocation	Two-Part (one segment displaced)	Three-Part (two segments displaced; one tuberosity remaining in continuity with the head)	Four-Part (three segments displaced)	Articular Surface
Anterior	fracture of greater tuberosity	fracture of surgical neck and greater tuberosity	fracture of surgical neck and both greater and lesser tuberosity	"head-splitting"
Posterior	fracture of lesser tuberosity	fracture of surgical neck and lesser tuberosity	fractures of surgical neck and both greater and lesser tuberosity	"impression"

may also be useful, particularly in fractures of the middle third of the clavicle.

FRACTURE OF THE SCAPULA Invariably resulting from direct trauma, frequently sustained in a motor vehicle accident or a fall from a height, fracture of the scapula may occasionally be evaluated on the anteroposterior view of the shoulder. More commonly the trans-scapular (or Y) view may be required, particularly in cases of comminution, because this projection better demonstrates displacement of the fragments (Fig. 5.24). CT scan may also effectively demon-strate the displacement of various segments. Complications, such as injury to the axillary artery or the brachial plexus, are rare.

Dislocations in the Glenohumeral Joint

ANTERIOR DISLOCATION Displacement of the humeral head anterior to the glenoid fossa, which usually results from indirect force applied to the arm—a combination of abduction, extension, and external rotation—accounts for about 97% of cases of glenohumeral disloca-tion. It is readily diagnosed on the anteroposterior view of the shoul-der (Fig. 5.25).

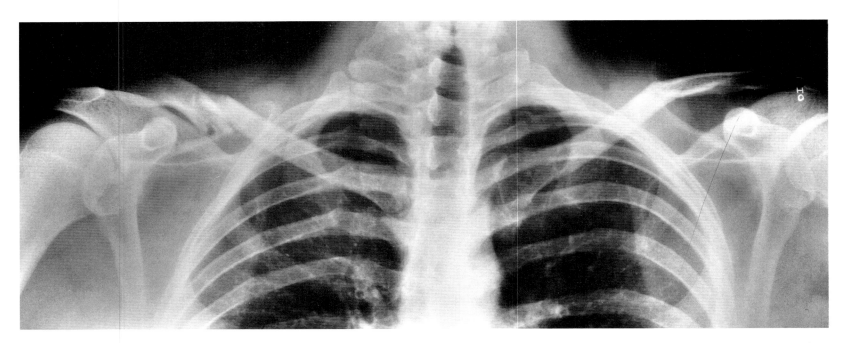

Figure 5.23 A 22-year-old man sustained multiple trauma in a motorcycle accident. Anteroposterior view of both shoulders demonstrates a comminuted fracture of the lateral third of the right clavicle and a simple fracture of the middle third of the left.

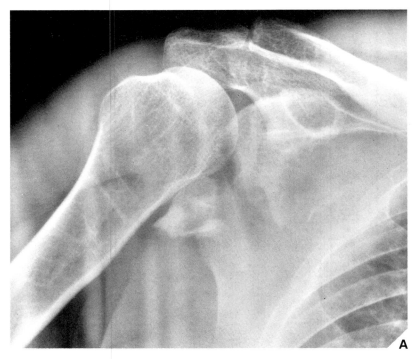

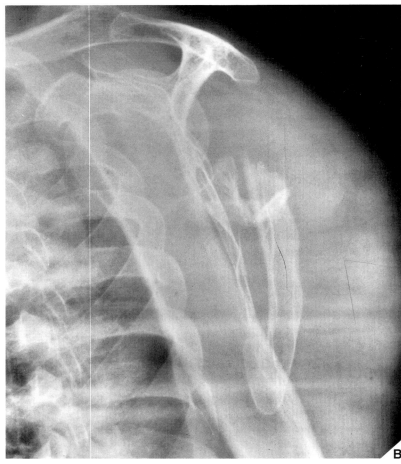

Figure 5.24 A 52-year-old man was injured in a motorcycle accident. (A) On the anteroposterior view of the right shoulder, a comminuted fracture of the scapula is evident. Displacement of the fragments, however, cannot be evaluated. (B) Trans-scapular (Y) view demonstrates lateral displacement of the body of the scapula.

At the time of dislocation, the humeral head strikes the inferior margin of the glenoid, and this may result in compression fracture of one or both of these structures. Fracture most frequently occurs in the posterolateral aspect of the humeral head at the junction with the neck, producing a "hatchet" defect called the *Hill-Sacks lesion*; it is best demonstrated on the anteroposterior projection of the shoulder with the arm internally rotated (Fig. 5.26). Fracture of the anterior aspect of the inferior rim of the glenoid, known as the *Bankart lesion*, is less commonly seen. It may occur secondary to the anterior movement of the humeral head in dislocation and is readily demonstrated on the anteroposterior projection with the arm in the neutral position (Fig. 5.27). When the site of the Bankart lesion is in the cartilaginous labrum, which at times may be detached, it may only be revealed by either computed arthrotomography (see Fig. 5.16) or MRI. The presence of either of these abnormalities is virtually diagnostic of previous anterior dislocation.

POSTERIOR DISLOCATION This type, which is much less commonly seen—accounting for only 2% to 3% of dislocations in the glenohumeral joint—results from either direct force, such as a blow to the anterior aspect of the shoulder, or indirect force applied to the arm combining adduction, flexion, and internal rotation. Posterior dislocation due to indirect force most often occurs secondary to accidental electric shock or convulsive seizures. In this type of dislocation, the humeral head lies posterior to the glenoid fossa and usually impacts on the posterior rim of the glenoid.

Making a correct diagnosis is often problematic, since the abnormality can easily be overlooked on the standard anteroposterior film of the shoulder, where the overlapping humeral head and glenoid fossa may be interpreted as normal. It is imperative in dealing with suspected posterior dislocation to demonstrate radiographically the glenoid fossa in profile. This can be done on the anteroposterior projection by rotating the patient 40° toward the affected side (see Fig. 5.7). Normally, the

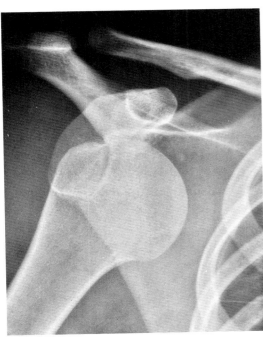

Figure 5.25 Anteroposterior film of the shoulder shows the typical appearance of anterior dislocation. The humeral head lies beneath the inferior rim of the glenoid.

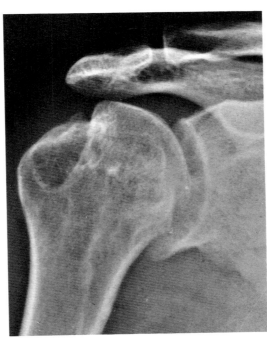

Figure 5.26 Anteroposterior view of the shoulder with the arm internally rotated demonstrates a "hatchet" defect, known as the Hill-Sacks lesion, on the posterolateral aspect of the humeral head.

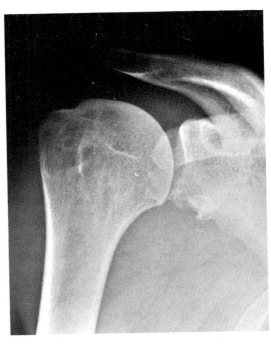

Figure 5.27 Anteroposterior view of the shoulder shows compression fracture of the anterior aspect of the inferior portion of the glenoid, known as the Bankart lesion.

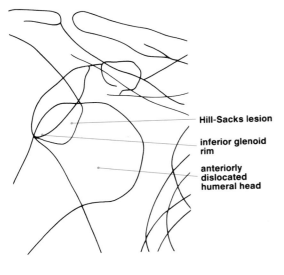

Hill-Sacks lesion
inferior glenoid rim
anteriorly dislocated humeral head

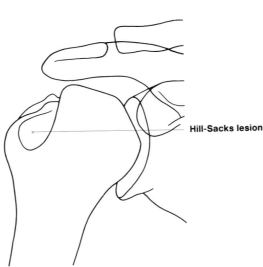

Hill-Sacks lesion

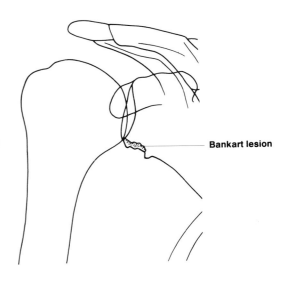

Bankart lesion

glenohumeral joint space is clear on this view. Obliteration of the space because of overlap of the humeral head with the glenoid is virtually diagnostic of posterior dislocation (Fig. 5.28). Diagnosis can also be made on the axillary projection, although limited abduction of the arm may make it impossible to obtain this view (Fig. 5.29).

Compression fracture of the anteromedial aspect of the humeral head, known as trough line impaction *(trough sign)*, commonly occurs in posterior dislocation secondary to the impaction of the humeral head on the posterior glenoid rim. The anteroposterior view of the shoulder with the arm externally rotated readily demonstrates this type of fracture (Fig. 5.30); it is also identifiable on the axillary projection (see Fig. 5.29).

COMPLICATIONS Anterior or posterior dislocation in the gleno-humeral joint may result in complications such as recurrent dislocations, posttraumatic arthritis, and injury to the axillary nerve and axillary artery.

Impingement Syndrome

The impingement syndrome of the shoulder refers to a condition in which the supraspinatus tendon and subacromial bursa are chronically entrapped between the humeral head inferiorly and either the anterior acromion itself, spurs of the anterior acromion or acromioclavicular joint, or the coracoacromial ligament superiorly (coracoacromial arch). Early diagnosis and treatment of the impingement syndrome are critical to prevent progression of this condition and improve shoulder function. Frequently, however, clinical signs and symptoms are nonspecific, and the diagnosis is often delayed until a full-thickness defect in the rotator cuff has developed. Only rarely can it be definitely diagnosed based on the clinical findings characterized by severe pain during abduction and external rotation of the arm. More reliable are radiographic findings associated with this syndrome, including subacromial proliferation of bone, spurring at the inferior aspect of the acromion, and degenerative changes of the humeral tuberosities at the insertion of the rotator cuff.

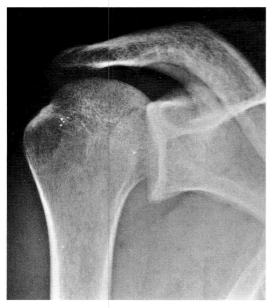

Figure 5.28 On the anteroposterior projection of the shoulder obtained by rotating the patient 40° toward the affected side, overlap of the medially displaced humeral head with the glenoid is virtually diagnostic of posterior dislocation.

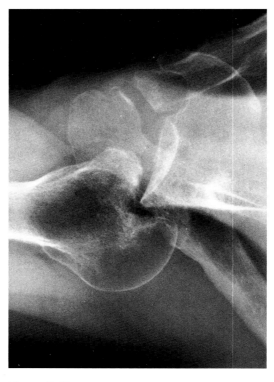

Figure 5.29 Axillary projection of the shoulder demonstrates posterior dislocation. Note the associated compression fracture of the anteromedial aspect of the humeral head.

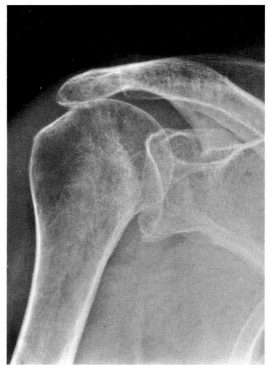

Figure 5.30 Anteroposterior view of the shoulder demonstrates posterior dislocation in the glenohumeral joint. Note the trough line impaction on the anteromedial aspect of the humeral head.

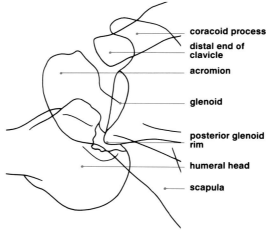

coracoid process
distal end of clavicle
acromion
glenoid
posterior glenoid rim
humeral head
scapula

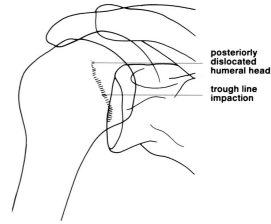

posteriorly dislocated humeral head
trough line impaction

Neer described three progressive stages of impingement syndrome apparent clinically and at surgery. Stage I consists of edema and hemorrhage and is reversible with conservative therapy. It typically occurs in young individuals engaged in sport activities requiring excessive use of the arm above the head (i.e., swimming). Stage II implies fibrosis and thickening of the subacromial soft tissue, rotator cuff tendinitis, and sometimes a partial tear of the rotator cuff. It is manifested clinically by recurrent pain and is often seen in patients 25 to 40 years old. Stage III represents complete rupture of the rotator cuff and is associated with progressive disability. It usually is seen in patients over 40 years old. Arthrography aids little in the early diagnosis of impingement syndrome, and other ancillary imaging techniques are also unsatisfactory for demonstration of the lesion in the early stages. Because of its high soft-tissue contrast resolution and multiplanar imaging capabilities, MRI is the only technique that can accurately image the early changes of this condition, in particular bursal thickening and effusion (subacromial bursitis), edema, and inflammatory changes of the rotator cuff and its tendons (Fig. 5.31).

Rotator Cuff Tear

The rotator cuff of the shoulder, a musculotendinous structure about the joint capsule, consists of four intrinsic muscles: the subscapularis, the supraspinatus, the infraspinatus, and the teres minor (see Fig. 5.3B). The tendinous portions of the cuff, which converge and fuse to form an envelope covering the humeral head, insert into the anatomic neck and tuberosities of the humerus. Tears usually occur in the supraspinatus portion of the cuff, about 1 cm from the insertion into the greater tuberosity of the humerus (known as a critical zone).

Injury to the rotator cuff may occur secondary to dislocation in the glenohumeral joint or to sudden abduction of the arm against resistance. It is most commonly seen in patients over 50 years of age due to normal degenerative changes in the cuff that predispose this structure to rupture after even minor shoulder injuries. Clinically, patients characteristically present with pain in the shoulder and inability to abduct the arm.

Although plain films of the shoulder are usually insufficient to demonstrate the tear, certain radiographic features characteristic of chronic rotator cuff tear may be present on the anteroposterior view. These include 1) narrowing of the acromiohumeral space to less than 6 mm, 2) erosion of the inferior aspect of the acromion secondary to cephalad migration of the humeral head, and 3) flattening and atrophy of the greater tuberosity of the humeral head due to the absence of traction stress by the rotator cuff (Fig. 5.32). Although these findings are usually diagnostic of chronic tear, contrast arthrography may be performed to confirm or exclude the suspected diagnosis. As the intact rotator cuff normally separates the subacromial-subdeltoid bursae complex from the joint cavity, only the glenohumeral joint, the axillary recess, the bursa subscapularis, and the bicipital tendon sheath should opacify on arthrographic

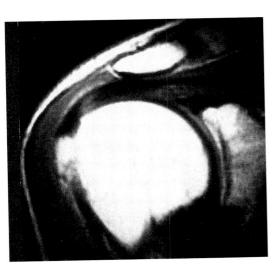

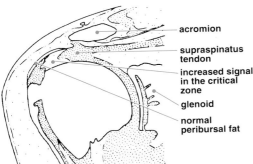

Figure 5.31 Oblique coronal T1-weighted MR image of early stage of the impingement syndrome. There is slightly increased signal in the critical zone of the supraspinatus tendon. Peribursal fat demarcating the subacromial-subdeltoid bursae complex is still intact. (Reprinted with permission of the authors and publisher from Holt RG, et al., 1990)

- acromion
- supraspinatus tendon
- increased signal in the critical zone
- glenoid
- normal peribursal fat

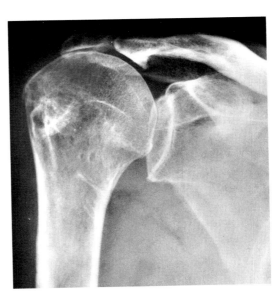

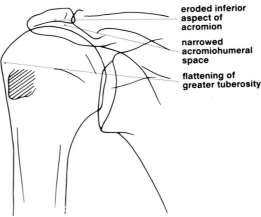

Figure 5.32 The plain-film characteristics of chronic rotator cuff tear are identifiable on the anteroposterior view of the shoulder.

- eroded inferior aspect of acromion
- narrowed acromiohumeral space
- flattening of greater tuberosity

examination (5.33A; see also Fig. 5.15B). Opacification of the sub-acromial–subdeltoid bursae is diagnostic of rotator cuff tear (Fig. 5.33B,C). Occasionally, contrast is seen only in the substance of the rotator cuff, while the subacromial–subdeltoid bursae complex remains unopacified, indicating a partial tear of the cuff (Fig. 5.34).

Although arthrography of the shoulder remains the gold-standard technique for evaluating a suspected rotator-cuff tear, MRI is being used more frequently as a noninvasive method to diagnose such a tear. The advantage of MRI over arthrography is not only that it is a noninvasive technique, but also that it allows visualization of the osseous and periarticular soft tissue of the shoulder in the coronal, sagittal, axial, and oblique planes. It has proved to be highly sensitive (75%–92%) and accurate (84%–94%) for diagnosing full–thickness rotator cuff disruption. Moreover, there is excellent

correlation between preoperative assessment of the size of rotator cuff tears by MRI and the measurement at surgery.

Visualization of the rotator cuff is optimal when oblique coronal images are obtained. The MRI findings for rotator cuff tear consist of focal discontinuity of the supraspinatus tendon, tendon and muscle retraction, abnormally increased signal within the tendon, and the presence of fluid in the subacromial-subdeltoid bursa complex (Fig. 5.35).

It must be noted, however, that the complex MRI appearance of the rotator cuff can be confounding in the diagnosis of a tear; experience and total knowledge of normal anatomy is required. Large tears are well visualized on MR images as areas of discontinuity and irregularity of the rotator cuff tendons, with joint fluid tracking through the cuff defect into the subacromial-subdeltoid bursa com-

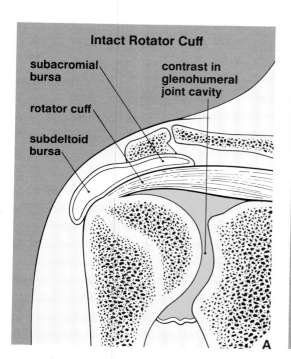

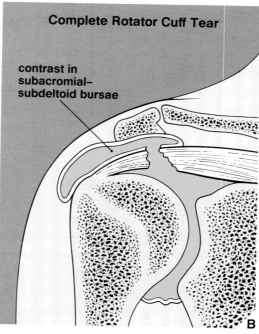

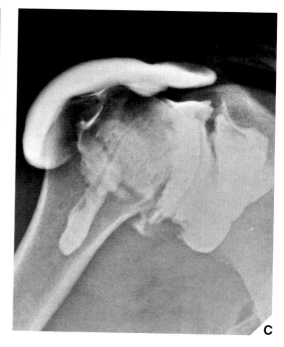

Figure 5.33 The intact rotator cuff (A) does not allow communication between the glenohumeral joint cavity and the subacromial-subdeltoid bursae complex. When arthrography is performed for suspected tear of the cuff, opacification of the bursae (B,C) indicates abnormal communication between them and the joint cavity, confirming the diagnosis.

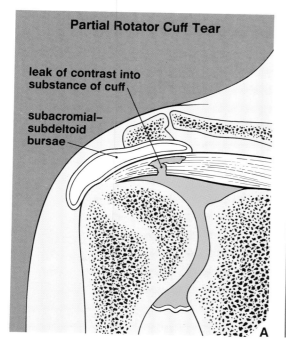

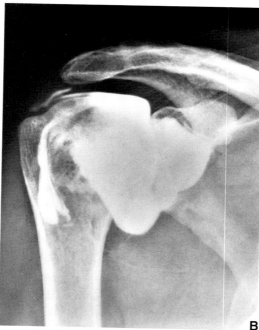

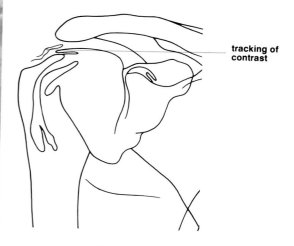

Figure 5.34 Partial tear of the rotator cuff (A) allows tracking of contrast into the substance of the cuff (B), while the subacromial-subdeltoid bursae remain free of contrast.

plex. With complete rotator cuff tears and retraction of the tendons, the corresponding muscle belly assumes a distorted globular shape that is easily recognized. Chronic tears may result in atrophy of the cuff musculature, manifested on T1-weighted images by a decrease in muscle size and bulk, and by infiltration of the muscle by a band of high-signal-intensity fat. Partial tears may be seen as various foci of high signal intensity within the homogeneous low signal intensity of the tendon or as irregularity or thinning of the tendon. Obscuration of the subacromial-subdeltoid fat line on T2-weighted images is a sensitive indicator of rotator cuff tears, and increased signal intensity in the same region on T2-weighted sequences corresponds to leakage of joint fluid into the subacromial-subdeltoid bursae complex.

MRI provides the surgeon with critical information regarding size and location of a tear, the specific tendons involved, the degree of musculature atrophy and tendon retraction, and the quality of the torn edges. Such information is invaluable for assessing the feasibility of surgery and the type of repair necessary.

Miscellaneous Abnormalities

ADHESIVE CAPSULITIS This condition, also referred to as "frozen shoulder," usually results from posttraumatic adhesive inflammation between the joint capsule and the peripheral articular cartilage of the shoulder. Clinically, it is characterized by pain, stiffness, and limitation of motion in the shoulder joint.

As plain-film radiography, which may only reveal disuse periarticular osteoporosis secondary to this condition, is insufficient to make a diagnosis, single- or double-contrast arthrography is the technique of choice when this abnormality is suspected. The arthrogram usually reveals decreased capacity of the joint capsule, or even complete obliteration of the axillary and subscapular recesses—findings diagnostic of this condition (Fig. 5.36).

ACROMIOCLAVICULAR SEPARATION Injuries to the acromioclavicular joint, which are commonly sustained during athletic activities by individuals between the ages of 15 and 40 years, often result in acromioclavicular separation. Various forces may cause injury to the acromioclavicular joint. The most common is a downward blow to the lateral aspect of the shoulder that drives the acromion inferiorly (caudad); others are traction on the arm pulling the shoulder away from the chest wall, and a fall on the outstretched hand or on the flexed elbow with the arm flexed forward 90°.

Whatever the mechanism of injury, the degree of damage to the acromioclavicular and coracoclavicular ligaments varies with the severity of the applied force and ranges from *mild sprain* of the acromioclavicular ligament, to *moderate sprain* involving tear of the acromioclavicular ligament and sprain of the coracoclavicular ligament, to *severe sprain* characterized by tear of the coracoclavicular ligament, with consequent dislocation in the acromioclavicular

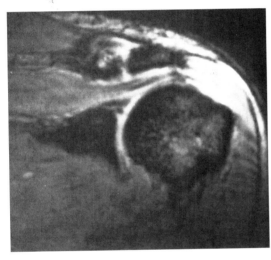

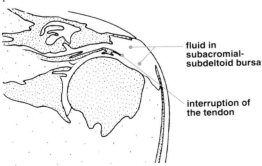

fluid in
subacromial-
subdeltoid bursa

interruption of
the tendon

Figure 5.35 Oblique coronal MR image of the left shoulder (MPGR T2*-weighted) demonstrates interruption of the supraspinatus tendon and fluid in the subacromial–subdeltoid bursae complex, diagnostic of complete rotator cuff tear. (Reprinted with permission of the authors and publishers from Holt RG et al., 1990)

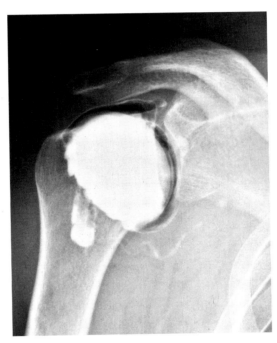

Figure 5.36 Double-contrast arthrogram of the shoulder demonstrates the characteristic findings of frozen shoulder. The capacity of the axillary pouch is markedly decreased and the subscapu-

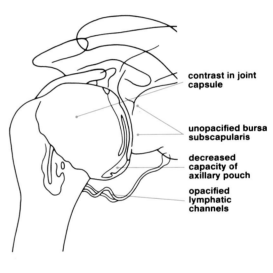

contrast in joint
capsule

unopacified bursa
subscapularis

decreased
capacity of
axillary pouch

opacified
lymphatic
channels

laris recess remains unopacified, while the lymphatic channels are filled with contrast secondary to increased intracapsular pressure.

joint (Fig. 5.37). It is important to bear in mind, as Rockwood and Green have pointed out, that the major deformity seen in this type of injury is not elevation of the clavicle, but rather downward displacement of the scapula and upper extremity (Fig. 5.38), although some degree of cephalad displacement of the distal end of the clavicle may accompany this type of injury. The clinical symptoms also vary with the severity of the injury; patients may present with complaints ranging from tenderness, swelling, and slight limitation of motion in the joint to complete inability to abduct the arm.

Suspected acromioclavicular dislocation is readily evaluated on the anteroposterior projection of the shoulder obtained with a 15° cephalad angulation of the radiographic tube (see Fig. 5.13). Often it is necessary to obtain a stress view in this projection by strapping a 5-to-10-pound weight to each forearm. A comparison study of the opposite shoulder is invariably helpful.

Radiographic studies can also be supplemented by quantitating acromioclavicular separation on the basis of the normal relations of the coracoid process, the clavicle, and the acromion (Fig. 5.39). Normally, the distance between the coracoid process and the inferior aspect of the clavicle, known as the coracoclavicular distance, ranges from 1.0 cm to 1.3 cm; and the joint space at the articulation of the clavicle with the acromion measures 0.3 cm to 0.8 cm. The degree of widening at these points helps to determine the severity of the injury. An increase, for example, of 0.5 cm in the coracoclavicular distance or a widening of the distance by 50% or more as compared with that in the opposite shoulder is characteristic of grade III acromioclavicular separation (Fig. 5.40).

POSTTRAUMATIC OSTEOLYSIS OF THE DISTAL CLAVICLE After injury to the shoulder, such as sprain of the acromioclavicular joint, resorption of the distal (acromial) end of the clavicle may occasionally occur. The osteolytic process, which is associated with mild to moderate pain, usually begins within two months following the injury. The initial radiographic findings consist of soft tissue swelling and periarticular osteoporosis. In its late stage, resorption of the distal end of the clavicle results in marked widening of the acromioclavicular joint (Fig. 5.41).

ELBOW

Trauma to the elbow is commonly encountered in all age groups, but is particularly common in childhood when, as toddlers, children often sustain elbow injuries. Play and athletic activities in childhood and young adolescence are also frequent occasions of trauma. Although history and clinical examination usually provide clues to the correct diagnosis, radiographic examination is indispensable in determining the type of fracture or dislocation, the direction of the fracture line, and the position of the fragments, as well as in evaluating concomitant soft tissue injuries.

Anatomic-Radiologic Considerations

The elbow articulation, a compound synovial joint, comprises the humeroulnar (ulnatrochlear), the humeroradial (radiocapitellar), and the proximal radioulnar joints. It is a hinged articulation with about 150° of flexion from a completely extended position. The flex-

Figure 5.37 Grades of Acromioclavicular Separation	
GRADE	RADIOGRAPHIC CHARACTERISTICS
I (Mild Sprain)	Minimal widening of acromioclavicular joint space, which normally measures 0.3–0.8 cm Coracoclavicular distance within normal range of 1.0–1.3 cm
II (Moderate Sprain)	Widening of acromioclavicular joint space to 1.0–1.5 cm Increase of 25% to 50% in coracoclavicular distance
III (Severe Sprain)	Marked widening of acromioclavicular joint space to 1.5 cm or more and of coracoclavicular distance by 50% or more Dislocation in acromioclavicular joint Apparent cephalad displacement of distal end of clavicle

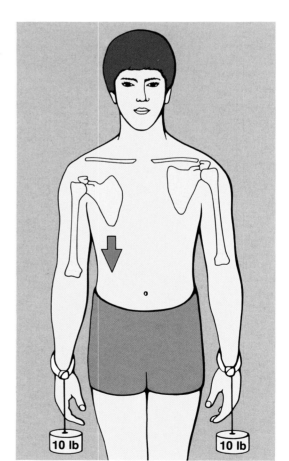

Figure 5.38 The major deformity seen in acromioclavicular separation is the downward displacement of the scapula and upper extremity, while the position of the clavicle in the affected side remains the same relative to the clavicle in the unaffected side. (Adapted from Rockwood CA Jr, Green DP, 1975)

ion and extension movements in the elbow occur in the ulna-trochlear and radiocapitellar joints. The biceps, brachioradialis, and brachialis muscles are the primary elbow flexors, while the triceps is the extensor of the elbow joint. Rotational movement occurs as the head of the radius, held tightly by the annular ligament of the ulna, rotates within the ulna's radial notch. The proximal and distal radioulnar joints allow 90° of pronation and supination of the fore-arm. The stability of the joint is ascertained by the group of ulnar-collateral ligaments medially, and radial-collateral ligaments later-ally. A fibrous capsule deep within the ligaments, structures sur-rounds the elbow joint.

When trauma to the elbow is suspected, radiographs are routinely obtained in the anteroposterior and lateral projections, occasionally supplemented by internal and external oblique views.

The *anteroposterior* projection usually suffices to demonstrate injury to the medial and the lateral epicondyles, the olecranon fossa, the

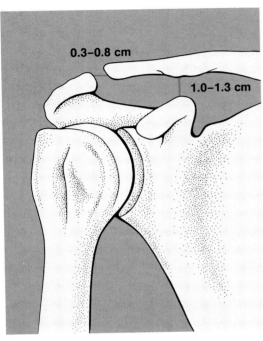

Figure 5.39 Schematic diagram shows the normal relation of the coracoid process to the inferior aspect of the clavicle and the normal width of the joint space at the acromioclavicular articulation.

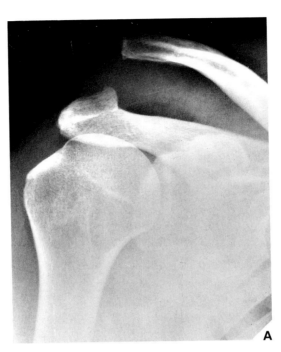

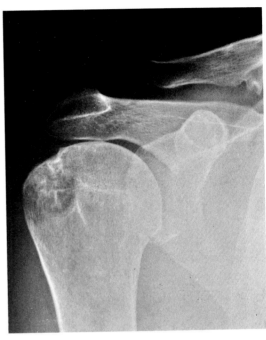

Figure 5.41 A 50-year-old man who five months previously had injured the right shoulder in a fall presented with complaints of pain while playing tennis. Anteroposterior view of the shoulder shows marked widening of the acromioclavicular joint secondary to resorption of the distal end of the clavicle—radiographic features typical of posttraumatic osteolysis. Note also the posttraumatic ossification at the attachment of the coraco-clavicular ligament.

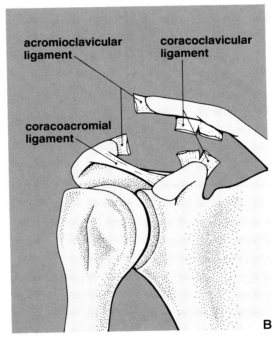

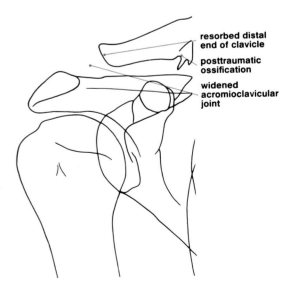

Figure 5.40 (A) Anteroposterior view of shoulder shows apparent cephalad displacement of the distal end of the clavicle and the widening of the acromioclavicular joint and the coracoclavicular distance. The marked deformities seen here, which are characteristic of grade III acromiocla-vicular separation (severe sprain), are the result of tear of the coracoclavicular and the acromio-clavicular ligaments with consequent dislocation in the acromioclavicular joint (B).

capitellum, the trochlea, and the radial head (Fig. 5.42). It also reveals an important anatomic relation of the forearm to the central axis of the arm known as the *carrying angle* (Fig. 5.43). Normally, the long axis of the forearm forms a valgus angle of 15° with the long axis of the arm; the forearm is thus angled laterally—that is, away from the central axis of the body.

On the anteroposterior view in children, it is essential to recognize the four secondary ossification centers of the distal humerus:

those of the capitellum, the medial and the lateral epicondyles, and the trochlea. The usual order in which these centers appear and the age at which they become radiographically visible are important factors in the evaluation of injuries to the elbow (Fig. 5.44). Displacement of any of these centers serves as a diagnostic indicator of the type of fracture or dislocation. For example, the medial epicondyle always ossifies before the trochlea. If radiographic examination in a child between 4 and 8 years of age reveals a bony structure

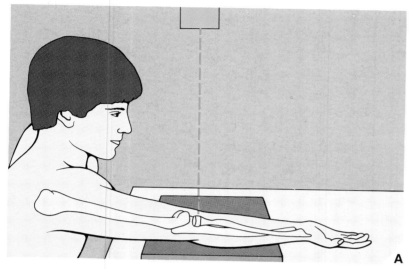

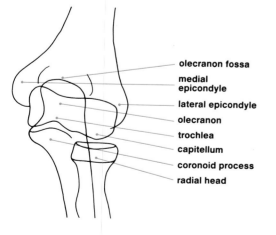

Figure 5.42 (A) For the anteroposterior view of the elbow, the forearm is positioned supine (palm up) on the radiographic table, with the elbow joint fully extended and the fingers slightly flexed. The central beam is directed perpendicularly toward the elbow joint. (B) The film in this projection demonstrates the medial and the lateral epicondyles, the olecranon fossa, the capitellum, and the radial head. The coronoid process is seen en face, and the olecranon overlaps the trochlea.

- olecranon fossa
- medial epicondyle
- lateral epicondyle
- olecranon
- trochlea
- capitellum
- coronoid process
- radial head

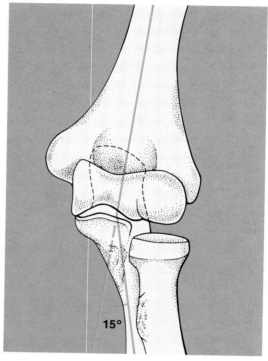

Figure 5.43 The angle formed by the longitudinal axes of the distal humerus and the proximal ulna constitutes the carrying angle of the forearm. Normally, there is a valgus angle of 15°.

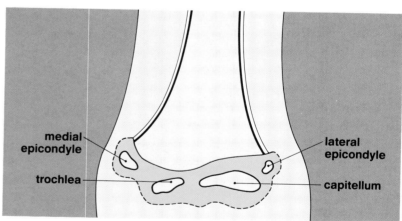

Figure 5.44 The secondary centers of ossification of the distal humerus usually appear in the following order: the capitellum at 1 to 2 years of age, the medial epicondyle at 4 years of age, the trochlea at 8 years of age, and the lateral epicondyle at 10 years of age.

in the region of the trochlea (that is, before this center of ossification should appear) and shows no evidence of the ossification center of the medial epicondyle, it must be assumed that the ossification center of the medial epicondyle has been avulsed and displaced into the joint (Fig. 5.45).

The *lateral* view of the elbow allows sufficient evaluation of the olecranon process, the anterior aspect of the radial head, and the humeroradial articulation. It is limited, however, in the information it can provide, particularly with respect to the posterior half of the radial head and the coronoid process, because of the overlap of bony structures (Fig. 5.46).

As with the anteroposterior projection, the lateral view in children reveals significant configurations and relations, which, if distorted, indicate the presence of abnormality. The distal humerus in children has an angular appearance resembling a hockey stick, the angle of which normally measures approximately 140°. Loss of this

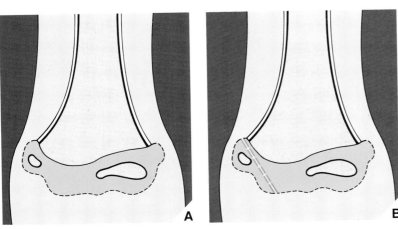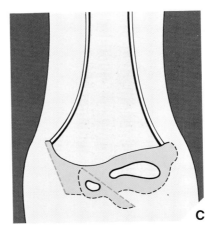

Figure 5.45 (A,B) Displacement of the ossification center of the medial epicondyle secondary to fracture may mimic the normal appearance of the ossification center of the trochlea (C).

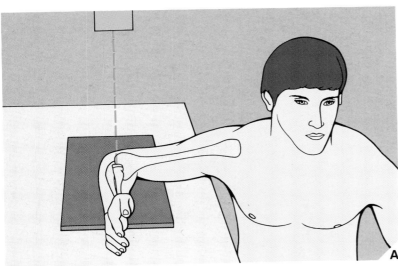

Figure 5.46 (A) For the lateral projection of the elbow, the forearm rests on its ulnar side on the radiographic cassette, with the joint flexed 90°, the thumb pointing upward, and the fingers slightly flexed. The central beam is directed vertically toward the radial head. (B) The film in this projection demonstrates the distal shaft of the humerus, the supracondylar ridge, the olecranon process, and the anterior aspect of the radial head. The articular surface and posterior aspect of the radial head are not well demonstrated on this view due to overlap by the coronoid process. The capitellum is also obscured by the overlapping trochlea.

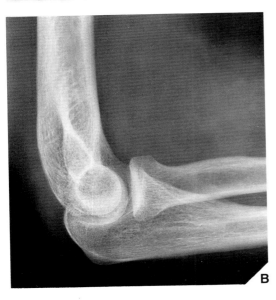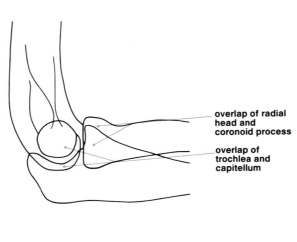

overlap of radial head and coronoid process

overlap of trochlea and capitellum

configuration occurs in supracondylar fracture (Fig. 5.47). Rogers has pointed out, in addition, the importance of the position of the capitellum relative to the distal humerus and the proximal radius. He found that a line drawn along the longitudinal axis of the proximal radius passes through the center of the capitellum and that a line drawn along the anterior cortex of the distal humerus and extended downward through the articulation intersects the middle third of the capitellum (Fig. 5.48). Disruption of this relation serves as an important indication of the possible presence of fracture or dislocation. Finally, regardless of the patient's age, displacement of the normal positions of the fat pads of the elbow also provides a useful diagnostic clue to the presence of fracture. Normally, the posterior fat pad, which lies deep in the olecranon fossa, is not visible on the lateral view. When it becomes visible and the anterior fat pad appears displaced—the positive fat-pad sign (see Fig. 4.30)—demonstration of the fracture line should be undertaken.

The *radial head-capitellum* view is a variant of the lateral projection, which was introduced by the author in 1982. As it overcomes the major limitation of the standard lateral view by projecting the radial head ventrad, free of overlap by the coronoid process, it has proved

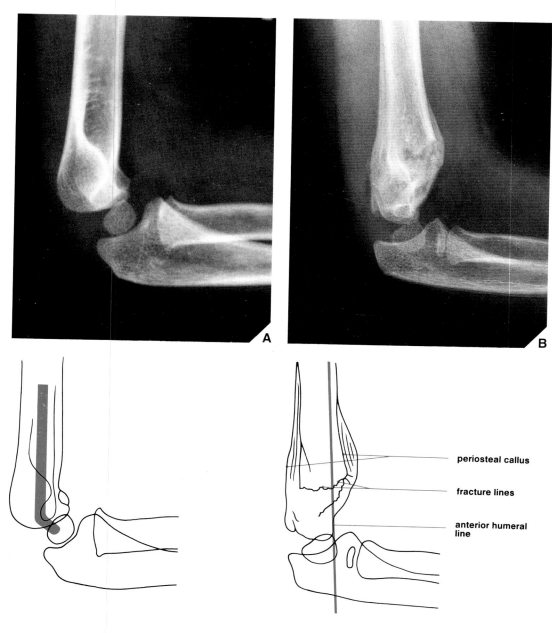

Figure 5.47 (A) Lateral view of the elbow joint in a 3-year-old child shows the normal hockey-stick appearance of the distal humerus. (B) Loss of this configuration, as seen in this film in a 3 ½-year-old girl who sustained trauma to the elbow four weeks prior to this radiographic examination, serves as an important landmark in recognizing supracondylar fracture of the distal humerus. Note also that the anterior humeral line falls anterior to the capitellum, indicating extension injury (see Fig. 5.48).

periosteal callus

fracture lines

anterior humeral line

to be a particularly effective technique. In addition to the radial head, it also clearly demonstrates the capitellum, the coronoid process, both the humeroradial and humeroulnar articulations (Fig. 5.49), as well as subtle fractures of these structures that may be obscure on other projections (see Figs. 5.64, 5.65, 5.67).

Other modalities may also be necessary for sufficient evaluation of injury to the elbow. Single- or, preferably, double-contrast arthrography, commonly combined with tomography *(arthrotomography)*, or CT has proved effective in visualizing subtle chondral fractures, osteochondritis dissecans, synovial and capsular abnormalities, and osteo-

chondral bodies in the joint. In general, indications for elbow arthrography include detection of the presence, size, and number of intra-articular osteochondral bodies; determination of whether calcifications around the elbow joint are intra- or extra-articular; evaluation of the articular cartilage; evaluation of juxta-articular cysts if they are communicating with the joint; evaluation of the joint capacity; and evaluation of various synovial and capsular abnormalities. Single-contrast arthrography is preferable when evaluating synovial abnormalities and intra-articular osteochondral bodies, since double contrast may result in air bubbles in the joint. Double contrast

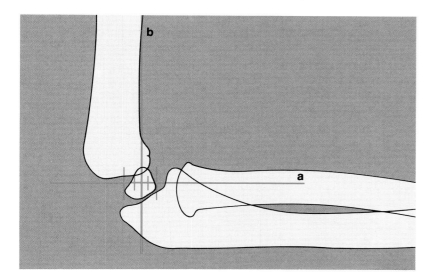

Figure 5.48 In children the normal position of the capitellum relative to the distal humerus and the proximal radius is determined by the portions of the capitellum intersected by two lines: Line (*a*) coincident with the longitudinal axis of the proximal radius passes through the center of the capitellum, and line (*b*) parallel to the anterior cortex of the distal humerus intersects the middle third of the capitellum. Disruption of this relation indicates the possible presence of abnormality (see Figs. 5.47B, 5.62B).

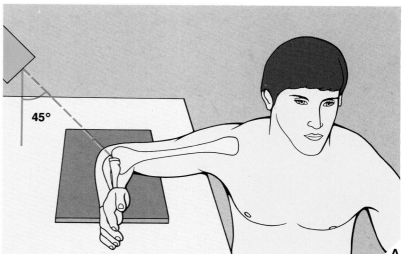

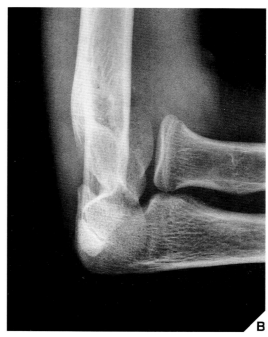

Figure 5.49 (A) For the radial head-capitellum view of the elbow, the patient is seated at the side of the radiographic table, with the forearm resting on its ulnar side, the elbow joint flexed 90°, and the thumb pointing upward. The central beam is directed toward the radial head at a 45° angle to the forearm. (B) The film in this projection shows the radial head projected ventrad, free of overlap by the coronoid process, which is also well demonstrated. This projection is also effective in evaluating the capitellum and the humeroradial and humeroulnar articulations.

arthrography, however, provides more detailed information; in particular, the articular surface and synovial lining are better delineated and the small details can be better visualized (Fig. 5.50). Frequently, in conjunction with elbow arthrography, conventional tomography may be used in a procedure called arthrotomography (Fig. 5.51) or CT examination (CT-arthrography) (Fig. 5.52) can be performed.

Axial CT images of the extended elbow are occasionally effective in demonstrating traumatic abnormalities. They are, however, difficult to obtain in the traumatized patient, and except for visual-ization of the proximal radioulnar joint and ulnatrochlear articula-tion, they are not frequently used. Occasionally, these sections can demonstrate osteochondral fractures of the radial head, and assess the integrity of the proximal radioulnar joint. On the other hand, Franklin and colleagues noted that axial CT images of the flexed elbow (so-called coronal sections) provide an ideal plane for evalua-tion of the olecranon fossa, the space between the trochlea and ole-cranon process posteriorly, as well as the radius and capitellum, and trochlea and coronoid process, anteriorly. Axial scans through the

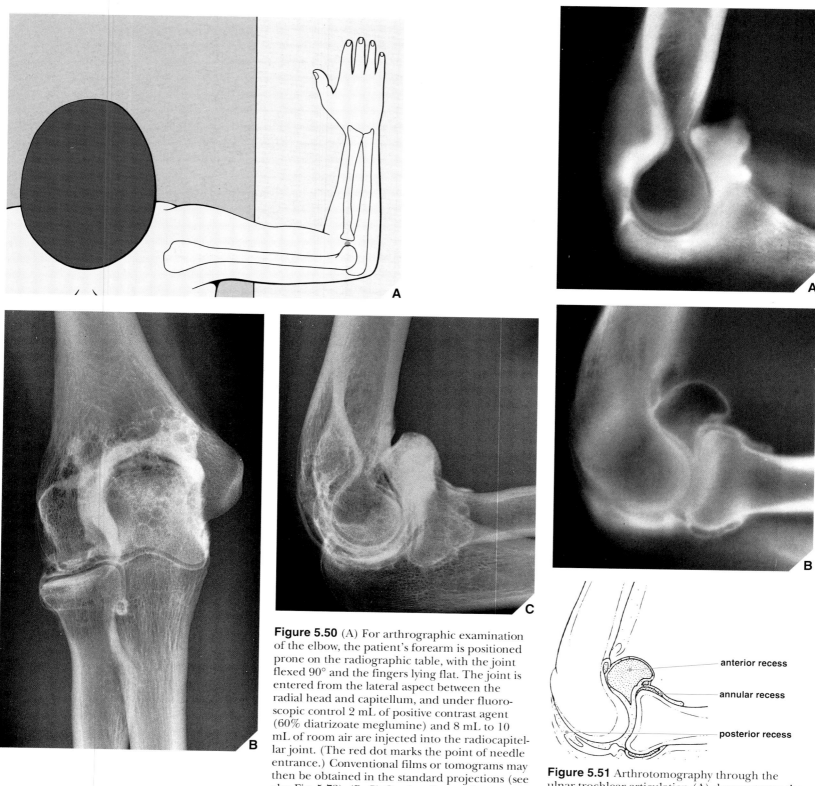

Figure 5.50 (A) For arthrographic examination of the elbow, the patient's forearm is positioned prone on the radiographic table, with the joint flexed 90° and the fingers lying flat. The joint is entered from the lateral aspect between the radial head and capitellum, and under fluoro-scopic control 2 mL of positive contrast agent (60% diatrizoate meglumine) and 8 mL to 10 mL of room air are injected into the radiocapitel-lar joint. (The red dot marks the point of needle entrance.) Conventional films or tomograms may then be obtained in the standard projections (see also Fig. 5.72). (B, C) On the elbow arthrogram, one can distinguish anterior, posterior, and annular recesses of the joint capsule. Also well demonstrated is articular cartilage of the radial head and capitellum.

anterior recess

annular recess

posterior recess

Figure 5.51 Arthrotomography through the ulnar-trochlear articulation (A) demonstrates the coronoid recess and through the radiocapitellar articulation (B) demonstrates the annular (peri-radial), anterior, and posterior recesses of the joint capsule.

flexed elbow also allow additional demonstration of the proximal radius in its long axis. If conventional tomographic examination alone is performed, trispiral cuts are preferred, as the thinner sections obtainable by this method provide overall better detail—as, for example, in localizing multiple fragments in comminuted fractures.

MRI examination effectively demonstrates traumatic abnormalities of the elbow joint and surrounding soft tissues. Axial, sagittal, and coronal planes are routinely used for elbow imaging. The axial plane is ideal to display the anatomic relationship of the proximal radioulnar joint and the head of the radius. On the sagittal plane, the ulnatrochlear and radiocapitellar articulations are well imaged and the biceps and brachialis muscle groups are well seen in their long axis. The biceps tendon and anconeus muscles are also well demonstrated (Fig. 5.53B,C). On coronal images, the trochlea, capitellum, and radial head are well demonstrated, as well as the various tendons and muscles around the elbow (Fig. 5.53A).

For a summary of the preceding discussion in tabular form, see Figures 5.54, 5.55, and 5.56.

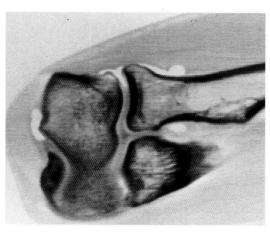
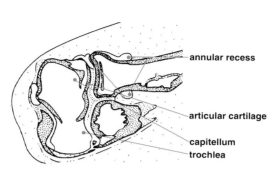

Figure 5.52 Postarthrography coronal CT scan of the elbow joint clearly demonstrates the annular recess and the outline of the lateral extension of the joint capsule. The articular cartilage is also well demonstrated.

- annular recess
- articular cartilage
- capitellum
- trochlea

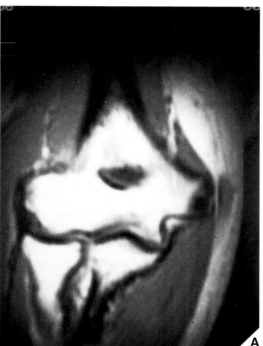
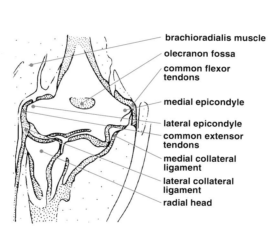
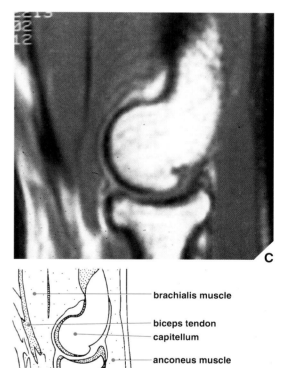

- brachioradialis muscle
- olecranon fossa
- common flexor tendons
- medial epicondyle
- lateral epicondyle
- common extensor tendons
- medial collateral ligament
- lateral collateral ligament
- radial head

- brachialis muscle
- biceps tendon
- capitellum
- anconeus muscle

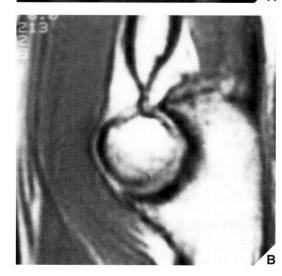
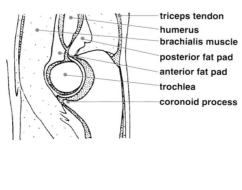
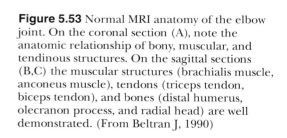

- triceps tendon
- humerus
- brachialis muscle
- posterior fat pad
- anterior fat pad
- trochlea
- coronoid process

Figure 5.53 Normal MRI anatomy of the elbow joint. On the coronal section (A), note the anatomic relationship of bony, muscular, and tendinous structures. On the sagittal sections (B,C) the muscular structures (brachialis muscle, anconeus muscle), tendons (triceps tendon, biceps tendon), and bones (distal humerus, olecranon process, and radial head) are well demonstrated. (From Beltran J, 1990)

FRACTURES OF THE DISTAL HUMERUS As the nomenclature of the various structures of the distal humerus used in different anatomy and surgery textbooks is not uniform, confusion has arisen regarding the classification of fractures of the distal humerus. To clarify the picture, a simplified anatomic division of the distal humerus is shown in Figure 5.57. The significance of the distinction

Table 5.54 Standard and Special Radiographic Projections for Evaluating Injury to the Elbow	
PROJECTION	DEMONSTRATION

Anteroposterior	Supra-, trans-, and intercondylar fractures of distal humerus
	Fractures of:
	  Medial and lateral epicondyles
	  Lateral aspect of capitellum
	  Medial aspect of trochlea
	  Lateral aspect of radial head
	Valgus and varus deformities
	Secondary ossification centers of distal humerus

Lateral	Supracondylar fracture of distal humerus
	Fractures of:
	  Anterior aspect of radial head
	  Olecranon process
	Complex dislocations in elbow joint
	Dislocation of radial head
	Fat-pad sign

External Oblique	Fractures of:
	  Lateral epicondyle
	  Radial head

Internal Oblique	Fractures of:
	  Medial epicondyle
	  Coronoid process

Radial Head-Capitellum	Fractures of:
	  Radial head
	  Capitellum
	  Coronoid process
	Abnormalities of humeroradial and humeroulnar articulations

Figure 5.55 Ancillary Imaging Techniques for Evaluating Injury to the Elbow	
TECHNIQUE	DEMONSTRATION

Tomography	Complex fractures about the elbow joint, particularly to assess position of fragments in comminution
	Healing process:
	  Nonunion
	  Secondary infection

Arthrography **Single- or double-contrast (usually augmented by tomography)**	Subtle abnormalities of articular cartilage Capsular ruptures Synovial abnormalities Chondral and osteochondral fractures Osteochondritis dissecans Osteochondral bodies in joint
Computed Tomography **Alone or combined with double-contrast arthrography**	Same as for arthrography
Magnetic Resonance Imaging	Abnormalities of the ligaments, tendons, and muscles Capsular ruptures Joint effusion Synovial cysts Hematomas Subtle abnormalities of bones (e.g., bone contusion) Osteochondritis dissecans Epiphyseal fractures (in children)

SPECTRUM OF RADIOLOGIC IMAGING TECHNIQUES
FOR EVALUATING INJURY TO THE ELBOW*

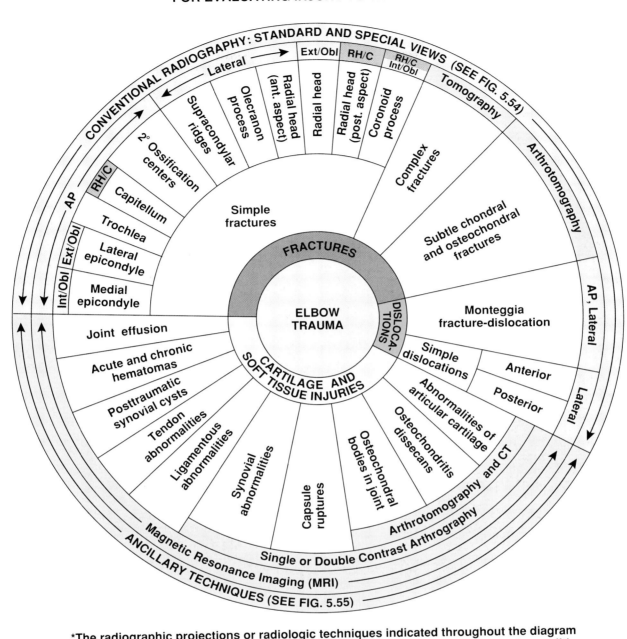

*The radiographic projections or radiologic techniques indicated throughout the diagram
are only those that are the most effective in demonstrating the respective traumatic conditions.

Figure 5.56 Spectrum of radiologic imaging techniques for evaluating injury to the elbow.

between the articular and extra-articular parts of the distal humerus lies in its importance to diagnosis, treatment, and prognosis. For example, as Rockwood and Green contended, fracture involving only the articular portion of the distal humerus usually results in loss of motion, but not loss of stability, whereas fracture of an entire condyle—that is, both articular and extra-articular portions—usually leads to restriction of motion and instability.

Based on the structure involved, fractures of the distal humerus can be classified as supracondylar, transcondylar, and intercondylar, as well as fractures of the medial and the lateral epicondyles, the capitellum, and the trochlea. The Müller classification is recommended, as it is a practical one based on a distinction between intra- and extra-articular fractures (Fig. 5.58). Usually, such injuries pose no diagnostic problems in adults and are readily evaluated on the

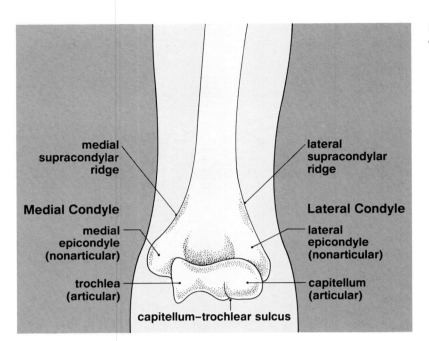

Figure 5.57 A simplified anatomic division of the structures of the distal humerus.

FRACTURES OF THE DISTAL HUMERUS

Extra-articular—Epicondylar, Supracondylar

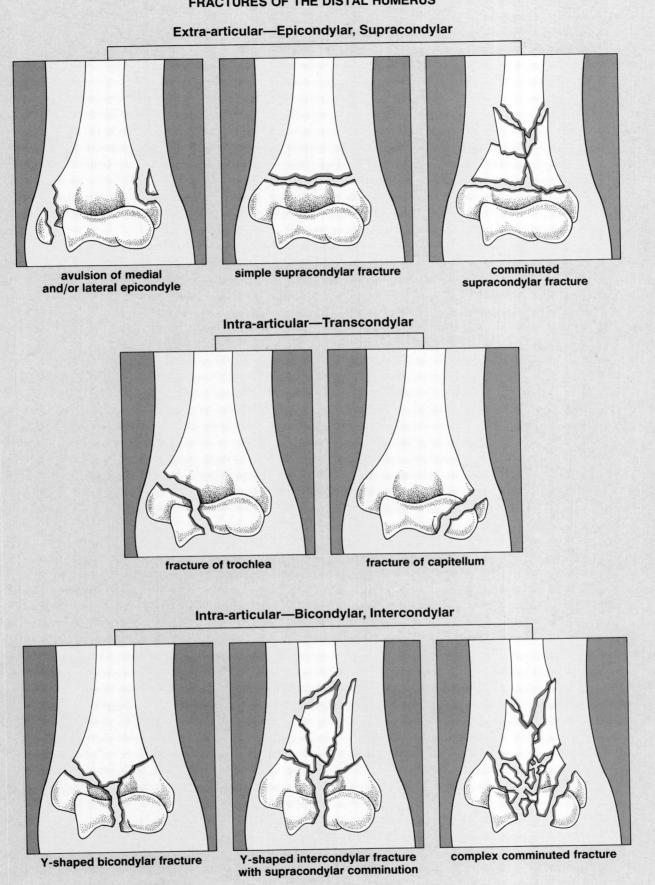

avulsion of medial
and/or lateral epicondyle

simple supracondylar fracture

comminuted
supracondylar fracture

Intra-articular—Transcondylar

fracture of trochlea

fracture of capitellum

Intra-articular—Bicondylar, Intercondylar

Y-shaped bicondylar fracture

Y-shaped intercondylar fracture
with supracondylar comminution

complex comminuted fracture

Figure 5.58 Classification of fractures of the distal humerus on the basis of extra- and intra-articular extension. (From Müller ME, et al., 1979)

anteroposterior and lateral projections of the elbow (Fig. 5.59). Only occasionally may tomographic examination need to be performed to localize comminuted fragments (Fig. 5.60).

In children, on the other hand, diagnosis may be problematic due to the presence of the secondary centers of ossification and their variability. Nevertheless, the anteroposterior and lateral projections usually suffice to demonstrate the abnormality, although the fracture line is occasionally more difficult to evaluate on the anteroposterior than on the lateral view. In children between the ages of 3 and 10 years, supracondylar fracture is the most common type of elbow fracture.

Extension injury, due to a fall on the outstretched hand with the elbow hyperextended, is present in 95% of such cases, and characteristically the distal fragment is posteriorly displaced (Fig. 5.61). In the flexion type of injury due to a fall on the flexed elbow, which occurs in only 5% of cases of supracondylar fracture, the distal fragment is anteriorly and upwardly displaced. Identifying supracondylar fracture on the lateral projection is usually facilitated by recognition of the loss of the normal hockey-stick appearance of the distal humerus and displacement of the capitellum relative to the line of the anterior cortex of the humerus. A positive fat-pad sign is invariably present (Fig. 5.62).

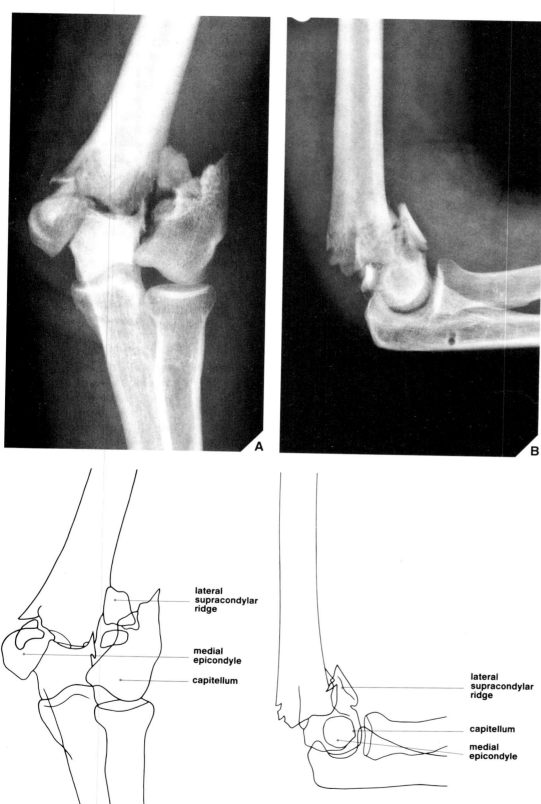

Figure 5.59 A 25-year-old man sustained a complex intra-articular fracture of the distal humerus in a motorcycle accident. Anteroposterior (A) and lateral (B) views clearly demonstrate the extension of the fracture lines and the position of the various fragments. The capitellum is separated, laterally displaced, and subluxed; the lateral supracondylar ridge is avulsed and anterolaterally displaced, and the medial epicondyle is externally rotated and medially displaced.

lateral
supracondylar
ridge

medial
epicondyle

capitellum

lateral
supracondylar
ridge

capitellum

medial
epicondyle

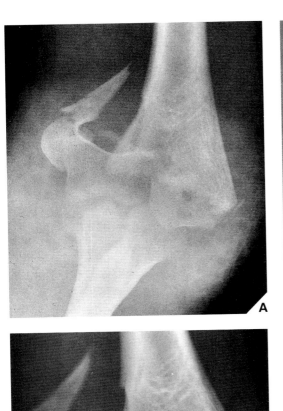

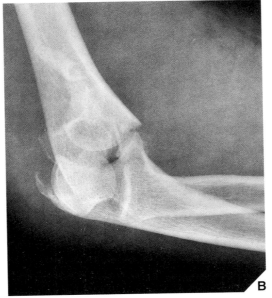

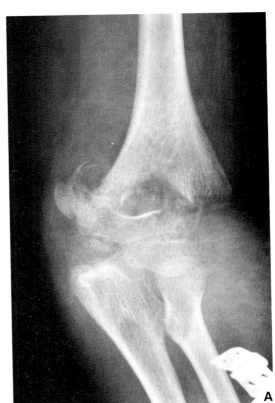

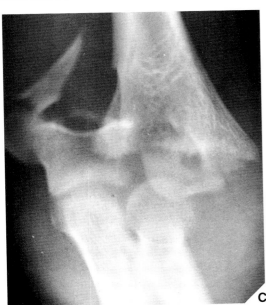

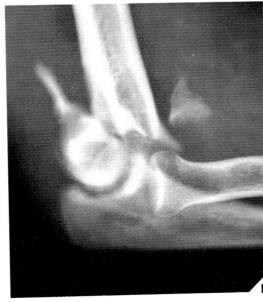

Figure 5.60 In a fall from a tree, a 20-year-old woman sustained a comminuted intra-articular fracture of the distal humerus, which was revealed on the standard anteroposterior (A) and lateral (B) projections of the elbow. However, the inadequate quality of the conventional studies due to marked soft tissue swelling, joint effusion, and the clinical condition of the patient (pain and limitation of motion in the joint) made full evaluation of the injury impossible.

Anteroposterior (C) and lateral (D) tomograms were obtained to evaluate the complex deformity. The capitellum is completely separated, medially rotated, and posteriorly displaced; the medial supracondylar ridge is avulsed; the trochlea and the medial epicondyle are separated from the distal humerus and medially displaced. A bony fragment from the ridge of the coronoid fossa is anteriorly displaced.

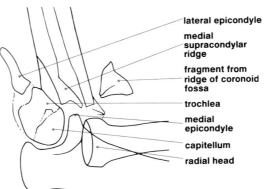
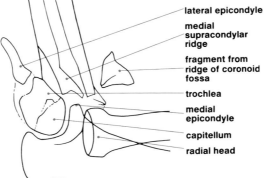

Figure 5.61 A 9-year-old boy fell off his bicycle on his outstretched hand. Anteroposterior (A) and lateral (B) views of the elbow show supracondylar fracture of the distal humerus with posteromedial displacement of the distal fragment. Note the increase in the valgus angle of the forearm on the anteroposterior view.

medial supracondylar ridge
medial epicondyle
fragment from ridge of coronoid fossa
lateral epicondyle
trochlea
capitellum
radial head

lateral epicondyle
medial supracondylar ridge
fragment from ridge of coronoid fossa
trochlea
medial epicondyle
capitellum
radial head

Whatever the age of the patient, it is important in fracture of the distal humerus to demonstrate and fully evaluate the type of injury, the extension of the fracture line, and the degree of displacement, since the method of treatment varies accordingly. When difficulties in interpretation of the type of fracture and the degree of displacement arise, it may be helpful to obtain films of the contralateral normal elbow for comparison.

COMPLICATIONS The most serious complications of supracondylar fracture are Volkmann ischemic contracture (see Fig. 4.48) and malunion. The latter commonly results in a varus deformity of the elbow, known as cubitus varus.

FRACTURE OF THE RADIAL HEAD   Fracture of the radial head is a common injury that results, in the majority of cases, from a fall on the outstretched arm and, only rarely, from a direct blow to the lateral aspect of the elbow.

Radial head fractures had been classified by Mason into three types: type I, undisplaced fractures; type II, marginal fractures with displacement (including impaction, depression, and angulation); type III, comminuted fractures involving the entire head. Later DeLee, Green, and Wilkins suggested adding type IV, fractures of the radial head in association with elbow dislocation (Fig. 5.63). All these fractures can be adequately demonstrated on the anteroposterior and lateral films of the elbow. However, as nondisplaced or minimally

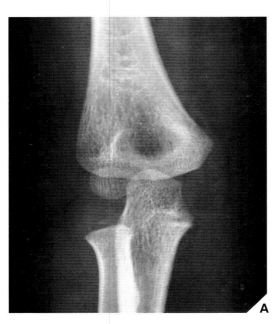 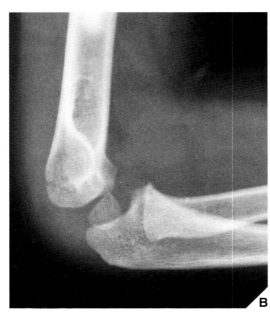 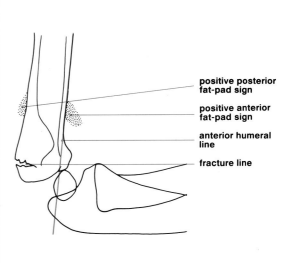

positive posterior
fat-pad sign

positive anterior
fat-pad sign

anterior humeral
line

fracture line

Figure 5.62 A 3-year-old girl fell on the street. On the anteroposterior view (A) the fracture line is practically invisible, while on the lateral view (B) it is more obvious. There is a positive posterior fat-pad sign, and the anterior fat pad is also clearly displaced. Note that the anterior humeral line intersects the posterior third of the capitellum, indicating slight anterior angulation of the distal fragment.

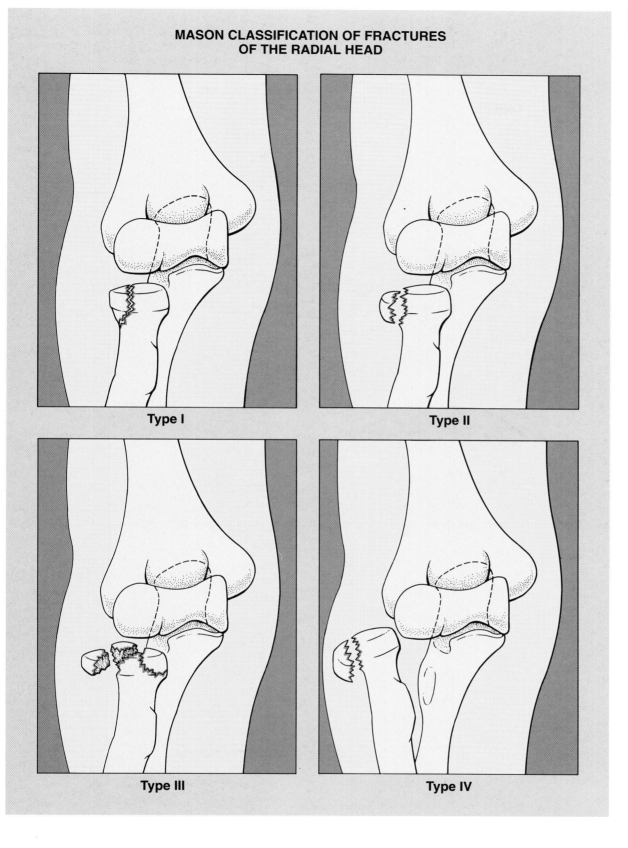

MASON CLASSIFICATION OF FRACTURES OF THE RADIAL HEAD

Type I

Type II

Type III

Type IV

Figure 5.63 Mason classification of fractures of the radial head.

displaced fractures may go undetected on these projections, the radial head-capitellum view should be included in the routine radiographic examination to detect occult injuries and to evaluate the degree of displacement (Fig. 5.64). Determination of the exact extension of the fracture line (that is, whether it is extra- or intra-articular) and the degree of displacement is crucial to deciding the course of treatment. Nondisplaced or minimally displaced fractures are usually treated conservatively by use of splints or casts, until healing allows active mobilization of the elbow. On the other hand, cleavage fracture of the radial articular surface involving one third or one half of the head with displacement greater than 3 mm to 4 mm usually indicates the need for open reduction and internal fixation (Fig. 5.65); this is particularly true in younger individuals. Excision of the radial head is the procedure of choice when comminution and displacement of the radial head are present (Fig. 5.66).

FRACTURE OF THE CORONOID PROCESS Rarely occurring as an isolated injury, fracture of the coronoid process is most often associated with posterior dislocation in the elbow joint. It is, therefore, important in cases of elbow injury to exclude the possibility of fracture of the coronoid process, since, undiagnosed, it may fail to unite, leading to instability and recurrent subluxation in the joint. The anteroposterior and lateral projections are usually insufficient to evaluate the coronoid process because of overlap of structures on these views. Demonstration of injury is best made on the radial head-capitellum projection (Fig. 5.67) and occasionally on the internal oblique view.

FRACTURE OF THE OLECRANON Olecranon fractures usually result from a direct fall on the flexed elbow, and this mechanism frequently produces comminution and marked displacement of the major fragments. An indirect mechanism, like a fall on the out-

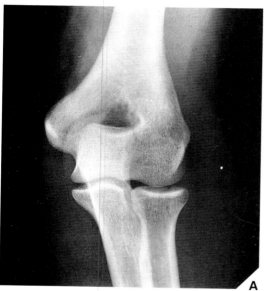

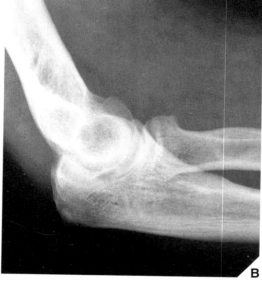

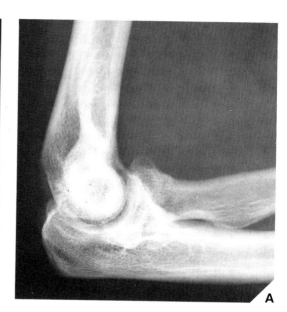

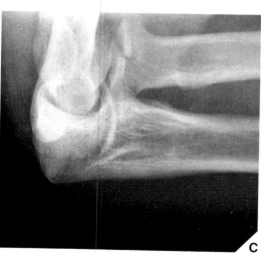

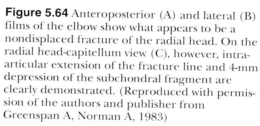

intraarticular extension of fracture

4-mm depression

positive fat-pad sign

fracture line

Figure 5.64 Anteroposterior (A) and lateral (B) films of the elbow show what appears to be a nondisplaced fracture of the radial head. On the radial head-capitellum view (C), however, intra-articular extension of the fracture line and 4-mm depression of the subchondral fragment are clearly demonstrated. (Reproduced with permission of the authors and publisher from Greenspan A, Norman A, 1983)

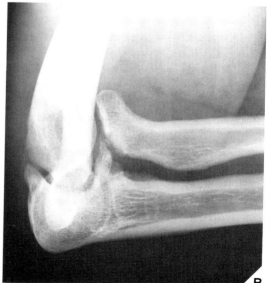

Figure 5.65 Standard lateral view of the elbow (A) demonstrates a fracture of the radial head, but bony overlap prevents exact evaluation of the extent of the fracture line and the degree of displacement. Radial head-capitellum view (B) reveals it to be a displaced articular fracture involving the posterior third of the radial head. (Reproduced with permission of the authors and publisher from Greenspan A, et al., 1984)

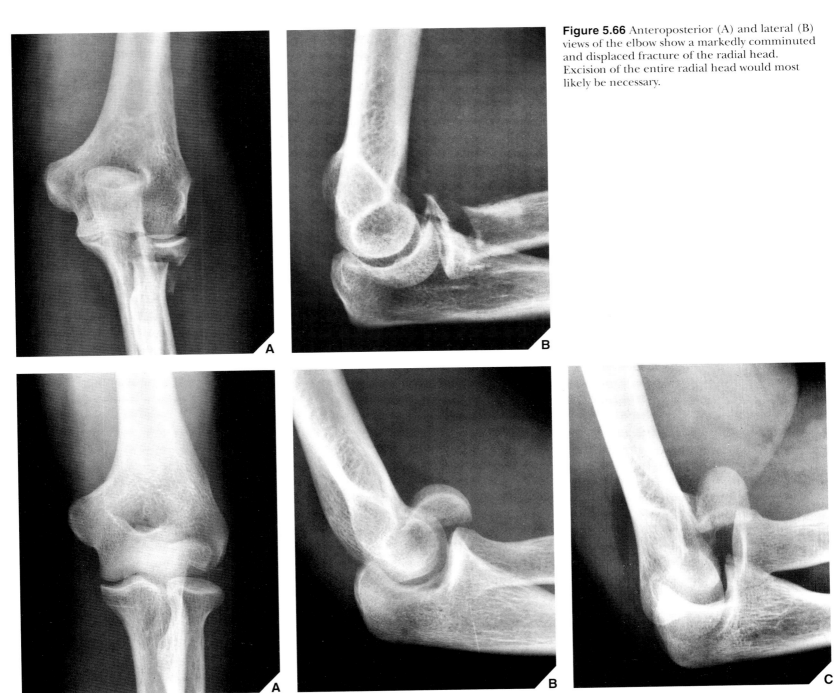

Figure 5.66 Anteroposterior (A) and lateral (B) views of the elbow show a markedly comminuted and displaced fracture of the radial head. Excision of the entire radial head would most likely be necessary.

Figure 5.67 While playing ice hockey, a 37-year-old man injured his right elbow in a fall. The initial anteroposterior (A) and lateral (B) studies show a fracture of the capitellum with anterior rotation and displacement. Note the typical "half-moon" appearance of the displaced capitellum on the lateral view. On the radial head-capitellum film (C), an unsuspected, nondisplaced fracture of the coronoid process is evident. (B,C: Reproduced with permission of the authors and publisher from Greenspan A, Norman A, 1982)

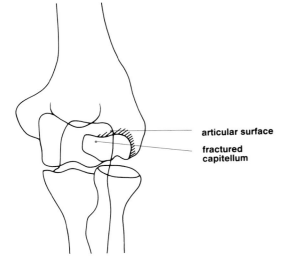

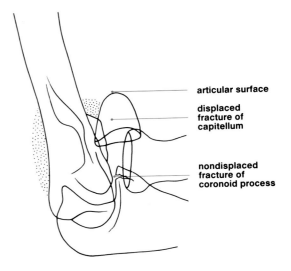

stretched arm, produces an oblique or transverse fracture with minimal displacement. The fracture is usually well demonstrated on a lateral projection of the elbow (Fig. 5.68).

A number of classifications have been developed to evaluate an olecranon fracture. Colton classified olecranon fractures as undisplaced, and displaced, the latter group being subdivided into avulsion fractures, oblique, and transverse fractures, comminuted fractures, and fracture-dislocations.

Another practical classification has been developed by Horne and Tanzer, who classified these fractures by their location apparent on the lateral radiographs (Fig. 5.69). Type I fractures are subdivided into two groups: A) oblique, extra-articular fractures of the olecranon tip, and B) transverse intra-articular fractures originating on the proximal third of the articular surface of olecranon fossa. Type II fractures are transverse or oblique fractures originating on the middle third of the articular surface of olecranon fossa. They also are subdivided into two groups: A) single fracture line, and B) two fracture lines, one proximal (transverse, or oblique) and the second, more distal, extending posteriorly. Type III fractures involve the distal third of the olecranon fossa and may be either transverse or oblique. The majority of fractures are type II.

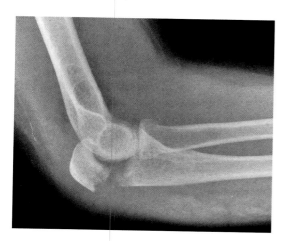

Figure 5.68 A 52-year-old woman fell on her outstretched arm and sustained a type III olecranon fracture, effectively demonstrated on the lateral view of the elbow. Note the positive anterior and posterior fat pad sign.

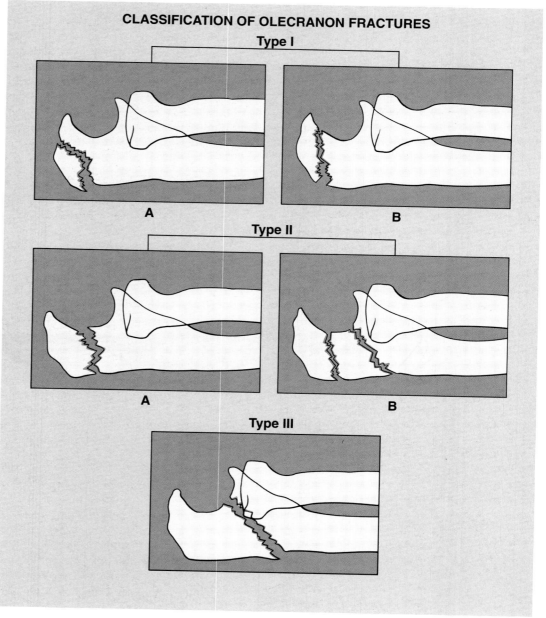

Figure 5.69 Classification of olecranon fractures. (Modified from Horne JG, Tanzer TL, 1981)

As far as treatment is concerned, nondisplaced fractures are usually treated conservatively, whereas displaced fractures are most often treated by open reduction and internal fixation.

Osteochondritis Dissecans of the Capitellum

This condition, also referred to as Panner disease, is considered to be related to trauma, namely to repeated exogenous injuries to the elbow. Valgus strain of the elbow in throwing sports such as baseball and football has been implicated as one etiologic factor. It most frequently affects the right elbow in right-handed children and adolescents, the vast majority of whom are males.

In the early stage of the disease, anteroposterior and lateral films may show no significant abnormality (Fig. 5.70A,B); the only radiographic sign of early-stage Panner disease may become apparent on the radial head-capitellum view with the finding of subtle flattening of the capitellum (Fig. 5.70C). As the condition progresses, the lesion, consisting of a detached segment of subchondral bone with overlying cartilage, gradually separates from its bed in the capitellum. Before separation the lesion is called "in situ"; after separation the osteochondral fragment becomes a "loose" body in the joint (Fig. 5.71). As sometimes more than one fragment is discharged into the joint, osteochondritis dissecans may be mistaken for idiopathic

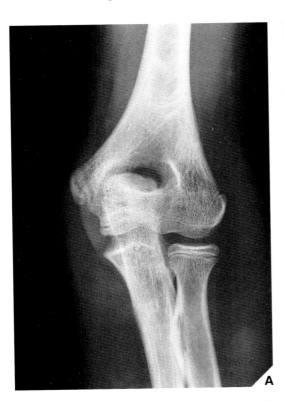

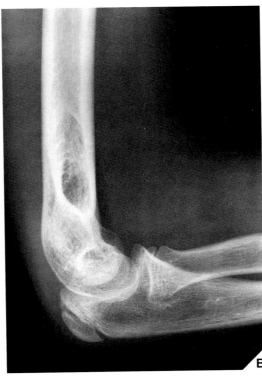

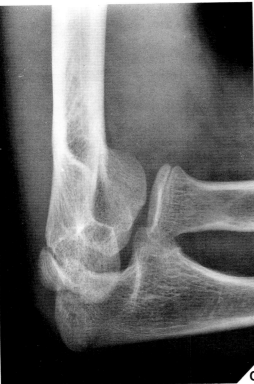

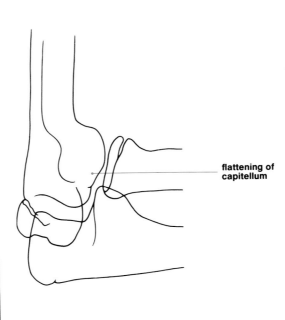

Figure 5.70 A 13-year-old boy who was very active in Little League baseball complained of pain in his right elbow for several months. Anteroposterior (A) and lateral (B) films of the elbow demonstrate no abnormalities. On the radial head-capitellum view (C), subtle flattening of the capitellum may indicate early-stage osteochondritis dissecans. (Reproduced with permission of the authors and publisher from Greenspan A, Norman A, 1982)

flattening of capitellum

synovial chondromatosis, a nontraumatic condition that is a form of synovial metaplasia. In this condition multiple cartilaginous bodies that are regular in outline and usually uniform in size are seen in the joint (see Fig. 15.72).

One of the most valuable radiologic procedures for evaluating osteochondritis dissecans is arthrotomography, which localizes the defect in the cartilaginous surface of the capitellum and distinguishes an in situ lesion from the more advanced stage of the disease (Fig. 5.72). This information is crucial for the orthopedic surgeon, since the in situ lesion may be treated conservatively, while surgical intervention

may be required if the osteochondral fragment has been partially separated from its bed or discharged into the joint. MRI may also effectively demonstrate the lesion (Fig. 5.73) and provide information about its stability.

Dislocations in the Elbow Joint

SIMPLE DISLOCATIONS The standard method of classifying elbow dislocations is based on the direction of displacement of the radius and the ulna in relation to the distal humerus. Three main types of dislocation can be distinguished as those affecting: 1) *both the radius and*

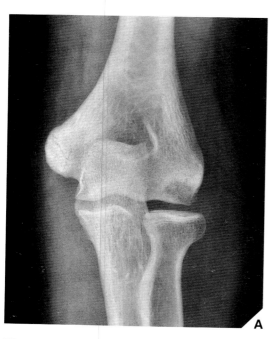
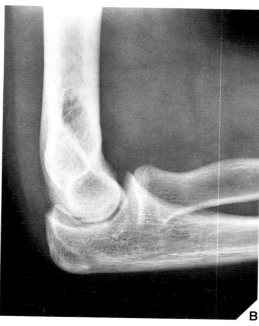
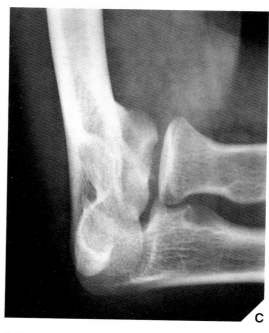

Figure 5.71 An active baseball player, a 15-year-old boy complained of pain in his right elbow for several months. Anteroposterior view of the elbow (A) reveals a radiolucent defect in the capitellum suggesting osteochondritis dissecans; the lateral view (B) is normal. Radial head-capitellum projection (C) demonstrates not only the full extent of the lesion in the capitellum but also osteochondral bodies in the joint—a sign of advanced-stage Panner disease. (Reproduced with permission of the authors and publisher from Greenspan A, et al., 1984)

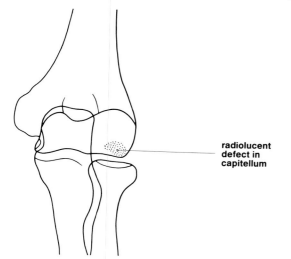

radiolucent defect in capitellum

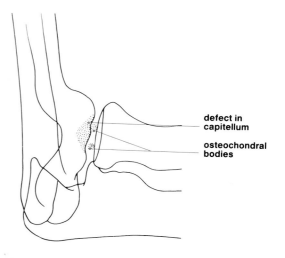

defect in capitellum

osteochondral bodies

the ulna, which may be dislocated posteriorly, anteriorly, medially, or laterally (or in a manner combining posterior or anterior with medial or lateral displacement); 2) *the ulna only*, which may be anteriorly or posteriorly displaced; and 3) *the radius only*, which may be anteriorly, posteriorly, or laterally dislocated.

Posterior and posterolateral dislocations of both the radius and the ulna are by far the most common types—they account for 80% to 90% of all dislocations in the joint. Isolated dislocation of the radial head, on the other hand, is a rare occurrence; it is more commonly associated with fracture of the ulna (see "Monteggia

Fracture-Dislocation" below). Dislocations are easily diagnosed on the standard anteroposterior and lateral films of the elbow.

The presence of dislocation should signal the possibility of an associated fracture of the ulna, which may be overlooked when radiographic examination is focused only on the elbow. For this reason, if dislocation in the elbow joint is suspected, it is mandatory to include the entire forearm on the anteroposterior and lateral films; and conversely, in cases of suspected ulnar fracture, radiographs should include the elbow joint. From a practical point of view, it is important, particularly in adults, to obtain two separate films: one

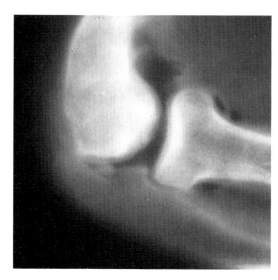
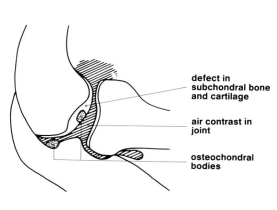

defect in subchondral bone and cartilage

air contrast in joint

osteochondral bodies

Figure 5.72 Lateral arthrotomogram of the elbow demonstrates defects in the subchondral segment of the capitellum and in the overlying cartilage. Loose osteochondral bodies are present, one located posteriorly in the ulnar-trochlear compartment and the other anteriorly in the radiocapitellar compartment. The findings represent advanced-stage osteochondritis dissecans.

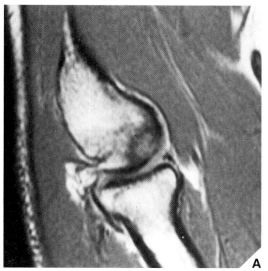
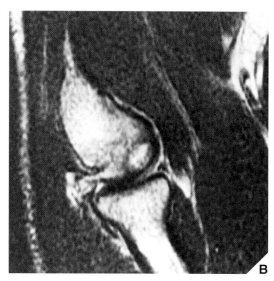

A   B

Figure 5.73 A 16-year-old baseball player presented with pain in the right elbow for six months. The MR sagittal sections (spin-echo sequences, TR 2000/TE 20 and TR 2000/TE 80) demonstrate an area of intermediate signal intensity on proton-weighted image (A) and high signal intensity on T2-weighted image (B), surrounded by a band of low signal intensity. The articular cartilage is intact. The findings are typical for in situ lesion of osteochondritis dissecans (Panner disease). (From Beltran J, 1990)

centered over the elbow joint and the other over the site of the suspected ulnar fracture. Care should be taken to center the films properly, since dislocation of the radial head can easily be missed on improperly centered films.

MONTEGGIA FRACTURE-DISLOCATION The association of fracture of the ulna with dislocation of the radial head is known by the eponym Monteggia fracture-dislocation. It usually results from forced prona-

tion of the forearm during a fall or a direct blow to the posterior aspect of the ulna. Four types of this abnormality have been described (Fig. 5.74), but the features of the classic description are most commonly (in 60% to 70% of cases) seen: fracture at the junction of the proximal and middle thirds of the ulna with anterior angulation associated with anterior dislocation of the radial head (type I). It is identifiable on physical examination by marked pain and tenderness about the elbow and displacement of the radial

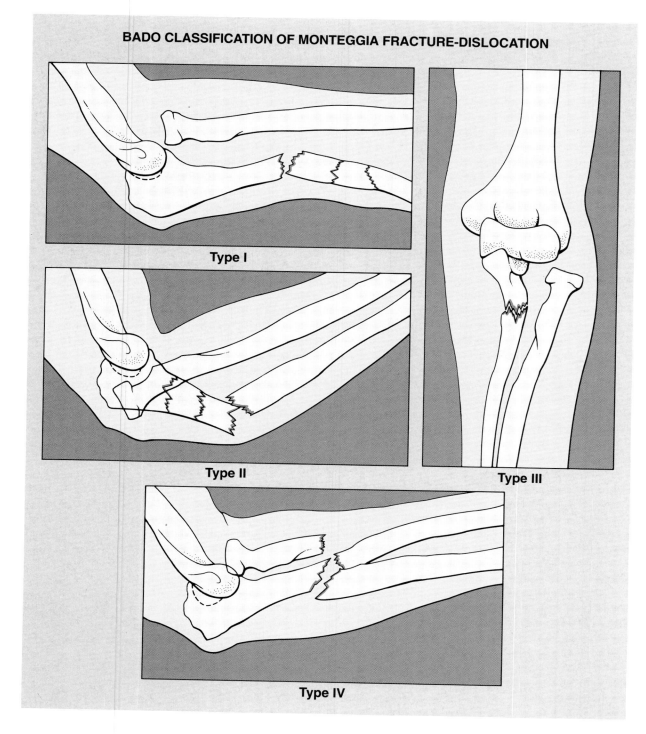

BADO CLASSIFICATION OF MONTEGGIA FRACTURE-DISLOCATION

Type I

Type II

Type III

Type IV

Figure 5.74 The Bado classification of Monteggia fracture-dislocation is based on the four types of abnormality usually resulting from forced pronation of the forearm. These may occur during a fall or direct blow to the posterior aspect of the ulna.

head into the antecubital fossa. The other types, which Bado has described, are as follows:

Type II   Fracture of the proximal ulna with posterior angulation and posterior or posterolateral dislocation of the radial head.

Type III Fracture of the proximal ulna with lateral or anterolateral dislocation of the radial head. Type II and III injuries

account for approximately 30% to 40% of Monteggia fractures.

Type IV   Fractures of the proximal ends of both the radius and the ulna with anterior dislocation of the radial head. (This is the least common type).

The anteroposterior and lateral projections are sufficient to provide a full evaluation of these abnormalities (Fig. 5.75).

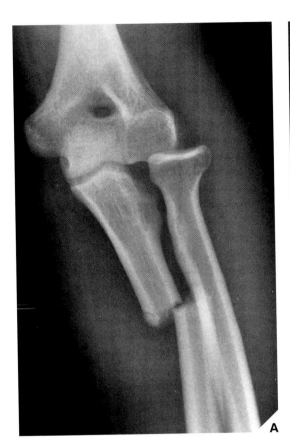

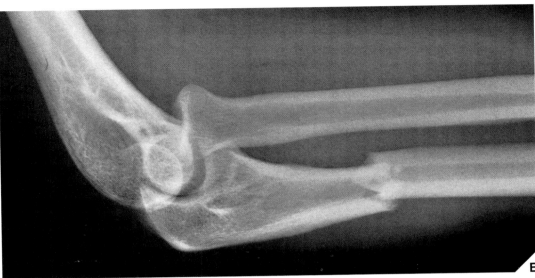

Figure 5.75 Anteroposterior (A) and lateral (B) views of the elbow that include the proximal third of the forearm demonstrate the typical appearance of type III Monteggia fracture-dislocation; fracture is at the proximal third of the ulna, associated with anterolateral dislocation of the radial head.

PRACTICAL POINTS TO REMEMBER

Shoulder Girdle

[1] Fractures of the proximal humerus may be evaluated on the anteroposterior, trans-scapular, and transthoracic lateral projections. The latter view:
- provides a true lateral image of the proximal humerus
- allows sufficient evaluation of the degree of displacement or angulation of the fragments.

[2] Fractures of the scapula, particularly if comminuted and displaced, are best evaluated on the trans-scapular (or Y) projection.

[3] For precise evaluation of the shoulder joint and better demonstration of the glenohumeral articulation, the anteroposterior projection obtained with the patient rotated about 40° toward the affected side (Grashey view):
- eliminates the overlap of the humeral head and the glenoid fossa
- allows visualization of the glenohumeral joint space and the glenoid in profile.

[4] The Hill-Sacks lesion, which is best demonstrated on the anteroposterior projection obtained with the arm internally rotated, and the Bankart lesion are virtually diagnostic of previous anterior dislocation.

[5] Compression fracture (trough line sign) of the anteromedial aspect of the humeral head is a common sequela of posterior dislocation. The anteroposterior projection obtained with the arm externally rotated readily demonstrates this finding.

[6] MRI characteristics of impingement syndrome include:
- cystic and sclerotic changes in the greater tuberosity
- perimuscular and peritendinous edema
- thickening of subacromial bursa (or effusion)
- thinning of the supraspinatus tendon
- increased signal intensity in the tendon (on T2-weighting)
- subacromial spur.

[7] Rotator cuff tear may effectively be evaluated by contrast arthrography. Opacification of the subacromial-subdeltoid bursae complex is diagnostic of this injury.

[8] MRI characteristics of rotator cuff tear include:
- discontinuity of the rotator cuff tendons
- high signal intensity within the tendon structure (on T2-weighted images)
- retraction of the musculotendinous junction of supraspinatus
- atrophy of the supraspinatus muscle and infiltration by fat
- obscuration of the subacromial-subdeltoid fat line (on T1-weighted images)
- fluid in the subacromial-subdeltoid bursae complex.

[9] Acromioclavicular separation is best demonstrated on the stress anteroposterior projection obtained with a 15° cephalad angulation of the radiographic tube and weights strapped to the patient's forearms. The radiographic characteristics of this condition include:
- width of the acromioclavicular joint space
- width of the coracoclavicular distance
- presence or absence of apparent cephalad displacement of the distal end of the clavicle.

Elbow

[1] On the anteroposterior projection of the elbow:
- observe the normal 15° valgus carrying angle formed between the arm and the forearm
- (in the child) recognize the four secondary ossification centers of the distal humerus and the age at which they appear: capitellum at 1–2 years, medial epicondyle at 4 years, trochlea at 8 years, and lateral epicondyle at 10 years.

[2] On the lateral view of the elbow:
- note the normal angular (hockey-stick) appearance of the distal humerus. The angle measures approximately 140°. Loss of this angle occurs in supracondylar fracture
- evaluate the position of the capitellum relative to the longitudinal axis of the proximal radius and the anterior humeral line
- pay attention to the presence or absence of the fat-pad sign. If this sign is positive in a patient with an elbow injury, fracture should always be considered.

[3] The radial head-capitellum projection is very useful in evaluating elbow trauma and should always be obtained as part of a routine study.

[4] Arthrotomography is an important technique in selected cases of elbow injury. The procedure helps to visualize:
- subtle chondral and osteochondral fractures
- osteochondritis dissecans
- synovial and capsular abnormalities
- osteochondral bodies in the joint.

[5] Supracondylar fracture of the distal humerus (usually of the extension type) is very common in children. The lateral film showing loss of the hockey-stick appearance of the distal humerus is diagnostic. If the lateral projection is equivocal, obtain a film of the contralateral (normal) elbow for comparison.

[6] Fracture of the radial head is common in adults. It is important to demonstrate:
- the type of fracture

- the extension of the fracture line
- the degree of articular displacement.

This information determines whether a conservative-versus-surgical course of treatment is indicated.

[7] Fracture of the coronoid process is usually occult and is most often associated with posterior dislocation in the elbow joint. If unrecognized, it may fail to unite, leading to recurrent subluxation or dislocation in the joint. The radial head-capitellum view is best suited to demonstrate it.

[8] Fractures of the olecranon are best demonstrated on the lateral view. They are classified into three types, according to the origin of the fracture line at the articular surface of the olecranon fossa.

[9] The orthopedic management of osteochondritis dissecans requires demonstrating the status of the articular cartilage of the capitellum. In this respect arthrotomography or MRI are the procedures of choice.

[10] In every case of ulnar fracture, look for associated dislocation of the radial head; and conversely, in every case of dislocation, look for fracture of the ulna (Monteggia fracture-dislocation). Proper radiographic technique for imaging these often missed injuries requires, in adults, obtaining two separate films that include the elbow joint and the forearm: one centered over the joint and the other over the mid-forearm. In children a single film that includes the elbow joint and the entire forearm suffices.

References

Adams JC: *Outline of Fractures Including Joint Injuries*, ed 4. Baltimore, Williams & Wilkins, 1964.

Anderson JE: *Grant's Atlas of Anatomy*, ed 8. Baltimore, Williams and Wilkins, 1983.

Arger PH, Oberkircher PE, Miller WT: Lipohemarthrosis. *Am J Radiol* 121:97, 1974.

Bado JL: *The Monteggia Lesion*. Springfield, IL, C.C. Thomas, 1962.

Bailey RW: Acute and recurrent dislocation of the shoulder. *J Bone Joint Surg* 49A:767, 1967.

Beltran J: The elbow. In: Beltran J: *MRI Musculoskeletal System*. Philadelphia, Lippincott, 1990.

Beltran J, Gray LA, Bools JC, Zuelzer W, Weis LD, Unverferth LJ: Rotator cuff lesions of the shoulder: Evaluating by direct sagittal CT arthrography. *Radiology* 160:161, 1986.

Bledsoe RC, Izenstark JL: Displacement of fat pads in disease and injury of the elbow: A new radiographic sign. *Radiology* 73:717, 1959.

Bohrer SP: The fat pad sign following elbow trauma: Its usefulness and reliability in suspecting "invisible" fractures. *Clin Radiol* 21:90, 1970.

Braunstein EM: Double contrast arthrotomography of the shoulder. *J Bone Joint Surg* 64A:192, 1982.

Brodeur AE, Silberstein MJ, Graviss ER: *Radiology of the Pediatric Elbow*. Boston, Hall Medical, 1981.

Chapman MW: Closed intramedullary nailing of the humerus. *Instructional Course Lectures AAOS* 32:324, 1983.

Cisternino SJ, Rogers LF, Stufflebam BC, Kruglik GD: The trough line: A radiographic sign of posterior shoulder dislocation. *Am J Roentgenol* 130:951, 1978.

Colton CL: Fractures of the olecranon in adults: Classification and management. *Injury* 5:121, 1973.

Cone RO, Szabo R, Resnick D, Gelberman R, Taleisnik J, Gilula LA: Computed tomography of the normal radioulnar joints. *Invest Radiol* 18:541, 1983.

DeLee JC, Green DP, Wilkins KE: Fractures and dislocations of the elbow. In: Rockwood CA Jr, Green DP: *Fractures in Adults*, ed 2, vol I. Philadelphia, Lippincott, 1984, pp 559-652.

Deutsch AL, Resnick D, Mink JH, Berman JL, Cone RO III, Resnik CS, Danzig L, Guerra J Jr: Computed and conventional arthrotomography of the glenohumeral joint: Normal anatomy and clinical experience. *Radiology* 153:603, 1984.

Eppright RH, Wilkins KE: Fractures and dislocations of the elbow. In: Rockwood CA Jr, Green DP (eds): *Fractures*, vol 1. Philadelphia, Lippincott, 1975.

Eto RT, Anderson PW, Harley JD: Elbow arthrography with application of tomography. *Radiology* 115:283, 1975.

Fowles JV, Sliman N, Kassab MT: The Monteggia lesion in children. Fracture of the ulna and dislocation of the radial head. *J Bone Joint Surg* 65A:1276, 1983.

Franklin PD, Dunlop RW, Whitelaw G, Jacques E Jr, Blickman JG, Shapiro JH: Computed tomography of the normal and traumatized elbow. *J Comput Assist Tomogr* 12:817, 1988.

Greenspan A, Norman A: The radial head-capitellum view: Useful technique in elbow trauma. *Am J Roentgenol* 138:1186, 1982.

Greenspan A, Norman A: The radial head-capitellum view: Another example of its usefulness (letter). *Am J Roentgenol* 139:193, 1982.

Greenspan A, Norman A: Letter to the editor (reply). *Am J Roentgenol* 140:1273, 1983.

Greenspan A, Norman A, Rosen H: Radial head-capitellum view in elbow trauma: Clinical application and radiographic-anatomic correlation. *Am J Roentgenol* 143:355, 1984.

Holt RG, Helms CA, Steinbach L, Neuman C, Munk PL, Genant HK: Magnetic resonance imaging of the shoulder: Rationale and current applications. *Skeletal Radiol* 19:5, 1990.

Horne JG, Tanzer TL: Olecranon fractures: A review of 100 cases. *J Trauma* 21:469, 1981.

Haynor DR, Shuman WP: Double contrast CT arthrography of the glenoid labrum and shoulder girdle. *RadioGraphics* 4:411, 1984.

Hill HA, Sachs MD: The grooved defect of the humeral head. A frequently unrecognized complication of dislocations of the shoulder joint. *Radiology* 35:690, 1940.

Kaplan PA, Resnick D: Stress-induced osteolysis of the clavicle. *Radiology* 158:139, 1986.

Kieft GJ, Bloem JL, Rozing PM, Oberman WR: Rotator cuff impingement syndrome: MR imaging. *Radiology* 166:211, 1988.

Kilcoyne RF, Shuman WP, Matsen FA III, Morris M, Rockwood CA: The Neer classification of displaced proximal humeral fractures: Spectrum of findings on plain radiographs and CT scans. *Am J Roentgenol* 173:70, 1983.

Killoran PJ, Marcove RC, Freiberger RH: Shoulder arthrography. *Am J Roentgenol* 103:658, 1968.

Kleinman PK, Kanzaria PK, Goss TP, Pappas AM: Axillary arthrotomography of the glenoid labrum. *Am J Roentgenol* 141:993, 1984.

Middleton WD, Lauson TL: *Anatomy and MRI of the Joints*. New York, Raven Press, 1989.

Kohn AM: Soft tissue alterations in elbow trauma. *Am J Roentgenol* 82:867, 1959.

Mitsunaga MM, Adishian DA, Bianco AJ Jr: Osteochondritis dissecans of the capitellum. *J Trauma* 22:53, 1982.

Murphy WA, Siegel MJ: Elbow fat pads with new signs and extended differential diagnosis. *Radiology* 124:659, 1977.

Neer CS: Displaced proximal humeral fractures. I. Classification and evaluation. *J Bone Joint Surg* 52A:1077, 1970.

Neer CS, Rockwood CA: Fractures and dislocations of the shoulder. In: Rockwood CA, Green DP (eds): *Fractures*, Philadelphia, Lippincott, 1973, p 585.

Neer CS II: Four-segment classification of displaced proximal humeral fractures. *Instructional Course Lectures AAOS* 24:160, 1975.

Neer CS II: Impingement lesions *Clin Orthoped* 173:70, 1983.

Neer CS II, Rockwood CA Jr: Fractures and dislocations of the shoulder. In: Rockwood CA, Green DP (eds): *Fractures in Adults*, Philadelphia, Lippincott, 1983, p 677.

Nelson SW: Some important diagnostic and technical fundamentals in the radiology of trauma, with particular emphasis on skeletal trauma. *Radiol Clin North Am* 4:241, 1966.

Norell HG: Roentgenologic visualization of the extracapsular fat. Its importance in the diagnosis of traumatic injuries to the elbow. *Acta Radiol* 42:205, 1954.

Pavlov H, Freiberger RH: Fractures and dislocations about the shoulder. *Semin Roentgenol* 13:85, 1978.

Reckling FW, Peltier L: Riccardo Galeazzi and Galeazzi's fracture. *Surgery* 58:453, 1965.

Resnick D: Shoulder pain. *Orthop Clin North Am* 14:81, 1983.

Rogers LF: Fractures and dislocations of the elbow. *Semin Roentgenol* 13:97, 1978.

Rogers LF, Malave S Jr, White H, Tachdjian MO: Plastic bowing, torus and greenstick supracondylar fractures of the humerus: Radiographic clues to obscure fractures of the elbow in children. *Radiology* 128:145, 1978.

Seeger LL, Gold RH, Bassett LW, Ellman H: Shoulder impingement syndrome: MR findings in 53 shoulders. *Am J Roentgenol* 150:343, 1988.

Singson RD, Feldman F, Rosenberg ZS: Elbow joint: Assessment with double-contrast CT arthrography. *Radiology* 160:167, 1986.

Slivka J, Resnick D: An improved radiographic view of the glenohumeral joint. *J Can Assoc Radiol* 30:83, 1979.

Smith FM: Children's elbow injuries: Fractures and dislocations. *Clin Orthop* 50: 7, 1967.

Wenzel WW: The FBI sign. *Rocky Mount Med J* 69:71, 1972.

Weston WJ: Elbow arthrography. In: Dalinka MK (ed): *Arthrography*. New York, Springer-Verlag, 1980.

Zlatkin, MB, Iannotti JP, Roberts MC, Esterhei JL, Dalinka MK, Kressel HY, Schwartz JS, Lenkinski RE: Rotator cuff tears: Diagnostic performance of MR imaging. *Radiology* 172:223, 1989.

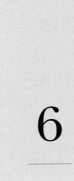

6

Upper Limb II: Distal Forearm, Wrist, and Hand

DISTAL FOREARM

INJURY TO THE DISTAL FOREARM, caused predominantly (90% of cases) by a fall on the outstretched hand, is common throughout life, but most common in the elderly. The type of injury usually sustained is fracture of the distal radius or ulna, the incidence of which substantially exceeds that of dislocation in the distal radioulnar and radiocarpal articulations. Although history and physical examination usually provide important information regarding the type of injury, radiographs are indispensable in determining the exact site and extent; and in several types of fractures only adequate radiographic examination can lead to a correct diagnosis.

Anatomic-Radiologic Considerations

Radiographs obtained in the posteroanterior and lateral projections are usually sufficient to evaluate most injuries to the distal forearm (Figs. 6.1, 6.2). On each of these views it is important to appreciate the normal anatomic relations of the radius and the ulna for a complete evaluation of trauma.

The posteroanterior view of the distal forearm reveals anatomic variations in the length of the radius and the ulna, known as *ulnar variance*. As a rule, the radial styloid process exceeds the length of the articular end of the ulna by 9 mm to 12 mm. At the site of articulation with the lunate, however, the articular surfaces of the radius and the ulna are on the same level, yielding *neutral ulnar variance* (Fig. 6.3). Occasionally, the ulna projects more proximally—*negative ulnar variance* (or ulna minus variant); or more distally—*positive ulnar variance* (or ulna plus variant) (Fig. 6.4). This view also reveals an important anatomic feature of the radius known as the *radial angle* (also called the *ulnar slant* of the articular surface of the radius), which normally ranges from 15° to 25° (Fig. 6.5).

The lateral view of the distal forearm demonstrates another significant feature, the *volar tilt* of the articular surface of the radius (known variously as *the dorsal angle, palmar facing,* or *palmar inclination*). The tilt normally ranges from 10° to 25° (Fig. 6.6).

Both these measurements have practical importance to the orthopedic surgeon in assessing displacement and the position of fragments after fracture of the distal radius. They can also help the surgeon to decide between closed and open reduction, as well as assist in follow-up examinations.

Ancillary imaging techniques do not play as great a role in evaluating trauma to the distal forearm as they do in injury to the wrist. Arthrographic examination (Fig. 6.7) may need to be performed in cases of suspected injury to the triangular fibrocartilage complex (TFCC), which consists of the triangular fibrocartilage (articular disk), the meniscus homologue, the dorsal and volar radioulnar ligaments, and the ulnar collateral ligament (Fig. 6.8). As the radiocarpal cavity into which contrast is injected normally does not communicate with the distal radioulnar joint, opacification of this compartment indicates a tear of the triangular fibrocartilage (see Fig. 6.20). In a small percentage of cases, a false-positive result may be due to a normal anatomic variant allowing communication between the radiocarpal compartment and the distal radioulnar joint.

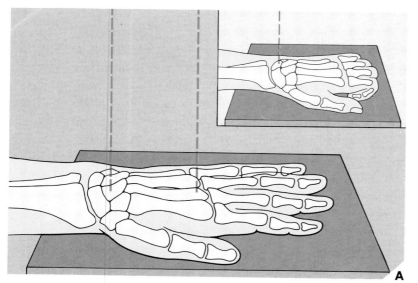

Figure 6.1 For the purpose of classification, a distinction is made between traumatic conditions involving the distal forearm, the wrist, and the hand. From a radiologic perspective, however, the positioning of the limb for posteroanterior and lateral films of the wrist area (that is, the distal forearm and the carpus) and the hand is essentially the same. (A) For the posteroanterior (dorsovolar) view of the wrist and the hand, the patient is seated with his or her arm fully extended on the radiographic table. The portion of the limb from the distal third of the forearm to the fingertips rests prone on the film cassette. Whether the wrist area or the hand is the focus of evaluation, the hand usually lies flat (palm down), with the fingers slightly spread. The point toward which the central beam is directed, however, varies: For the wrist the beam is directed toward the center of the carpus; for the hand, toward the head of the third metacarpal bone. For better demonstration of the wrist area, the patient's fingers may be flexed to cause the carpus to lie flat on the film cassette (inset). (B) On the film in this projection, the distal radius and the ulna, as well as the carpal and metacarpal bones and phalanges, are well demonstrated. The thumb, however, is seen in an oblique projection; and the bases of the second to fifth metacarpals partially overlap. In the wrist there is also overlap of the pisiform and the triquetrum, as well as the trapezium and trapezoid bones. (C) On this projection a carpal angle can be determined. It is formed by two tangents, the first drawn against the proximal borders of the scaphoid and lunate (1), the second drawn against the proximal borders of the triquetrum and lunate (2). The angle measures normally between 110° and 150°, showing considerable deviation with age, sex, and race.

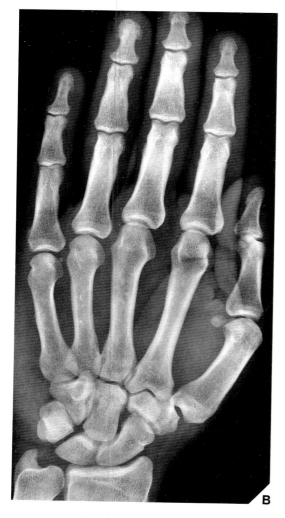

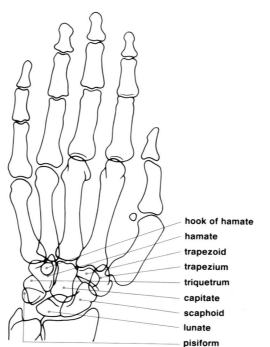

hook of hamate
hamate
trapezoid
trapezium
triquetrum
capitate
scaphoid
lunate
pisiform

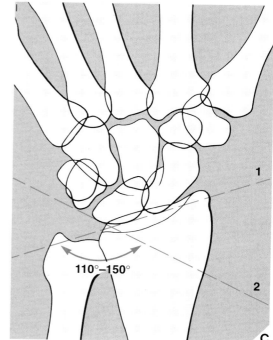

110°–150°

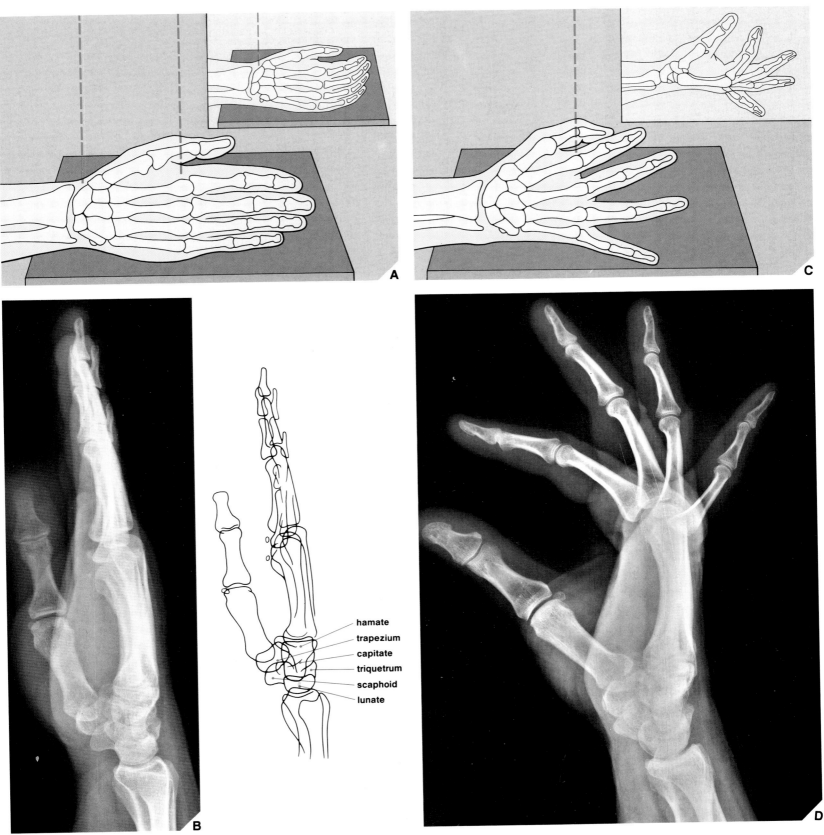

Figure 6.2 (A) For the lateral projection of the wrist area and the hand, the patient's arm is fully extended and resting on its ulnar side. The fingers may be *fully extended* or, preferably, *slightly flexed (inset)*, with the thumb slightly in front of the fingers. For evaluation of the wrist area, the central beam is directed toward the center of the carpus, while for the hand it is directed toward the head of the second metacarpal. (B) On the film in this projection, the distal radius and the ulna overlap, but the relation of the longitudinal axes of the capitate, the lunate, and the radius can sufficiently be evaluated (see Fig. 6.51). Although the metacarpals and the phalanges also overlap, dorsal or volar displacement of a fracture of these bones can easily be detected (see Fig. 4.1). The thumb is imaged in true dorsovolar projection. (C) A more effective way of imaging the fingers in the lateral projection is to have the patient spread the fingers in a fan-like manner, with the ulnar side of the fifth phalanx resting on the film cassette. The central beam is directed toward the heads of the metacarpals. (D) On the film in this projection, the overlap of the phalanges commonly seen on the standard lateral view is eliminated. The interphalangeal joints can readily be evaluated.

Labels in figure B: hamate, trapezium, capitate, triquetrum, scaphoid, lunate

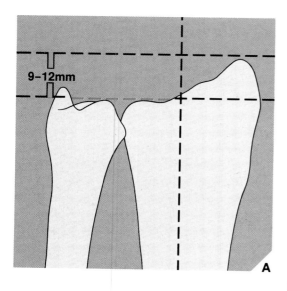

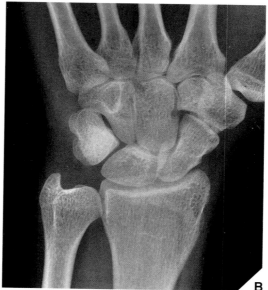

Figure 6.3 Neutral ulnar variance. (A) As a rule, the radial styloid process rises 9 mm to 12 mm above the articular surface of the distal ulna. (B) At the site of articulation with the lunate, the articular surfaces of the radius and the ulna are on the same level.

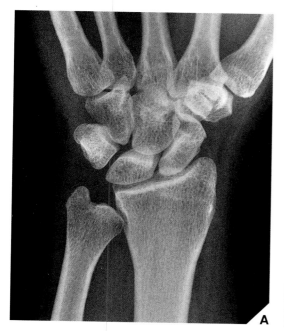

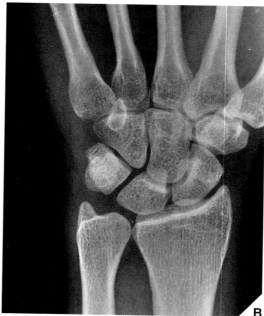

Figure 6.4 (A) Negative ulnar variance. The articular surface of the ulna projects 5 mm proximal to the site of radiolunate articulation. (B) Positive ulnar variance. The articular surface of the ulna projects 5 mm distal to the site of radiolunate articulation.

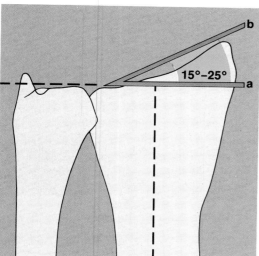

Figure 6.5 The ulnar slant of the articular surface of the radius is determined, with the wrist in the neutral position, by the angle formed by two lines: one perpendicular to the long axis of the radius at the level of the radioulnar articular surface (a), and a tangent connecting the radial styloid process and the ulnar aspect of the radius (b).

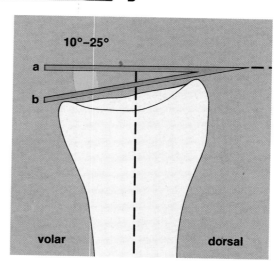

Figure 6.6 The palmar inclination of the radial articular surface is determined by measuring the angle formed by a line perpendicular to the long axis of the radius at the level of the styloid process (a), and a tangent connecting the dorsal and volar aspects of the radial articular surface (b).

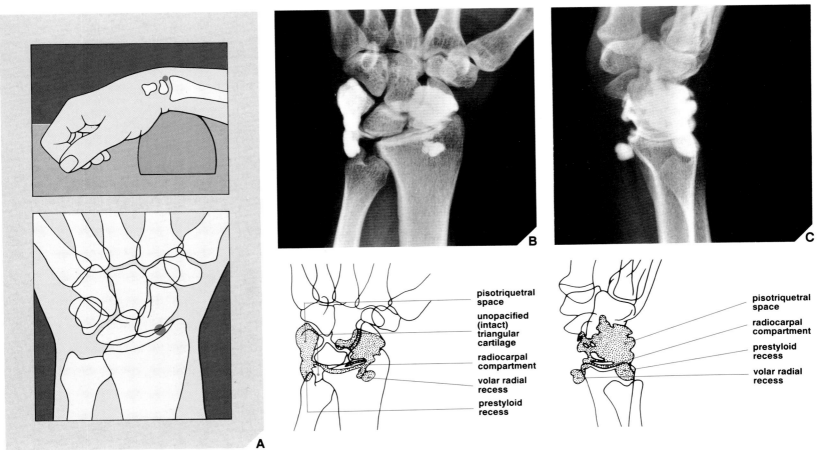

Figure 6.7 (A) For arthrographic examination of the radiocarpal joint, the wrist is positioned prone on a radiolucent sponge to open the joint for needle insertion. Under fluoroscopic control the joint is entered, using a 22-gauge needle, at a point lateral to the scapholunate ligament. (The red dot marks the site of puncture.) Two or 3 mL of contrast (60% diatrizoate meglumine) are injected, and posteroanterior (dorsovolar), lateral, and oblique films are obtained. Posteroanterior (B) and lateral (C) views show contrast filling the radiocarpal compartment, the prestyloid and volar radial recesses, and the pisotriquetral space. Intact triangular fibrocartilage does not allow contrast to enter the distal radioulnar joint, and intact intercarpal ligaments prevent leak of contrast into the intercarpal articulations.

Figure 6.8 The triangular fibrocartilage complex (TFCC) includes the triangular fibrocartilage, radioulnar ligament, ulnocarpal ligament, extensor carpi ulnaris sheath, and meniscus homologue. It stabilizes the distal radioulnar joint and functions as a cushion of compressing axial forces. The triangular fibrocartilage attaches medially to the fovea of the ulna and laterally to the lunate fossa of the radius.

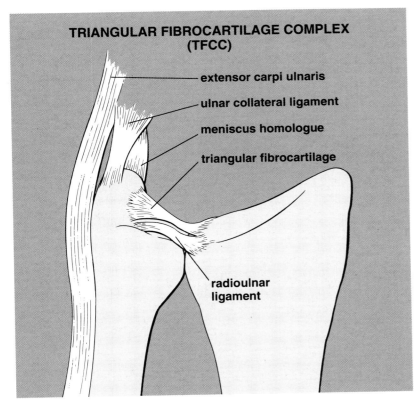

TRIANGULAR FIBROCARTILAGE COMPLEX (TFCC)

- extensor carpi ulnaris
- ulnar collateral ligament
- meniscus homologue
- triangular fibrocartilage
- radioulnar ligament

For a summary in tabular form of the standard radiographic projections and ancillary imaging techniques used to evaluate trauma to the distal forearm, see Figures 6.9 and 6.10.

Injury to the Distal Forearm
Fractures of the Distal Radius
COLLES FRACTURE The most frequently encountered injury to the distal forearm, Colles fracture usually results from a fall on the outstretched hand with the forearm pronated in dorsiflexion. It is most commonly seen in adults over 50 years of age and more often in women than in men. In the classic description of this injury, known in the European literature as the *Pouteau fracture*, the fracture line is extra-articular, usually occurring about 2 cm to 3 cm from the articular surface of the distal radius. In many cases the distal fragment is radially and dorsally displaced and shows dorsal angulation, although other variants in the alignment of fragments may also be seen (Fig. 6.11). Frequently, there is an associated fracture of the

Figure 6.9 Standard Radiographic Projections for Evaluating Injury to the Distal Forearm

PROJECTION	DEMONSTRATION
Posteroanterior	Ulnar variance
	Carpal angle
	Radial angle
	Distal radioulnar joint
	Colles fracture
	Hutchinson fracture
	Galeazzi fracture-dislocation
Lateral	Palmar facing of radius
	Pronator quadratus fat stripe
	Colles fracture
	Smith fracture
	Barton fracture
	Galeazzi fracture-dislocation

Figure 6.10 Ancillary Imaging Techniques for Evaluating Injury to the Distal Forearm

TECHNIQUE	DEMONSTRATION
Arthrography	Radiocarpal articulation
	Tear of triangular fibrocartilage
Arteriography	Concomitant injury to the arteries of the forearm
Radionuclide Imaging (scintigraphy, bone scan)	Subtle fractures of radius and ulna
Computed Tomography	Fracture healing and complications of healing
	Soft tissue injury (muscles, tendons)
Magnetic Resonance Imaging	Soft tissue injury
	Subtle fractures and bone contusion of radius and ulna
	Tear of triangular fibrocartilage

COLLES FRACTURE: VARIANTS IN ALIGNMENT OF FRAGMENTS

volar   dorsal

impaction without displacement

simple dorsal displacement

dorsal displacement and dorsal angulation

radial (lateral) displacement

radial (lateral) displacement and radial angulation

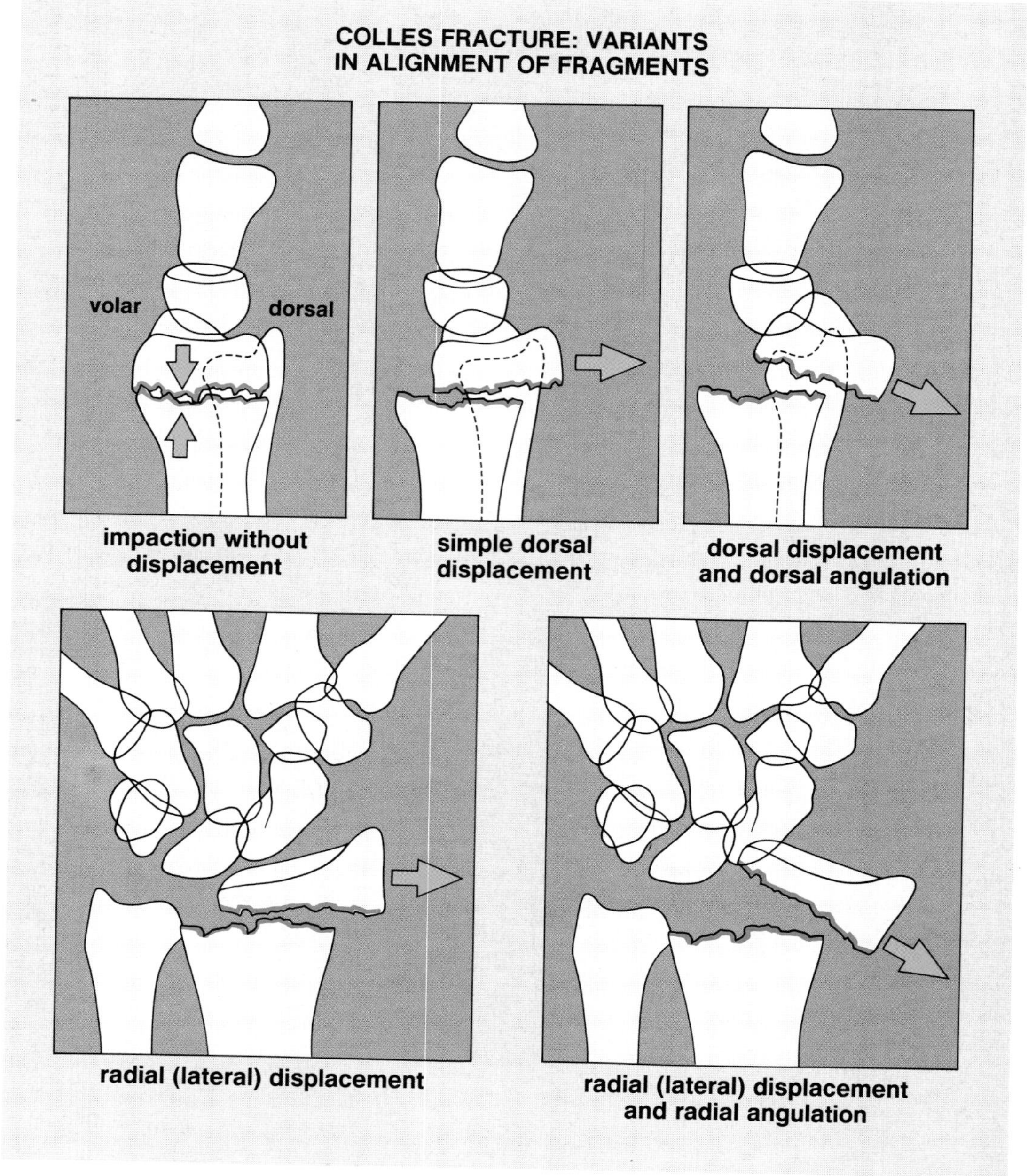

Figure 6.11 Five variants of displacement and angulation of the distal fragment in Colles fracture. Some of these patterns may occur in combinations, yielding complex deformity.

ulnar styloid process. It should be noted that some authors (e.g., Frykman) include intra-articular extension of the fracture line, as well as an associated fracture of the distal end of the ulna, under this eponym (Fig. 6.12).

Films in the posteroanterior and lateral projections are sufficient to demonstrate Colles fracture. The complete evaluation on both views should take note of the status of the radial angle and the palmar inclination, as well as the degree of foreshortening of the radius secondary to impaction or bayonet-type displacement (Fig. 6.13).

COMPLICATIONS At the time of fracture concomitant injury to the median and ulnar nerves may occur. Lack of stability of the fragments during healing may result in loss of reduction, but delayed union and nonunion are very rarely seen. As a sequela, posttraumatic arthritis may develop in the radiocarpal articulation.

Figure 6.12 Frykman Classification of Colles Fractures

RADIUS FRACTURE	DISTAL ULNA FRACTURE	
Location	*Absent*	*Present*
Extra-articular	I	II
Intra-articular (radiocarpal joint)	III	IV
Intra-articular (radioulnar joint)	V	VI
Intra-articular (radiocarpal and radioulnar joints)	VII	VIII

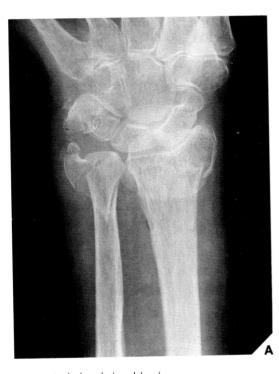
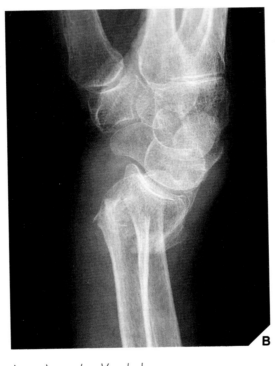

Figure 6.13 Posteroanterior (A) and lateral (B) views of the distal forearm demonstrate the features of Colles fracture. On the posteroanterior projection a decrease in the radial angle and an associated fracture of the distal ulna are evident. The lateral view reveals the dorsal angulation of the distal radius, as well as a reversal of the palmar inclination. On both views the radius is foreshortened secondary to bayonet-type displacement.

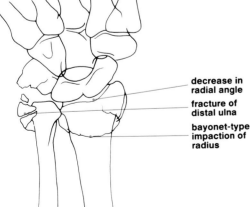

decrease in radial angle

fracture of distal ulna

bayonet-type impaction of radius

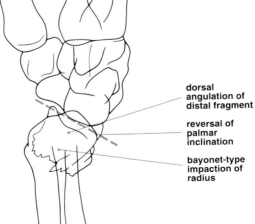

dorsal angulation of distal fragment

reversal of palmar inclination

bayonet-type impaction of radius

BARTON AND HUTCHINSON FRACTURES Both these fractures are intra-articular fractures of the distal radius. The classic *Barton fracture* affects the dorsal margin of the distal radius and extends into the radiocarpal articulation (Fig. 6.14); occasionally, there may also be an associated dislocation in the joint. When the fracture involves the volar margin of the distal radius with intra-articular extension, it is known as a *reverse* (or *volar*) *Barton fracture* (Fig. 6.15). Since in both variants the fracture line is oriented in the coronal plane, it is best demonstrated on the lateral projection.

The *Hutchinson fracture* (also known as chauffeur's fracture—a name derived from the era of hand-cranked automobiles when direct trauma to the radial side of the wrist was often sustained from recoil of the crank) involves the radial (lateral) margin of the distal radius, extending through the radial styloid process into the radiocarpal articulation.

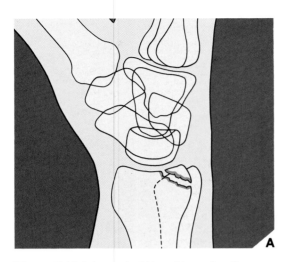

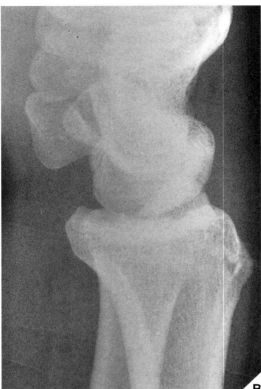

Figure 6.14 Schematic (A) and lateral radiograph (B) show the typical appearance of Barton fracture. The fracture line in the coronal plane extends from the dorsal margin of the distal radius into the radiocarpal articulation.

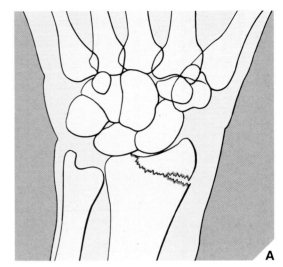

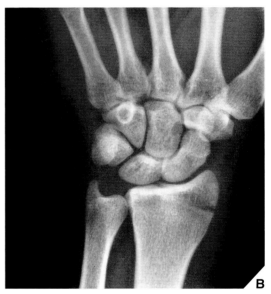

Figure 6.16 Schematic (A) and dosovolar radiograph (B) showing classic appearance of Hutchinson fracture. The fracture line in the sagittal plane extends through the radial margin of the radial styloid process into the radiocarpal articulation.

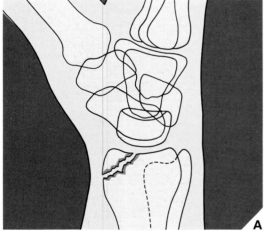

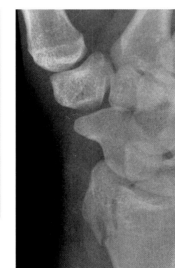

Figure 6.15 Schematic (A) and oblique radiograph (B) show the reverse (or volar) Barton fracture; the fracture line is also oriented in the coronal plane, but extends from the volar margin of the radial styloid process into the radiocarpal joint.

Because of the sagittal orientation of the fracture line, the posteroanterior view is better suited to diagnose this type of injury (Fig. 6.16).

SMITH FRACTURE Usually resulting from a fall on the back of the hand or a direct blow to the dorsum of the hand in palmar flexion, a Smith fracture consists of a fracture of the distal radius, which sometimes extends into the radiocarpal joint, with volar displacement and angulation of the distal fragment (Fig. 6.17). Because the deformity in this fracture is the opposite of that seen in a Colles injury, it is often referred to as a reverse Colles fracture; it is, however, much less common than Colles. There are three types of Smith fracture, defined on the basis of the obliquity of the fracture line (Fig. 6.18), which is best assessed on the lateral projection. Types II and III are usually unstable and may require surgical intervention.

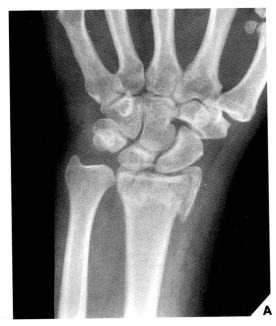
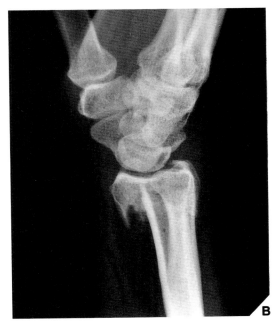

Figure 6.17 Posteroanterior (A) and lateral (B) films of the distal forearm show the typical appearance of Smith fracture. Volar displacement of the distal fragment is clearly evident on the lateral view.

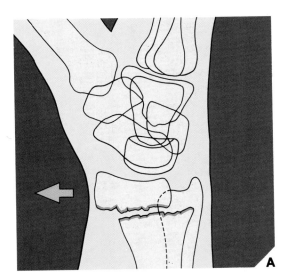
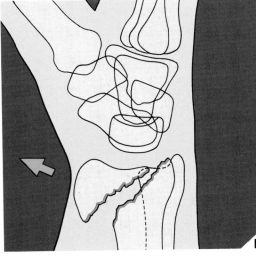
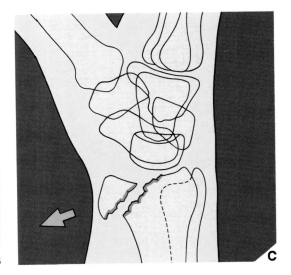

Figure 6.18 The three types of Smith fracture are distinguished by the obliquity of the fracture line. Volar displacement of the distal fragment is characteristic of all three types. (A) In Smith type I, the fracture line is transverse, extending from the dorsal to the volar cortices of the radius. (B) The oblique fracture line in type II extends from the dorsal lip of the distal radius to the volar cortex. (C) Type III, which is almost identical to the reverse Barton fracture (see Figure 6.15), is an intra-articular fracture with extension to the volar cortex of the distal radius.

GALEAZZI FRACTURE–DISLOCATION This abnormality, which may result indirectly, from a fall on the outstretched hand combined with marked pronation of the forearm, or directly, from a blow to the dorsolateral aspect of the wrist, consists of a fracture of the distal third of the radius, sometimes extending into the radiocarpal articulation, and an associated dislocation in the distal radioulnar joint. Characteristically, the proximal end of the distal fragment is dorsally displaced, with dorsal angulation at the fracture site; the ulna is dorsally and ulnarly (medially) dislocated. Posteroanterior and lateral films are routinely obtained when this injury is suspected, but the lateral view clearly reveals its nature and extent (Fig. 6.19).

Injury to the Soft Tissue at the Distal Radioulnar Articulation
One of the most common sequelae of injury to the distal radioulnar articulation is tear of the triangular fibrocartilage complex. Tear may occur as the result of fractures such as those described in the preceding sections, or independently, following injury to the distal forearm and wrist.

Plain films in the standard projections are invariably normal regarding the status of the triangular cartilage, particularly if there is no evidence of fracture or dislocation on which to base suspicion of soft tissue injury. When it is suspected, however, a single-contrast arthrogram of the wrist can confirm or exclude the diagnosis.

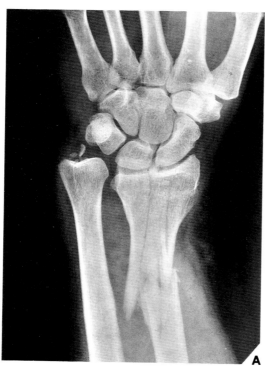
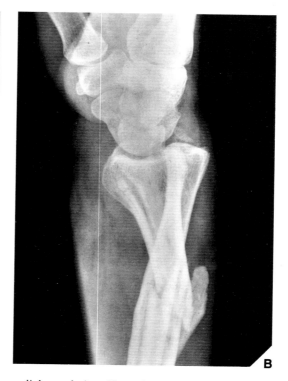

Figure 6.19 Posteroanterior (A) and lateral (B) projections of the distal forearm demonstrate the two components of Galeazzi fracture-dislocation. The posteroanterior view clearly reveals the fracture of the distal radius, which in this case is a comminuted fracture extending into the radiocarpal joint. The distal fragment has a slight radial angulation. Note also the associated comminuted fracture of the ulnar styloid process and the dislocation in the radioulnar joint. These features are also seen on the lateral projection, but this view provides in addition a better demonstration of the dorsal dislocation of the distal ulna.

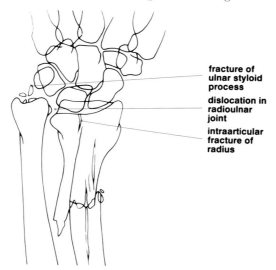
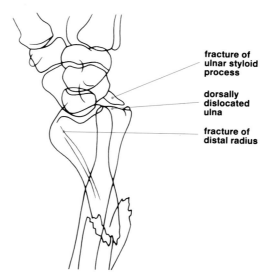

fracture of
ulnar styloid
process

dislocation in
radioulnar
joint

intraarticular
fracture of
radius

fracture of
ulnar styloid
process

dorsally
dislocated
ulna

fracture of
distal radius

Normally, contrast fills the radiocarpal compartment, the prestyloid and volar radial recesses, and the pisotriquetral space (see Fig. 6.7). The presence of contrast in the distal radioulnar compartment or at the site of the triangular cartilage indicates a tear (Fig. 6.20).

WRIST AND HAND

Considered as a functional unit, the wrist and hand are the most common sites of injury in the skeletal system. Fractures of the metacarpals and phalanges, however, by far predominate in incidence over fractures and dislocations in the carpal bones and joints, which constitute approximately 6% of all such injuries. In most instances history and physical examination provide valuable information on which to base a suspected diagnosis, but radiographic findings derived from films obtained in at least two projections at 90° to each other (see Fig. 4.1) are essential to determine a specific diagnosis of injury to these sites.

Anatomic–Radiologic Considerations

Trauma to the wrist and hand usually can be sufficiently evaluated on plain-film studies in the dorsovolar (posteroanterior) and lateral projections (see Figs. 6.1, 6.2). However, determination of the exact extent of damage to the different carpal bones forming the complex structure of the wrist may require supplemental studies specific for the various anatomic sites. These special views include the following:

1. the dorsovolar obtained in ulnar deviation of the wrist for evaluation of the scaphoid bone, which appears foreshortened on the standard dorsovolar projection as a result of its normal volar tilt (Fig. 6.21)

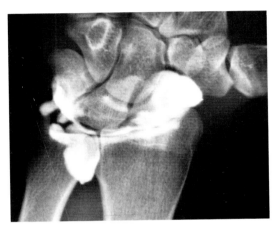

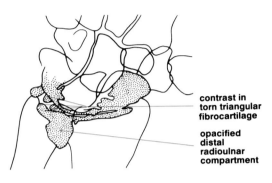

contrast in torn triangular fibrocartilage

opacified distal radioulnar compartment

Figure 6.20 A single-contrast arthrogram of the wrist shows leak of contrast into the space occupied by the triangular cartilage, with characteristic filling of the distal radioulnar compartment, confirming a tear of the triangular fibrocartilage complex (compare with Figure 6.7B).

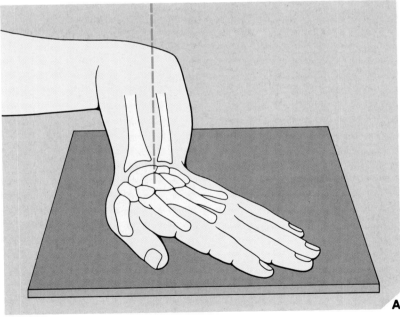

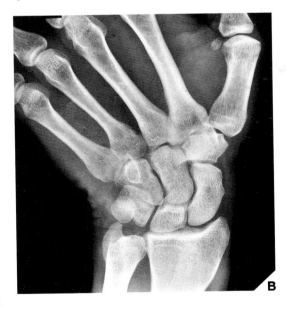

Figure 6.21 (A) For the dorsovolar view of the wrist in ulnar deviation, the forearm rests flat on the radiographic table with the anterior surface down and the elbow flexed 90°. The hand, lying flat on the film cassette, is ulnarly deviated. The central beam is directed toward the carpus. (B) The film in this projection demonstrates the scaphoid, free of the distortion caused by its normal volar tilt when the wrist is in the neutral position.

2. the supinated oblique for visualizing the pisiform bone and the pisotriquetral joint (Fig. 6.22)
3. the pronated oblique for imaging the triquetral bone, the radio-volar aspect of the scaphoid, and the radial styloid process (Fig. 6.23)
4. the carpal-tunnel for demonstrating the hook of the hamate, the pisiform, and the volar aspect of the trapezium (Fig. 6.24).

A full assessment of traumatic conditions and their sequelae may also require ancillary imaging techniques. Among the most commonly performed are conventional tomography, most often in the form of thin-section trispiral cuts, for detecting occult fractures; fluoroscopy combined with videotaping for evaluation of wrist kinematics and joint instability; arthrography and MRI for determining soft tissue injuries such as capsular and tendinous ruptures; and radionuclide bone scan for detecting subtle fractures and early complications of fracture healing. Computed tomography (CT) may also occasionally be performed to evaluate the so-called humpback deformity of the scaphoid or to detect fracture of the hook of the hamate.

Arthrography still remains the best procedure for evaluating the triangular fibrocartilage complex abnormalities and tears of various intercarpal ligaments. In general, single-contrast arthrography using

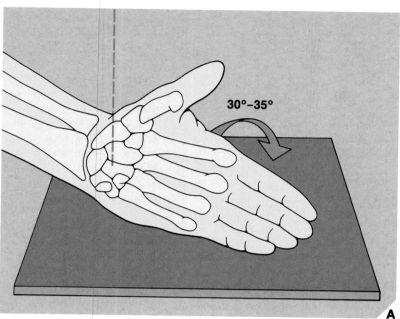

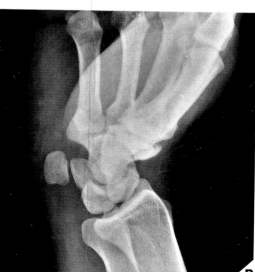

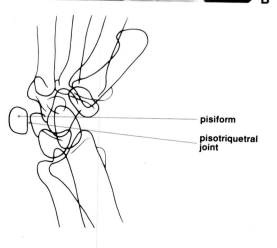

Figure 6.22 (A) For the supinated oblique view of the wrist, the hand, resting on its ulnar side on the film cassette, is tilted about 30° to 35° toward its dorsal surface. The outstretched fingers are held together, with the thumb slightly abducted. The central beam is directed toward the center of the wrist. (B) The film in this projection demonstrates the pisiform bone and the pisotriquetral joint.

pisiform
pisotriquetral joint

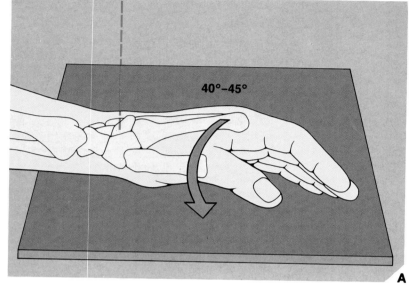

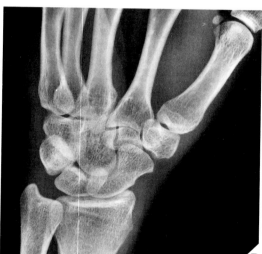

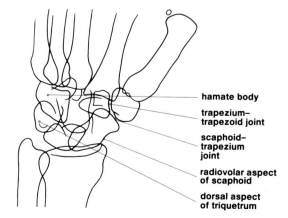

Figure 6.23 (A) For the pronated oblique view of the wrist, the hand, resting on its ulnar side on the film cassette, is tilted about 40° to 45° toward its palmar surface. The slightly flexed fingers are held together, with the thumb in front of them. The central beam is directed toward the center of the carpus. (B) The film in this projection demonstrates the dorsal aspect of the triquetrum, the body of the hamate, the radiovolar aspect of the scaphoid, and the scaphoid-trapezium and trapezium-trapezoid articulations.

hamate body
trapezium–trapezoid joint
scaphoid–trapezium joint
radiovolar aspect of scaphoid
dorsal aspect of triquetrum

positive contrast agents is performed. However, if post-arthrographic CT examination is to be done, double-contrast arthrography using air is preferable. The introduction of the three compartment injection technique and combining the arthrographic wrist examination with digital technique and post-arthrographic CT examination make this modality a procedure of choice in evaluating a painful wrist. A complete arthrographic evaluation of the wrist requires opacification of the mid-carpal compartment, radiocarpal compartment and distal radiounar joint. These three compartments are normally separated from one another by various interosseous ligaments and in the case

of distal radioulnar joint, the triangular fibrocartilage complex (Fig. 6.25). Flow of contrast from one compartment to another indicates a defect in one of these ligaments. Unidirectional contrast flow through the ligament defects, associated with a small flap acting as a valve, has been reported, and may be overlooked if the contrast is injected only on one side of the defect. For this reason, the separate injection of all three compartments is preferable. It has to be stressed, however, that defects in the ligaments may occasionally be found in normal, asymptomatic subjects; therefore, their significance remains uncertain.

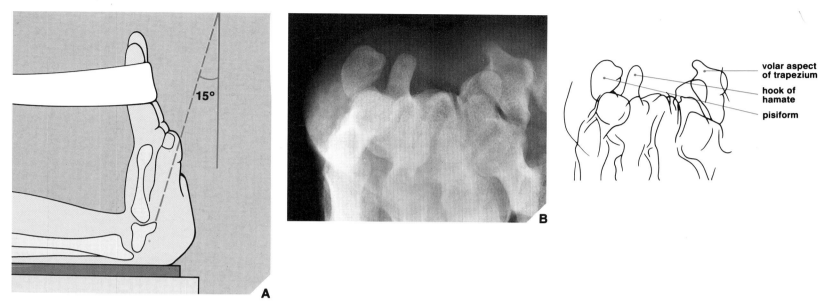

Figure 6.24 (A) For the carpal-tunnel view of the wrist, the hand is maximally dorsiflexed by means of the patient's opposite hand or a strap, with the palmar surface of the wrist resting on the film cassette. The central

beam is directed toward the cup of the palm at about a 15° angle. (B) The film in this projection demonstrates an axial view of the hook of the hamate, as well as the pisiform bone and the volar margin of the trapezium.

Figure 6.25 Carpal joint compartments are separated from one another by various interosseous ligaments.

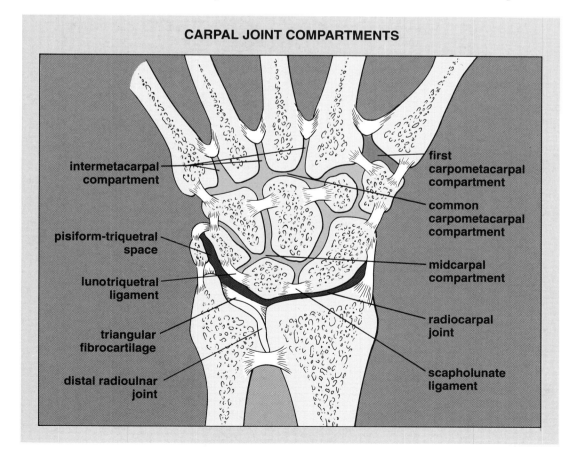

CARPAL JOINT COMPARTMENTS

intermetacarpal compartment

first carpometacarpal compartment

common carpometacarpal compartment

pisiform-triquetral space

midcarpal compartment

lunotriquetral ligament

radiocarpal joint

triangular fibrocartilage

distal radioulnar joint

scapholunate ligament

More recently, digital subtraction arthrography has been advocated by Resnick and Manaster as an effective way to demonstrate subtle leaks of contrast. The advantages of digital subtraction arthrography include not only shortening of examination time but also a decrease in concentration of contrast agent and more precise localization of defects in intercarpal ligaments, particularly when the defects are multiple (see Fig. 2.1).

Magnetic resonance imaging (MRI) has become a very promising imaging modality for evaluation of the wrist and hand (Fig. 6.26). This technique may image not only abnormalities of the soft tissues, including interosseous ligaments and triangular fibrocartilage, but also bony abnormalities such as occult fractures and early osteonecrosis, particularly of the lunate and scaphoid. It is also very useful in imaging the carpal tunnel (Fig. 6.27) and detecting the subtle abnormalities of carpal tunnel syndrome (Fig. 6.28).

Ancillary techniques such as stress films and arthrography may also need to be employed for evaluation of disruption or displacement of the ligaments of the hand, particularly in gamekeeper's thumb.

For a summary in tabular form of the standard and special radiographic projections, as well as the ancillary techniques used to evaluate trauma to the wrist and hand, see Figures 6.29, 6.30, and 6.31.

Injury to the Wrist
Fractures of the Carpal Bones
FRACTURE OF THE SCAPHOID BONE Fractures of the scaphoid (or carpal navicular) are the second most common injuries of the upper limb, exceeded in frequency only by fractures of the distal radius, and they comprise 2% of all fractures. Of all fractures and disloca-

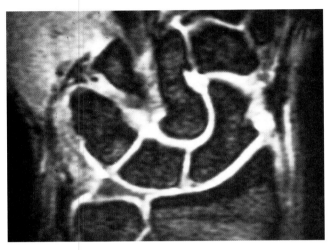

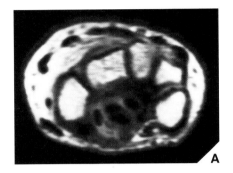

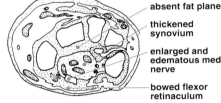

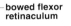

Figure 6.26 Coronal T2-weighted MR image (gradient echo pulse sequence) of the wrist demonstrates distal radius and ulna and carpal bones. The proximal interosseous ligaments and the triangular fibrocartilage are clearly delineated. (From Beltran J, 1990)

- lunotriquetral interosseous ligament
- scapholunate interosseous ligament
- triangular fibrocartilage

- absent fat plane
- thickened synovium
- enlarged and edematous median nerve
- bowed flexor retinaculum

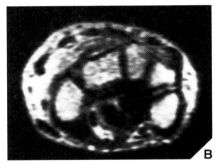

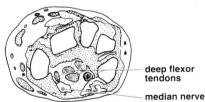

- deep flexor tendons
- median nerve

Figure 6.27 Proton density-weighted spin echo axial MR image (TR 2000/TE 20) through the carpal tunnel demonstrates the various structures. Note the median nerve, displaying intermediate signal intensity and flexor retinaculum imaged with low signal intensity. (From Beltran J, 1990)

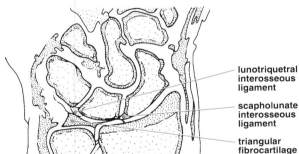

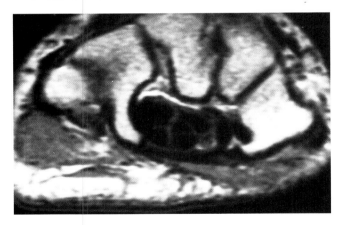

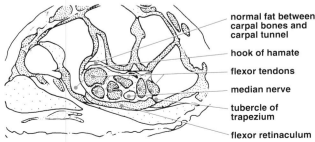

- normal fat between carpal bones and carpal tunnel
- hook of hamate
- flexor tendons
- median nerve
- tubercle of trapezium
- flexor retinaculum

Figure 6.28 A 21-year-old woman with clinically diagnosed carpal tunnel syndrome underwent MRI examination of her right wrist. (A) Proton density- and (B) T2-weighted axial images demonstrate an increased signal of the median nerve and thickened synovium surrounding the flexor tendons in the carpal tunnel. Note the volar bowing of the flexor retinaculum and the absent fat plane between the deep flexor tendons and the more dorsal radiolunatotriquetral ligament. (From Beltran J, 1990)

tions in the carpus, this fracture is the most common, accounting for 50% to 60% of such injuries. They frequently occur in young adults (ages 15 to 30) following falls on the outstretched palm of the hand. Scaphoid fractures can be classified according to direction of the fracture line, the degree of stability of the fragments, and the location of the fracture line. From a diagnostic perspective the latter is a more practical way of classifying fractures of the scaphoid (5% to 10% of which occur in the tuberosity and distal pole, 15% to 20% in the proximal pole, and 70% to 80% in the waist), since it has prognostic value (Fig. 6.32). Fractures of the tuberosity (extra-articular)

and distal pole usually result from a direct trauma and rarely cause any significant clinical problems. Fractures of the waist, if there is no displacement or carpal instability, display a good healing pattern in more than 90% of cases. Fractures involving the proximal pole have a high incidence of nonunion and osteonecrosis.

When fracture of the scaphoid is suspected, plain films are routinely obtained in the dorsovolar, dorsovolar in ulnar deviation, oblique, and lateral projections, and these conventional studies usually suffice to demonstrate the abnormality. When they fail to do so, however, thin-section trispiral tomography has proven very effective (Fig. 6.33).

Figure 6.29 Standard and Special Radiographic Projections for Evaluating Injury to the Wrist and Hand

PROJECTION	DEMONSTRATION	PROJECTION	DEMONSTRATION

Dorsovolar	Carpal bones
	Three carpal arcs
	Eye of the hamate
	Scaphoid fat stripe
	Radiocarpal articulation
	Metacarpals
	Phalanges
	Carpometacarpal, metacarpophalangeal, and interphalangeal joints
	Scapholunate dissociation:
	    Terry-Thomas sign
	    Scaphoid signet-ring sign
	Fractures of:
	    Scaphoid
	    Capitate
	    Lunate
	    Metacarpals
	    Phalanges
	Bennett and Rolando fractures
		Oblique (hand)	Fractures of:
			    Metacarpals
			    Phalanges
			Boxer's fracture

		Supinated Oblique (wrist)	Pisotriquetral joint Pisiform fractures

		Pronated Oblique (wrist)	Dorsal aspect of triquetrum and triquetral fractures
			Body of hamate fractures
			Radiovolar aspect of scaphoid
			Articulations between:
			    Scaphoid and trapezium
			    Trapezium and trapezoid

		Carpal-Tunnel	Volar aspect of trapezium
			Fractures of:
			    Hook of the hamate
			    Pisiform

In ulnar deviation	Scaphoid fractures	*Abduction-Stress* (thumb)	Gamekeeper's thumb

Lateral	Longitudinal axial alignment of third metacarpal, capitate, lunate, and radius
	Fractures of:
	    Triquetrum
	    Metacarpals
	    Phalanges
	Carpal dislocations:
	    Lunate
	    Perilunate
	    Midcarpal
	Dislocations of metacarpals and phalanges		

Figure 6.30 Ancillary Imaging Techniques for Evaluating Injury to the Wrist and Hand

TECHNIQUE	DEMONSTRATION	TECHNIQUE	DEMONSTRATION

Fluoroscopy/Videotaping	Kinematics of wrist and hand
	Carpal instability
	Transient carpal subluxations
		Tomography (usually trispiral)
		Projections:
		    Dorsovolar
		    Lateral
		    Oblique
			Fractures of carpal bones, particularly scaphoid and lunate
			Rolando fracture
			Keinböck disease
			Fracture healing and complications (e.g., nonunion and osteonecrosis)

Radionuclide Imaging (scintigraphy, bone scan)	Subtle chondral and osteochondral fractures Fracture healing and complications (e.g., infection, osteonecrosis)		

Arthrography (single-contrast)	Tear of:
	    Intercarpal ligaments
	    Ulnar collateral ligament (gamekeeper's thumb)
		Lateral
		Carpal-tunnel
			Fractures of hook of the hamate

		Flexion-extension	Stability of scaphoid fracture
Magnetic Resonance Imaging	Carpal tunnel syndrome Injury to the soft tissues Subtle fractures Osteonecrosis	*Computed Tomography*	Subtle fractures, particularly of hook of the hamate Humpback deformity of scaphoid

SPECTRUM OF RADIOLOGIC IMAGING TECHNIQUES FOR EVALUATING INJURY TO THE DISTAL FOREARM, WRIST, AND HAND*

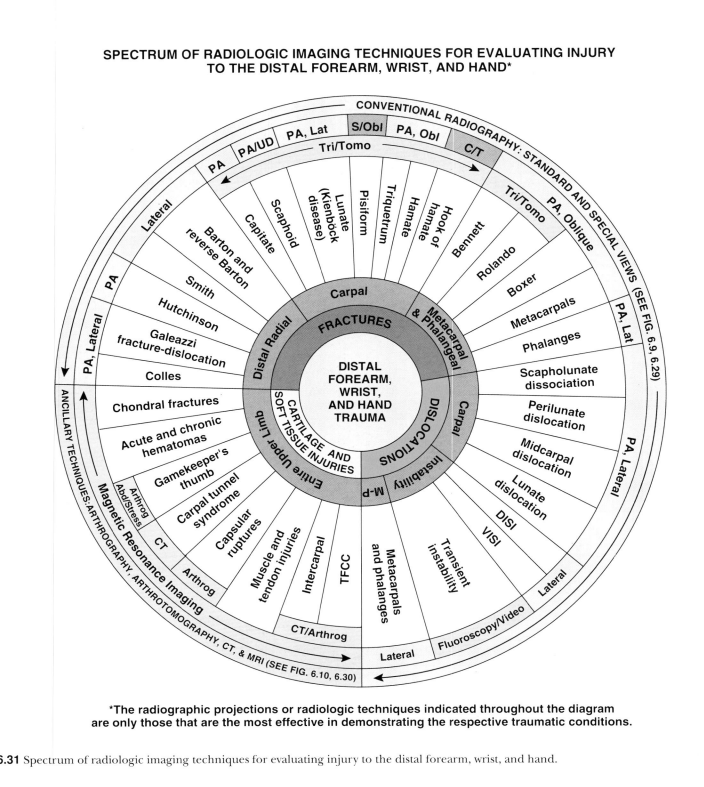

*The radiographic projections or radiologic techniques indicated throughout the diagram are only those that are the most effective in demonstrating the respective traumatic conditions.

Figure 6.31 Spectrum of radiologic imaging techniques for evaluating injury to the distal forearm, wrist, and hand.

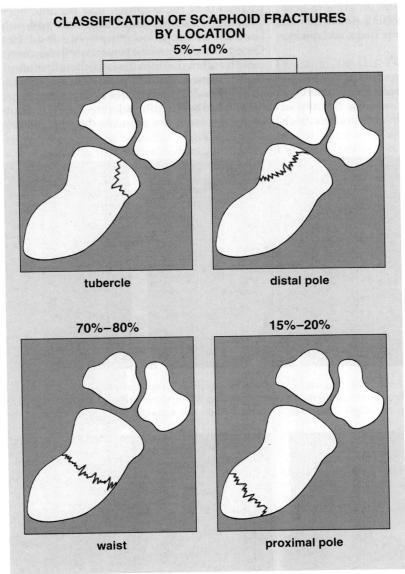

CLASSIFICATION OF SCAPHOID FRACTURES BY LOCATION

5%–10%

tubercle

distal pole

70%–80%

15%–20%

waist

proximal pole

Figure 6.32 Classification of scaphoid fractures by location of the fracture line.

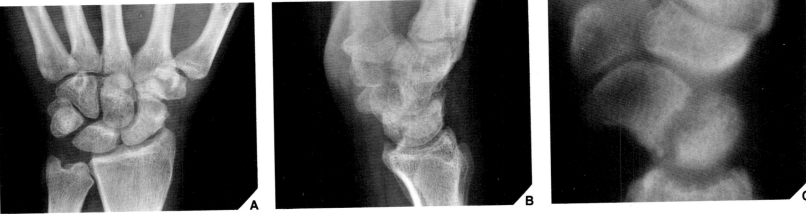

Figure 6.33 A 28-year-old man sustained an injury to his left wrist; pain persisted for three weeks. Dorsovolar (A) and lateral (B) films show periarticular osteoporosis, but no fracture line is evident. On a thin-section trispiral tomogram in the lateral projection (C), a fracture of the scaphoid becomes apparent.

When plain-film findings are normal in cases of suspected injury to the intercarpal ligament complex, fluoroscopy combined with videotaping can sometimes contribute to an evaluation of wrist kinematics and to the diagnosis of carpal instability or transient subluxation (Fig. 6.56). Arthrographic examination of the wrist (see Fig. 6.7) is effective when neither routine radiographic nor video-fluoroscopic findings are conclusive. A wrist arthrogram can reveal abnormal communication between the radiocarpal and midcarpal compartments that indicates a tear in the scapholunate or lunotriquetral interosseous ligament complex (Fig. 6.57).

LUNATE AND PERILUNATE DISLOCATIONS Dorsovolar and lateral plain films of the wrist in the neutral position are usually sufficient to diagnose suspected lunate and perilunate dislocations. As the lateral view clearly demonstrates the normal alignment of the longitudinal axes of the lunate, the capitate, and the third metacarpal over the distal radial surface, a break at any point in this line is pathognomonic of subluxation or dislocation. Lunate dislocation can thus be recognized when its axis is angled away from the distal radial surface, while the capitate remains in its normal alignment (Fig. 6.58A). Similarly, lunate dislocation can also be identified on the dorsovolar projection

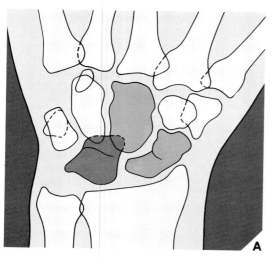
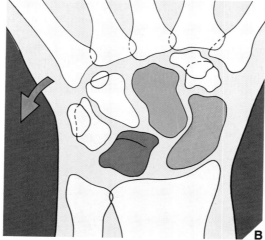

Figure 6.56 Having sustained an injury to the wrist three months previously, a patient presented with pain and an audible click on ulnar deviation of the wrist. Routine films in the dorsovolar, dorsovolar in ulnar deviation, and oblique projections were normal. Fluoroscopy combined with videotaping confirmed suspected lunate-capitate instability. On ulnar deviation transient scapholunate dissociation and lunate-capitate subluxation became apparent. Schematic diagrams based on the video sequence show the relationship of the carpal bones before (A) and after (B) the click. In part (B) note the small gap between the lunate and the capitate due to transient dorsal subluxation of the capitate.

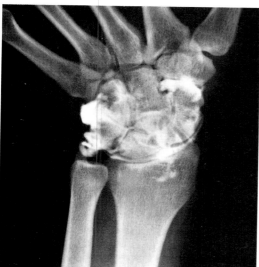

Figure 6.57 A 21-year-old man injured his right wrist during a wrestling competition. Standard views, including ulnar deviation of the wrist, were unremarkable. Likewise, video-fluoroscopic examination did not reveal significant abnormalities. A wrist arthrogram, however, shows leak of contrast into the midcarpal articulations, indicating a tear in the scapholunate interosseous ligament complex. Note also that the triangular fibrocartilage complex is intact.

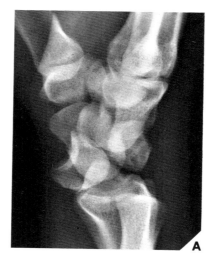
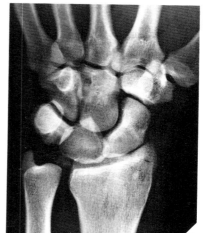

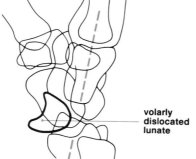

volarly dislocated lunate

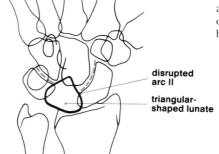

disrupted arc II

triangular-shaped lunate

Figure 6.58 (A) On the lateral view of the wrist, lunate dislocation is evident from the break in the longitudinal alignment of the third metacarpal and the capitate over the distal radial surface at the site of the lunate, which is volarly rotated and displaced. (B) Dorsovolar projection shows a disrupted arc II at the site of the lunate, indicating malalignment. Note also the triangular appearance of the lunate, which is virtually pathognomonic of dislocation of this bone.

by disruption of arc II described by the distal concave surfaces of the scaphoid, the lunate, and the triquetrum, as well as the concomitant triangular appearance of the lunate (Fig. 6.58B).

Perilunate dislocation can be recognized on the lateral view of the wrist by the dorsal or volar angulation of the longitudinal axis of the capitate away from its normal central alignment with the lunate and the distal radial surface. The lunate in this case remains in articulation with the radius, although there may be some degree of tilt of the lunate due to subluxation associated with perilunate dislocation (Fig. 6.59A). On the dorsovolar view, the overlapping of the proximal and distal carpal rows and a break in arcs II and III at the site of the capitate indicate the presence of perilunate dislocation (Fig. 6.59B).

TRANS-SCAPHOID PERILUNATE DISLOCATION When dislocation of the carpal bones is associated with a fracture, the prefix *trans-* indicates which bone is fractured. The most common fracture associated with carpal dislocation is trans-scaphoid perilunate dislocation. As in the preceding types of carpal dislocations, plain films in the standard dorsovolar, dorsovolar in ulnar deviation, and lateral projections usually suffice to lead to a firm diagnosis. The normal relations of the carpal bones seen on these views should help to identify the type of abnormality. Although rarely effective in evaluating carpal dislocations, tomographic examination may be indicated when plain films of the wrist are equivocal as to which carpal bones are dislocated (Fig. 6.60). Other types of associated fractures are less commonly seen (Fig. 6.61).

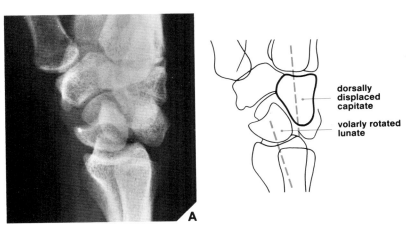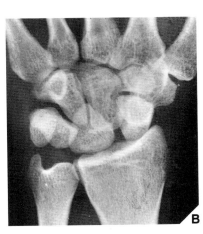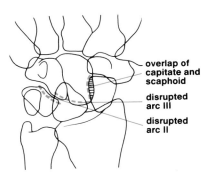

Figure 6.59 (A) Lateral view of the wrist demonstrates perilunate dislocation characterized by displacement of the capitate dorsal to the lunate, which, though slightly volarly rotated, remains in articulation with the distal radius. Note the break in the longitudinal alignment of the third

metacarpal and the capitate with the lunate and the distal radial surface. On the dorsovolar projection (B) perilunate dislocation is evident from the overlapping proximal and distal carpal rows and the resulting disruption of arcs II and III.

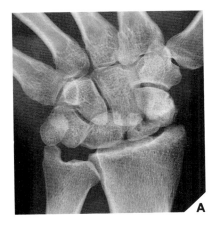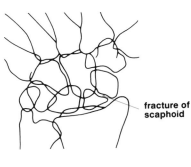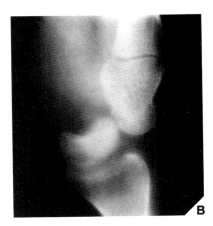

Figure 6.60 (A) Dorsovolar view of the wrist in ulnar deviation clearly shows scaphoid fracture, but the disruptions in the distal carpal arcs are unclear as to the type of dislocation. The lateral view was also inconclusive. (B) Lateral tomogram demonstrates that the capitate is displaced dorsal to the lunate, which remains in articulation with the distal radius—the classic appearance of perilunate dislocation.

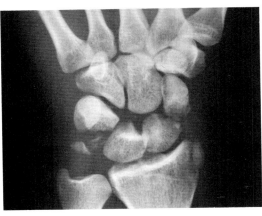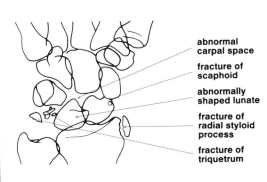

Figure 6.61 Dorsovolar view of the wrist clearly reveals fractures of the radial styloid process, the scaphoid, and the triquetrum. The wide space separating the proximal and distal carpal rows and the triangular shape of the lunate indicate the possibility of lunate dislocation. Note the disruption in arcs I and II. The lateral view confirmed volar displacement of the lunate and the normal position of the capitate. This abnormality can be described as transradial, trans-scaphoid, transtriquetral lunate dislocation.

Carpal Instability

Various carpal instabilities have been described. The most common include dorsal-intercalated-segment instability (DISI) and volar-intercalated-segment instability (VISI).

To explain the carpal instability, Lichtman and colleagues developed the carpal ring theory. The proximal carpal row, which represents intercalated segment, moves as a unit firmly stabilized by interosseous ligaments. Controlled mobility occurs at the scapho-trapezial (radial link) and triquetrohamate (ulnar link) joints (Fig. 6.62). With a break in the ring, either within bony structures or ligaments, the proximal carpal row no longer moves as a unit. The lunate will then tilt either dorsally or volarly in response to this uncontrolled mobility, manifested by either dorsal intercalated segment instability (DISI) or volar intercalated segment instability (VISI) (Fig. 6.63). DISI is the most common deformity. It is recognized on the true lateral view of the wrist by dorsal tilt of the lunate, frequently associated with volar (palmar) tilt of the scaphoid (the capitolunate angle measures more than 30°, and the scapholunate angle more than 60°) (Fig. 6.63C). It may be caused by either bony or ligamentous disruption in the ring on the radial side of the wrist. Most commonly, scaphoid fracture, with or without nonunion, and scapholunate ligamentous dissociation may be the cause of this deformity. VISI is recognized when volar tilt of the lunate is noted on the true lateral view frequently accompanied by dorsal tilt of capitate (the capitolunate angle measures more than 30° and the scapholunate angle less than 30°) (Fig. 6.63D). It is caused by a break in the ring on the ulnar side of the wrist. Most frequently it is ligamentous dissociation and triquetro-hamate joint disruption that leads to this deformity. According to McNiesh, when breaks in the ring occur on both the radial and ulnar side as, for instance, in concurrent scapholunate and lunotriquetral ligamentous dissociation, the VISI pattern predominates.

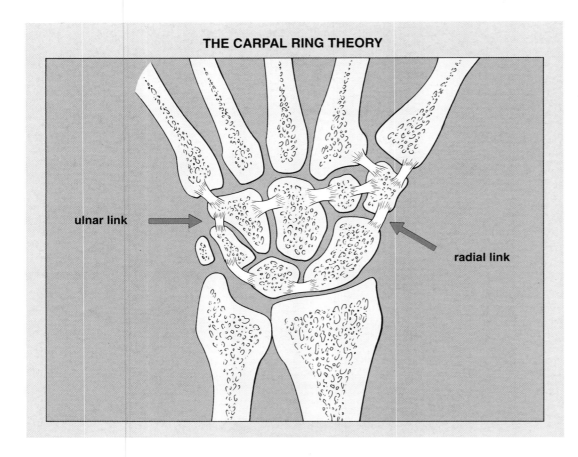

THE CARPAL RING THEORY

ulnar link

radial link

Figure 6.62 The carpal ring theory. The proximal carpal row (intercalated segment) moves as a unit firmly stabilized by interosseous ligaments. *Controlled* mobility occurs at the scaphotrapezial (radial link) and triquetrohamate (ulnar link) joints. Break in the ring, either bony or ligamentous, can produce *uncontrolled* mobility, manifested by either dorsal intercalated segment instability (DISI) or volar intercalated segment instability (VISI). (Modified from Lichtman DM, et al., 1981)

Injury to the Hand
Fractures of the Metacarpal Bones
BENNETT AND ROLANDO FRACTURES Both these fractures are *intra-articular* fractures that occur at the base of the first metacarpal bone. From the perspective of orthopedic management, it is important to dis-tinguish these from the *extra-articular* types, which are transverse or oblique fractures of the first metacarpal just distal to the carpometacarpal joint (Fig. 6.64). Failure to diagnose and properly treat intra-articular metacarpal fractures may result in protracted pain, stiffness, and posttraumatic arthritis due to incongruity of articular surfaces.

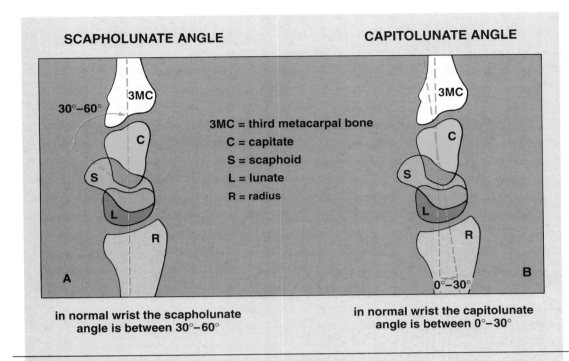

SCAPHOLUNATE ANGLE

CAPITOLUNATE ANGLE

3MC = third metacarpal bone
C = capitate
S = scaphoid
L = lunate
R = radius

in normal wrist the scapholunate angle is between 30°–60°

in normal wrist the capitolunate angle is between 0°–30°

DISI AND VISI DEFORMITIES

DISI
Dorsal Intercalated Segment Instability
(Dorsiflexion Carpal Instability)

VISI
Volar Intercalated Segment Instability
(Volarflexion Carpal Instability)

1. dorsal tilt of lunate
2. volar tilt of scaphoid

1. volar tilt of lunate
2. dorsal tilt of capitate

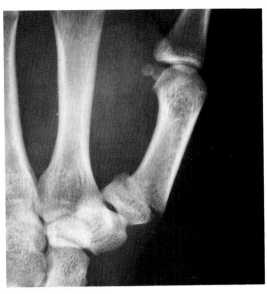

Figure 6.64 An extra-articular fracture at the base of the first metacarpal should not be confused with Bennett and Rolando fractures, which are intra-articular.

Figure 6.63 Dorsal intercalated segment instability (DISI) and volar intercalated segment instability (VISI). (A) Normal scapholunate angle. The scapholunate angle is formed by the intersection of longitudinal axes of scaphoid and lunate and normally measures from 30° to 60°. (B) Normal capitolunate angle. The capitolunate angle is formed by the intersection of the capitate axis (drawn from the midpoint of its head to the center of its distal articular surface) and the lunate axis (drawn through the center of its proximal and distal poles) and normally measures from 0° to 30°. (C) In dorsal intercalated segment instability (DISI), the scapholunate angle measures more than 60° and the capitolunate angle more than 30°. (D) In volar intercalated segment instability (VISI), the scapholunate angle measures less-than 30°, and the capitolunate angle much more than 30° (Modified from Gilula LA, Weeks PM, 1978)

The *Bennett fracture* is a fracture of the proximal end of the first metacarpal that extends into the first carpometacarpal joint. Usually, a small fragment on the volar aspect of the base of the first metacarpal remains in articulation with the trapezium bone, while the rest of the first metacarpal is dorsally and radially dislocated as the result of pull of the abductor pollicis longus (Fig. 6.65). For this reason the injury should properly be called a fracture-dislocation. Diagnosis and evalua-

tion of the Bennett fracture are readily made on plain films of the hand in the dorsovolar, oblique, and lateral projections.

The *Rolando fracture* is a comminuted Bennett fracture; the fracture line may have a Y, V, or T configuration. As there may be multiple fragments, the routine radiographic projections used to diagnose the Bennett fracture usually need to be supplemented by trispiral tomographic examination to localize comminuted fragments and to

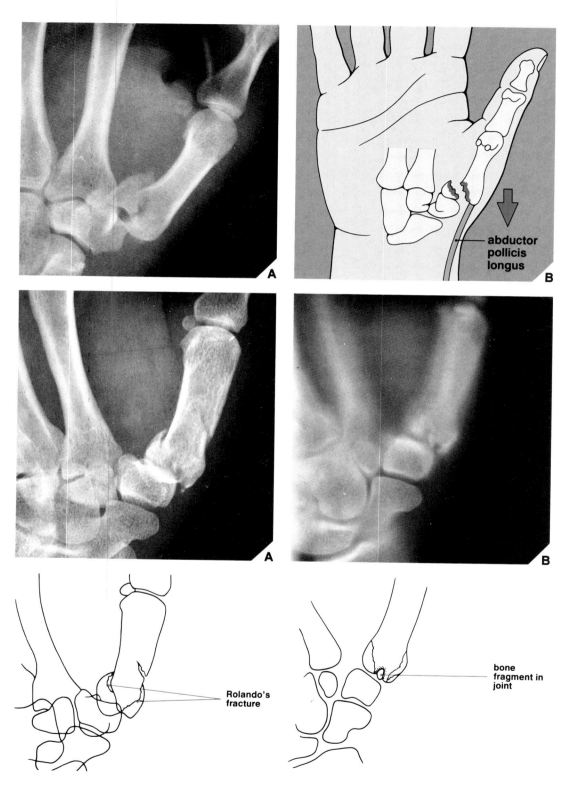

Figure 6.65 A 27-year-old man who was involved in a fist fight presented with pain localized in the right thenar. Dorsovolar plain film of the hand (A) shows the typical appearance of Bennett fracture. A small fragment at the base of the first metacarpal remains in articulation with the trapezium, while the rest of the bone is dorsally and radially dislocated. The accompanying schematic diagram (B) shows the patho-mechanics of this injury.

Figure 6.66 (A) Oblique view of the right hand shows a comminuted intra-articular fracture of the proximal end of the first metacarpal—Rolando fracture. To localize the fragments, trispiral tomographic examination (B) was performed, revealing a small bone chip entrapped in the trapeziometacarpal joint.

exclude the possibility of entrapment of a small bony fragment in the first carpometacarpal joint (Fig. 6.66).

BOXER'S FRACTURE   Boxer's fracture is a fracture of the metacarpal neck with volar angulation of the distal fragment. It may occur in any of the metacarpal bones, but is most commonly seen in the fifth metacarpal. The fracture and deformity are sufficiently demonstrated on plain films of the hand in the dorsovolar and oblique projections (Fig. 6.67A). As comminution frequently accompanies this type of fracture, it is important to determine its extent. Comminution may predispose the fracture after reduction to settle into an angular deformation. The oblique projection usually suffices to determine the extent of comminution (Fig. 6.67B), although tomography may occasionally be required.

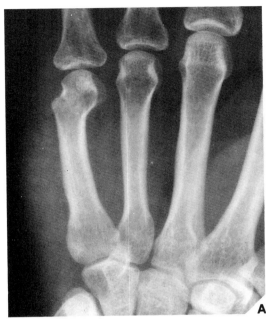
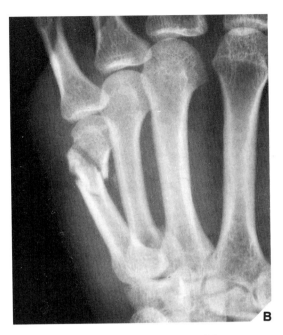

Figure 6.67 (A) Dorsovolar view of the right hand demonstrates a fracture of the fifth metacarpal with volar angulation of the distal fragment—a simple boxer's fracture. When comminution is present, it is essential for its prognostic value to demonstrate the extent of fracture lines, as such fractures are frequently unstable. The oblique projection (B) usually suffices to determine the extent of comminution.

Injury to the Soft Tissue of the Hand

GAMEKEEPER'S THUMB Gamekeeper's thumb results from disruption of the ulnar collateral ligament of the first metacarpophalangeal joint, often accompanied by fracture of the base of the proximal phalanx. Standard dorsovolar and oblique films of the thumb usually suffice to demonstrate the associated fracture (Fig. 6.68A,B), but full evaluation requires an abduction-stress film of the thumb when this condition is suspected. An increase to more than 30° in the angle between the first metacarpal and the proximal phalanx is a characteristic finding in gamekeeper's thumb, indicating subluxation (Fig. 6.68C,D). Arthrographic examination of the thumb may also be performed to assess disruption, displacement, or entrapment of the ulnar collateral ligament (Fig. 6.69).

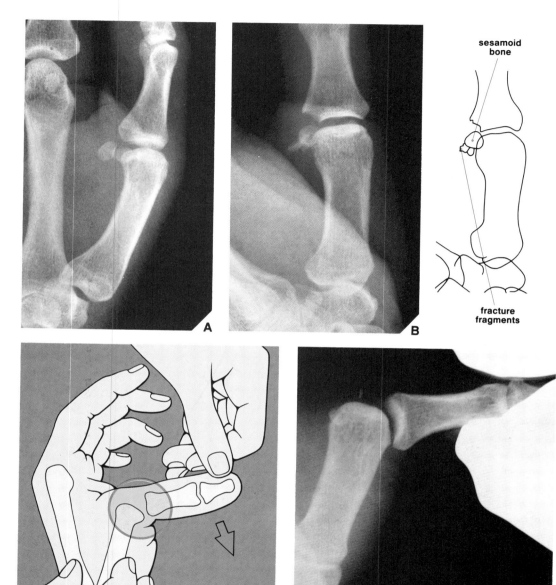

Figure 6.68 Having fallen on his hand on the ski slopes, a 38-year-old man presented with pain at the base of his right thumb. Physical examination revealed instability in the first metacarpophalangeal joint. Oblique (A) and dorsovolar (B) films of the right thumb show a fracture of the base of the proximal phalanx and local soft tissue swelling—findings associated with gamekeeper's thumb. In another patient dorsovolar and lateral films of the first phalanx did not show evidence of fracture; but as instability of the first metacarpophalangeal joint was indicated on physical examination, an abduction-stress film of the thumb was obtained (C). The film (D) demonstrates subluxation of the joint by the increase to more than 30° in the angle between the first metacarpal and the proximal phalanx of the thumb, confirming gamekeeper's thumb.

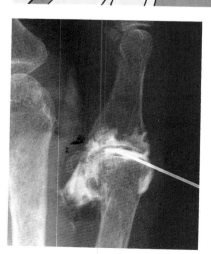

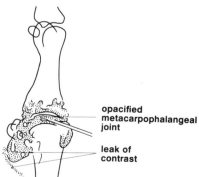

Figure 6.69 An arthrogram of the thumb demonstrates the characteristic findings in gamekeeper's thumb. The leak of contrast along the ulnar side of the head of the first metacarpal indicates a tear of the ulnar collateral ligament. (Courtesy of Dr. D. Resnick, San Diego, California)

PRACTICAL POINTS TO REMEMBER

Distal Forearm

[1] For a full evaluation of trauma on the posteroanterior view of the distal forearm, it is important to recognize:
- ulnar variance—neutral, negative, and positive
- the radial angle, which normally ranges from 15° to 25°.

[2] For a full evaluation of trauma on the lateral view of the distal forearm, it is important to recognize the volar tilt of the articular surface of the radius, which normally ranges from 10° to 25°.

[3] A complete evaluation of the Colles fracture should take into consideration:
- the degree of foreshortening of the radius
- the direction of displacement of the distal fragment
- intra-articular extension of the fracture line
- associated fracture of the ulna.

[4] Learn to distinguish the Colles fracture from the:
- Barton fracture, dorsal and volar types, which are best demonstrated on the lateral projection
- Hutchinson (or chauffeur's) fracture, which is best seen on the posteroanterior view
- Smith fracture, which is best evaluated on the lateral projection.

[5] With the finding of dislocation in the distal radioulnar articulation, look for an associated radial fracture—Galeazzi fracture–dislocation.

[6] A common sequela of trauma to the distal radioulnar joint, tear of the triangular fibrocartilage complex can be confirmed or excluded by single-contrast arthrogram of the wrist or MRI examination.

Wrist

[1] If clinical history and physical examination are consistent with scaphoid fracture and routine radiographs appear normal, trispiral tomography is the next logical step.

[2] Delayed diagnosis and treatment of scaphoid fracture may result in nonunion, osteonecrosis, and post-traumatic arthritis.

[3] Triquetral fracture is best diagnosed on the lateral and pronated oblique views of the wrist. If plain films appear normal, tomography in the lateral projection can confirm or exclude the diagnosis.

[4] Fractures of the hamate body are best demonstrated on the lateral and pronated oblique projections.

[5] In suspected fracture of the hook of the hamate, look for the oval cortical ring shadow projecting over the hamate on the dorsovolar view of the wrist. If this "eye" of the hamate is absent, indistinctly outlined, or sclerotic, hamulus fracture is highly probable. Trispiral tomography in the lateral and carpal-tunnel projections is a useful technique in evaluating the hamulus.

[6] Fracture of the pisiform is best demonstrated on the supinated oblique and carpal-tunnel projections.

[7] In Kienböck disease the choice of surgical procedures depends on a demonstration of the integrity of the lunate. Tomography, preferably trispiral, in two planes is usually indicated. MRI may demonstrate osteonecrosis in the early stages.

[8] Lunate and perilunate dislocations are readily identified on the lateral view by disruption of the normal central alignment of the longitudinal axes of the capitate and lunate over the distal radial surface:
- in lunate dislocation disruption of the alignment occurs at the lunate
- in perilunate dislocation it occurs at the capitate
- in midcarpal dislocation it occurs at the site of both bones.

[9] In any type of carpal dislocation, look for an associated fracture.

[10] If intercarpal instability is suspected and routine radiographs are normal, fluoroscopy combined with videotaping should be the next examination. If ligament tear is suspected, arthrography should be performed.

Hand

[1] Learn to distinguish the Bennett and Rolando fractures—intra-articular fractures occurring at the base of the first metacarpal bone—from extra-articular fractures.

[2] The Bennett fracture involves a dislocation of most of the first metacarpal and is, therefore, a fracture-dislocation.

[3] When evaluating the Rolando fracture—really a comminuted Bennett fracture—exclude the possibility of entrapment of a fragment in the first carpometacarpal joint. Tomography is an essential technique in evaluating comminution.

[4] In the boxer's fracture, comminution of the volar cortex is often present. It is essential to demonstrate its presence radiographically.

[5] In suspected gamekeeper's thumb, obtain an abduction-stress film of the thumb.

[6] Disruption, displacement, or entrapment of the ulnar collateral ligament in gamekeeper's thumb can be evaluated on an arthrogram of the first metacarpophalangeal joint.

References

Adkinson JW, Chapman MW: Treatment of acute lunate and perilunate dislocations. *Clin Orthop* 164:199, 1982.

Arkless R: Cineradiography in normal and abnormal wrist. *Am J Roentgenol* 96:837, 1966.

Armistead RB, Linscheid RL, Dobyns JH, Beckenbaugh RD: Ulnar lengthening in the treatment of Kienböck's disease. *J Bone Joint Surg* 64A:170, 1982.

Aufranc OE, Jones WN, Turner RH: Anterior marginal articular fracture of distal radius. *JAMA* 196:106, 1966.

Bado JL: The Monteggia lesion. *Clin Orthop* 50:71, 1967.

Beckenbaugh RD, Shives TC, Dobyns JH, Linscheid RL: Kienböck's disease: The natural history of Kienböck's disease and consideration of lunate fractures. *Clin Orthop* 149:98, 1980.

Beltran J: *MRI: Musculoskeletal System.* Philadelphia, Lippincott, 1990.

Bennett EH: On fracture of the metacarpal bone of the thumb. *Br Med J* 11:12, 1886.

Berger RA, Blair WF, El-Khoury GY: Arthrotomography of the wrist: The triangular fibrocartilage complex. *Clin Orthop* 172:257, 1983.

Bishop AT, Beckenbaugh RD: Fracture of the hamate hook. *J Hand Surg* 13A:135, 1988.

Blair WF, Berger RA, El-Khoury GY: Arthrotomography of the wrist: An experimental and preliminary clinical study. *J Hand Surg* 10A:350, 1985.

Brown P, Dameron T: Surgical treatment for nonunion of the scaphoid. *South Med J* 68:415, 1975.

Bryan RS, Dobyns JH: Fractures of the carpal bones other than lunate and navicular. *Clin Orthop* 149:107, 1980.

Campbells CS: Gamekeeper's thumb. *J Bone Joint Surg* 37B:148, 1955.

Crittenden JJ, Jones DM, Santarelli AG: Bilateral rotational dislocation of the carpal navicular. *Radiology* 94:629, 1970.

Curtis DJ, Downey EF Jr: A simple first metacarpophalangeal stress test. *Radiology* 148:855, 1983.

Dalinka MK, Osterman AL, Kricun ME: Trauma to the carpus. *Contemporary Diagnostic Radiology* 5:1, 1982.

De Palma AF, Gartland JJ, Dowling JJ: Colles' fracture. *Pa Med* 69:72, 1966.

Dobyns JH, Linscheid RL: Fractures and dislocations of the wrist. In: Rockwood CA Jr, Green DP (eds): *Fractures.* Philadelphia, Lippincott, 1975.

Downey EF Jr, Curtis DJ: Patient-induced stress test of the first metacarpophalangeal joint: A radiographic assessment of collateral ligament injuries. *Radiology* 158:679, 1986.

Egawa M, Asai T: Fracture of the hook of the hamate: Report of six cases and the suitability of computerized tomography. *J Hand Surg* 8:393, 1983.

Ellis K: Smith's and Barton's fractures. *J Bone Joint Surg* 47B:724, 1965.

Epner RA, Bowers WH, Guilford WB: Ulnar variance—the effect of wrist positioning and roentgen filming technique. *J Hand Surg* 7:298, 1982.

Fisher MR, Rogers LF, Hendrix RW: A systematic approach to the diagnosis of carpometacarpal dislocations. *RadioGraphics* 2:612, 1982.

Gelberman RH, Salamon PB, Jurist JM, Posch JL: Ulnar variance in Kienböck's disease. *J Bone Joint Surg* 57A:674, 1975.

Gilula LA: Carpal injuries: Analytic approach and case exercises. *Am J Roentgenol* 133:503, 1979.

Gilula LA: Roentgenographic evaluation of the hand and wrist, In: Weeks PM (ed): *Acute Bone and Joint Injuries of the Hand and Wrist.* . St. Louis, Mosby, 1981, p 3.

Gilula LA, Weeks PM: Post-traumatic ligamentous instabilities of the wrist *Radiology* 129:641, 1978.

Gold RH: Arthrography of the wrist. In: Arndt R-D, Horns JW, Gold RH (eds): *Clinical Arthrography.* Baltimore, Williams & Wilkins, 1981.

Goldman AB: The wrist. In: Freiberger RH, Kaye JJ (eds): *Arthrography.* New York, Appleton-Century-Crofts, 1979, p 277.

Green DP, O'Brien ET: Classification and management of carpal dislocations. *Clin Orthop Rel Res* 149:55,1980.

Green SM, Greenspan A: An expanded imaging approach for diagnosing tears of the triangular fibrocartilage complex. *Bull Hospital Joint Dis Orthop Inst* 48:187, 1988.

Greenspan A, Posner MA, Tucker M: The value of carpal tunnel trispiral tomography in the diagnosis of fracture of the hook of the hamate. *Bull Hosp Jt Dis Orthop Inst* 45:74, 1985.

Howard FM: Fractures of the basal joint of the thumb. *Clin Orthop* 220:46, 1987.

Johnson RP: The acutely injured wrist and its residuals. *Clin Orthop* 149:33, 1980.

Kleinert JM, Zenni EJ Jr: Nonunion of the scaphoid. Review of literature and current treatment. *Orthop Rev* 13:125, 1984.

Levinsohn EM, Palmer AK: Arthrography of the traumatized wrist. *Radiology* 146:647, 1983.

Levinsohn EM, Palmer AK: Arthrography of the traumatized wrist. Correlation with radiography and the carpal instability series. *Radiology* 146:647, 1983.

Levinsohn EM, Palmer AK, Coren AB, Zinberg E: Wrist arthrography: The value of the three compartment injection technique. *Skeletal Radiol* 16:539, 1987.

Lichtman DM, Alexander AH, Mack GR, Gunther SF: Kienböck's disease: Update on silicone replacement arthroplasty. *J Hand Surg* 7:343, 1982.

Lichtman DM, Schneider JR, Swafford AR, et al: Ulnar midcarpal instability—clinical and laboratory analysis. *J Hand Surg* 6:515, 1981.

Linscheid RL: Arthrography of the metacarpophalangeal joint. *Clin Orthop* 103:91, 1974.

Linscheid RL, Dobyns JH, Beabout JW, Bryan RS: Traumatic instability of the wrist: Diagnosis, classification, and pathomechanics. *J Bone Joint Surg* 54A:1612, 1972.

Linscheid RL, Dobyns JH, Younge DK: Trispiral tomography in the evaluation of wrist injury. *Bull Hosp Jt Dis Orthop Inst* 44:297, 1984.

Manaster BJ: Digital wrist arthrography: Precision in determining the site of radiocarpal-midcarpal communication. *Am J Roentgenol* 147:563, 1986.

Mayfield JK: Mechanism of carpal injuries. *Clin Orthop* 149:45, 1980.

Mayfield JK, Johnson RP, Kilcoyne RK: Carpal dislocations: Patho-mechanics and progressive perilunar instability. *J Hand Surg* 5:226, 1980.

McNiesh LM: Unique musculoskeletal trauma. *Rad Clin North Am* 25:1107, 1987.

Middleton WD, Kneeland JB, Kellman GM, Cates JD, Sanger JR, Jesmanowicz A, Froncisz W, Hyde JS: MR Imaging of the carpal tunnel: Normal anatomy and preliminary findings in the carpal tunnel syndrome. *Am J Roentgenol* 148:307, 1987.

Mazet R Jr, Hohl M: Fractures of the carpal navicular. *J Bone Joint Surg* 45A:82, 1963.

McDonald G, Petrie D: Ununited fracture of the scaphoid. *Clin Orthop* 108:110, 1975.

Mino DE, Palmer AK, Levinsohn EM: The role of radiography and computerized tomography in the diagnosis of subluxation and dislocation of the distal radioulnar joint. *J Hand Surg* 8:23, 1983.

Murray WT, Meuller PR, Rosenthal DI, Javernek RR: Fracture of the hook of the hamate. *Am J Roentgenol* 133:899, 1979.

Norman A, Nelson JM, Green SM: Fractures of the hook of the hamate: Radiographic signs. *Radiology* 154:49, 1985.

Palmer AK, Glisson RR, Werner FW: Ulnar variance determination. *J Hand Surg* 7:376, 1982.

Palmer AK, Levinsohn M, Kuzma GR: Arthrography of the wrist. *J Hand Surg* 8:15, 1983.

Peltier LF: Eponymic fractures: John Rhea Barton and Barton's fractures. *Surgery* 34:960, 1953.

Posner MA: Injuries to the hand and wrist in athletes. *Orthop Clin North Am* 8:593, 1977.

Posner MA, Greenspan A: Trispiral tomography for the evaluation of wrist problems. *J Hand Surg* 13A:175, 1988.

Protas JM, Jackson WR: Evaluating carpal instabilities with fluoroscopy. *Am J Roentgenol* 135:137, 1980.

Quinn SF, Belsole RS, Greene TL, Rayhack JM: Work in progress: Postarthrography computed tomography of the wrist: Evaluation of the triangular fibrocartilage complex. *Skeletal Radiology* 17:565, 1989.

Resnick D: Arthrography and tenography of the hand and wrist. In: Dalinka MK (ed): *Arthrography.* New York, Springer-Verlag, 1980.

Resnick D, Danzig LA: Arthrographic evaluation of injuries of the first metacarpophalangeal joint: Gamekeeper's thumb. *Am J Roentgenol* 126:1046, 1976.

Ruby LK, Cooney WP III, An KN, Linscheid RL, Chao EYS: Relative motion of selected carpal bones: A kinematic analysis of the normal wrist. *J Hand Surg* 13A:1, 1988.

Russell TB: Inter-carpal dislocations and fracture-dislocations. A review of fifty-nine cases. *J Bone Joint Surg* 31B:524, 1949.

Sanders WE: Evaluation of the humpback scaphoid by computed tomography in the longitudinal axial plane of the scaphoid. *J Hand Surg*

13A:182, 1988.

Sarmiento A, Pratt GW, Berry NC, Sinclair WF: Colles' fracture. *J Bone Joint Surg* 57A:311, 1975.

Schwartz AM, Ruby LK: Wrist arthrography revisited. *Orthopaedics* 5:883, 1982.

Sherman SB, Greenspan A, Norman A: Osteonecrosis of the distal pole of the carpal scaphoid following fracture—a rare complication. *Skeletal Radiol* 9:189, 1983.

Stark HH, Jobe FW, Boyes JH, Ashworth CR: Fracture of the hook of the hamate in athletes. *J Bone Joint Surg* 59A:575, 1977.

Taleisnick J: Classifications of carpal instability. *Bull Hosp Jt Dis Orthop Inst* 44:511, 1984.

Taleisnik J: Post-traumatic carpal instability. *Clin Orthop* 149:73, 1980.

Tehranzadeh J, Davenport J, Pais MJ: Scaphoid fracture: Evaluation with flexion-extension tomography. *Radiology* 176:167, 1990.

Yeager B, Dalinka M: Radiology of trauma to the wrist: Dislocations, fracture dislocations and instability patterns. *Skeletal Radiol* 13:120, 1985.

White SJ, Louis DS, Braunstein EM, Hankin FM, Greene TL: Capitate–lunate instability: Recognition by manipulation under fluoroscopy. *Am J Roentgenol* 143:361, 1984.

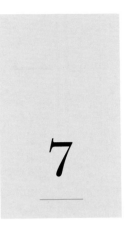

Lower Limb I: Pelvic Girdle and Proximal Femur

FRACTURES INVOLVING THE STRUCTURES of the pelvic girdle, which are usually sustained in motor vehicle accidents or falls from heights, represent only a small percentage of all skeletal injuries. Their importance, however, lies in the significant morbidity and mortality associated with them, which is usually due to accompanying injury to the major blood vessels, nerves, and lower urinary tract. Since the clinical signs of pelvic trauma may not always be obvious, radiographic examination is essential to establish a correct diagnosis. Fractures of the acetabulum constitute approximately 20% of all pelvic fractures, and they may or may not be associated with dislocation in the hip joint. Fractures of the proximal (upper) femur, occasionally referred to as hip fractures, occur frequently in the elderly, often as a result of minimal injury. They are seen more frequently in women than in men (2:1), intracapsular fractures of the proximal femur having an even higher female-to-male ratio (5:1).

Anatomic–Radiologic Considerations

The main radiologic modalities used in evaluation of traumatic conditions of the pelvic girdle, acetabulum, and proximal femur include plain-film radiography and conventional as well as computed tomography (CT). Other ancillary techniques are also essential for a complete evaluation of concomitant soft tissue and pelvic-organ injuries: angiography for the pelvic blood vessels and cystourethrography for the lower urinary tract. Radionuclide bone scan and magnetic resonance imaging (MRI) may also be necessary to disclose subtle fractures of the femoral neck and early stages of posttraumatic osteonecrosis of the femoral head.

The standard and special radiographic projections used to evaluate injury to the pelvic girdle and proximal femur include the anteroposterior view of the pelvis, the anterior and posterior oblique views of the pelvis, the anteroposterior view of the hip, and the frog-lateral view of the hip. At times the groin-lateral or other special projections may also be required.

Most traumatic conditions involving the sacral wings, the iliac bones, the ischium, the pubis, and the femoral head and neck can sufficiently be evaluated on the *anteroposterior* projection of the pelvis and hip (Fig. 7.1). This view also demonstrates an important anatomic relation of the longitudinal axes of the femoral neck and shaft. Normally, the angle formed by these axes ranges from 125° to 135°. This measurement is valuable in determining displacement in femoral neck fractures. A varus configuration is characterized by a

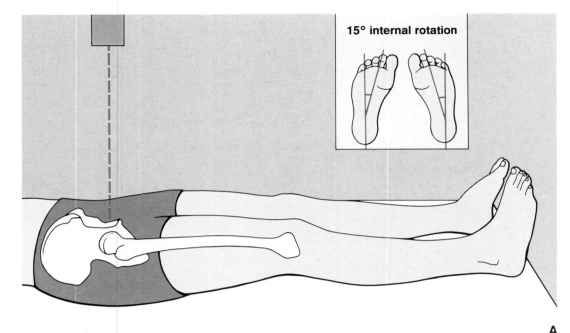

15° internal rotation

Figure 7.1 (A) For the anteroposterior view of the pelvis and hip, the patient is supine with the feet in slight (15°) internal rotation *(inset)*, which compensates for the normal anteversion of the femoral neck (see Fig. 7.7B), elongating its image. For a view of the entire pelvis, the central beam is directed vertically toward the midportion of the pelvis; for selective examination of either hip joint, it is directed toward the affected femoral head. (B) The radiograph in this projection demonstrates the iliac bones, the sacrum, the pubis, and the ischium, as well as the femoral heads and necks and both the greater and the lesser trochanters. The acetabula are partially obscured by the overlying femoral heads, and the sacroiliac joints are seen en face.

A

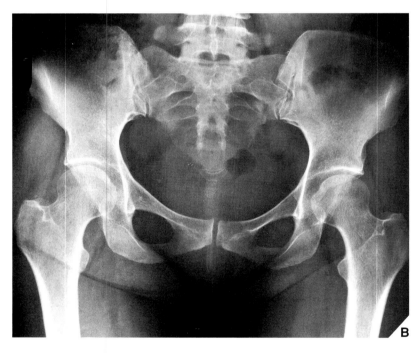

B

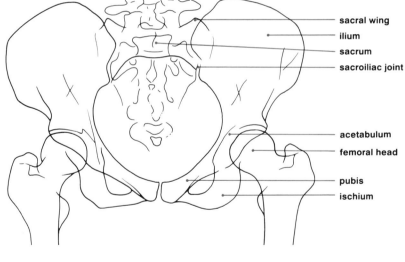

sacral wing
ilium
sacrum
sacroiliac joint

acetabulum
femoral head

pubis
ischium

decrease in this angle, and a valgus configuration by an increase in this angle (Fig. 7.2). The anteroposterior view, however, is frequently not sufficient to provide adequate evaluation of the entire sacral bone, the sacroiliac joints, and the acetabulum. Demonstration of the sacroiliac joints requires either a posteroanterior projection, which is obtained to greater advantage with 25° to 30° caudal angulation of the radiographic tube, or an anteroposterior view with 30° to 35° cephalad angulation. The latter projection, known as the *Ferguson* view, is also helpful in more effectively evaluating injury to the sacral bone and the pubic and ischial rami (Fig. 7.3). Oblique

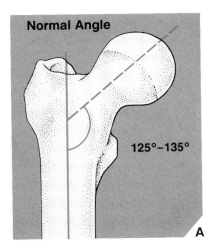
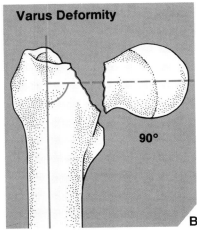
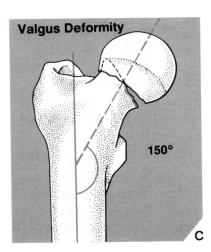

Figure 7.2 (A) The angle formed by the longitudinal axes of the femoral neck and shaft normally ranges from 125° to 135°. In the evaluation of displacement in femoral neck fractures, a decrease in this angle (B) is known as a varus deformity, while an increase (C) characterizes a valgus deformity.

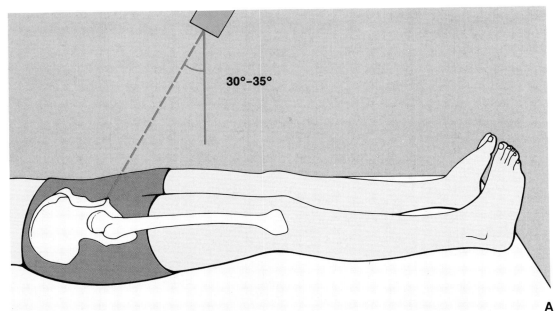

Figure 7.3 (A) For the angled anteroposterior (Ferguson) view of the pelvis, the patient is in the same position as for the standard anteroposterior projection. The radiographic tube, however, is angled about 30° to 35° cephalad, and the central beam is directed toward the midportion of the pelvis. (B) The radiograph in this projection provides a tangential view of the sacroiliac joints and the sacral bone. The pubic and ischial rami are also well demonstrated.

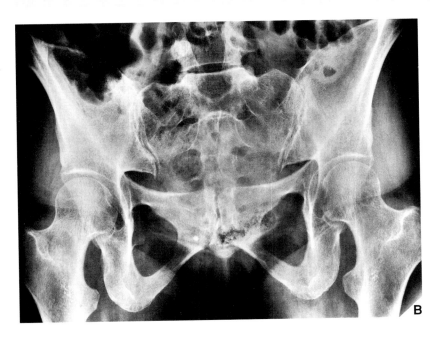

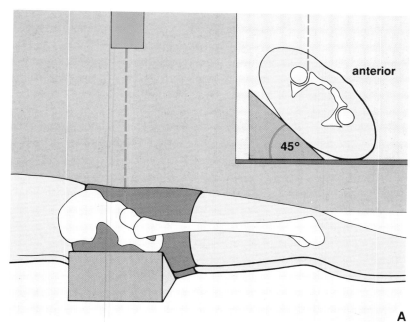

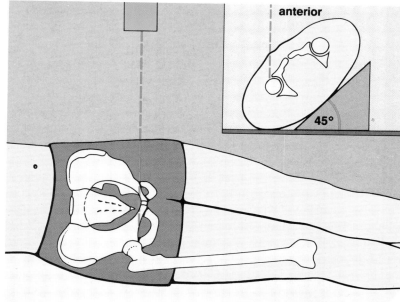

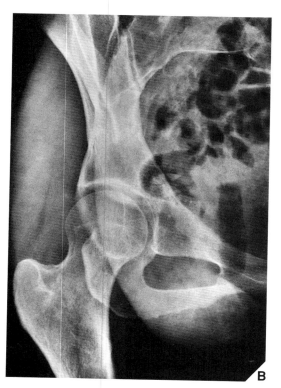

Figure 7.4 (A) For the anterior oblique (Judet) view of the pelvis, the patient is supine and anteriorly rotated, the affected hip elevated 45° *(inset)*. The central beam is directed vertically toward the affected hip. (B) On the radiograph in this projection, the iliopubic (anterior) column (see Fig. 7.20) and the posterior lip of the acetabulum are well delineated.

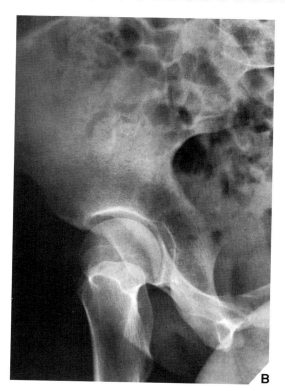

Figure 7.5 (A) For the posterior oblique (Judet) view of the pelvis, the patient is supine and anteriorly rotated, the unaffected hip elevated 45° *(inset)*. The central beam is directed vertically through the affected hip. (B) On the film in this projection, the ilioischial (posterior) column (see Fig. 7.20) and the anterior acetabular rim are well demonstrated.

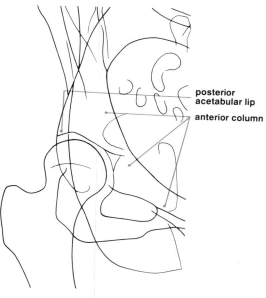

posterior acetabular lip

anterior column

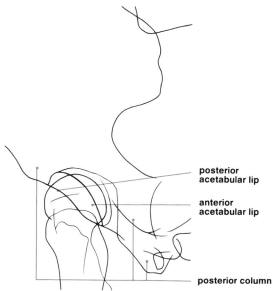

posterior acetabular lip

anterior acetabular lip

posterior column

projections, known as *Judet* views, are necessary to evaluate the acetabulum. The *anterior (internal) oblique* projection helps delineate the iliopubic (anterior) column and the posterior lip (rim) of the acetabulum (Fig. 7.4). The *posterior (external) oblique* projection delineates the ilioischial (posterior) column and the anterior acetabular rim (Fig. 7.5). Of value in demonstrating the structures of the proximal femur and hip, the *frog-lateral* projection allows adequate evaluation of fractures of the femoral head and the greater and the lesser trochanters (Fig. 7.6). Demonstration of the anterior and posterior aspects of the femoral head as well as the anterior rim of the acetab-

ulum may require a *groin-lateral* projection of the hip, which is particularly useful in evaluating anterior or posterior displacement of fragments in proximal femoral fractures as well as the degree of rotation of the femoral head. This projection, by providing an almost true lateral image of the proximal femur, also demonstrates an important anatomic feature, the angle of anteversion of the femoral neck, which normally ranges from 25° to 30° (Fig. 7.7).

Ancillary imaging techniques play a crucial role in the evaluation of traumatic conditions of the pelvis and acetabulum, providing essential and often otherwise unobtainable information that helps

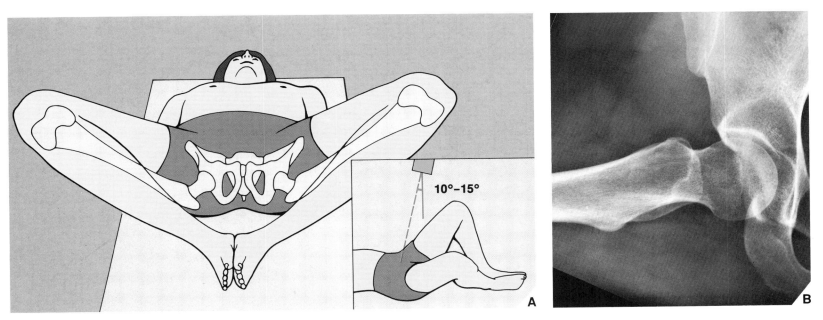

Figure 7.6 (A) For the frog-lateral view of the proximal femur and hip, the patient is supine with the knees flexed, the soles of the feet together, and the thighs maximally abducted. For simultaneous imaging of both hips, the central beam is directed vertically or with 10° to 15° cephalad angulation to a point slightly above the pubic symphysis *(inset)*; for selective examination of one hip, it is directed toward the affected hip joint. (B) The film in this projection demonstrates the lateral aspect of the femoral head and both trochanters.

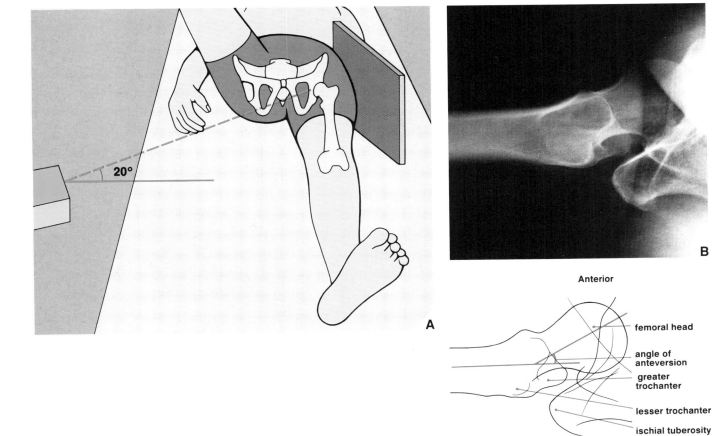

Figure 7.7 (A) For the groin-lateral view of the hip, the patient is supine with the affected extremity extended and the opposite leg elevated and abducted. The cassette is placed against the affected hip on the lateral aspect, and the central beam is directed horizontally toward the groin with about 20° cephalad angulation. (B) The film in this projection provides almost a true lateral image of the femoral head, thereby allowing evaluation of its anterior and posterior aspects. It also demonstrates the anteversion of the femoral neck, which normally ranges from 25° to 30°.

the orthopedic surgeon determine the method of treatment and assess the prognosis of pelvic and acetabular fractures. Conventional tomography utilizing multidirectional motion is particularly helpful in ascertaining the size, number, and position of the major fragments in pelvic and acetabular fractures. However, since the surgical management of such fractures is based on the stability of the fragments as well as on the presence or absence of intra-articular extension of the fracture line and intra-articular fragments, CT

examination may be necessary to provide information that is not available from the standard and special projections of conventional radiography or conventional tomographic techniques (Fig. 7.8; see also Figs. 7.22B–D, 7.23B,C, 7.24B–D). In addition to data about the condition of the weight-bearing parts of the joint and the configuration of the fracture fragments, CT can delineate soft tissue and concomitant injury to soft tissue structures. However, in cases of severe injury when immediate surgical intervention is required, obtaining

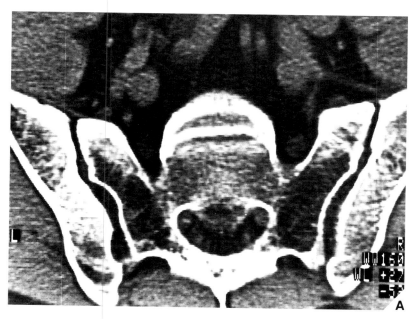

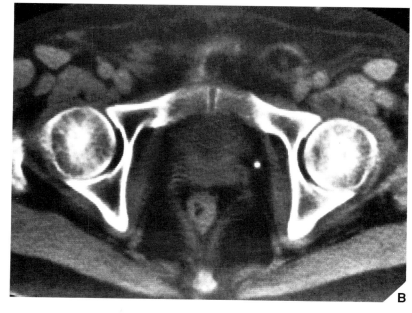

Figure 7.8 (A) CT section at the level of S-2 demonstrates the true (synovial) sacroiliac joints. (B) In this section through the hip joints the relation of the femoral heads to the acetabula can sufficiently be evaluated. The pubic bone and the pubic symphysis are also well delineated.

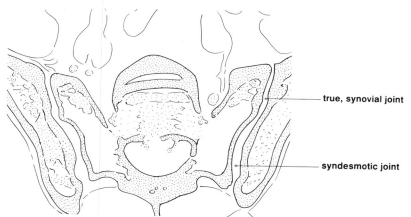

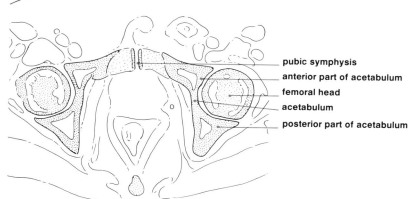

CT scans may be time consuming and impractical. In such cases plain-film radiographs can be obtained more quickly, allowing more rapid recognition of the type of injury. CT is particularly effective in the postsurgical assessment of the alignment of fragments and fracture healing.

The urinary system is frequently at risk in pelvic fractures. Bladder injuries have been reported in 6% and urethral injuries in 10% of patients with pelvic fractures. The evaluation of such conditions requires contrast examination of the urinary system by means of intravenous urography (IVP) and cystourethrography. Pelvic arteriography and venography may also be required to evaluate injury to the vascular system. In addition to its diagnostic value, arteriography can be combined with an interventional procedure, such as embolization, to control hemorrhage.

For a summary of the preceding discussion in tabular form, see Figures 7.9, 7.10, and 7.11.

Figure 7.9 Standard and Special Radiographic Projections for Evaluating Injury to the Pelvis, Acetabulum, and Proximal Femur

PROJECTION	DEMONSTRATION	PROJECTION	DEMONSTRATION

Anteroposterior	Angle of femoral neck
	Radiographic landmarks
	  (lines) relating to
	    acetabulum:
	      Iliopubic (iliopectineal)
	      Ilioischial
	      Teardrop
	      Acetabular roof
	      Anterior acetabular rim
	      Posterior acetabular rim
	Varus and valgus deformities
	Avulsion fractures
	Malgaigne fracture
	Fractures of:
	    Ilium (Duverney)
	    Ischium
	    Pubis
	    Sacrum (in some cases)
	    Femoral head and neck
	Dislocations in hip joint
		Oblique
		  (Judet views)
		
		  Anterior (internal)
		
		  Posterior (external)
		
		Frog-Lateral
		
		Groin-Lateral
			Iliopubic line
			Fractures of:
			    Anterior (iliopubic) column
			    Posterior acetabular rim
			
			Quadrilateral plate
			Fractures of:
			    Posterior (ilioischial) column
			    Anterior acetabular rim
			
			Fractures of:
			    Femoral head and neck
			    Greater and lesser trochanters
			Angle of anteversion of
			    femoral head
			Anterior and posterior cortices
			    of femoral neck
			Ischial tuberosity
			Rotation and displacement of
			    femoral head in subcapital
			    fractures

With 30°–35° cephalad
  angulation (Ferguson)
  (or posteroanterior
  with or without 25°–30°
  caudal angulation)
	Fractures of:
	    Sacrum
	    Pubic ramus
	    Ischial ramus
	Injury to sacroiliac joints		

Figure 7.10 Ancillary Imaging Techniques for Evaluating Injury to the Pelvis, Acetabulum, and Proximal Femur

TECHNIQUE	DEMONSTRATION	TECHNIQUE	DEMONSTRATION

Tomography
  (multidirectional)
	Position of fragments and
	  extension of fracture line
	  in complex fractures,
	  particularly of pelvis
	  and acetabulum
		Radionuclide Imaging
		  (scintigraphy, bone scan)
			Occult fractures
			Stress fractures
			Posttraumatic osteonecrosis

Computed Tomography	Same features as above
	Weight-bearing parts of joints
	Sacroiliac joints
	Intra-articular fragments
	Soft-tissue injuries
		Intravenous Urography (IVP)
		Cystourethrography
		
		Angiography
		  (arteriography, venography)
			Concomitant injury to ureters,
			  urinary bladder, and urethra
			
			Injury to vascular system

MRI	Soft tissue injuries Posttraumatic osteonecrosis		

Injury to the Pelvis and Acetabulum

The pelvis is a nearly rigid ring essentially comprising three elements: the sacrum and two paired lateral components, each composed of the ilium, the ischium, and the pubis. Because of this configuration and the interrelationship of its components, identification of an apparently solitary fracture should not end the process of radiographic examination. The pelvis should carefully be scrutinized for other fractures of the ring or diastasis in the sacroiliac joints or the pubic symphysis (see Fig. 4.5).

CLASSIFICATION OF PELVIC FRACTURES Various classification systems have been proposed not only to identify the distinctive appearances of pelvic injuries as an aid to radiographic recognition and diagnosis but also to categorize such injuries as an aid to orthopedic management and prognosis. The latter point is particularly important in pelvic fractures because of the inherent instability of the structures

composing the pelvic girdle, their integrity depending entirely on ligamentous support and the stabilizing influence of the sacroiliac joints. Thus, pelvic fractures can be grouped according to whether or not they significantly detract from the stability of the pelvic ring, with the orthopedic management and prognosis of those fractures identified as stable (Fig. 7.12) differing considerably from that of unstable fractures (Fig. 7.13).

Systems that classify pelvic injuries for the purpose of radiographic diagnosis and orthopedic management using categories other than stable and unstable have also been suggested. Pennal, Tile, and their colleagues have elaborated a system based on the direction of the force that produces pelvic injuries. They identified four patterns of force as underlying mechanisms of injury that produce distinctive radiographic appearances:

1. *Anteroposterior compression* in which the force vector in the antero-posterior or posteroanterior direction produces vertically ori-

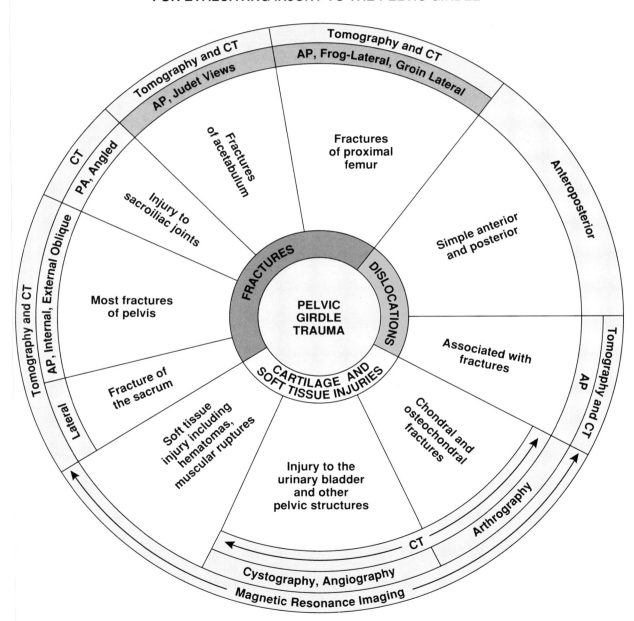

SPECTRUM OF RADIOLOGIC IMAGING TECHNIQUES FOR EVALUATING INJURY TO THE PELVIC GIRDLE*

*The radiographic projections or radiologic techniques indicated throughout the diagram are only those that are the most effective in demonstrating the respective traumatic conditions.

Figure 7.11 Spectrum of radiologic imaging techniques for evaluating injury to the pelvic girdle.

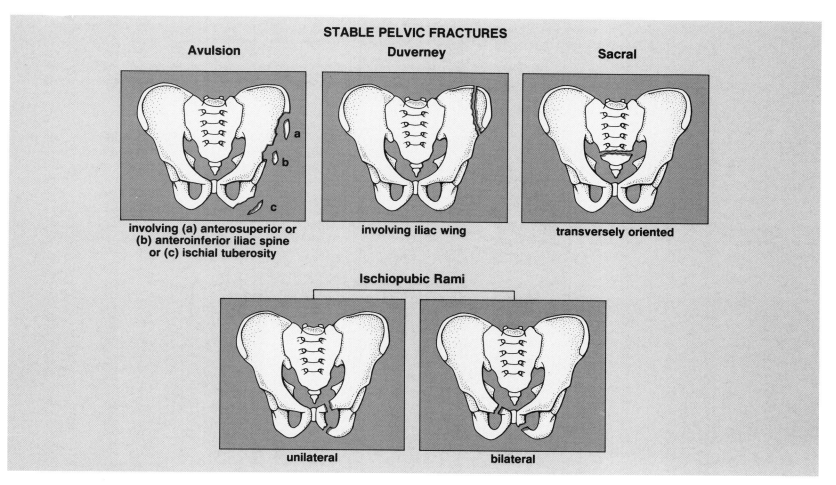

Figure 7.12 Stable pelvic fractures. (Adapted from Dunn AW, Morris HD, 1968)

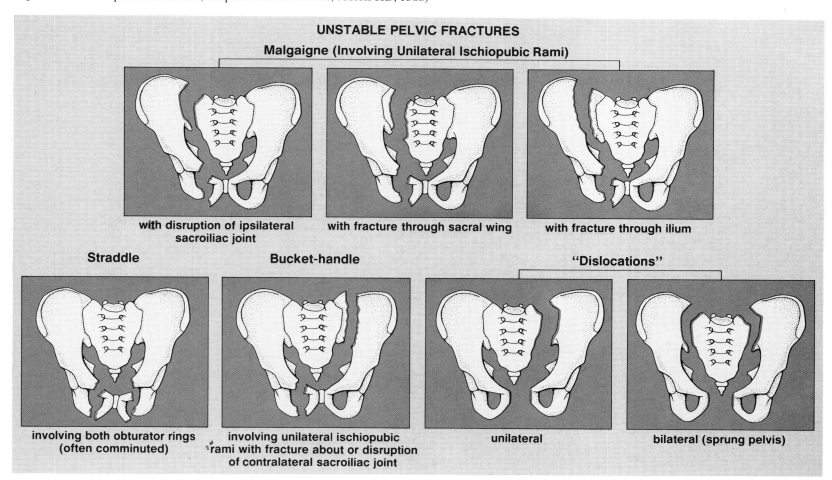

Figure 7.13 Unstable pelvic fractures. (Adapted from Dunn AW, Morris HD, 1968)

ented fractures of the pubic rami and disruption of the pubic symphysis and sacroiliac joints, which often results in bilateral pelvic "dislocation" (sprung pelvis).

2. *Lateral compression* in which the lateral force vector often results in horizontally or coronally oriented fractures of the pubic rami, compression fractures of the sacrum, fractures of the iliac wings, and central dislocation in the hip joint as well as varying degrees of pelvic instability due to displacement or rotation of one or both hemipelves, depending on whether the compressive force is applied more anteriorly or more posteriorly.

3. *Vertical shear* in which the inferosuperiorly oriented disruptive force, delivered to one or both sides of the pelvis lateral to the midline often as a result of a fall from a height, frequently produces vertically oriented fractures of the pubic rami, sacrum, and iliac wings. Because of significant ligamentous disruption, this type of force is associated with injuries producing severe pelvic instability.

4. *Complex patterns* in which at least two different force vectors have been delivered to the pelvis, the patterns produced by anteroposterior and lateral compression being the most commonly encountered.

This system, which corresponds to the more traditional categorization of pelvic fractures into stable and unstable, has practical value in allowing sufficient evaluation of pelvic injuries to be made on the anteroposterior projection in patients requiring immediate surgical intervention when CT scans would be impractical to obtain. It also provides correlations between the type of force delivered to the pelvis and the concomitant ligamentous and pelvic-organ injury that can be expected. In anteroposterior compression-type injuries, for example, the anterior sacroiliac ligaments, the sacrotuberous-sacroiliac ligament complex, and the symphysis ligaments are damaged. This type of injury may also be associated with urethral and urinary bladder rupture and damage to the pelvic blood vessels. In lateral-compression injuries, rupture of the posterior sacroiliac liga-

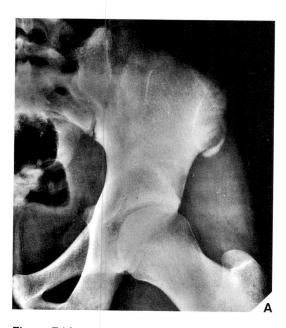 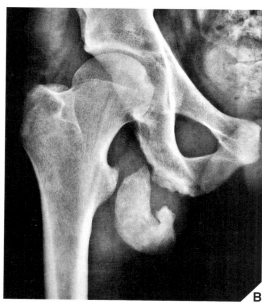 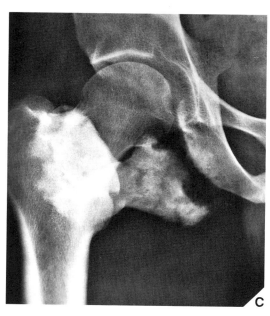

Figure 7.14 A 16-year-old boy was injured during an athletic activity. (A) Anteroposterior view of the pelvis shows a crescent-shaped fragment adjacent to the lateral aspect of the iliac wing, which represents the avulsed apophysis of the anterosuperior iliac spine. (B) Anteroposterior view of the hip in a 26-year-old runner clearly demonstrates avulsion of the ischial tuberosity. (C) As a sequela of avulsion of the ischial tuberosity and injury to the soft tissue in the region, a 28-year-old athlete developed ossification of the obturator externus muscle.

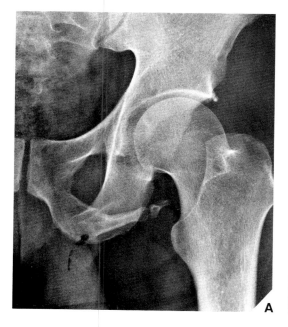 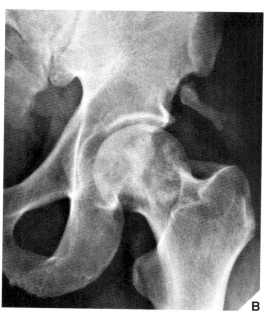

Figure 7.15 A rare congenital anomaly, the pelvic digit may occasionally be mistaken for avulsion fracture. (A) Anteroposterior view of the left hip shows a finger-like, jointed structure attached to the caudal portion of the left ischium. (B) Anteroposterior view of the hip in a 55-year-old man with no history of trauma demonstrates a well formed digit at the site of the anteroinferior iliac spine. (Reproduced with permission of the authors and publisher from Greenspan A, Norman A, 1982)

ment and/or the sacrospinous-sacrotuberous ligament complex may result. Injury to the urinary tract may or may not be present. In vertical shear injuries, the ipsilateral posterior and anterior sacroiliac, the sacrospinous-sacrotuberous, and the anterior symphysis ligaments are usually ruptured. Vertical shear injuries are frequently accompanied by damage to the sciatic nerve and pelvic blood vessels, often resulting in massive hemorrhage. The discussion that follows, however, focuses on the more traditional pedagogical categories of pelvic trauma.

Fractures of the Pelvis

AVULSION FRACTURES   Usually involving the anterosuperior or anteroinferior iliac spine or the ischial tuberosity, avulsion fractures, which are classified as stable fractures (see Fig. 7.12), most commonly occur in athletes as a result of forcible muscular contraction: the *sartorius muscle* in avulsion of the anterosuperior iliac spine; the *rectus femoris muscle* in avulsion of the anteroinferior iliac spine; and the *hamstrings* in avulsion of the ischial tuberosity. Most fractures of these structures are apparent on a single anteroposterior view of the pelvis (Fig. 7.14). However, confusion in diagnosis may arise when healing occurs by exuberant callus formation, at which time or after full ossification such fractures may be mistaken for neoplasms. Another entity that may mimic avulsion injury to the pelvis is the so-called pelvic digit, a congenital anomaly characterized by a bony formation in the soft tissue about the pelvic bones (Fig. 7.15).

MALGAIGNE FRACTURE   This unstable injury, involving one hemipelvis, most commonly consists of unilateral fractures of the superior and inferior pubic rami and disruption of the ipsilateral sacroiliac joint (see Fig. 7.13). In the variants of this type of injury, the unilateral fractures of the pubic rami may be accompanied by a fracture through the sacral wing near the sacroiliac joint or through the ilium (see Fig. 7.13). Separation of the pubic symphysis may coexist with such injuries, and cephalad or posterior displacement of the entire pelvis may occur. The Malgaigne fracture, which is recognized clinically by shortening of the lower extremity, is readily demonstrated on the anteroposterior view of the pelvis (Fig. 7.16).

MISCELLANEOUS PELVIC FRACTURES   Injuries other than the Malgaigne fracture are also easily evaluated on plain films of the pelvis in the standard and special projections or on CT examination. The *Duverney fracture* is a stable fracture of the wing of the ilium without interruption of the pelvic ring (see Fig. 7.12). The *straddle fracture* consists of comminuted fractures of both obturator rings (that is, all four ischiopubic rami) (see Fig. 7.13). In one third of patients with this unstable fracture, bladder rupture or urethral injuries occur. The *bucket-handle* or *contralateral double vertical fracture* involves both the superior and inferior ischiopubic rami on one side combined with fracture about or disruption of the sacroiliac joint on the opposite side (see Fig. 7.13). *Fractures of the sacrum*, which may be either transversely or vertically oriented (see Fig. 7.12), may occur alone or, more often, in association with other pelvic injuries, such as the so-called *pelvic "dislocations."* The latter are characterized by disruption in one or both sacroiliac joints (unilateral or bilateral "dislocation") associated with separation of the pubic symphysis (Fig. 7.17; see also Fig. 7.13). The anteroposterior projection obtained with 30° cephalad angulation, as well as conventional or computed tomography, is helpful in disclosing sacral fractures, which are frequently overlooked.

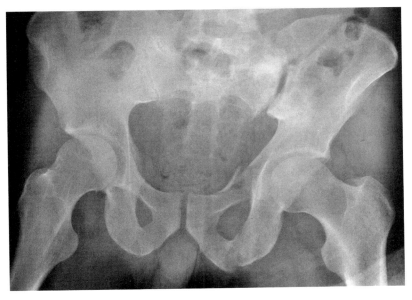

Figure 7.16 A 35-year-old man who was involved in an automobile accident sustained vertical fractures of the left obturator ring and fracture of the ipsilateral iliac bone—a typical Malgaigne injury.

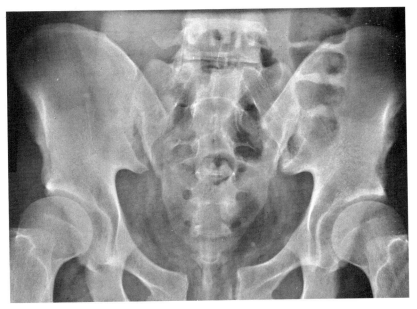

Figure 7.17 A 25-year-old man was involved in a motorcycle accident. Anteroposterior view of the pelvis reveals the typical appearance of pelvic "dislocation." The pubic symphysis is disrupted and markedly widened, and there is widening of both sacroiliac joints.

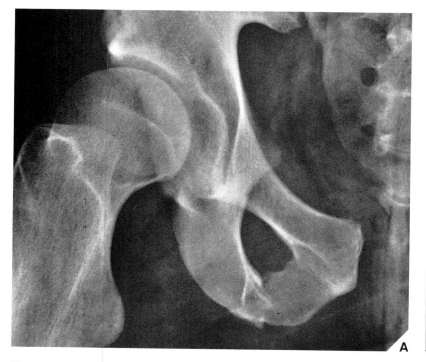

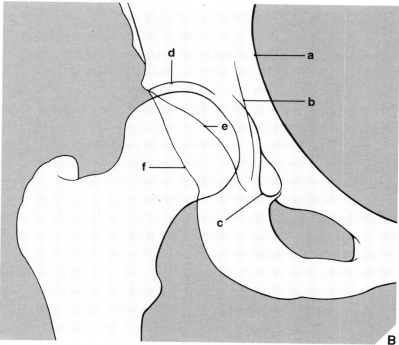

Figure 7.18 (A, B) On the anteroposterior view of the hip, six lines relating to the acetabulum and its surrounding structures can be distinguished: *a*, iliopubic or iliopectineal (arcuate) line; *b*, ilioischial line, formed by the posterior portion of the quadrilateral plate (surface) of the iliac bone; *c*, teardrop, formed by the medial acetabular wall, the acetabular notch, and the anterior portion of the quadrilateral plate; *d*, roof of the acetabulum; *e*, anterior rim of the acetabulum; *f*, posterior rim of the acetabulum. Distortion of any of these normal radiographic landmarks indicates the possible presence of abnormality.

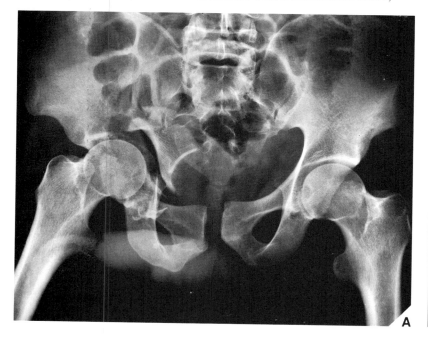

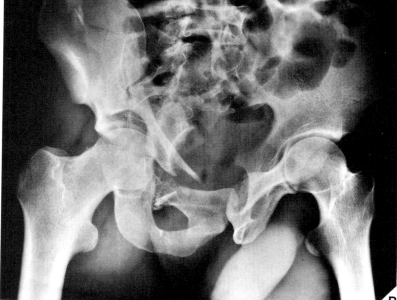

Figure 7.19 A 32-year-old drug addict was hit by a car. (A) Anteroposterior view of the pelvis shows a comminuted fracture of the right acetabulum, fracture of the right ilium, and diastasis in the pubic symphysis. There is also a fracture of the sacrum with diastasis in the left sacroiliac joint. (B) On the anterior oblique projection, the acetabular fracture is seen to involve mainly the anterior pelvic column.

Fractures of the Acetabulum

Evaluation of the acetabulum on plain films may be difficult because of obscuring overlying structures (see Fig. 7.18A). If acetabular fracture is suspected, radiographs in at least four projections should be obtained: the anteroposterior view of the pelvis, the anteroposterior view of the hip, and the anterior and posterior oblique (Judet) views. Plain-film radiography may also need to be supplemented by conventional tomography or CT, as discussed earlier.

As an aid to recognizing the presence of abnormality on the anteroposterior projection of the pelvis and hip, Judet, Judet, and Letournel have identified six lines relating to the acetabulum and its

immediately surrounding structures (Fig. 7.18). Fracture of the acetabulum usually distorts these radiographic landmarks, allowing a diagnosis to be made on the anteroposterior projection; but an accurate and complete evaluation of the fracture requires that oblique views be obtained (Fig. 7.19). As mentioned earlier, the anterior (internal) oblique projection demonstrates the iliopubic column and the posterior lip of the acetabulum (see Fig. 7.4), and the posterior (external) oblique view images the ilioischial column and the anterior rim of the acetabulum (see Fig. 7.5). These projections, together with the division of the pelvic bone into anterior and posterior columns (Fig. 7.20), provide the basis for the traditional classifi-

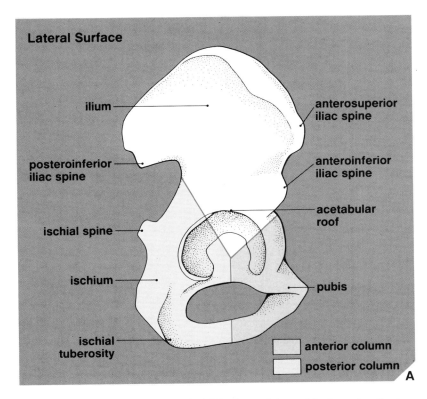

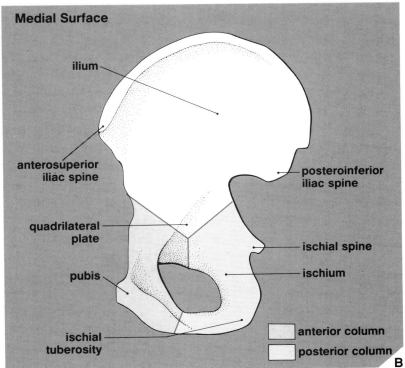

Figure 7.20 Lateral (A) and medial (B) views of the pelvis show the division of the bone into anterior and posterior columns, which provides the basis for the traditional classification of acetabular fractures. (Adapted from Judet R, et al., 1964)

cation of acetabular fractures. This classification has been modified by Letournel to include the following types of fractures (Fig. 7.21):

1. Fracture of the iliopubic (anterior) column; (this is a rare type of fracture)
2. Fracture of the ilioischial (posterior) column; (this is a common type of fracture)
3. Transverse fracture through the acetabulum involving both pelvic columns; (this is a common type of fracture)
4. Complex fractures, including T-shaped and stellate fractures, in

which the acetabulum is broken into three or more fragments; (this is the most common type of fracture).

CT plays a leading role in the evaluation of acetabular and pelvic fractures because of its capability of demonstrating the exact position of displaced fragments, which may be trapped within the hip joint, as well as allowing adequate assessment of concomitant soft tissue injury (Figs. 7.22–7.24). It also requires less manipulation of the patient than the standard radiographic views or conventional tomography—a fact especially important in patients with multiple injuries.

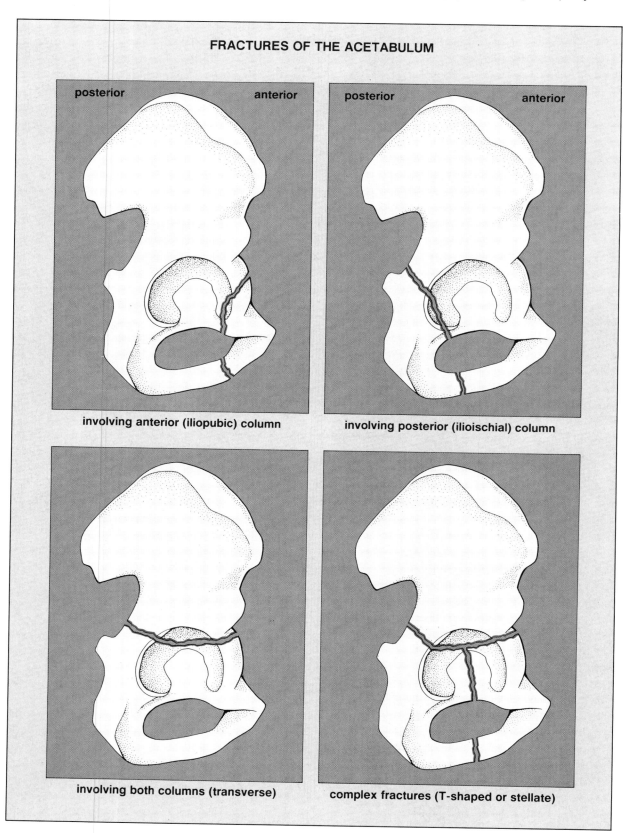

FRACTURES OF THE ACETABULUM

posterior anterior
involving anterior (iliopubic) column

posterior anterior
involving posterior (ilioischial) column

involving both columns (transverse)

complex fractures (T-shaped or stellate)

Figure 7.21 In the traditional classification of acetabular fractures, the fracture may involve the anterior column, the posterior column, or both columns. In complex acetabular fractures both columns are involved and the fracture line may be T- shaped or stellate. (Adapted from Letournel E, 1980)

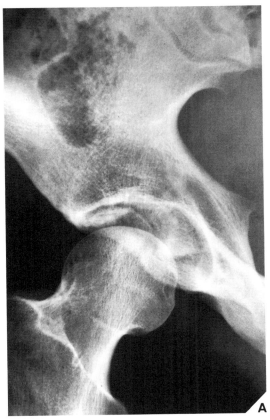

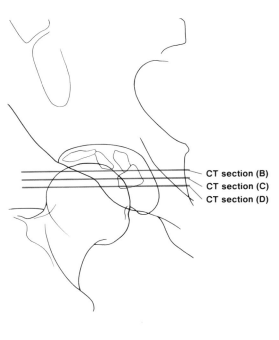

Figure 7.22 As a result of an automobile accident, a 30-year-old woman sustained an injury that was diagnosed on the standard projections as a fracture of the acetabular roof. (A) On the posterior oblique projection, the fracture is shown to be comminuted. CT examination was performed, and a series of sections (B, C, D) shows the topographic distribution of the various intra-articular fragments and evidence of inferolateral subluxation of the femoral head—important information not appreciated on the standard projections.

CT section (B)
CT section (C)
CT section (D)

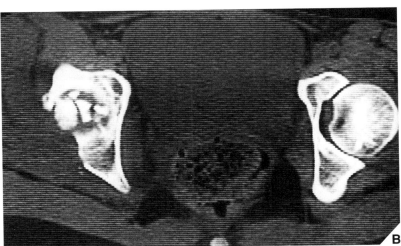

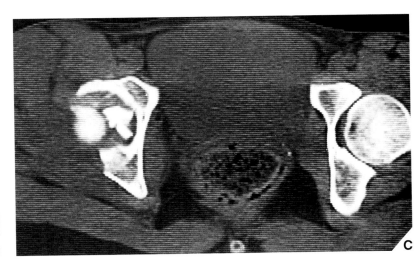

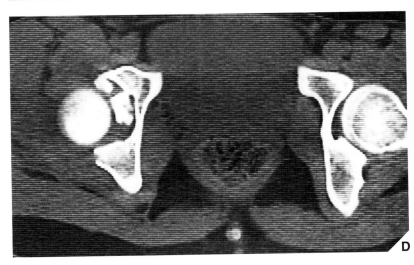

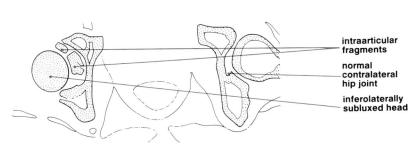

intraarticular fragments

normal contralateral hip joint

inferolaterally subluxed head

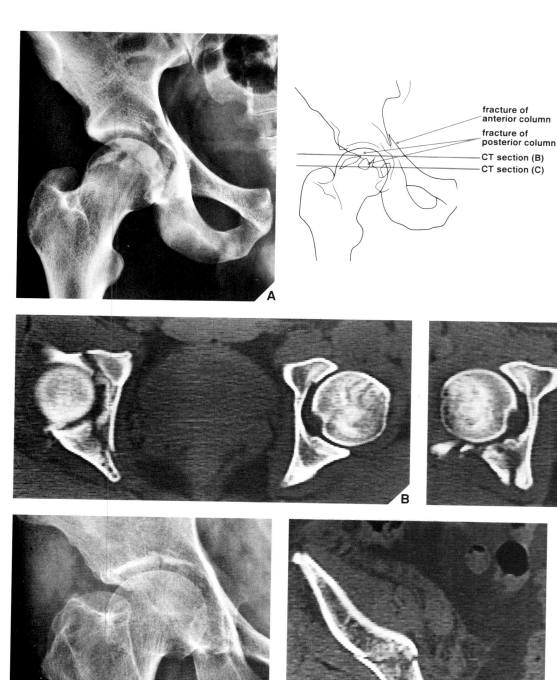

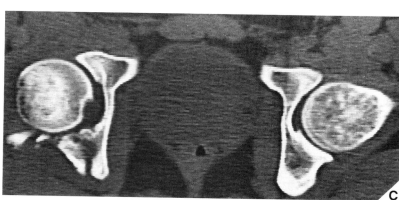

Figure 7.23 A 22-year-old man sustained a dashboard injury in an automobile accident. (A) Standard anteroposterior film of the hip shows fractures of the anterior and posterior columns. (B, C) On CT examination, demonstration of the exact extent of the fracture lines and the spatial relationships between the fragments provides crucial information for the orthopedic surgeon in planning open reduction and internal fixation.

fracture of anterior column
fracture of posterior column
CT section (B)
CT section (C)

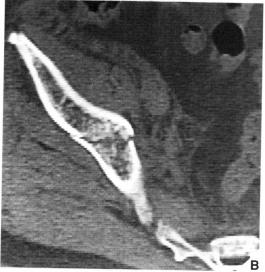

Figure 7.24 After a fall on the street, a 63-year-old man experienced discomfort while walking. (A) Standard anteroposterior view of the right hip shows a radiolucent line in the acetabular roof but no other findings indicative of abnormality. Other views of the pelvis were not obtained because the patient refused. With his consent the next day, multiple CT sections (B, C, D) were obtained, confirming fracture of the acetabular roof. They reveal in addition completely unsuspected fractures of the anterior column and iliac bone, with marked thickening of the obturator internus muscle secondary to hemorrhage and edema.

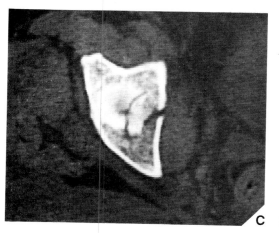

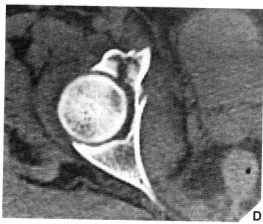

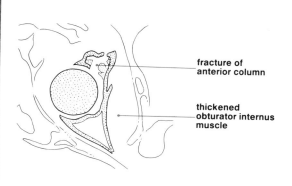

fracture of anterior column

thickened obturator internus muscle

Injury to the Proximal Femur
Fractures of the Proximal Femur

When fracture of the proximal femur is suspected, the standard radiographic examination should include at least two projections: the anteroposterior and the frog-lateral views of the hip (see Figs. 7.1, 7.6); the groin-lateral view of the hip is also frequently required (see Fig. 7.7). For many nondisplaced and displaced fractures, however, a single anteroposterior view of the hip may suffice (Fig. 7.25). In cases of subtle or impacted fractures, tomographic examination may be necessary and is particularly helpful in determining the type and degree of displacement (Fig. 7.26). Radionuclide bone scan may also need to be called upon in questionable cases (see Fig. 4.6).

Traditionally, fractures of the proximal femur (so-called hip fractures) are divided into two groups: 1) *intracapsular fractures* involving the femoral head or neck, which may be capital, subcapital, transcervical, or basicervical and 2) *extracapsular fractures* involving the trochanters, which may be intertrochanteric or subtrochanteric (Fig. 7.27). The significance of this distinction lies in the greater incidence of posttraumatic complications following intracapsular fracture of the upper femur. The most common complication, osteonecrosis (ischemic or avascular necrosis), occurs in 15% to 35% of patients sustaining intracapsular fractures, but the percentage varies according to the reported series.

The reason for the high incidence of the development of osteonecrosis following fracture of the femoral neck lies in the nature of the blood supply to the proximal femur. The capsule of the hip joint arises from the acetabulum and attaches to the anterior aspect of the femur along the intertrochanteric line at the

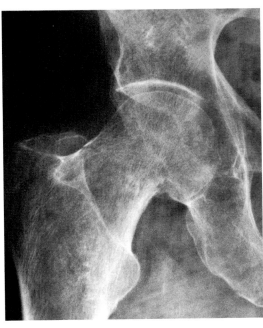

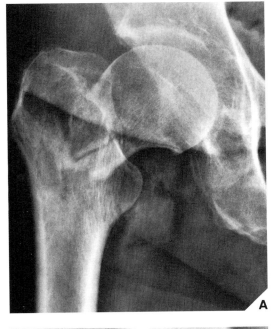

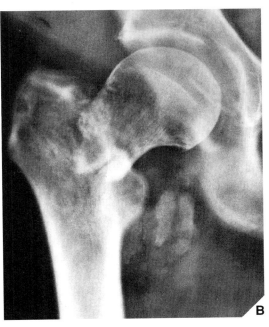

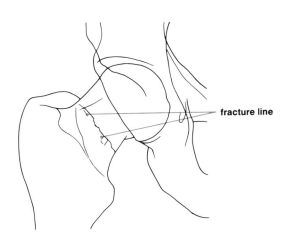

Figure 7.25 In a fall in her bathroom, an 83-year-old woman sustained a typical nondisplaced midcervical fracture of the femoral neck, as demonstrated on this anteroposterior view.

fracture line

Figure 7.26 A 37-year-old man fell from a ladder. (A) On the anteroposterior view of the right hip, a displaced basicervical fracture of the femoral neck is evident. The type of displacement, however, cannot be determined with certainty on this film. To obtain this crucial information, tomography was performed. (B) On the anterior cut (obtained 14 cm above the level of the radiographic table), the femoral head is sharply outlined. (C) On the posterior cut (obtained 7 cm above the table), in contrast to the indistinct contour of the femoral head, the sharp outline of the femoral shaft indicates its posterior displacement.

FRACTURES OF THE PROXIMAL FEMUR

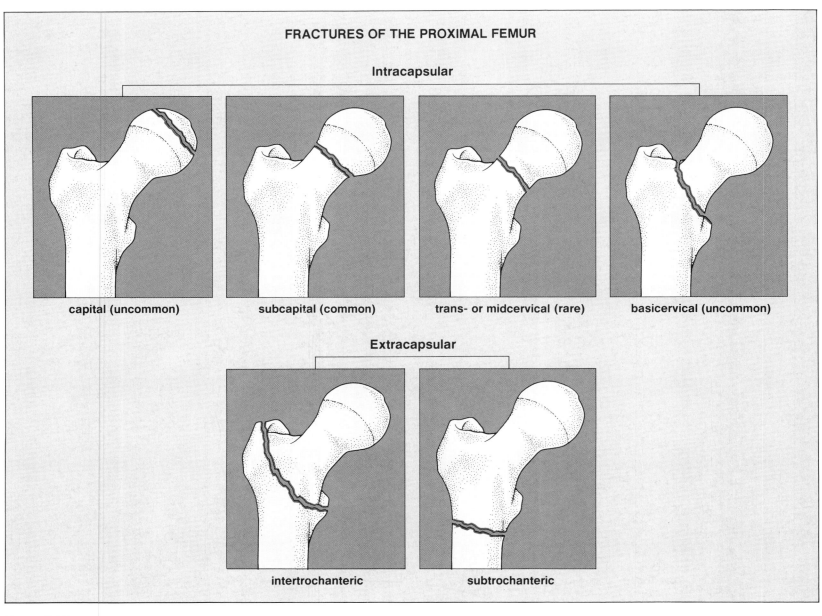

Intracapsular

capital (uncommon)   subcapital (common)   trans- or midcervical (rare)   basicervical (uncommon)

Extracapsular

intertrochanteric   subtrochanteric

Figure 7.27 Fractures of the proximal femur are traditionally classified as intracapsular and extracapsular.

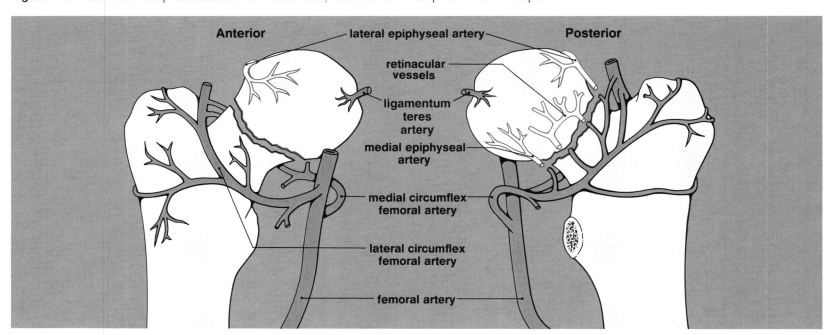

Anterior   lateral epiphyseal artery   **Posterior**

retinacular vessels

ligamentum teres artery

medial epiphyseal artery

medial circumflex femoral artery

lateral circumflex femoral artery

femoral artery

Figure 7.28 The proximal femur is supplied with blood mainly by the circumflex femoral arteries, branches of which ascend subcapsularly along the femoral neck to the femoral head. Intracapsular fracture of the proximal femur may so severely interrupt the blood supply that osteonecrosis results.

base of the femoral neck. Posteriorly, the capsule envelops the femoral head and proximal two thirds of the neck. Most of the blood supply to the femoral head is derived from the circumflex femoral arteries, which form a ring at the base of the neck, sending off branches that ascend subcapsularly along the femoral neck to the femoral head. Only a very small portion of the femoral head is supplied by arteries in the ligamentum teres (ligamentum capitis femoris) (Fig. 7.28). Because of this vascular configuration, intracapsular fractures tend to tear the vessels, interrupting the blood supply and leading eventually to osteonecrosis. The trochanteric region, on the other hand, is extracapsular and receives an excellent supply of blood from branches of the circumflex femoral arteries and from muscles that attach around both trochanters. Thus, as a rule, intertrochanteric fractures do not lead to osteonecrosis of the femoral head.

Nonunion is also a common complication following fracture of the femoral neck, occurring in 10% to 44% of patients with such fractures. According to Pauwels, the obliquity of the fracture line determines the prognosis. The more oblique the fracture line is, the more likely nonunion will occur (see Fig. 7.29).

INTRACAPSULAR FRACTURES Of the many classifications of femoral neck fractures that have been proposed, the Pauwels and Garden classifications are useful from a practical point of view because they take into consideration the stability of the fracture—an important factor in orthopedic management and prognosis.

Pauwels classifies femoral neck fractures according to the degree of angulation of the fracture line from the horizontal plane on the postreduction anteroposterior radiograph, stressing that the closer the fracture line approximates the horizontal, the more stable the fracture and the better the prognosis (Fig. 7.29). Garden, however, proposed a staging system of femoral neck fractures based on displacement of the femoral head before reduction. Displacement in the Garden system is graded according to the position of the principal (medial) compressive trabeculae (Fig. 7.30). His classification of such fractures is divided into four stages (Fig. 7.31):

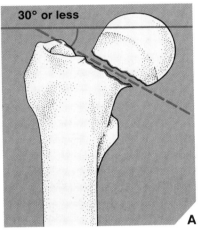
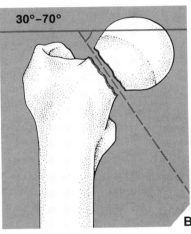
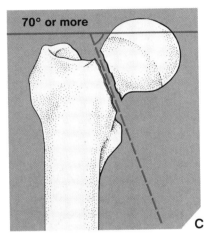

Figure 7.29 (A–C) The Pauwels classification of intracapsular fractures is based on the obliquity of the fracture line: the more the fracture line approaches the vertical, the less stable the fracture, and consequently the greater the chances for nonunion. (Adapted from Pauwels F, 1976)

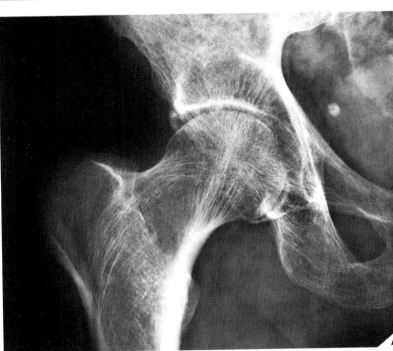

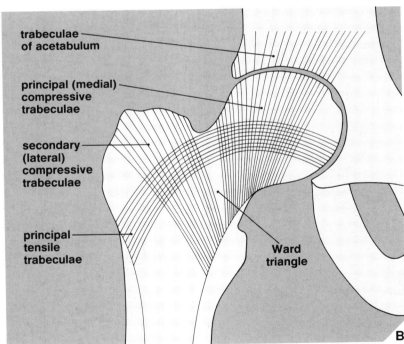

Figure 7.30 (A, B) The Garden staging system of femoral neck fractures is based on the three groups of trabeculae that are demonstrable within the femoral head and neck. The principal tensile trabeculae form an arc, extending from the lateral margin of the greater trochanter, through the superior cortex of the neck and across the femoral head, ending at its inferior aspect below the fovea. The principal (medial) compressive trabeculae are vertically oriented, extending from the medial cortex of the neck into the femoral head in a triangular configuration. They are normally aligned with the trabeculae seen in the acetabulum. The secondary (lateral) compressive trabeculae extend from the calcar and lesser trochanter to the greater trochanter in a fanlike pattern. The central area bounded by this trabecular system is known as Ward triangle.

Stage I Incomplete subcapital fracture. In this so-called impacted or abducted fracture, the femoral shaft is externally rotated and the femoral head is in valgus. The medial trabeculae of the femoral head and neck form an angle greater than 180° (Fig. 7.32). This is a stable fracture with a good prognosis.

Stage II Complete subcapital fracture without displacement. In this complete fracture through the neck, the femoral shaft remains in normal alignment with the femoral head, which is not displaced, but tilted in a varus deformity so that its medial trabeculae do not align with those of the pelvis. The medial trabeculae of the head form an angle of approximately 160° with those of the femoral neck. This is also a stable fracture with a good prognosis.

Stage III Complete subcapital fracture with partial displacement. In this category the femoral shaft is externally rotated. The femoral head is medially rotated, abducted, and tilted in a varus deformity. The medial trabeculae of the head are out of alignment with those

of the pelvis. This fracture is usually unstable, but it may be converted to a stable fracture by proper reduction. The prognosis is not as good as that for stage I and II fractures.

Stage IV Complete subcapital fracture with full displacement. In this type the femoral shaft, in addition to being externally rotated, is upwardly displaced and lies anterior to the femoral head. Although the head is completely detached from the shaft, it remains in its normal position in the acetabulum. The medial trabeculae are in alignment with those of the pelvis (Fig. 7.33). This is an unstable fracture with a poor prognosis.

This staging of femoral neck fractures has important prognostic value. In following 80 patients over one year, Garden found complete union in all those graded stages I and II, 93% in those graded stage III, and only 57% in those graded stage IV. Osteonecrosis occurred in only 8% of nondisplaced stage I or II fractures but in 30% of displaced stage III or IV fractures.

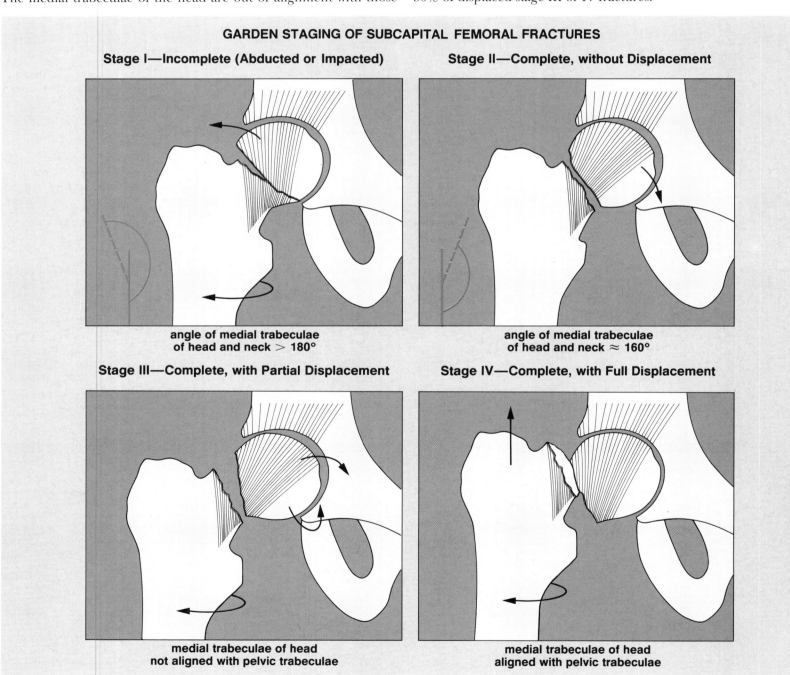

GARDEN STAGING OF SUBCAPITAL FEMORAL FRACTURES

Stage I—Incomplete (Abducted or Impacted)

angle of medial trabeculae
of head and neck > 180°

Stage II—Complete, without Displacement

angle of medial trabeculae
of head and neck ≈ 160°

Stage III—Complete, with Partial Displacement

medial trabeculae of head
not aligned with pelvic trabeculae

Stage IV—Complete, with Full Displacement

medial trabeculae of head
aligned with pelvic trabeculae

Figure 7.31 The Garden staging of subcapital femoral fractures is based on displacement of the femoral head before reduction. Displacement is graded according to the position of the medial compressive trabeculae. (Adapted from Garden RS, 1974)

EXTRACAPSULAR FRACTURES Frequently resulting from direct injury in a fall, extracapsular fractures occur in an even older age group than do intracapsular fractures. Most of these fractures are inter-trochanteric, the major fracture line extending from the greater to the lesser trochanter, and they are usually comminuted. Radiographic diagnosis can usually be made on a single anteroposterior projection of the hip (Fig. 7.34). Rarely, the fracture line may be obscure, requiring oblique projections or even tomography for its demonstration.

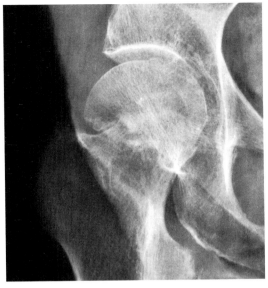
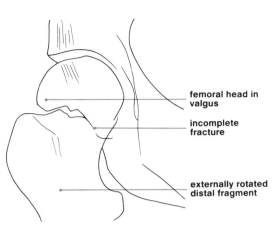

Figure 7.32 In a fall to the floor, a 72-year-old woman sustained a fracture of the right femoral neck. Anteroposterior projection demonstrates a subcapital fracture, which appears to be impacted. The femoral head is in valgus, the distal fragment is externally rotated, and the medial trabeculae of the femoral head and neck form an angle greater than 180°. These features characterize a Garden stage I fracture.

femoral head in valgus
incomplete fracture
externally rotated distal fragment

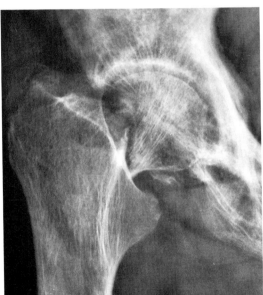
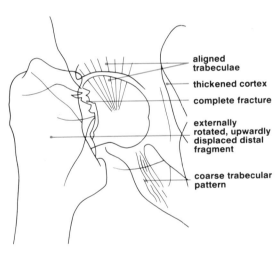

Figure 7.33 In a fall on a subway platform, a 77-year-old woman sustained a fracture of the right femoral neck. Anteroposterior view of the hip shows a complete subcapital fracture with full displacement. The head, which is detached from the neck, is in its normal position in the acetabulum. Note the alignment of the trabeculae in the head and acetabulum. The femoral shaft is upwardly displaced and externally rotated. These features identify this injury as a Garden stage IV fracture. As an incidental finding, note the thickening of the cortex and the coarse trabecular pattern characteristic of Paget disease.

aligned trabeculae
thickened cortex
complete fracture
externally rotated, upwardly displaced distal fragment
coarse trabecular pattern

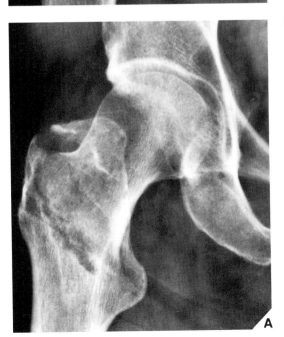
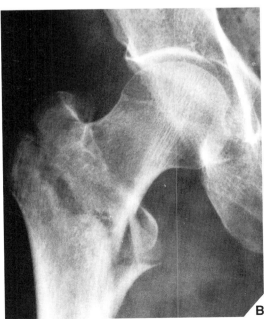

Figure 7.34 (A) Anteroposterior view of the right hip demonstrates a comminuted, three-part intertrochanteric fracture, which can be classified as a Boyd-Griffin type II fracture. (B) Anteroposterior projection of the right hip shows a comminuted, multipart intertrochanteric fracture associated with a subtrochanteric component. This fracture can be classified as a Boyd-Griffin type III fracture. (For the Boyd-Griffin classification of intertrochanteric fractures, see Figure 7.36.)

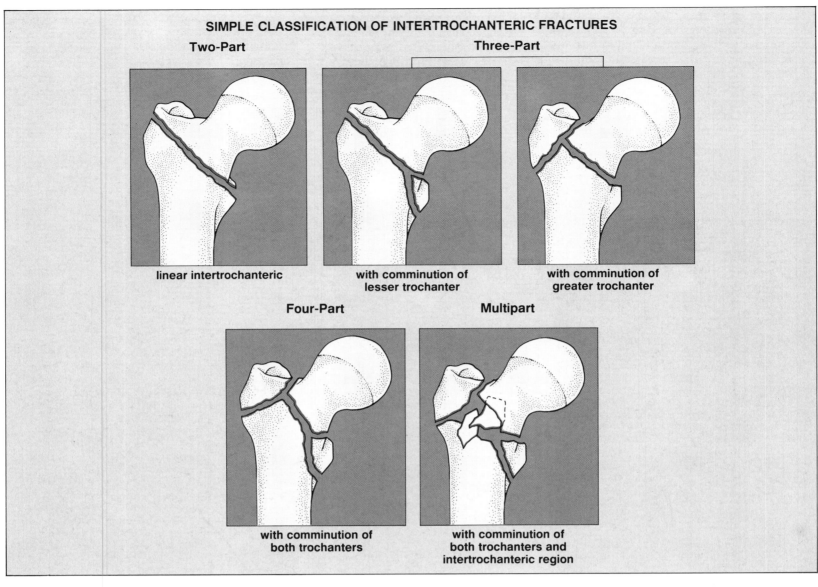

Figure 7.35 The simple classification of intertrochanteric fractures is based on the number of bony fragments.

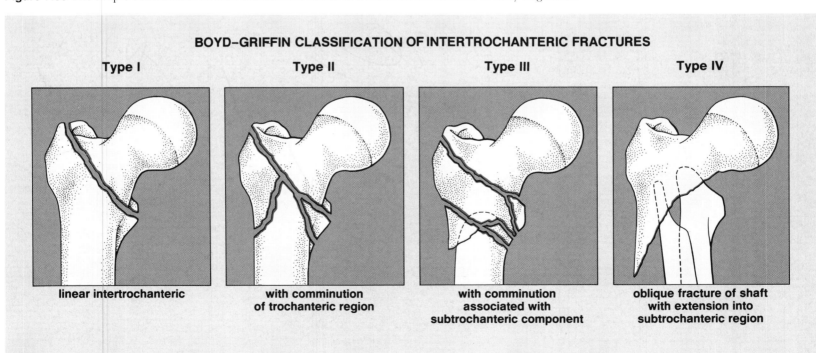

Figure 7.36 The Boyd-Griffin classification of intertrochanteric fractures takes into consideration the presence or absence of comminution and the involvement of the subtrochanteric region. (Adapted from Boyd HB, Griffin LL, 1949)

As mentioned earlier, extracapsular fractures of the proximal femur, for which several classifications have been developed, can generally be divided into two major subgroups: intertrochanteric and subtrochanteric. Intertrochanteric fractures can be further subdivided according to the number of fragments or the extension of the fracture line. A simple classification of such fractures has been proposed that takes into consideration the number of fragments (Fig. 7.35). The two-part fracture in this system is stable, while the four- and multipart fractures are unstable. Boyd and Griffin have proposed a classification of intertrochanteric fractures according to the presence or absence of comminution and involvement of the subtrochanteric region (Fig. 7.36). Comminution of the posterior and medial cortices has important prognostic value. If comminuted, the fracture is unstable and

may require a displacement osteotomy, a procedure particularly important in the treatment of four-part fractures when both trochanters are involved. If there is no comminution, the fracture is stable and treatment involves fixation with a compression screw.

Subtrochanteric fractures have been classified by Fielding according to the level of the fracture line and by Zickel according to their level, obliquity, and comminution (Fig. 7.37). An important fact about subtrochanteric fractures is their relatively benign course due to the good supply of blood and adequate collateral circulation to this region of the femur. The occurrence of osteonecrosis of the femoral head and the incidence of nonunion as a result of intertrochanteric and subtrochanteric fractures are very low. The only serious complication to watch for is postoperative infection.

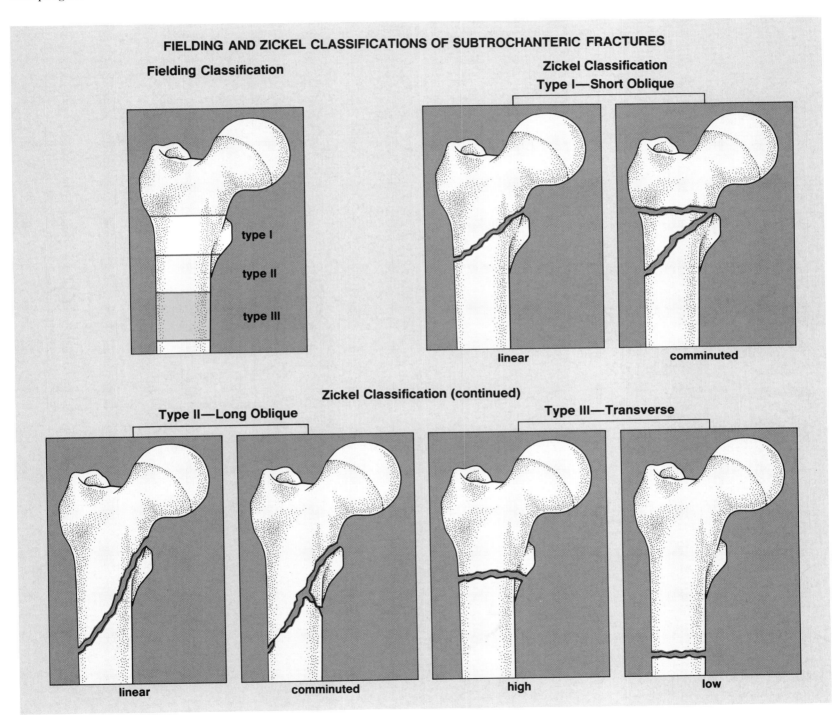

Figure 7.37 The Fielding classification of subtrochanteric fractures *(top left)* is based on the level of the subtrochanteric region in which the fracture occurs. Type I fractures, the most common type, occur at the level of the lesser trochanter; type II, within the region 2.5 cm below the lesser trochanter; and type III, the least common type, occurs within the region 2.5 cm to 5 cm below the lesser trochanter. The Zickel classification of subtrochanteric fractures takes into consideration the level and obliquity of the fracture line as well as the presence or absence of comminution. (Adapted from Fielding JW, 1973; Zickel RE, 1976)

Dislocations in the Hip Joint

Generally, dislocations in the hip joint can be classified as anterior, posterior, or central (medial). They are readily identified on plain films of the hip in the anteroposterior projection. In *anterior dislocation*, which accounts for only 13% of all hip dislocations, the femoral head is displaced into the obturator, pubic, or iliac region. On the anteroposterior film, the femur is abducted and externally rotated and the femoral head lies medial and inferior to the acetabulum (see Fig. 4.36). In *posterior dislocation*, which is the most common type of dislocation, the anteroposterior view reveals the femur to be internally rotated and adducted, while the femoral head lies lateral and superior to the acetabulum (Fig. 7.38). *Central dislocation* (or *central protrusio*) is always associated with an acetabular fracture, the femoral head protruding into the pelvic cavity (Fig. 7.39).

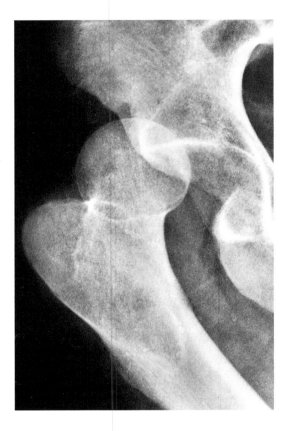

Figure 7.38 A 30-year-old woman sustained a typical posterior hip dislocation in an automobile accident. Note on this anteroposterior projection that the extremity is adducted and the femoral head overlaps the posterior lip of the acetabulum.

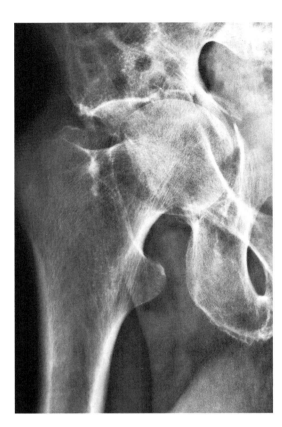

Figure 7.39 While riding a bicycle, a 43-year-old man was hit by a truck. Anteroposterior view of the right hip shows a typical central dislocation in the hip associated with a comminuted fracture of the medial acetabular wall. Note the protrusio of the femoral head into the pelvic cavity.

PRACTICAL POINTS TO REMEMBER

Pelvis and Acetabulum

[1] Fractures of the pelvis are important because of the high incidence of concomitant injury to:
- major blood vessels
- nerves
- lower urinary tract.

[2] Pelvic fractures can be classified for the purposes of radiographic diagnosis and orthopedic management:
- into stable and unstable injuries on the basis of the stability of the fragments
- according to the direction of the force delivered to the pelvis as injuries resulting from anteroposterior compression, lateral compression, vertical shear, or complex pattern.

[3] Fractures of the acetabulum are best demonstrated on the anterior and posterior oblique projections (Judet views).

[4] In acetabular fractures it is important to distinguish between:
- fractures of the anterior pelvic column
- fractures of the posterior pelvic column.

[5] CT plays an important role in the evaluation of fractures of both the pelvis and acetabulum because of its capability of demonstrating:
- the exact position and configuration of comminuted fragments
- the presence or absence of intra-articular fragments
- injury to the soft tissues.

[6] Intravenous urography (IVP) and cystourethrography are essential in the evaluation of concomitant injury to the lower urinary system.

Proximal Femur

[1] The importance of distinguishing between intracapsular and extracapsular fractures of the proximal femur (hip fractures) lies in the possible complications. Intracapsular fractures of the femoral neck are associated with a higher incidence of nonunion and osteonecrosis of the femoral head.

[2] The Garden staging of intracapsular fractures of the femoral neck has practical value in determining stability and prognosis.

[3] The Boyd-Griffin classification of intertrochanteric fractures according to the presence or absence of comminution and involvement of the subtrochanteric region has important prognostic value and serves as a guide to operative management.

[4] Subtrochanteric fractures are classified by:
- Fielding according to the level of the fracture line
- Zickel according to the level, obliquity, and comminution of the fracture.

[5] Magnetic resonance imaging is the ideal modality to detect and evaluate early changes of posttraumatic osteonecrosis of the femoral head.

References

Berquist TH, Coventry MB: The pelvis and hips. In: Berquist TH (ed): *Imaging of Orthopedic Trauma and Surgery.* Philadelphia, Saunders, 1986, p 181.

Boyd HB, Griffin LL: Classification and treatment of trochanteric fractures. *Arch Surg* 58:853, 1949.

Bray TJ, Chapman MW: Fractures of the hip. *Instructional Course Lectures AAOS.* 33:168, 1984.

Bucholz RW: The pathological anatomy of Malgaigne fracture-dislocation of the pelvis. *J Bone Joint Surg* 63A:400, 1981.

Clawson DK, Melcher PJ: Fractures and dislocations of the hip. In: Rockwood CA Jr, Green DP (eds): *Fractures.* Philadelphia, Lippincott, 1975.

Coleman BG, Kressel HY, Dalinka MK, et al: Radiographically negative avascular necrosis: Detection with MR imaging. *Radiology* 168:525, 1988.

Dunn AW, Morris HD: Fractures and dislocations of the pelvis. *J Bone Joint Surg* 50A:1639, 1968.

Fernbach SK, Wilkinson RH: Avulsion injuries of the pelvis and proximal femur. *Am J Roentgenol* 137:581, 1981.

Fielding JW: Subtrochanteric fractures. *Clin Orthop* 92:86, 1973.

Fishman EK, Magid D, Mandelbaum BR, Scott WW, Weiss P, Hadfield R, Mudge B, Kopits SE, Brooker AF, Siegelman SS: Multiplanar (MPR) imaging of the hip. *RadioGraphics* 6:7, 1986.

Garden RS: The structure and function of the proximal end of the femur. *J Bone Joint Surg* 43B:576, 1961.

Garden RS: Low-angle fixation in fractures of the femoral neck. *J Bone Joint Surg* 43B:647, 1961.

Garden RS: Reduction and fixation of subcapital fractures of the femur. *Orthop Clin North Am* 5:683–712, 1974.

Gertzbein SD, Chenoweth DR: Occult injuries of the pelvic ring. *Clin Orthop* 128:202, 1977.

Greenspan A, Norman A: The pelvic digit. *Bull Hosp Jt Dis Orthop Inst* 44:72, 1984.

Greenspan A, Norman A: The "pelvic digit"—an unusual developmental anomaly. *Skeletal Radiol* 9:118, 1982.

Griffith HJ, Standertskjöld-Nordenstam CG, Burke J, Lamont B, Kimmel J: Computed tomography in the management of acetabular fractures. *Skeletal Radiol* 11:22, 1984.

Gylling SF, Ward RE, Holcroft JW, Bray TJ, Chapman MW: Immediate external fixation of unstable pelvic fractures. *Am J Surg* 150:721, 1985.

Hamilton S: Pelvic digit. *Br J Radiol* 58:1010, 1985.

Harley JD, Mack LA, Winquist RA: Computed tomography of acetabular fractures: Comparison with conventional radiography. *Am J Roentgenol* 138:413, 1982.

Huittinen VM, Slatis P: Fractures of the pelvis. Trauma mechanism, types of injury and principles of treatment. *Acta Chir Scand* 138:563, 1972.

Judet R, Judet J, Letournel E: Fractures of the acetabulum: Classification and surgical approaches for open reduction. *J Bone Joint Surg* 46A:1615, 1964.

Kane WJ: Fractures of the pelvis. In: Rockwood CA Jr, Green DP (eds): *Fractures*. Philadelphia, Lippincott, 1975.

Letournel E: Acetabulum fractures: Classification and management. *Clin Orthop* 151:81, 1980.

Levitt RG, Sagel SS, Stanley RJ, Evens RG: Computed tomography of the pelvis. *Semin Roentgenol* 13:193, 1978.

Malgaigne JF: The classic-double vertical fractures of the pelvis. *Clin Orthop* 151: 8, 1980.

Mitchell DG Rao VM, Dalinka MK, et al: Femoral head avascular necrosis: Correlation of MR imaging, radiographic staging, radionuclide imaging, and clinical findings. *Radiology* 162:709,1987.

Pauwels F: *Biomechanics of the Normal and Diseased Hip*. New York, Springer-Verlag, 1976.

Peltier LF: Complications associated with fractures of the pelvis. *J Bone Joint Surg* 47A:1060, 1965.

Pennal GF, Davidson J, Garside H, Plewes J: Results of treatment of acetabular fractures. *Clin Orthop* 151:115, 1980.

Pennal GF, Tile M, Waddell JP, Garside H: Pelvic disruption: Assessment and classification. *Clin Orthop* 151:12, 1980.

Rogers LF: The pelvis. In: Rogers LF (ed): *Radiology of Skeletal Trauma*. New York, Churchill Livingstone, 1982, p 601.

Rosenthal D, Scott JA: Biomechanics important to interpret radiographs of the hip. *Skeletal Radiol* 9:185, 1983.

Sauser DD, Billimoria PE, Rouse GA, Mudge K: CT evaluation of hip trauma. *Am J Roentgenol* 135:269, 1980.

Seiler JG III, Christie MJ, Homra L: Correlation of the findings of magnetic resonance imaging with those of bone biopsy in patients who have stage I or II ischemic necrosis of the femoral head. *J Bone Joint Surg* 71A:28, 1989.

Shirkhoda A, Brashear HR, Staab EV: Computed tomography of acetabular fractures. *Radiology* 134:683, 1980.

Stoller DW, Genant HK: The hip. In: Stoller, DW (ed): *Magnetic Resonance Imaging in Orthopaedics and Rheumatology*. Philadelphia, Lippincott, 1989.

Sullivan JD, Kahn DS: Formation of a bone and joint following blunt injury to the pelvis. *Clin Orthop* 140:80, 1979.

Thaggard A III, Harle TS, Carlson V: Fractures and dislocations of bony pelvis and hip. *Semin Roentgenol* 13:117, 1978.

Vas WG, Wolverson MK, Sundaram M, Heiberg E, Pilla T, Shields JB, Crepps L: Role of computed tomography in pelvis fractures. *J Comput Assist Tomogr* 6:796, 1982.

Young JWR, Burgess AR, Brumback RJ, Poka A: Lateral compression fractures of the pelvis: The importance of plain radiographs in the diagnosis and surgical management. *Skeletal Radiol* 15:103, 1986.

Young JWR, Burgess AR, Brumback RJ, Poka A: Pelvic fractures: Value of plain radiography in early assessment and management. *Radiology* 160:445, 1986.

Young JWR, Resnik CS: Fracture of the pelvis: Current concepts of classification. *Am J Roentgenol* 155:1169, 1990.

Zickel RE: An intramedullary fixation device for the proximal part of the femur. *J Bone Joint Surg* 58A:866, 1976.

8

Lower Limb II:
Knee

THE VULNERABILITY OF THE KNEE, the largest joint in the body, to direct trauma makes knee injuries very common throughout life. Most acute injury to the knee is sustained during adolescence and adulthood, motor vehicle accidents and athletic activities being the major etiologic factors. Fractures are much more common than dislocations, but injuries to the cartilaginous and soft tissue structures, such as tears of the menisci and ligaments, are the most common types of injuries, particularly in older adolescents and younger adults. The symptoms accompanying knee trauma vary according to the specific site of injury and thus constitute important indications of the type of injury. However, clinical history and physical examination are rarely sufficient for making a precise diagnosis. Radiologic examination plays a determining role in diagnosing the various traumatic conditions involving the knee joint.

Anatomic-Radiologic Considerations

Plain-film radiographs are the first line of approach to the traumatized knee, and often they are sufficient for evaluating many traumatic conditions of the joint. However, the great incidence of cartilaginous and soft tissue injuries, occurring either as isolated conditions or in association with fractures, requires the use of ancillary imaging techniques for adequate evaluation of the joint capsule, articular cartilage, menisci, and ligaments.

The standard radiographic examination usually consists of obtaining films of the knee in four projections: the anteroposterior, the lateral, and the tunnel projections, as well as an axial view of the patella. The *anteroposterior* view of the knee allows sufficient evaluation of many of the most important aspects of the distal femur and proximal tibia: the medial and lateral femoral and tibial condyles, the medial and lateral tibial plateaus and tibial spines, as well as the medial and lateral joint compartments and the head of the fibula (Fig 8.1). However, the patella is not well demonstrated on this view because it appears superimposed on the distal femur. Proper evaluation of this structure requires a *lateral* projection (Fig. 8.2) on which the relationship of the patella and femur can also be assessed. Proximal (superior) displacement of the patella is called patella alta; distal (inferior) displacement is called patella baja. The length of the patella is measured from its upper pole (base) to the apex. The length of the patellar ligament is measured from its proximal attachment, just above the apex, to the notch on the proximal margin of the tibial tubercle. These two measurements are approximately equal and the normal variation does not exceed 20% (Fig. 8.3). In addition to imaging the patella in profile, the lateral view of the knee allows evaluation of the femoropatellar compartment, the suprapatellar bursa (pouch), and the quadriceps tendon. The femoral condyles overlap on this projection, and the tibial plateaus are demonstrated in profile. Occasionally, a cross-table lateral view of the knee—obtained with the patient supine, the affected leg extended, and the central beam directed horizontally—may be

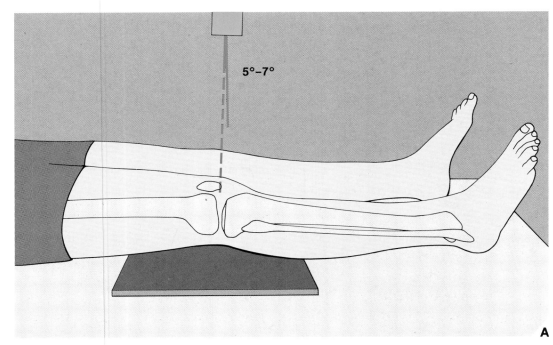

5°–7°

A

Figure 8.1 (A) For the anteroposterior view of the knee, the patient is supine, with the knee fully extended and the leg in the neutral position. The central beam is directed vertically to the knee with 5° to 7° cephalad angulation. (B) The radiograph in this projection sufficiently demonstrates the medial and lateral femoral and tibial condyles, the tibial plateaus and spines, and both the medial and lateral joint compartments. The patella is seen *en face* as an oval-shaped structure between the femoral condyles.

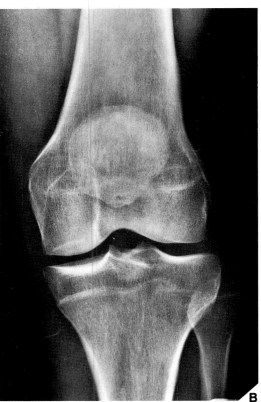

B

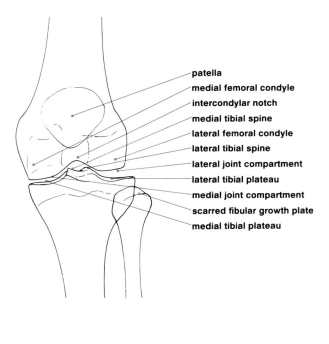

patella
medial femoral condyle
intercondylar notch
medial tibial spine
lateral femoral condyle
lateral tibial spine
lateral joint compartment
lateral tibial plateau
medial joint compartment
scarred fibular growth plate
medial tibial plateau

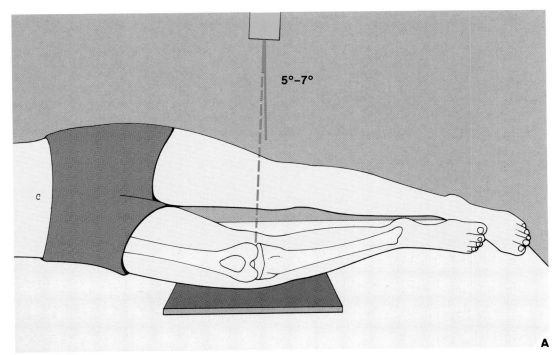

Figure 8.2 (A) For the lateral view of the knee, the patient is lying flat on the same side as the affected knee, which is flexed about 25° to 30°. The central beam is directed vertically toward the medial aspect of the knee joint with about 5° to 7° cephalad angulation. (B) The film in this projection demonstrates the patella in profile, as well as the femoropatellar joint compartment and a faint outline of the quadriceps tendon. The femoral condyles are seen overlapping, and the tibial plateaus are imaged in profile. Note the slight posterior tilt of the tibial plateaus, which normally measures about 10°.

5°–7°

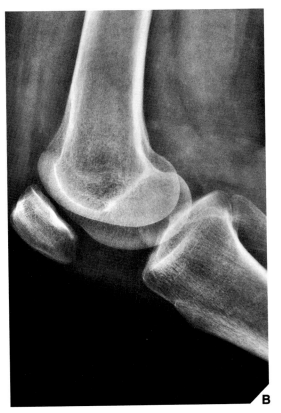

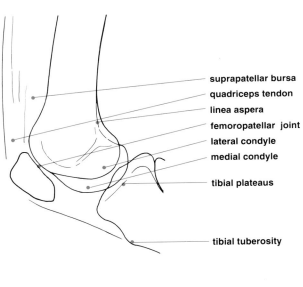

suprapatellar bursa
quadriceps tendon
linea aspera
femoropatellar joint
lateral condyle
medial condyle
tibial plateaus

tibial tuberosity

required to demonstrate the intracapsular fat-fluid level (FBI sign of lipohemarthrosis; see Fig. 4.31). An angled posteroanterior projection of the knee, known as the *tunnel* (or *notch*) view, is also obtained as part of the standard radiographic examination (Fig. 8.4). This view is useful in visualizing the posterior aspect of the femoral condyles, the intercondylar notch, and the intercondylar eminence of the tibia.

To demonstrate an *axial* view of the patella, various techniques are available. The one most commonly used provides what has been called the *sunrise* view (Fig. 8.5). However, the degree of flexion required to obtain this view results in depressing the patella more deeply within the intercondylar fossa and, consequently, the articular surfaces of the femoropatellar joint are not well demonstrated. To overcome this limitation, Merchant and his colleagues have described a technique for obtaining an axial view of the patella that demonstrates the femoropatellar joint to better advantage (Fig. 8.6). It is particularly effective in detecting subtle subluxations of the patella, because it allows specific measurements to be made of the

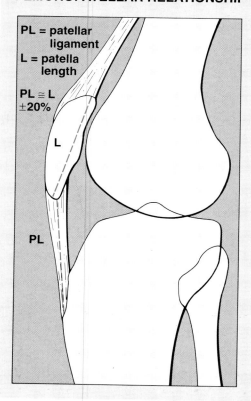

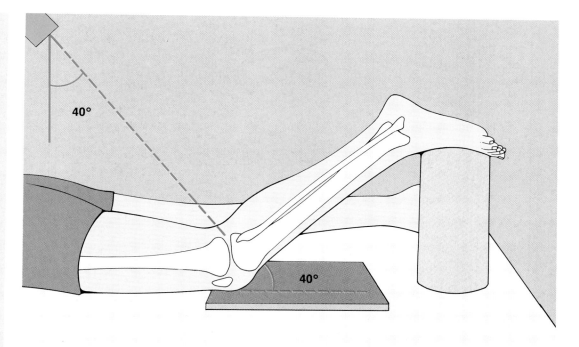

Figure 8.3 Femoropatellar relationship. The length of the patella and the patellar ligament are approximately equal; normal variability does not exceed 20%.

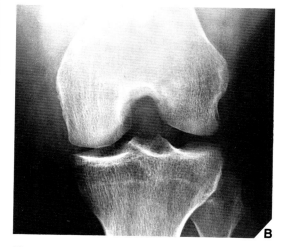

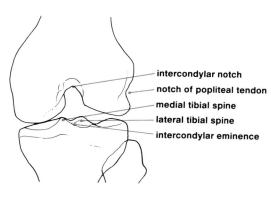

Figure 8.4 (A) For the tunnel (or notch) projection of the knee, the patient is prone with the knee flexed about 40°, the foot supported by a cylindrical sponge. The central beam is directed caudally toward the knee joint at a 40° angle from the vertical. (B) The film in this projection demonstrates the posterior aspect of the femoral condyles, the intercondylar notch, and the intercondylar eminence of the tibia.

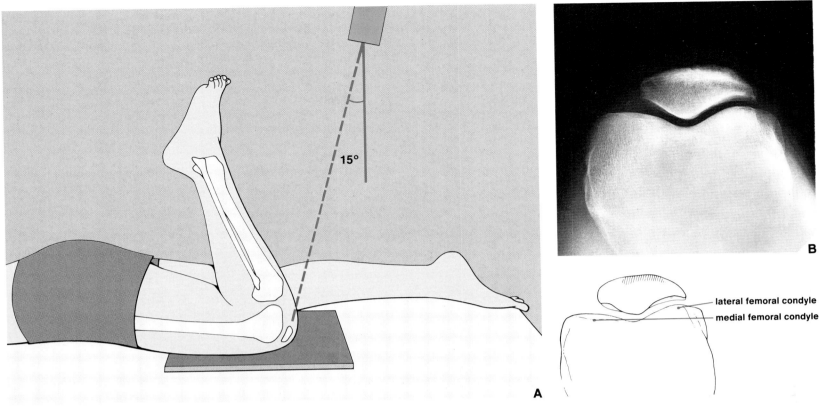

Figure 8.5 (A) For an axial (sunrise) view of the patella, the patient is prone, with the knee flexed 115°. The central beam is directed toward the patella with about 15° cephalad angulation. (B) The radiograph in this projection demon- strates a tangential (axial) view of the patella. Note the deep position of this structure in the intercondylar fossa. The femoropatellar joint compartment is well demonstrated.

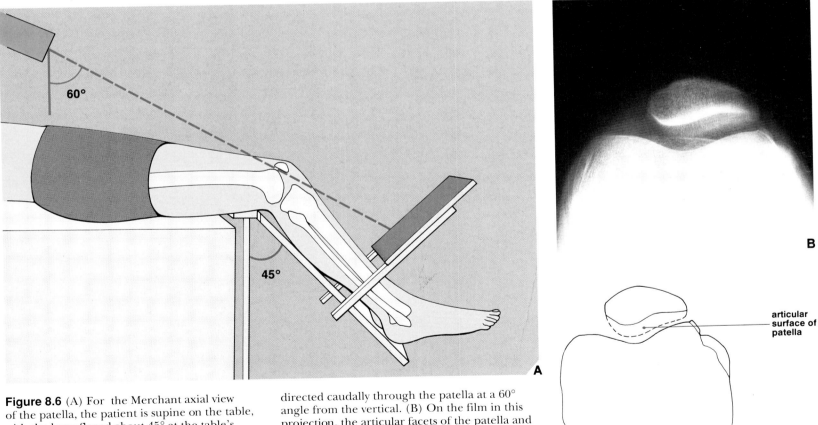

Figure 8.6 (A) For the Merchant axial view of the patella, the patient is supine on the table, with the knee flexed about 45° at the table's edge. A device keeping the knee at this angle also holds the film cassette. The central beam is directed caudally through the patella at a 60° angle from the vertical. (B) On the film in this projection, the articular facets of the patella and femur are well demonstrated.

normal relations of the patella to the femoral condyles. Subtle abnormalities in these relations may not be seen on the standard axial view due to the degree of knee flexion required for that view, which prevents the patella from subluxing.

The measurements of the femoropatellar relations obtainable from Merchant axial projection concern the sulcus angle and the congruence angle (Fig. 8.7). Normally, the *sulcus angle,* which is described by the highest points of the femoral condyles and the deepest point of the intercondylar sulcus, measures approximately 138°. By dissecting this angle with two lines—a reference line drawn from the apex of the patella to the deepest point of the sulcus and a second line from the lowest point of the patellar articular ridge to the deepest point of the sulcus—Merchant and co-workers were able to determine the degree of congruence, or the *congruence angle,* of

the femoropatellar joint. When the deepest point of the patellar articular ridge fell medial to the reference line, the angle formed was assigned a negative value; when it fell lateral to the reference line, the angle was designated with a positive value. In 100 normal subjects included in their study, the average congruence angle was -6°. An angle of +16° or greater was found to be associated with various patellofemoral disorders, particularly lateral patellar subluxation (see Fig. 8.34). On occasion, patellofemoral disorders that are more difficult to diagnose may require, as Ficat and Hungerford recommended, additional tangential views obtained with 30°, 60°, and 90° of knee flexion.

Among the ancillary techniques available for the evaluation of injuries to the knee, tomography, arthrography, and MRI provide crucial information. Tomography is especially useful in the evalua-

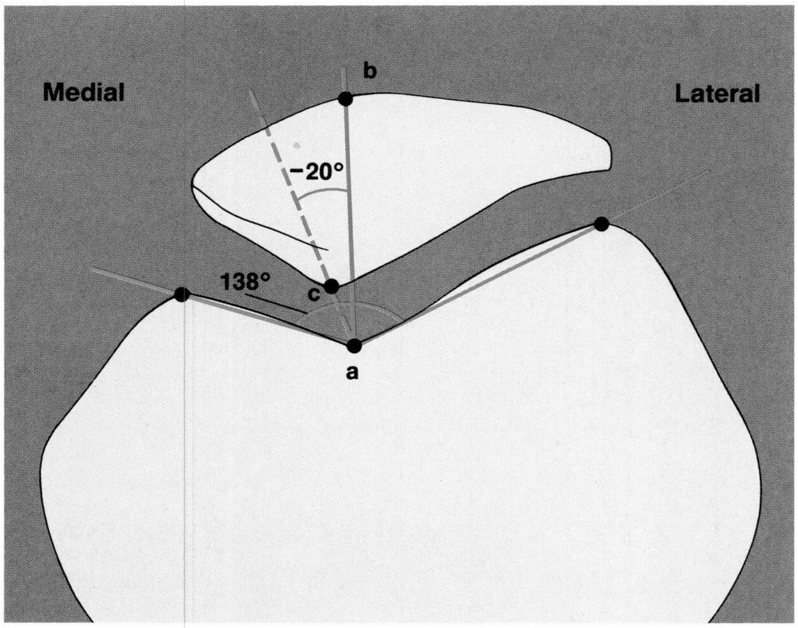

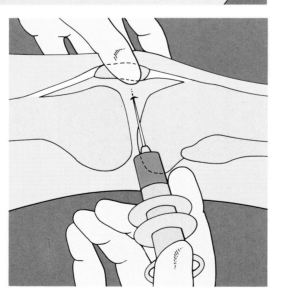

Figure 8.7 Two specific measurements can be obtained from the Merchant axial view: the sulcus angle and the congruence angle. The sulcus angle, formed by lines extending from the deepest point of the intercondylar sulcus (*a*) medially and laterally to the tops of the femoral condyles, normally measures approximately 138°. To determine the congruence angle, the sulcus angle is bisected to establish a reference line (*ba*), which is drawn to connect the apex of the patella (*b*) with the deepest point of the sulcus (*a*). In normal individuals this line is close to vertical. A second line (*ca*) is then drawn from the lowest point on the articular ridge of the patella (*c*) to the deepest point of the sulcus (*a*). The angle formed by this line and the reference line is the congruence angle. If the lowest point on the patellar articular ridge is lateral to the reference line, the congruence angle has a positive value; if it is medial to the reference line, as in the present example, the angle has a negative value. In Merchant's study, the average congruence angle in normal subjects was -6° (SD, ± 11°). (Adapted from Merchant AC, et al., 1974)

Figure 8.8 For arthrographic examination of the knee, the patient is supine on the radiographic table, with both legs fully extended and in the neutral position. The patella is pulled laterally and rotated anteriorly, and the joint is entered from the lateral aspect at the midpoint of the patella. Before injection of contrast, the joint should be aspirated to avoid dilution of the contrast medium by joint fluid. For a double contrast study, 40 mL to 50 mL of room air are injected into the joint, followed by 5 mL to 7 mL of positive contrast agent (usually 60% diatrizoate meglumine mixed with 0.3 mL of epinephrine 1:1000, which delays absorption of the contrast). Radiographs are then obtained in the prone position using the spot-film technique (see Fig. 8.10).

tion of complex fractures of the distal femur, the tibial plateaus, and the patella. In fractures of the tibial plateaus, it is effective in determining the amount of depression of the articular surface and in identifying small comminuted fragments that may be displaced into the joint, as well as comminution about the tibial spines, which may indicate avulsion of the cruciate ligaments. Tomography, by its ability to demonstrate the integrity of the anterior cortex, is also helpful in planning a surgical approach to the treatment of tibial plateau fractures.

Arthrography used to be the procedure of choice in evaluating injuries to the soft tissue structures of the knee, such as the joint capsule, menisci, and ligaments (Fig. 8.8). It is still valuable in examination of the articular cartilage, particularly when subtle chondral or osteochondral fracture is suspected, or when confirmation of the

presence or absence of osteochondral bodies in the knee joint is required in suspected osteochondritis dissecans. However, in the evaluation of the menisci, cruciate ligaments, and collateral ligaments, arthrographic examination has been almost completely replaced by magnetic resonance imaging (MRI).

The medial and lateral menisci (or semilunar cartilages) of the knee are crescent-shaped fibrocartilaginous structures attached, respectively, to the medial and lateral aspects of the superior articular surface of the tibia (Fig. 8.9). Normally, the medial meniscus is visualized on arthrography as a triangular structure intimately attached to the joint capsule and tibial (medial) collateral ligament; its smooth borders are coated by positive contrast medium and surrounded by injected air. The normal arthrogram shows no air or contrast within the substance of the meniscus or at its periphery

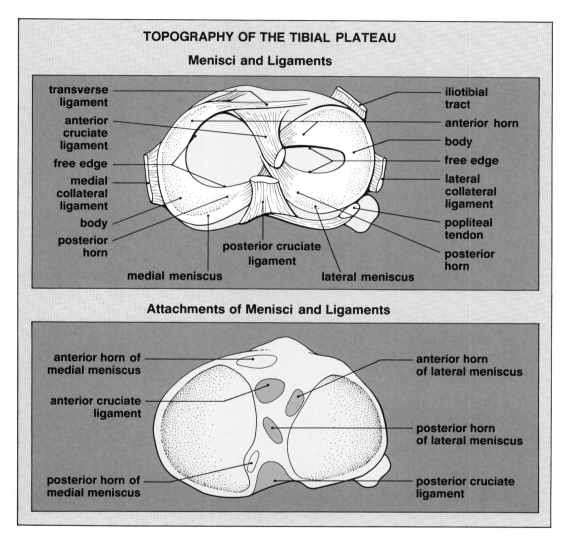

Figure 8.9 In the topography of the tibial plateau, the medial meniscus is a C-shaped fibrocartilaginous structure whose anterior horn attaches anteriorly to the intercondylar eminence of the tibia and whose posterior horn inserts into the intercondylar area in front of the attachment of the posterior cruciate ligament. The anterior horn of the lateral meniscus, which is an O-shaped structure, is attached in front of the lateral intercondylar tubercle, and the posterior horn inserts medially into the lateral intercondylar tubercle, in front of the attachment of the posterior horn of the medial meniscus.

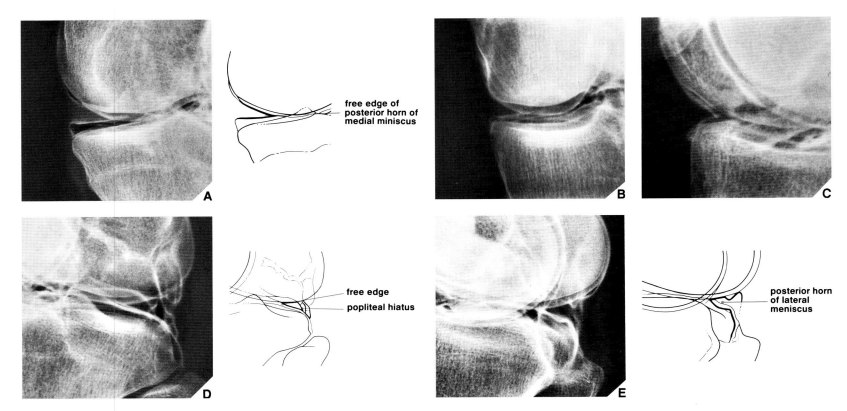

Figure 8.10 Multiple spot films obtained during arthrographic examination of the knee demonstrate the normal appearance of the medial (A-C) and lateral (D,E) semilunar cartilages. The contrast-outlined margins of the medial meniscus show its triangular shape. The posterior horn (A) is longer than the body (B) and the anterior horn (C), and the free edge of the meniscus is sharply pointed. Features of the normal lateral meniscus include the gap of the popliteal hiatus, which separates the meniscus from the joint capsule (D). The posterior horn reattaches to the capsule more posteriorly (E). No contrast should be seen within the substance of any aspect of the menisci.

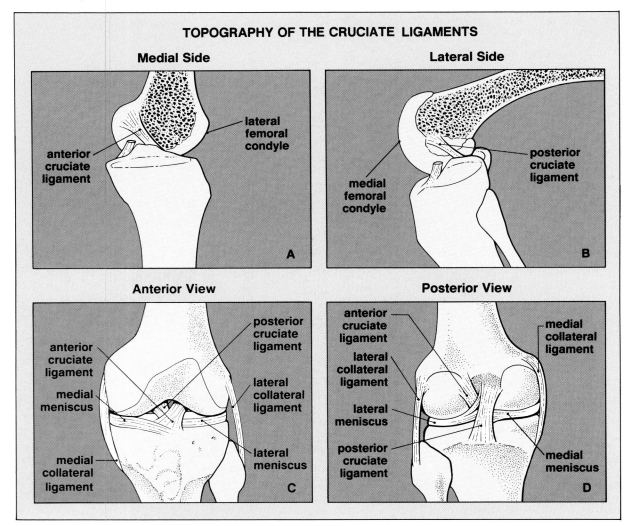

Figure 8.11 In the topography of the cruciate ligaments of the knee, the anterior cruciate ligament arises on the medial surface of the lateral femoral condyle at the intercondylar notch (A) and attaches on the anterior portion of the intercondylar eminence of the tibia (C) (see also Fig. 8.9). The posterior cruciate ligament originates on the lateral surface of the medial femoral condyle within the intercondylar notch (B) and inserts on the posterior surface of the intercondylar eminence (D) (see also Fig. 8.9). Neither cruciate ligament is attached to the tibial tubercles.

(Fig. 8.10A-C). Although the lateral meniscus is structurally very similar to the medial meniscus, it has a very important distinguishing feature. The popliteal muscle's tendon and its sheath pass through a portion of the posterior horn of the lateral meniscus, separating it from the joint capsule. This anatomic site, known as the *popliteal hiatus*, gives an arthrographic impression of separation of the periphery of the lateral meniscus from the capsule; it should not be mistaken for a tear (Fig. 8.10D,E). An important fact to remember is that not all areas of the menisci are well demonstrated by knee arthrography. Only the parts seen tangentially can accurately be assessed. For example, the posterior part of the posterior horn of the lateral meniscus constitutes a blind spot, because it extends deeply into the knee joint (see Fig. 8.9).

The cruciate ligaments of the knee are also structures commonly subject to injury (Fig. 8.11). In the evaluation of these ligaments, arthrography was the procedure of choice before the MRI era, and even now is occasionally performed. The radiograph is obtained to best advantage in the lateral projection with 60° to 80° of knee flexion and with the examiner applying pressure to the posterior aspect of the proximal tibia. When tensed, the anterior cruciate ligament normally projects as a straight line extending from the intercondylar notch to a point approximately 8 mm posterior to the anterior margin of the tibia. The posterior cruciate ligament is seen as a straight or slightly bulging line extending to the posterior margin of the tibial plateau (Fig. 8.12).

In the past few years, MRI of the knee has gained wide acceptance in the diagnosis of traumatic abnormalities, and currently is the method of choice in evaluating various knee structures, particularly the menisci, cruciate ligaments, and collateral ligaments. Routinely, T1- and T2-weighted images are obtained in the sagittal, coronal, and axial planes. The sagittal plane is generally the most effective for evaluation of the cruciate ligaments, menisci, patellar ligament and quadriceps tendon. Coronal sections are needed for evaluation of the medial and lateral collateral ligaments, as well as the menisci. The axial plane is best to evaluate the patellofemoral joint compartment. The axial plane is also helpful in evaluating the popliteal cysts and their relationship to the surrounding structures of the popliteal fossa.

The menisci are seen on MRI as wedged-shaped or bow-tie-shaped structures of uniformly low signal intensity in practically all pulse sequences (Fig. 8.13). The anterior and posterior cruciate ligaments, like the menisci, are seen as low-signal intensity structures on all spin echo sequences. The anterior cruciate ligament is straight and fan-shaped (slightly wider at its femoral attachment) and

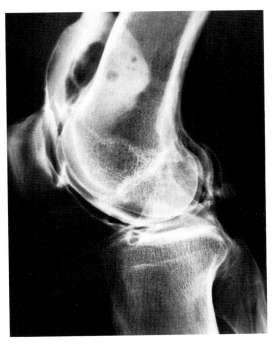

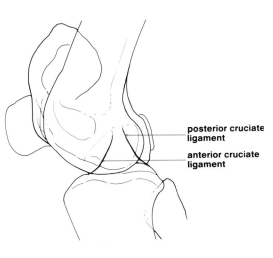

posterior cruciate ligament

anterior cruciate ligament

Figure 8.12 Double-contrast arthrogram of the knee demonstrates the normal appearance of the cruciate ligaments. Note the angle formed by their projectional intersection and their taut appearance. Each ligament can be traced from its origin in the femur to its insertion in the tibia. The boundaries of the cruciate ligaments are sharply outlined because the contrast medium coats their synovial reflexions. The cruciate ligaments are extrasynovial structures; only the anterior surface of the anterior cruciate ligament and the posterior surface of the posterior cruciate ligament are covered by synovium.

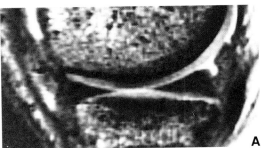

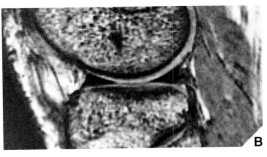

A   **B**

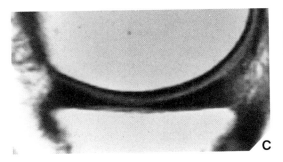

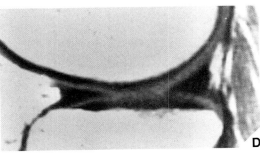

C   **D**

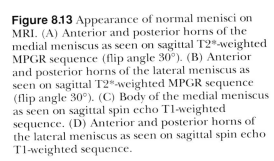

Figure 8.13 Appearance of normal menisci on MRI. (A) Anterior and posterior horns of the medial meniscus as seen on sagittal T2*-weighted MPGR sequence (flip angle 30°). (B) Anterior and posterior horns of the lateral meniscus as seen on sagittal T2*-weighted MPGR sequence (flip angle 30°). (C) Body of the medial meniscus as seen on sagittal spin echo T1-weighted sequence. (D) Anterior and posterior horns of the lateral meniscus as seen on sagittal spin echo T1-weighted sequence.

demonstrates low-to-intermediate signal intensity (Fig. 8.14A). The posterior cruciate ligament is arcuate in shape when the knee is in extension or mild flexion and becomes increasingly taut as the knee is flexed. Normally, it has a very low signal intensity (Fig. 8.14B).

The medial and lateral collateral ligaments are best demonstrated on the images obtained in the coronal plane. Like the menisci and cruciate ligaments, they also display low signal intensity (Fig. 8.15).

Evaluation of knee instability due to ligament injuries may require obtaining stress views. These techniques are most commonly performed in cases of suspected injury to the medial collateral ligament (Fig. 8.16; see also Fig. 8.56B). They are less frequently performed during the evaluation of insufficiency of the anterior and posterior cruciate ligaments (Fig. 8.17). These examinations should preferably be performed under local anesthesia.

Arteriography and venography may need to be employed in the evaluation of concomitant injury to the vascular system. Computed tomography (CT) has a limited application in knee injuries, although it is occasionally used to evaluate injury to the cartilage and soft tissues, particularly the menisci and cruciate ligaments. CT used in conjunction with arthrography (computed arthrotomography) is useful in the evaluation of osteochondritis dissecans (see Fig. 8.43) and in detecting non-opaque osteochondral bodies in the knee joint.

For a summary of the preceding discussion in tabular form see Figures 8.18, 8.19, and 8.20.

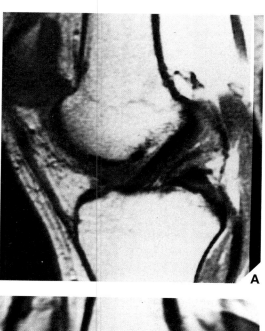
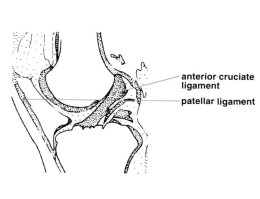

anterior cruciate ligament

patellar ligament

A

Figure 8.14 Spin echo sagittal MR images (TR 2000/TE 20) of the normal cruciate ligaments. (A) Anterior margin of the anterior cruciate ligament is straight and well-defined; the posterior margin is ill-defined due to the oblique orientation of the ligament. (B) The posterior cruciate ligament is seen in its entirety, in one plane, from the femoral to the tibial attachments. Observe the small bulge anteriorly produced by the anterior meniscofemoral ligament. (From Beltran J, 1990)

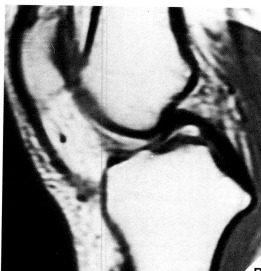
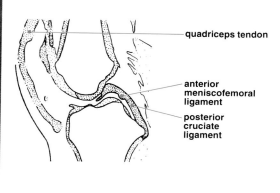

quadriceps tendon

anterior meniscofemoral ligament

posterior cruciate ligament

B

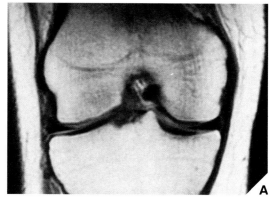
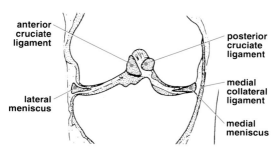

Figure 8.15 (A) Spin echo coronal MR image (TR 2000/TE 20) of the normal medial collateral ligament. The medial collateral ligament is well defined in this section through the intercondylar notch. The insertion of the posterior cruciate ligament in the inner aspect of the medial femoral condyle is well demonstrated. The menisci are seen as small triangles of low signal intensity. (B) Spin echo coronal MR image (TR 2000/TE 20) of the lateral (fibular) collateral ligament. On this posterior section note the meniscofemoral ligament, which extends from the posterior horn of the lateral meniscus to the inner surface of the medial femoral condyle. The lateral and medial menisci and posterior cruciate ligament are well demonstrated. (From Beltran J, 1990)

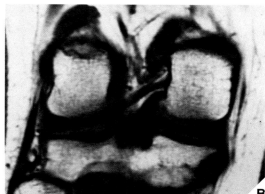
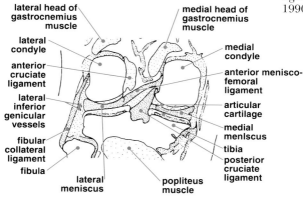

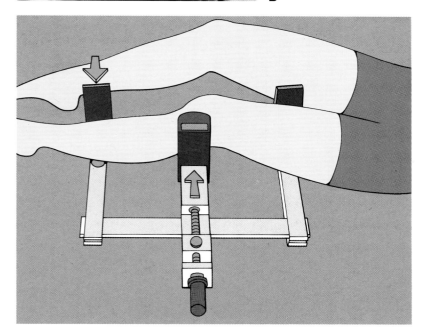
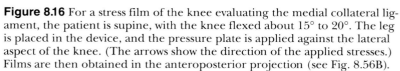

Figure 8.16 For a stress film of the knee evaluating the medial collateral ligament, the patient is supine, with the knee flexed about 15° to 20°. The leg is placed in the device, and the pressure plate is applied against the lateral aspect of the knee. (The arrows show the direction of the applied stresses.) Films are then obtained in the anteroposterior projection (see Fig. 8.56B).

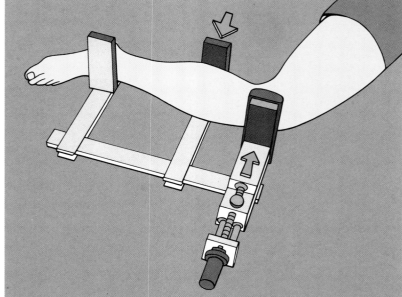

Figure 8.17 For a stress film of the knee evaluating the anterior cruciate ligament, the patient is placed in the device on his or her side, with the knee flexed 90°. The pressure plate is applied against the anterior aspect of the knee. (The arrows show the direction of the applied stresses.) Films are then obtained in the lateral projection.

Figure 8.18 Standard and Special Radiographic Projections for Evaluating Injury to the Knee

PROJECTION	DEMONSTRATION	PROJECTION	DEMONSTRATION

Anteroposterior	Medial and lateral joint compartments
	Varus and valgus deformities
	Fractures of:
	    Medial and lateral femoral condyles
	    Medial and lateral tibial plateaus
	    Tibial spines
	    Proximal fibula
	Osteochondral fracture
	Osteochondritis dissecans (late stage)
	Spontaneous osteonecrosis
	Pellegrini-Stieda lesion
		Lateral (continued)	Sinding-Larsen-Johansson disease*
			Osgood-Schlatter disease*
			Osteochondral fracture
			Osteochondritis dissecans (late stage)
			Spontaneous osteonecrosis
			Joint effusion
			Tears of:
			    Quadriceps tendon
			    Patellar ligament

Overpenetrated	Bi- or multipartite patella Fractures of patella	Stress	Tears of cruciate ligaments
Stress	Tear of collateral ligaments	Cross-table	FBI sign of lipohemarthrosis

Lateral	Femoropatellar joint compartment
	Patella in profile
	Suprapatellar bursa
	Fractures of:
	    Distal femur
	    Proximal tibia
	    Patella
		Tunnel
		(posteroanterior)
			Posterior aspect of femoral condyles
			Intercondylar notch
			Intercondylar eminence of tibia

		Axial **(sunrise and Merchant)**	Articular facets of patella† Sulcus angle† Congruence angle† Fractures of patella Subluxation and dislocation of patella†

* These conditions are best demonstrated using a low kilovoltage/soft tissue technique.
† These features are better demonstrated on Merchant axial view.

Figure 8.19 Ancillary Imaging Techniques for Evaluating Injury to the Knee

TECHNIQUE	DEMONSTRATION	TECHNIQUE	DEMONSTRATION

Tomography	Position of fragments and extension of fracture line in complex fractures of:
	    Distal femur
	    Proximal tibia
	    Patella
	Quantification of depression in tibial plateau fractures
	Healing process:
	    Nonunion
	    Secondary infection
		Arthrography (continued)	Osteochondral bodies in joint
			Subtle abnormalities of articular cartilage
			Spontaneous osteonecrosis

		Computed Tomography and Computed Arthrotomography	Injuries to:
			    Articular cartilage
			    Cruciate ligaments
			    Menisci
			Osteochondral bodies in joint
			Osteochondritis dissecans

Arthrography
(usually double-contrast; occasionally single-contrast using air only)
	Meniscal tears
	Injuries to:
	    Cruciate ligaments
	    Medial collateral ligament
	    Quadriceps tendon
	    Patellar ligament
	    Joint capsule
	Chondral and osteochondral fractures
	Osteochondritis dissecans (early and late stages)
		Radionuclide Imaging
		(scintigraphy, bone scan)
		
		Angiography
		(arteriography, venography)
		
		Magnetic Resonance Imaging
			Subtle fractures not demonstrated on standard studies
			Early and late stages of:
			    Osteochondritis dissecans
			    Spontaneous osteonecrosis
			
			Concomitant injury to arteries and veins
			
			Same as arthrography, computed tomography, and radionuclide imaging

SPECTRUM OF RADIOLOGIC IMAGING TECHNIQUES
FOR EVALUATING INJURY TO THE KNEE*

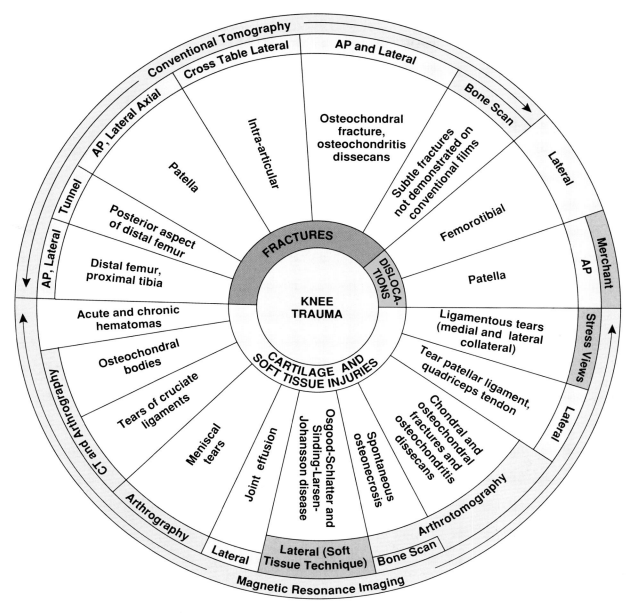

*The radiographic projections or radiologic techniques indicated throughout the diagram
are only those that are the most effective in demonstrating the respective traumatic conditions.

Figure 8.20 Spectrum of radiologic imaging techniques for evaluating injury to the knee.

Injury to the Knee

Fractures about the Knee

FRACTURES OF THE DISTAL FEMUR Most often sustained in motor vehicle accidents or falls from heights, fractures of the distal femur are classified according to the site and extension of the fracture line as supracondylar, condylar, and intercondylar. Supracondylar fractures can be further classified as nondisplaced, impacted, displaced, and comminuted (Fig. 8.21). These injuries are usually well demonstrated on the standard anteroposterior and lateral projections of the knee (Fig. 8.22), although in rare instances an oblique view of the knee may be needed to evaluate an obliquely oriented fracture

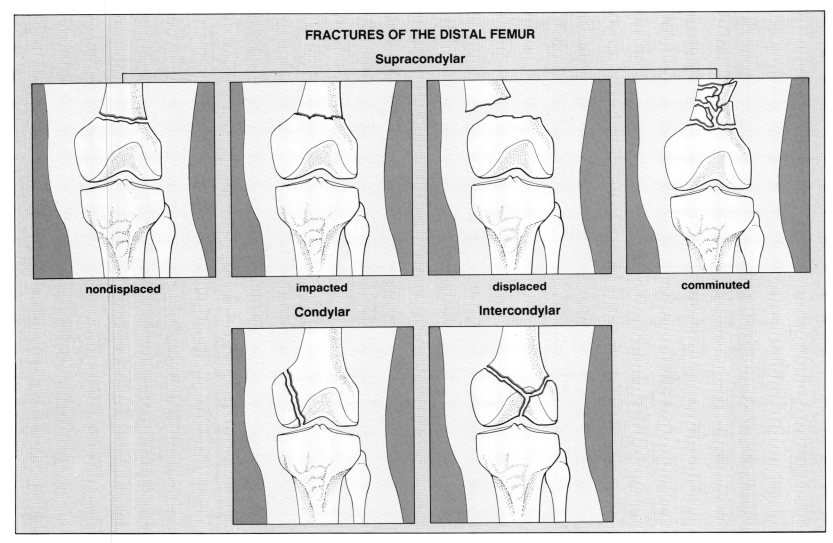

FRACTURES OF THE DISTAL FEMUR

Supracondylar

nondisplaced   impacted   displaced   comminuted

Condylar   **Intercondylar**

Figure 8.21 Fractures of the distal femur can be classified according to the site and extension of the injury as supracondylar, condylar, and intercondylar fractures.

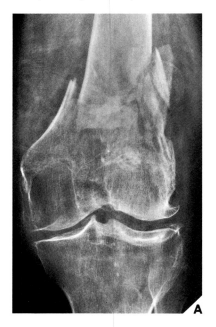
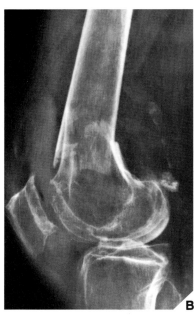
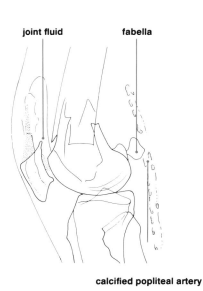

joint fluid   fabella

calcified popliteal artery

Figure 8.22 A 58-year-old man was involved in a motorcycle accident. Anteroposterior (A) and lateral (B) views of the knee demonstrate a comminuted supracondylar fracture of the distal femur. The extension of the fracture lines and the position of the fragments can adequately be assessed on these standard studies.

line. Tomography may also be required in cases of comminution for a full evaluation of the fracture lines and localization of the fragments (Fig. 8.23).

FRACTURES OF THE PROXIMAL TIBIA The medial and lateral tibial plateaus are the most common sites of fractures of the proximal tibia.

Because they usually result when the knee is struck by a moving vehicle, they are also called "fender" or "bumper" fractures; some, however, may be the result of twisting falls. The Hohl classification gives an overview of six different types of tibial plateau fractures and is useful in correlating the various types of injuries with the applied forces causing them (Fig. 8.24). In the Hohl classification, pure abduction

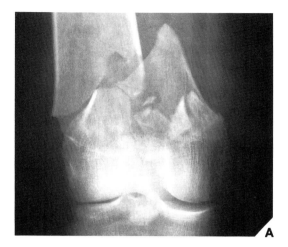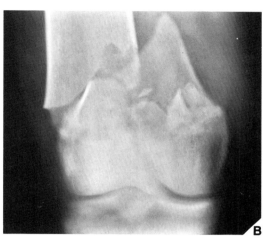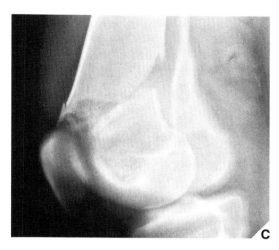

Figure 8.23 A 22-year-old racing car driver was injured in an accident on the track. (A) Anteroposterior view of the right knee shows a comminuted fracture of the distal femur. Tomography was performed, and sections in the anteroposterior (B) and lateral (C) projections demonstrate intra-articular extension of the fracture lines, with split of the condyles and posterior displacement of the distal fragments. The multiple comminuted fragments can be localized.

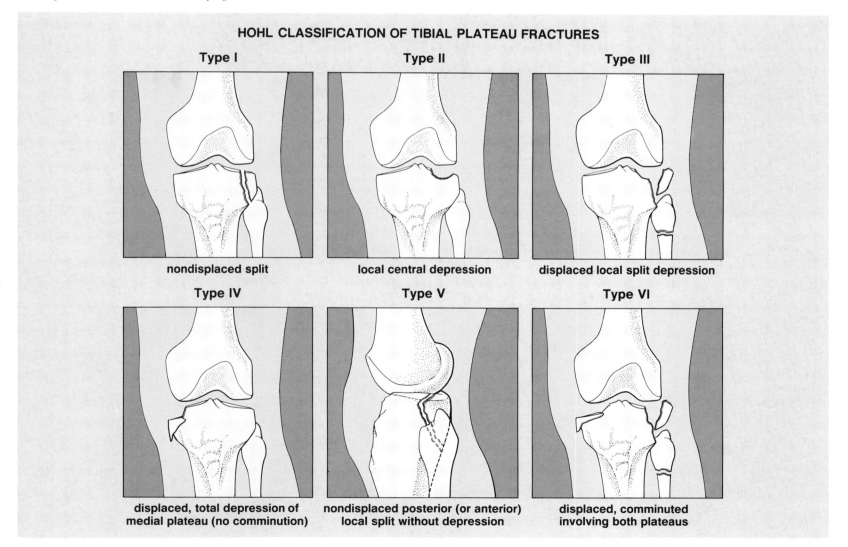

Figure 8.24 The Hohl classification of fractures of the tibial plateau. (Adapted from Hohl M, 1967)

injury results in a nondisplaced split fracture of the lateral tibial plateau (type I) (Fig. 8.25). When axial compression is combined with abduction force, local central depression (type II) and local split depression (type III) fractures occur (Fig. 8.26). Total depression fractures (type IV), which are more commonly seen in the medial tibial plateau because of its anatomic configuration (absence of the fibula), are characterized by lack of comminution of the articular surface. Type V fractures in the Hohl classification, which are infrequently encountered, are local split fractures without central depression involving the anterior or posterior aspects of the tibial plateau. Comminuted fractures involving both tibial plateaus and having a Y or T configuration (type VI) usually result from vertical compression, such as a fall on the extended leg (Fig. 8.27). Types III and VI are frequently associated with fracture of the proximal fibula.

Fractures of the tibial plateau may not be obvious on the routine radiographic examination of the knee, particularly if there is no depression (Fig. 8.28A,B). In such cases, however, the cross-table lateral projection often reveals the FBI sign, which indicates the presence of an intra-articular fracture (Fig. 8.28C). Demonstration of an obscure fracture line may require oblique projections, but tomographic examination may reveal the fracture line and demonstrate its extension (Fig. 8.28D). If the fracture is depressed, tomography can also help quantify the degree of depression (Fig. 8.29).

An important feature of tibial plateau fractures is their association with injury to ligaments and the menisci. The structures most at risk are the medial collateral and the anterior cruciate ligaments (see Fig 8.11) and the lateral meniscus (see Fig. 8.9), since lateral tibial plateau fractures usually result from valgus stress (Fig. 8.30).

Moreover, damage to the anterior cruciate ligament may be associated with avulsion of the lateral tibial spine or the anterior intercondylar eminence. Stress views and MRI usually reveal these associated abnormalities. If clinical examination and radiologic studies, including stress views, show ligamentous structures to be intact, nondisplaced fractures of the tibial plateau can be treated conservatively. In depression-type fractures, however, Larson recommends open reduction in patients whose fractures show 8 mm of articular depression. Generally, surgery is indicated for fractures of the tibial plateau showing articular depression of 10 mm or more.

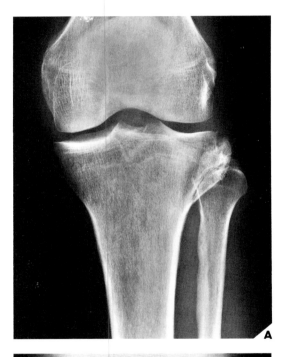

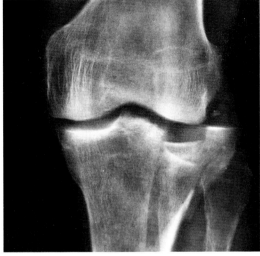

Figure 8.26 Anteroposterior view of the knee shows the appearance of a tibial plateau fracture, which is a combination of wedge and central depression fractures involving the lateral tibial condyle.

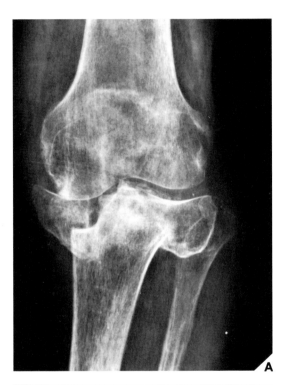

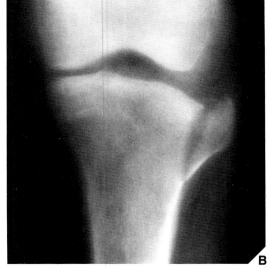

Figure 8.25 A 30-year-old alcoholic was hit by a car while he was crossing the street. Anteroposterior plain film (A) and tomogram (B) show a wedge fracture of the lateral tibial plateau.

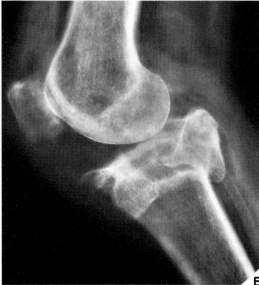

Figure 8.27 Anteroposterior plain film (A) and lateral tomogram (B) demonstrate the characteristic appearance of the Y-type bicondylar tibial fracture.

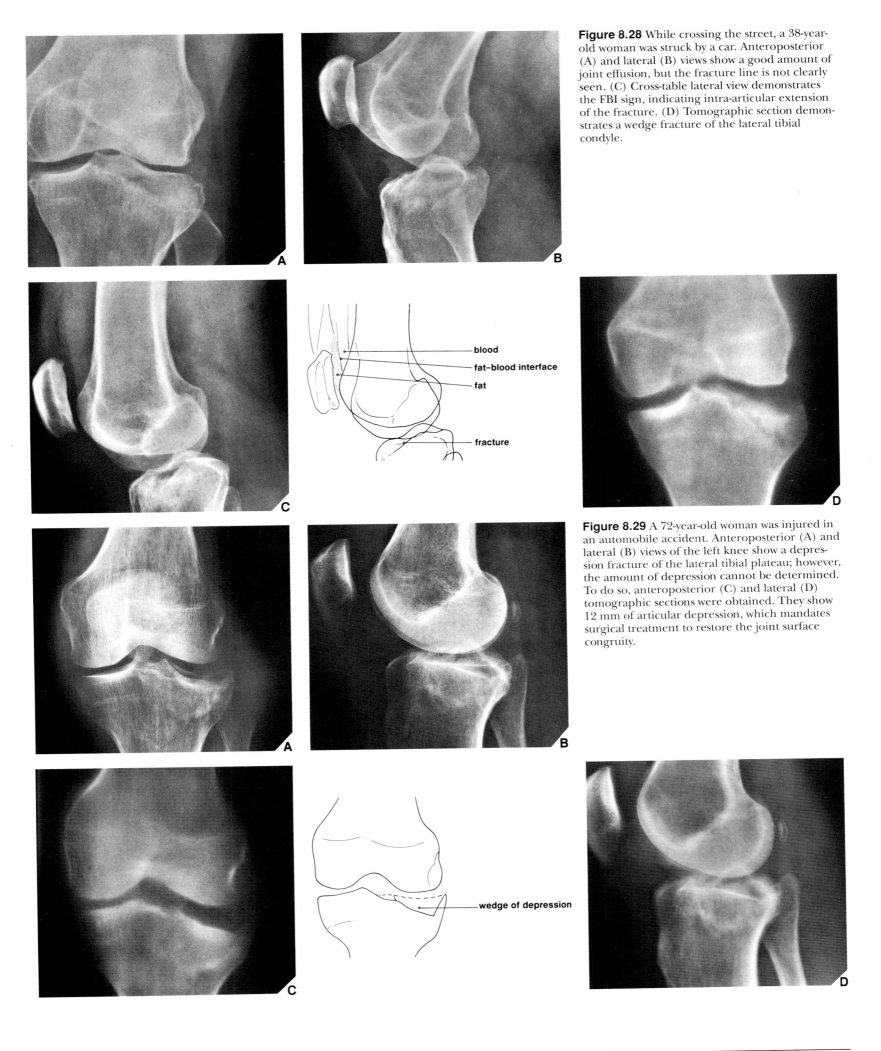

Figure 8.28 While crossing the street, a 38-year-old woman was struck by a car. Anteroposterior (A) and lateral (B) views show a good amount of joint effusion, but the fracture line is not clearly seen. (C) Cross-table lateral view demonstrates the FBI sign, indicating intra-articular extension of the fracture. (D) Tomographic section demonstrates a wedge fracture of the lateral tibial condyle.

Figure 8.29 A 72-year-old woman was injured in an automobile accident. Anteroposterior (A) and lateral (B) views of the left knee show a depression fracture of the lateral tibial plateau; however, the amount of depression cannot be determined. To do so, anteroposterior (C) and lateral (D) tomographic sections were obtained. They show 12 mm of articular depression, which mandates surgical treatment to restore the joint surface congruity.

COMPLICATIONS The most frequent complications of fractures of the distal femur and the proximal tibia are malunion and posttraumatic arthritis.

FRACTURES AND DISLOCATIONS OF THE PATELLA Fractures of the patella, which may result from a direct blow to the anterior aspect of the knee or from indirect tension forces generated by the quadriceps tendon, constitute about 1% of all skeletal injuries. Generally, patellar fractures may be longitudinal (vertical), transverse, or comminuted (Fig. 8.31). In the most commonly encountered patellar injury, seen in 60% of cases, the fracture line is transverse or slightly oblique, involving the midportion of the patella. In evaluation of such injury, it is important to recognize what has been called the bipartite or multipartite patella. This anomaly represents a developmental variant of the accessory ossification center or centers of the superolateral margin of the patella and should not be mistaken for a fracture (Fig. 8.32). Tomography may help distinguish this developmental anomaly from patellar fracture. As an aid to avoid misdiagnosing a bipartite or multipartite patella as a fracture, it is important to keep in mind that the accessory ossification centers are invariably in the upper lateral quadrant of the patella and, if the apparent fragments are put together, they do not form a normal patella. Fracture fragments, on the other hand, form a normal patella if they are replaced. Injury to the patella is usually sufficiently demonstrated on the overpenetrated anteroposterior and lateral views of the knee (Fig. 8.33).

Dislocations of the patella, which are usually lateral, result from acute injury and are easily diagnosed on the standard projections of the knee. Subluxations of the patella, on the other hand, are much more common than true dislocations and usually result from chronic injury. The best radiographic examination for demonstrating patellar subluxation, particularly in subtle cases, is the Merchant axial view (Fig. 8.34).

Sinding-Larsen-Johansson and Osgood-Schlatter Diseases
These conditions, which are seen predominantly in adolescents, are now considered to be related to trauma. They occur at either end of the patellar ligament: Sinding-Larsen-Johansson disease at its proximal end, where it attaches to the lower pole (apex) of the patella;

Figure 8.30 Lateral tibial plateau fractures, which result from valgus stress, are often associated with tears of the lateral meniscus and the medial collateral and anterior cruciate ligaments.

torn anterior cruciate ligament

torn lateral meniscus

torn medial collateral ligament

wedge fracture of tibial plateau

Figure 8.31 Classification of patellar fractures. (Adapted from Hohl M, Larson RL, 1975)

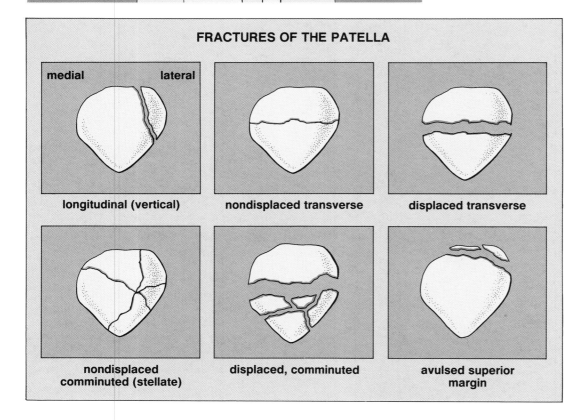

FRACTURES OF THE PATELLA

medial   lateral

longitudinal (vertical)

nondisplaced transverse

displaced transverse

nondisplaced comminuted (stellate)

displaced, comminuted

avulsed superior margin

and Osgood-Schlatter disease at its distal end, where it attaches to the tibial tubercle (tuberosity).

Sinding-Larsen-Johansson disease is characterized clinically by local pain and tenderness on palpation and radiographically by separation and fragmentation of the lower pole of the patella, associated with soft tissue swelling and, occasionally, calcifications at the site of the patellar ligament. The lateral radiograph, obtained with a low-kilovoltage/soft tissue technique, is the single most important examination (Fig. 8.35); in combination with a positive clinical examination, it usually establishes the diagnosis.

Osgood-Schlatter disease, which occurs three times more frequently in adolescent boys than in adolescent girls, is characterized by fragmentation of the tibial tubercle and soft tissue swelling anterior to it. In 25% to 33% of all reported cases, the condition is bilateral. As in Sinding-Larsen-Johansson disease, the lateral film, obtained using a soft tissue technique, is most effective in demonstrating this condition (Fig. 8.36). However, an accurate diagnosis is based on both radiographic and clinical findings. Soft tissue swelling is a fundamental diagnostic feature.

Occasionally, Sinding-Larsen-Johansson and Osgood-Schlatter diseases may coexist. It is important to remember that the presence of multiple ossification centers in the tibial tuberosity and lower pole of the patella may at times mimic these conditions. However, the absence of soft tissue swelling in such cases allows the distinction to be made.

Injuries to the Cartilage of the Knee

Osteochondral (or chondral) fracture, osteochondritis dissecans, and spontaneous osteonecrosis are three conditions with similar radiologic appearances. They are invariably confused with each other, and in many instances the terms are used interchangeably. They represent, however, three separate orthopedic entities, each with a specific etiology and each requiring a specific treatment. Usually,

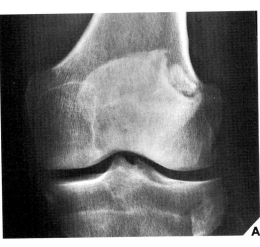
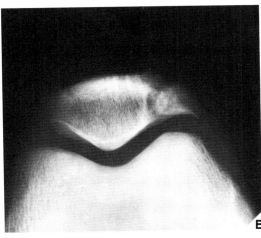
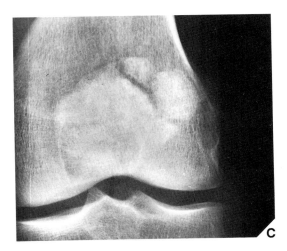

Figure 8.32 Anteroposterior (A) and axial (B) views demonstrate the typical appearance of a bipartite patella. Note the position of the accessory ossification center at the superolateral margin of the patella. (C) A tripartite patella was an incidental finding on this overpenetrated anteroposterior film, which was obtained to exclude the possibility of gouty arthritis.

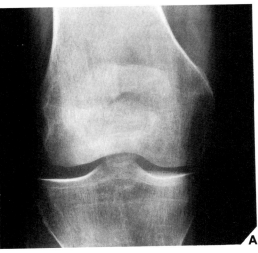
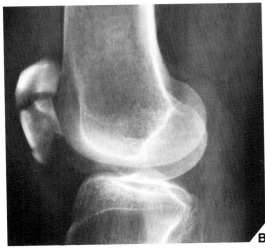

Figure 8.33 After a fall on the stairs, a 63-year-old man presented with severe pain in the anterior aspect of the right knee. Anteroposterior (A) and lateral (B) films show the typical appearance of fracture of the patella. Note the large amount of suprapatellar joint effusion.

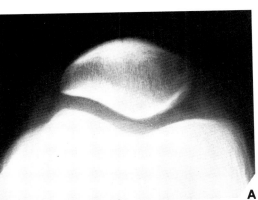
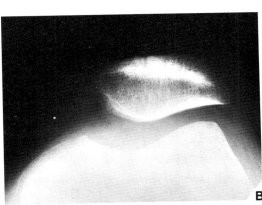

Figure 8.34 A 23-year-old woman complained of occasional knee pain and buckling, particularly while jogging. (A) Standard axial view of the patella shows no apparent abnormalities. (B) Merchant axial view, however, demonstrates lateral subluxation of the patella. Note the positive congruence angle (see Fig. 8.7).

history, physical examination, and radiographic presentation can help distinguish these conditions from one another.

OSTEOCHONDRAL (OR CHONDRAL) FRACTURE Shearing, rotary, or tangentially aligned impaction forces directed to the knee joint may result in acute injury to the articular end of the femur. The resulting fracture may involve cartilage only—chondral fracture—or cartilage and the underlying subchondral segment of bone—osteochondral fracture (Fig. 8.37). These fractures, which may occur in either of the femoral or tibial condyles, the tibial plateau, and the patella, may range in severity from minimal indentation of the articular surface to displacement of an osteochondral fragment into the joint. Since a chondral fracture involves only articular cartilage, it can be demonstrated either by arthrography or MRI. An osteochondral fracture, on the other hand, may be seen on a plain-film radiograph, particularly if the fragment has been dislodged. The presence of such a fragment in the joint may be indistinguishable from the radiographic appearance of osteochondritis dissecans (see below). However, a clinical history of acute injury sustained in sports-related activities, such as football, soccer, or skiing, and associated with symptoms such as severe pain, local tenderness, and often joint effusion, is invariably helpful in making a distinction between these similar conditions (Fig. 8.38).

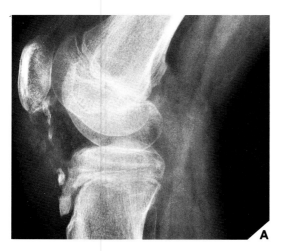
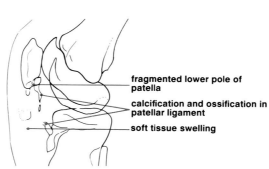
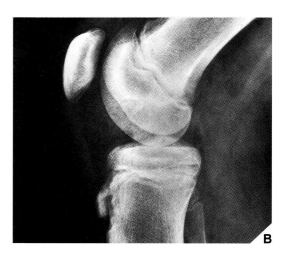

Figure 8.35 A 13-year-old boy complained of pain and swelling at the site of the patellar ligament. He had no history of acute trauma. (A) Lateral view of the right knee, obtained with a low kilovoltage/soft-tissue technique, shows fragmentation of the lower pole of the patella and significant soft tissue swelling associated with calcifications and ossifications of the patellar ligament—findings characteristic of Sinding-Larsen-Johansson disease. (B) The normal left knee is shown for comparison.

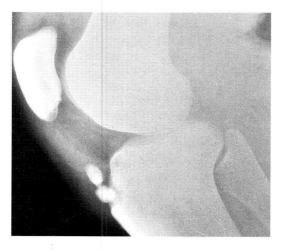
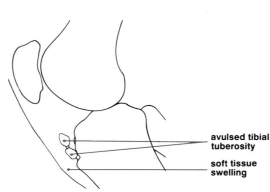

Figure 8.36 A 12-year-old boy had severe tenderness over the left tibial tuberosity. The lateral film, obtained with a soft tissue technique, reveals fragmentation of the tibial tuberosity in association with soft tissue swelling—characteristic findings in Osgood-Schlatter disease.

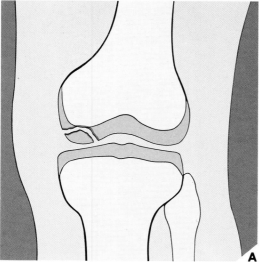
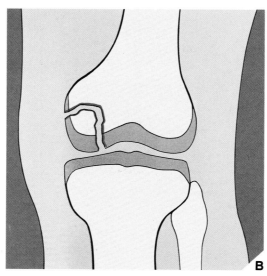

Figure 8.37 A chondral fracture (A) affects only the cartilage, whereas an osteochondral fracture (B) involves both the cartilage and the subchondral segment of bone.

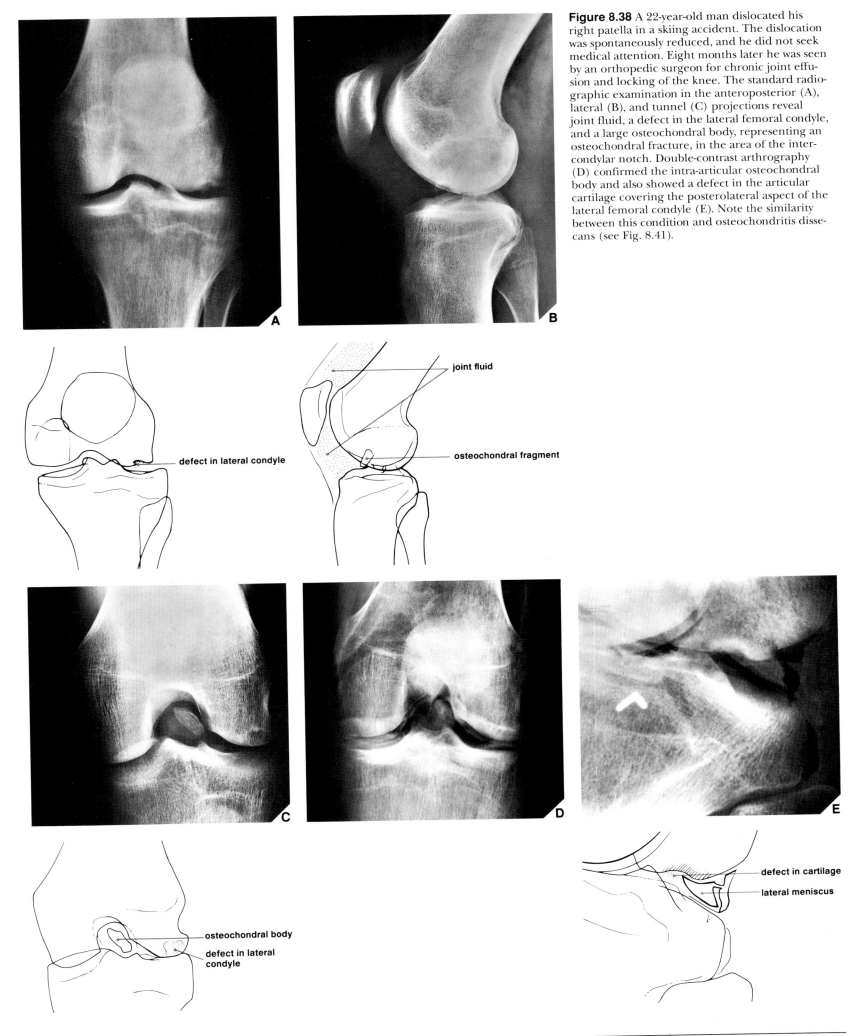

Figure 8.38 A 22-year-old man dislocated his right patella in a skiing accident. The dislocation was spontaneously reduced, and he did not seek medical attention. Eight months later he was seen by an orthopedic surgeon for chronic joint effusion and locking of the knee. The standard radiographic examination in the anteroposterior (A), lateral (B), and tunnel (C) projections reveal joint fluid, a defect in the lateral femoral condyle, and a large osteochondral body, representing an osteochondral fracture, in the area of the intercondylar notch. Double-contrast arthrography (D) confirmed the intra-articular osteochondral body and also showed a defect in the articular cartilage covering the posterolateral aspect of the lateral femoral condyle (E). Note the similarity between this condition and osteochondritis dissecans (see Fig. 8.41).

joint fluid

defect in lateral condyle

osteochondral fragment

osteochondral body

defect in lateral condyle

defect in cartilage

lateral meniscus

OSTEOCHONDRITIS DISSECANS This relatively common condition, seen predominantly in adolescents and young adults and more often in males than in females, has recently come to be considered a form of osteochondral fracture caused not by acute, but by chronic injury. As in acute osteochondral fractures, shearing or rotary forces applied to the articular surface of the femur result in detachment of a fragment of articular cartilage, often together with a segment of subchondral bone.

Aichroth has pointed out that the separated segment is avascular and this feature distinguishes osteochondritis dissecans from acute osteochondral fracture. In a clinical survey of osteochondritis dissecans in 200 patients, he also determined the distribution of the lesion. The most common location was the lateral aspect of the medial femoral condyle, a nonweight-bearing segment; other sites were less commonly affected (Fig. 8.39). The degree of damage to the articular cartilage, as in acute osteochondral fractures, varies from an in situ osteochondral body, to an osteocartilaginous flap, to complete detachment of an osteochondral segment (Fig. 8.40).

In the early stages of the disease, plain radiographs in the standard projections usually show no abnormality. The only positive finding may be joint effusion. In more advanced stages of the disease, a radiolucent line is seen separating the osteochondral body from the femoral condyle (Fig. 8.41). For the orthopedic management of this condition, it is important to evaluate the status of the articular cartilage. Double-contrast arthrography can differentiate an in situ lesion from a more advanced lesion, where the osteochondral body is partially or completely detached from its bed (Fig. 8.42). Separation of the fragment mandates surgical intervention. Sometimes, other special techniques may need to be employed, such as using only air as a contrast medium, combining arthrogra-

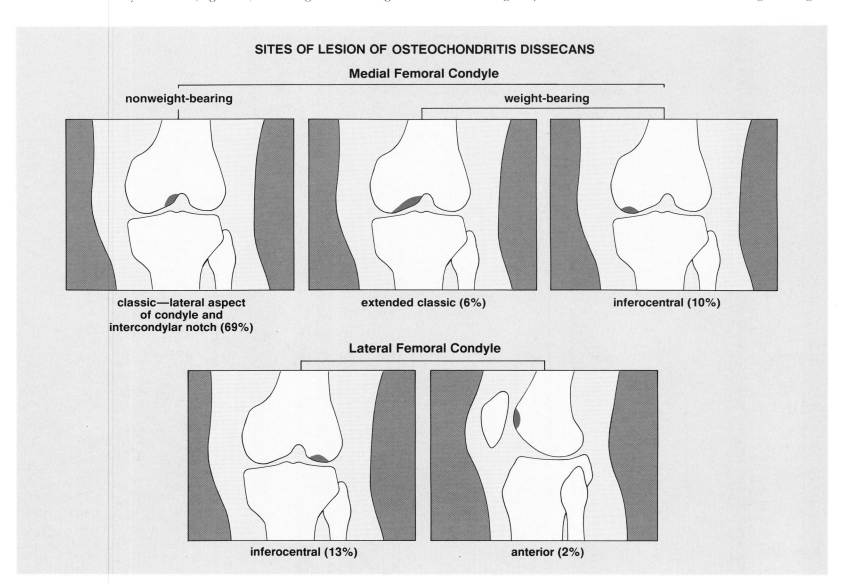

Figure 8.39 Osteochondritis dissecans most frequently affects the medial femoral condyle, the nonweight-bearing portion (the lateral aspect of the condyle and the intercondylar notch), which is the most common site of the lesion. The lateral femoral condyle is much less commonly involved. (Adapted from Aichroth P, 1971)

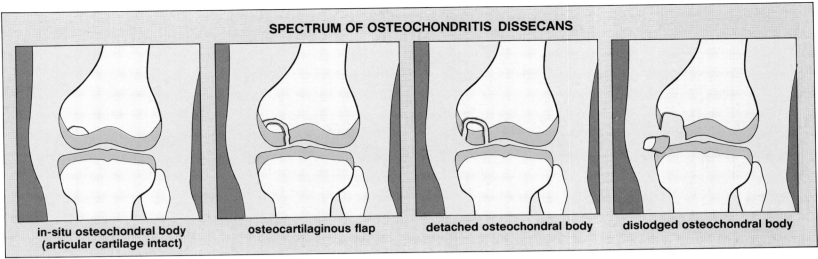

SPECTRUM OF OSTEOCHONDRITIS DISSECANS

in-situ osteochondral body (articular cartilage intact)

osteocartilaginous flap

detached osteochondral body

dislodged osteochondral body

Figure 8.40 The spectrum of chronic injury to the articular end of the distal femur (osteochondritis dissecans) ranges from an in situ lesion to a defect in the subchondral bone associated with a dislodged osteochondral body.

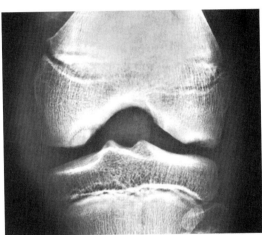

Figure 8.41 An ll-year-old boy complained of pain in his right knee for three months. Anteroposterior view of the knee shows the typical lesion of osteochondritis dissecans in the medial femoral condyle. A radiolucent line separates the oval-shaped, in situ body from the femoral condyle. Incidentally, the lateral femoral condyle shows an irregular outline of the weightbearing segment. This finding represents a developmental variant in ossification and is of no further consequence.

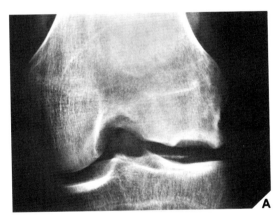
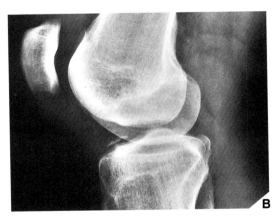
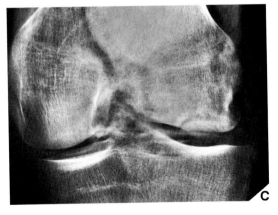

Figure 8.42 A 23-year-old man presented with complaints of chronic pain in the knee for four months. He had no history of acute trauma in recent years. Tunnel (A) and lateral (B) views show a defect in the subchondral bone at the inferocentral aspect of the lateral femoral condyle and an osteo- chondral fragment that has been discharged into the joint. Arthrography was performed to evaluate the articular cartilage. The arthrogram (C) shows contrast filling the subchondral defect, indicating damage to the articular cartilage.

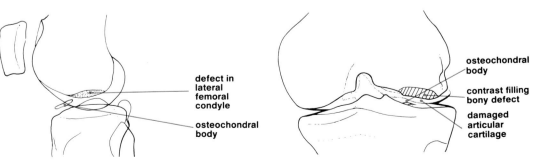

defect in lateral femoral condyle

osteochondral body

osteochondral body

contrast filling bony defect

damaged articular cartilage

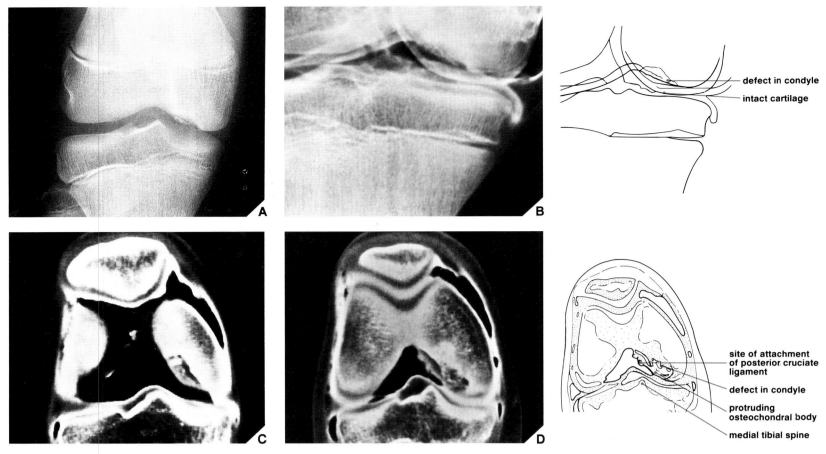

defect in condyle
intact cartilage

site of attachment
of posterior cruciate
ligament

defect in condyle

protruding
osteochondral body

medial tibial spine

Figure 8.43 A 13-year-old boy complained of pain in his right knee for eight months. (A) Anteroposterior film shows the lesion of osteochondritis dissecans in its classic location, the lateral aspect of the medial femoral condyle. The lesion appears to be still in situ. (B) On contrast arthrography, the lesion is shown to be covered by intact articular cartilage from the inferior aspect of the femoral condyle, but computed arthrotomographic sections (C,D) demonstrate that the lesion, located in the anterolateral aspect of the femoral condyle (a portion not protected by articular cartilage), is partially discharged into the joint at the site of the attachment of the posterior cruciate ligament.

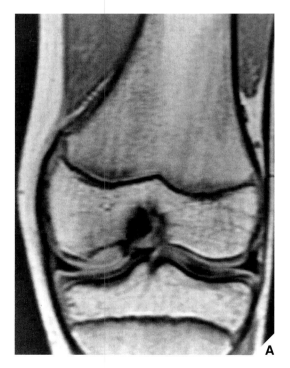

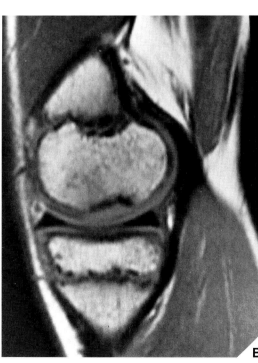

Figure 8.44 An 11-year-old boy experienced knee pain for three months. (A) MR image in the coronal plane (SE TR 1800/TE 20) shows bony fragment well-separated from the medial femoral condyle by the low signal intensity line. (B) Image in the sagittal plane (SE TR 800/TE 20) demonstrates intact articular cartilage overlying the separated fragment, indicating an in situ lesion.

phy with tomography or CT to demonstrate the presence and distribution of the osteochondral bodies (Fig. 8.43), or performing MRI examination of the knee (Fig. 8.44).

Occasionally, a small, disk-shaped secondary ossification center is present on the posterior portion of the femoral condyle; this normal variant should not be mistaken for osteochondritis dissecans. Similarly, during normal ossification of the distal femoral epiphysis, developmental changes may appear as irregularities in the outline of the condyle. The appearance of these irregularities, which are usually posteriorly located and hence best seen on the tunnel projection, may mimic osteochondritis dissecans (see Fig. 8.41).

SPONTANEOUS OSTEONECROSIS Characterized by acute onset of pain, spontaneous osteonecrosis of the knee is a distinct clinicopathologic entity with a predilection for the weight-bearing segment of the medial femoral condyle. It occurs in older adults, frequently in their sixth and seventh decades, and should not be mistaken for adult onset of osteochondritis dissecans. Although the etiology is obscure, certain factors, such as trauma, intra-articular injection of steroids, and possibly tear of the meniscus, as Norman and Baker have pointed out, may play a role in the pathogenesis of this condition.

The earliest radiologic sign of this condition is an increased uptake of isotope on radionuclide bone scan; radiographically, the earliest indication is a minimal degree of flattening of the femoral condyle (Fig. 8.45). Later, usually one to three months after the sudden onset of symptoms, radiographs may show a subchondral focus of radiolucency. As the condition progresses, the lesion may be seen radiographically as a subchondral osteolytic (necrotic) focus surrounded by a sclerotic margin representing a zone of repair (Fig. 8.46). Frequently, these lesions are accompanied by meniscal tears and, for this reason, either contrast arthrography or MRI should always be performed if spontaneous osteonecrosis is suspected (Fig. 8.47). Some authors postulate that the concentration of stress of the torn meniscus on the articular cartilage may result in local ischemia, thus predisposing to the development of osteonecrosis.

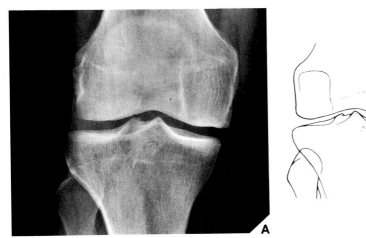
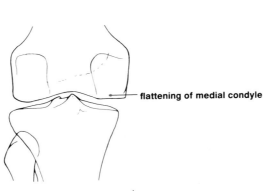

flattening of medial condyle

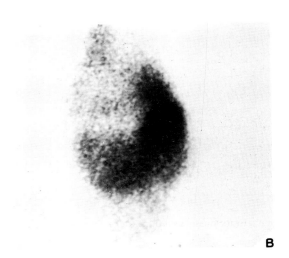

B

Figure 8.45 Four weeks before this radiographic examination, a 58-year-old man felt a sharp pain in the right knee when he stepped off a curb. The pain subsided after one week but recurred shortly afterward. (A) Anteroposterior view of the knee shows flattening of the medial aspect of the medial femoral condyle. (B) Radionuclide bone scan was performed, and it shows a marked increase in uptake of the tracer in the area of the medial femoral condyle. The features seen in both studies characterize an early stage of spontaneous osteonecrosis.

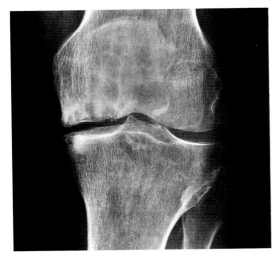
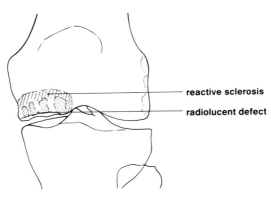

reactive sclerosis
radiolucent defect

Figure 8.46 A 74-year-old man stepped off a curb and felt a sharp pain in the left knee. Radiographs obtained on the following day were normal. The pain in the knee subsided after ten days, but two months later he developed joint effusion, which was aspirated. He was given a series of three intra-articular injections of steroids (hydrocortisone), after which most of the symptoms subsided. Four months after the initial injury the symptoms recurred, and at this time the standard radiographic examination was repeated. Anteroposterior projection shows a large radiolucent defect surrounded by a zone of sclerosis in the weight-bearing segment of the medial femoral condyle. The lesion represents spontaneous osteonecrosis.

Injury to the Soft Tissues about the Knee

KNEE JOINT EFFUSION Normally, the suprapatellar bursa is apparent on a plain film of the knee in the lateral projection as a thin, radiodense strip just posterior to the quadriceps tendon (Fig. 8.48). In knee joint effusion, which often occurs secondary to injury elsewhere in the knee, the suprapatellar bursa fills with fluid. Distention of the bursa is evident radiographically as an oval-shaped density that obliterates the fat space anterior to the femoral cortex (Fig. 8.49). If there is an associated intra-articular fracture of either the distal femur or the proximal tibia, a cross-table lateral view may demonstrate the FBI sign (see Fig. 8.28C).

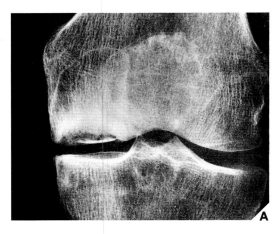 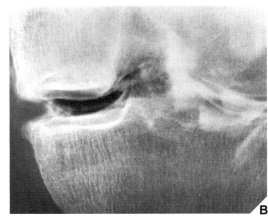 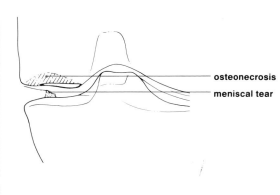

Figure 8.47 A 63-year-old woman missed a step while descending the staircase and felt a sharp pain in the left knee. The radiographic examination performed three days later showed only moderate osteoporosis, which was not related to trauma. Three months later she was re-examined for persistent pain and accumulation of fluid in the joint. (A) Anteroposterior view of the knee shows spontaneous osteonecrosis in the weight-bearing portion of the medial femoral condyle. Double-contrast arthrography was performed to evaluate any possible injury to the menisci. The arthrogram (B) demonstrates a vertical tear of the medial meniscus at the site of the osteonecrotic lesion.

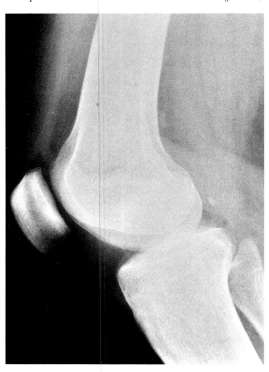 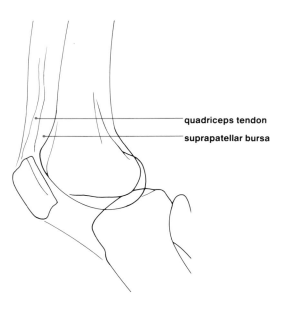

Figure 8.48 The suprapatellar bursa normally appears on the lateral view of the knee as a radiodense strip just posterior to the quadriceps tendon.

MENISCAL INJURY As fibrocartilaginous structures, the menisci of the knee (see Fig. 8.9) are not visible on plain-film radiographs. Contrast arthrography may demonstrate these structures, although recently MRI has become a standard procedure for evaluating the menisci.

Tear of the medial meniscus is a common injury resulting from physical and sports-related activities. Various types of tears may be encountered (Fig. 8.50). The most common type is a vertical tear, which may be simple or bucket-handle; horizontal tears usually occur in an older age group. The patient usually complains of pain and locking of the knee, and on clinical examination there is tenderness along the medial joint line. On arthrography, meniscal tear is recognized as a projection of positive contrast medium or air into

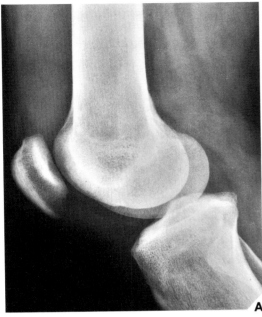

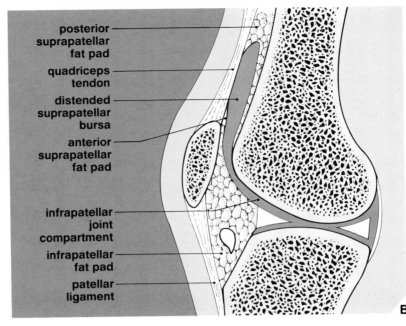

posterior suprapatellar fat pad
quadriceps tendon
distended suprapatellar bursa
anterior suprapatellar fat pad
infrapatellar joint compartment
infrapatellar fat pad
patellar ligament

Figure 8.49 (A,B) In knee joint effusion the suprapatellar bursa distends with fluid, thus obliterating the fat space posterior to the quadriceps tendon. (Adapted from Hall FM, 1978)

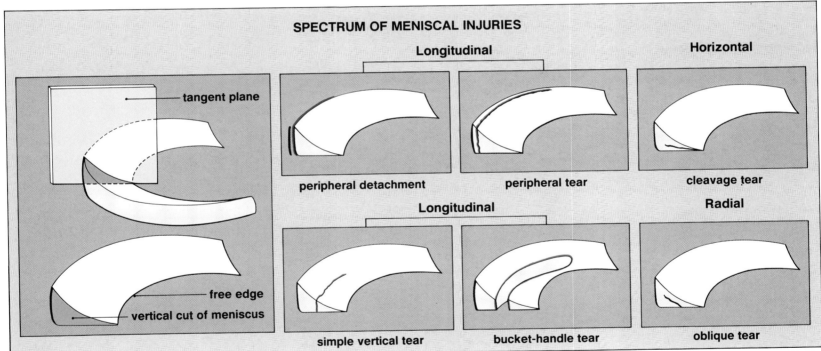

SPECTRUM OF MENISCAL INJURIES

Longitudinal

Horizontal

tangent plane

peripheral detachment

peripheral tear

cleavage tear

Longitudinal

Radial

free edge
vertical cut of meniscus

simple vertical tear

bucket-handle tear

oblique tear

Figure 8.50 Meniscal injuries can be broadly classified as longitudinal, horizontal, and radial, depending on the plane in which they occur. The left panel represents diagrammatically the radiologic image of the meniscus; the right panel, various tears.

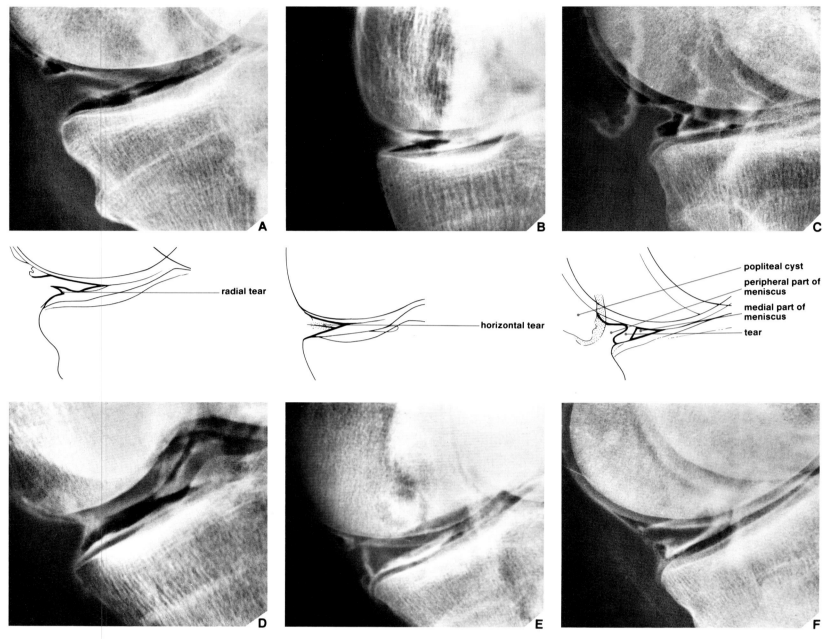

Figure 8.51 Arthrographically, meniscal tears are recognized by a projection of contrast medium or air into the substance of the structure or at its periphery. The following spot films demonstrate some of the various types of tears that may affect the medial meniscus: (A) radial (oblique) tear of the posterior horn; (B) horizontal tear of the body; (C) bucket-handle tear of the posterior horn; (D) bucket-handle tear of the body with displacement of the fragment into the intercondylar notch; (E) peripheral tear of the posterior horn; and (F) peripheral detachment of the posterior horn.

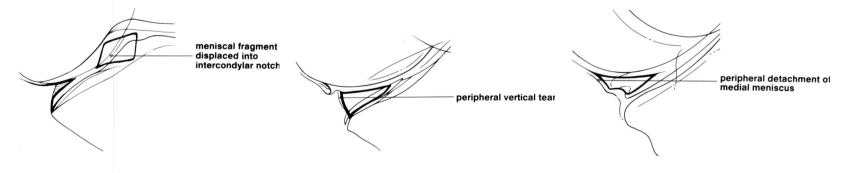

the substance of the meniscus or at its periphery (Fig. 8.51). On MRI the menisci are seen as structures of uniformly low signal intensity. A meniscal tear is identified by the presence of an increased intrameniscal signal that extends to the surface of this structure (Fig. 8.52). A globular or linear focus of increased signal intensity in the meniscus that does not extend to the surface does not represent a tear. The significance of this finding is still unclear. Stoller, Genant, and Beltran believe that these findings represent an area of hyaline or myxoid degeneration within the substance of the meniscus. These abnormalities, known as type I (round focus) and type II (linear area) meniscal lesions (Fig. 8.53A,B), are not seen on arthroscopic examination of the knee. The true tears are designated as type III and type IV lesions (Fig. 8.53C; see also Fig. 8.52).

Tears of the lateral meniscus are less common. This has been attributed to the greater degree of mobility of the lateral meniscus because of its rather loose peripheral attachment to the synovium and lack of attachment to the fibular (lateral) collateral ligament. Lateral meniscal tears, however, commonly accompany a developmental anomaly, the so-called discoid meniscus, which according to Kaplan is probably related to an abnormal attachment of its posterior horn to the tibial plateau and repetitive abnormal movements, with subsequent enlargement and thickening of meniscal tissue. The discoid meniscus is recognized clinically by a loud clicking sound on flexion and extension of the knee joint and radiographically on the plain-film anteroposterior view by an abnormally wide lateral joint compartment (Fig. 8.54A). Its arthro-

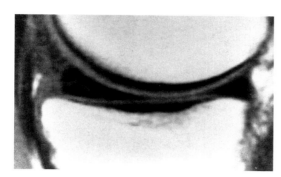

Figure 8.52 Sagittal spin echo T1-weighted MR image (TR 700/TE 20) shows a tear of the medial meniscus. Note the high-intensity signal of the tear, which extends into the inferior surface of the meniscus.

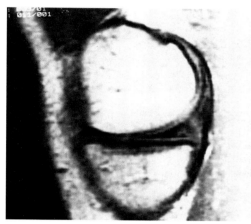

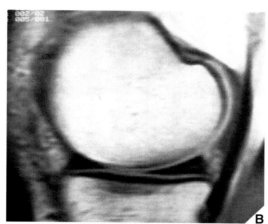

A

B

Figure 8.53 (A) Sagittal spin echo MR image (TR 2000/TE 20) shows a type I lesion of the posterior horn of the medial meniscus. The intrameniscal lesion does not extend to the articular surface. (B) In a type II lesion of the posterior horn of the medial meniscus, the configuration is linear, and as with a type I, the lesion does not extend into the articular surface. (C) Schematic representation of various types of meniscal lesions.

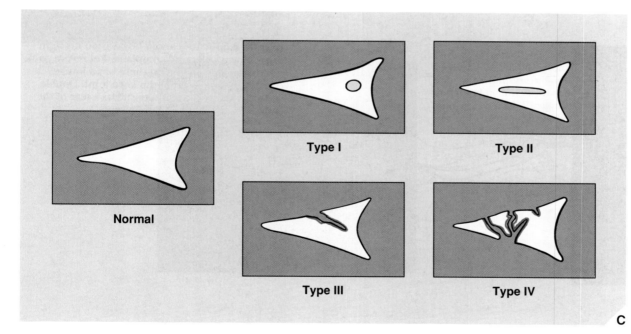

Normal

Type I

Type II

Type III

Type IV

C

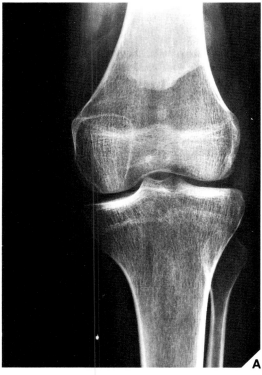
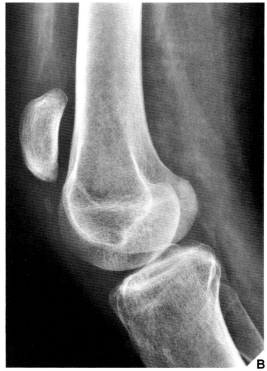

Figure 8.64 A 38-year-old woman athlete was injured during a running competition. Antero-posterior (A) and lateral (B) views of the knee demonstrate an abnormally high position of the patella, a finding suggesting tear of the patellar ligament. The diagnosis was confirmed on surgical exploration.

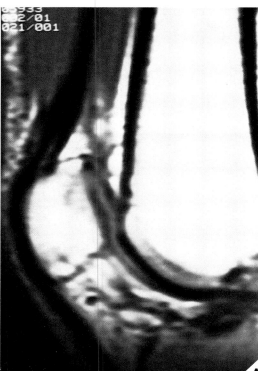
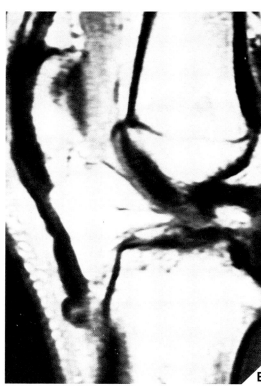

Figure 8.65 (A) Sagittal spin echo proton density MR image (TR 2000/TE 20) shows partial rupture of the quadriceps tendon, represented by edema and hemorrhage (intermediate signal intensity) between the tendon fibers (low signal intensity). (B) Sagittal spin echo proton density MR image (TR 2000/TE 20) demonstrates evulsion of the patellar ligament at the insertion into the tibial tuberosity. (From Beltran J, 1990)

PRACTICAL POINTS TO REMEMBER

[1] The posterior aspect of the femoral condyles and the intercondylar notch are best shown on the tunnel projection of the knee.

[2] Merchant axial projection of the patella, rather than the standard sunrise view, is better suited to evaluate:
• the articular facets of the patellofemoral joint
• subtle patellar subluxations.

[3] In arthrographic examination of the menisci, be aware of:
• the popliteal hiatus at the posterior horn of the lateral meniscus, a normal feature that may be confused with a tear
• a blind spot involving the posterior portion of the posterior horn of the lateral meniscus, where a tear can be overlooked.

[4] Magnetic resonance imaging is the modality of choice to evaluate soft-tissue injury around the knee, in particular to the menisci and the cruciate and collateral ligaments. It is also the best modality to image posttraumatic joint effusion, acute and chronic hematomas, and other traumatic abnormalities of the muscular, ligamentous, and tendinous structures.

[5] Tomographic examination is very useful in evaluating the amount of depression in tibial plateau fractures.

[6] Tibial plateau fractures are often accompanied by meniscal tear and ligament injury.

[7] The bipartite or multipartite patella may mimic patellar fracture. To avoid misdiagnosing these developmental anomalies as a fracture, remember that:
• the bipartite or multipartite patella is seen at the superolateral margin of the patella
• the apparent comminuted fragments do not form a whole, as they would in patellar fracture.

[8] Sinding-Larsen-Johansson and Osgood-Schlatter diseases are conditions related to trauma. In both entities soft tissue swelling on clinical and radiographic examination is a fundamental diagnostic feature.

[9] Learn to distinguish three conditions that have very similar radiologic presentations:
• osteochondral fracture, which is an acute injury to the articular cartilage and subchondral bone
• osteochondritis dissecans, which is the result of chronic injury
• spontaneous osteonecrosis, which is characterized by acute onset of pain and has been linked to trauma, corticosteroid injections, and meniscal tear.
Contrast arthrography, arthrotomography, computed arthrotomography, and MRI are essential techniques in the evaluation of the status of the articular cartilage in each of these conditions.

[10] Tears of the menisci and ligaments of the knee are best demonstrated by magnetic resonance imaging. Tears of the medial meniscus are much more common than tears of the lateral semilunar cartilage. The discoid lateral meniscus predisposes this structure to injury.

[11] The "unhappy O'Donoghue triad," resulting from valgus stress forces applied to the knee joint, consists of tears of the:
• medial meniscus
• medial collateral ligament
• anterior cruciate ligament.

References

Ahlback S, Bauer GCH, Bohne WH: Spontaneous osteonecrosis of the knee. *Arthritis Rheum* 11:705, 1968.

Aichroth P: Osteochondritis dissecans of the knee. A clinical survey. *J Bone Joint Surg* 53B:440, 1971.

Aichroth P: Osteochondral fractures and their relationship to osteochondritis dissecans of the knee. *J Bone Joint Surg* 53B:448, 1971.

Bassett LW, Grover JS, Seeger LL: Magnetic resonance imaging of knee trauma. *Skeletal Radiol* 19:401, 1990.

Bellon EM, Keith MW, Coleman PE, Shah ZR: Magnetic resonance imaging of internal derangements of the knee. *RadioGraphics* 8:95, 1988.

Beltran J: *MRI: Musculosketal System.* Philadelphia, Lippincott, 1990.

Chand K: Horizontal (cleavage) tears of the knee-joint menisci in the elderly. *J Am Geriatr Soc* 20:430, 1972.

Dalinka MK: Knee arthrography. In: Dalinka MK (ed): *Arthrography.* New York, Springer-Verlag, 1980, pp 1-88.

Dalinka MK, Gohel VK, Rancier L: Tomography in the evaluation of the anterior cruciate ligament. *Radiology* 108:31, 1973.

Elstrom J, Pankovich A, Sassoon H, et al: The use of tomography in the assessment of fractures of the tibial plateau. *J Bone Joint Surg* 58:551, 1976.

Ficat RP, Hungherford DS: Disorders of the patello-femoral joint. Baltimore, Williams & Wilkins, 1977.

Freiberger RH: Technique of knee arthrography. In: Freiberger RH, Kaye JJ, Spiller J (eds): *Arthrography.* New York, Appleton-Century-Crofts, 1979, pp 5–30.

Freiberger RH, Pavlov H: Knee arthrography. *Radiology* 166:489, 1988.

Ghelman B: Meniscal tears of the knee: Evaluation by high-resolution CT combined with arthrography. *Radiology* 157:23, 1985.

Gilley JS, Gelman Edson M, Metcalf RW: Chondral fractures of the knee: Arthrographic, arthroscopic, and clinical manifestations. *Radiology* 138:51, 1981.

Hall FM: Radiographic diagnosis and accuracy in knee joint effusions. *Radiology* 115:49, 1975.

Hall FM: Further pitfalls in knee arthrography. *J Can Assoc Radiol* 97:179, 1970.

Harris RD, Hecht HL: Suprapatellar effusions: A new diagnostic sign. *Radiology* 97:1, 1970.

Hohl M: Tibial condylar fractures. *J Bone Joint Surg* 49A:1455, 1967.

Hohl M, Larson RL: Fractures and dislocations of the knee. In: Rockwood CA Jr, Green DP (eds): *Fractures.* Philadelphia, Lippincott, 1975.

Hohl M, Luck JV: Fractures of the tibial condyle. A clinical and experimental study. *J Bone Joint Surg* 38A:1001, 1956.

Insall J, Salvati E: Patella position in the normal knee joint. *Radiology* 101:101, 1971.

Kaplan EB: Discoid lateral meniscus of the knee joint. Nature, mechanism and operative treatment. *J Bone Joint Surg* 39A:77, 1957.

Kaye JJ: Knee arthrography today. *Radiology* 157:265, 1985.

Lotke PA, Ecker ML: Osteonecrosis of the medial tibial plateau. *Contemp Orthop* 10:47, 1985.

Merchant AC, Mercer RL, Jacobson RH, Cool CR: Roentgenographic analysis of patello-femoral congruence. *J Bone Joint Surg* 56A:1391, 1974.

Mesgarzadeh M, Sapega AA, Bonakdarpour A, et al: Osteochondritis dissecans: Analysis of mechanical stability with radiography, scintigraphy, and MR imaging. *Radiology* 165:775, 1987.

Milgram JW: Radiological and pathological manifestation of osteochondritis dissecans of the distal femur: A study of 50 cases. *Radiology* 126:305, 1978.

Milgram JW, Rogers LF, Miller JW: Osteochondral fractures: Mechanism of injury and fate of fragments. *Am J Roentgenol* 130:651, 1978.

Moore T, Harvey JP Jr: Roentgenographic measurement of tibial plateau depression due to fracture. *J Bone Joint Surg* 56A:155, 1974.

Muheim G, Bohne WH: Prognosis in spontaneous osteonecrosis of the knee. Investigation by radionuclide scintimetry and radiography. *J Bone Joint Surg* 52B:605, 1970.

Munk PL, Helms CA, Genant HK, Holt G: Magnetic resonance imaging of the knee: Current status, new directions. *Skeletal Radiol* 18:569, 1989.

Nachlas IW, Olpp JL: Para-articular calcification (Pellegrini-Stieda) in affections of the knee. *Surg Gynecol Obstet* 81:206, 1945.

Nance EP Jr, Kaye JJ: Injuries of the quadriceps mechanism. *Radiology* 142:301, 1982.

Newberg AH, Greenstein R: Radiographic evaluation of tibial plateau fractures. *Radiology* 126:319, 1978.

Newberg AH, Seligson D: Patellofemoral joint: 30-, 60-, and 90-degree views. *Radiology* 137:57, 1980.

Nicholas JA, Freiberger RH, Killoran PJ: Double-contrast arthrography of the knee joint: Its value in the management of two hundred and twenty-five knee derangements. *J Bone Joint Surg* 52A:203, 1970.

Norman A, Baker ND: Spontaneous osteonecrosis of the knee and medial meniscal tears. *Radiology* 129:653, 1978.

O'Donoghue DH: *Chondral and osteochondral fractures*, ed 4. Philadelphia, Saunders, 1984.

O'Donogue DH: *Treatment of Injuries to Athletes*, ed 4. Philadelphia, Saunders, 1984.

Ogden JA, Southwick WO: Osgood-Schlatter's disease and tibial tuberosity development. *Clin Orthop* 116:180, 1976.

Osgood RB: Lesions of the tibial tubercle occurring during adolescence. *Boston Med Surg* 1148:114, 1903.

Pavlov H, Freiberger RH: An easy method to demonstrate the cruciate ligaments by double-contrast arthrography. *Radiology* 126:817, 1978.

Pavlov H, Schneider R: Extrameniscal abnormalities as diagnosed by knee arthrography. *Radiol Clin North Am* 19:287, 1981.

Pavlov H, Ghelman B, Vigorita V: *Atlas of Knee Menisci: An Arthrographic-Pathologic Correlation.* New York, Appleton-Century-Crofts, 1983.

Roberts J: Fractures of the condyles of the tibia. Anatomical and clinical end-result study of 100 cases. *J Bone Joint Surg* 50A:1505, 1968.

Sartoris DJ, Kursunoglu S, Pineda C, Kerr R, Pate D, Resnick D: Detection of intra-articular osteochondral bodies in the knee using computed arthrotomography. *Radiology* 155:447, 1985.

Schulak D, Gunn D: Fractures of the tibial plateaus. A review of the literature *Clin Orthop* 100:166, 1975.

Schwimmer M, Edelstein G, Heiken JP, Gilula LA: Synovial cysts of the knee: CT evaluation. *Radiology* 154:175, 1985.

Smillie IS: Congenital discoid meniscus. *J Bone Joint Surg* 30:671, 1948.

Smillie IS: *Injuries of the Knee Joint*, ed 4. Baltimore, Williams & Wilkins, 1970.

Stoller DW, Martin C, Crues JV III, Kaplan L, Mink JH: Meniscal tears: Pathologic consideration with MR imaging. *Radiology* 163:731, 1987.

Wershba B, Dalinka MK, Coren GS: Double-contrast knee arthrography in the evaluation of osteochondritis dissecans. *Clinic Orthop* 107:81, 1975.

Wickstrom KT, Spitzer RM, Olsson HE: Roentgen anatomy of the posterior horn of the lateral meniscus. *Radiology* 116:617, 1975.

Williams JL, Cliff MM, Bonakdarpour A: Spontaneous osteonecrosis of the knee. *Radiology* 107:15, 1973.

Wolfe RD, Dieden JD: Cruciate ligament injury: Diagnostic difficulties in the presence of meniscal injury. *Radiology* 157:19, 1985.

Lower Limb III: Ankle and Foot

THE ANKLE IS THE MOST frequently injured of all the major weight-bearing joints in the body. Most victims are young adults injured while participating in athletic activities such as running, skiing, and soccer. Ankle structures susceptible to injury include bones, ligaments, tendons, and syndesmoses; ligaments can be damaged in the absence of fractures. When this occurs, damage to ligaments may go unrecognized on plain radiographs, with the result that the patient is not properly treated.

The type of fracture usually indicates the mechanism of injury, determined, as Kleiger has pointed out, by the position of the foot, the direction and intensity of the applied force, and the resistance of the structures making up the joint. The mechanism of injury may in turn serve as an indicator of which ligament structures are damaged.

Although occasionally meticulous history-taking and clinical examination can help determine the mechanism of trauma and predict damage to the various structures, radiologic examination is the key to reliable evaluation of the site and extent of injury. There are two basic types of ankle trauma: inversion injuries and eversion injuries. These, however, may be complicated by internal or external rotation, hyperflexion or hyperextension, and vertical compression forces.

Foot injuries are also common and usually result from direct trauma, such as a blow or a fall from a height; only rarely do such injuries result from indirect forces such as abnormal stress or strain of muscles or tendons. Foot fractures, accounting for 10% of all fractures, are more common than dislocations, which usually are associated with fractures, and occur at the midtarsal, tarsometatarsal, and metatarsophalangeal articulations.

Anatomic-Radiologic Considerations

The ankle joint proper consists of the tibiotalar and distal tibiofibular articulations, the latter a syndesmotic joint rather than a true synarthrodial one. In matters of injury, however, one must consider that the ankle joint acts as a unit with other joints of the foot, particularly the talocalcaneal (subtalar) articulation, where application of stress can have great impact on ankle injuries.

The ankle joint is formed by three bones—the distal tibia and fibula and the talus—and three principal sets of ligaments—the medial collateral (deltoid) ligament; the lateral collateral ligament, consisting of the anterior talofibular, posterior talofibular, and calcaneofibular ligaments; and the syndesmotic complex, a fibrous joint between the distal tibia and fibula (Fig. 9.1). The distal tibiofibular syndesmotic complex, one of the most important anatomic structures in maintaining ankle integrity and stability, consists of three elements: the distal anterior tibiofibular ligament, the distal posterior tibiofibular ligament, and the interosseous membrane.

From the viewpoint of anatomy and kinetics, the foot is divided into three distinct sections: hindfoot, midfoot, and forefoot. The hindfoot, separated from the midfoot by the midtarsal (or Chopart) joint, includes the talus and calcaneus; the midfoot, separated from the forefoot by the tarsometatarsal (Lisfranc) joint, includes the navicular, cuboid, and three cuneiform bones; and the forefoot includes the metatarsals and phalanges (Fig. 9.2).

A word about terminology is in order, because the terminology describing motion of the ankle and foot in the literature is not uniform and confusion has been created about the various mechanisms of ankle and foot injuries. Frequently, but incorrectly, the terms adduction, inversion, varus, and supination have been used interchangeably, as have their counterparts abduction, eversion, valgus, and pronation. However, supination and pronation are more appropriately applied to compound motion. *Supination* consists of adduc-

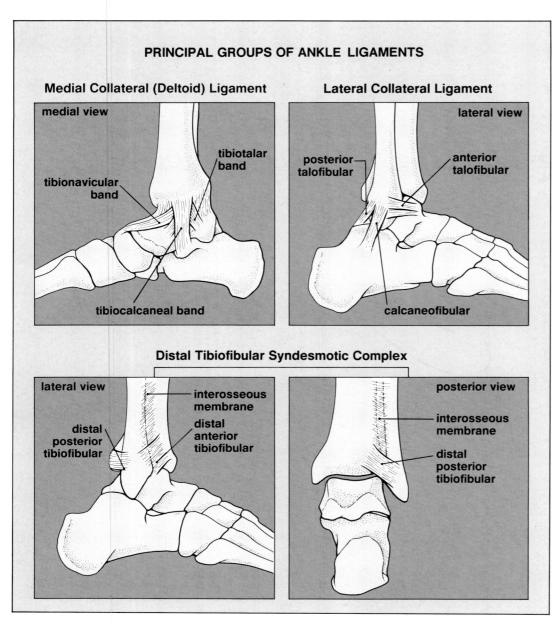

Figure 9.1 Three principal sets of ligaments form the ankle joint: the medial collateral (deltoid) ligament, the lateral collateral ligament, and the distal tibiofibular syndesmotic complex, which is important for maintaining ankle integrity and stability.

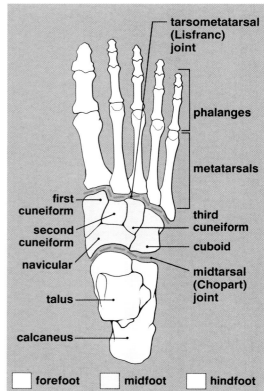

Figure 9.2 The foot can be viewed as comprising three anatomic divisions: the hindfoot, midfoot, and forefoot, separated respectively by the midtarsal (Chopart) and tarsometatarsal (Lisfranc) joints.

tion and inversion of the forefoot (motion in the tarsometatarsal and midtarsal joints) and inversion of the heel, which assumes a varus configuration (motion in subtalar joint), as well as slight plantar flexion of the ankle (tibiotalar) joint. In *pronation*, compound motion consists of abduction and eversion of the forefoot (motion in the tarsometatarsal and midtarsal joints) and eversion of the heel, which assumes a valgus configuration (motion in the subtalar joint), together with slight dorsiflexion (or dorsal extension) of the ankle (Fig. 9.3).

Adduction properly applies to medial deviation of the forefoot, and *abduction* to lateral deviation of the forefoot, both motions occurring in the tarsometatarsal (Lisfranc) joint; *adduction of the heel* refers to inversion of the calcaneus, and *abduction of the heel* to eversion of the calcaneus, both motions occurring in the subtalar joint.

Plantar flexion refers to caudad (downward) foot motion, *dorsiflexion* to cephalad (upward) foot motion—motions occurring in the ankle (tibiotalar) joint. Varus and valgus should not be used to describe motion but should be reserved for description of ankle or foot position in case of deformity. Occasionally, varus and valgus are used interchangeably with inversion and eversion to describe the applied stress.

Imaging of the Ankle and Foot

The standard radiographic examination of the ankle, as a rule, includes the anteroposterior (including the mortise), lateral, and oblique projections. Stress views are also frequently obtained for evaluating ankle injuries. These may also need to be supplemented with special projections.

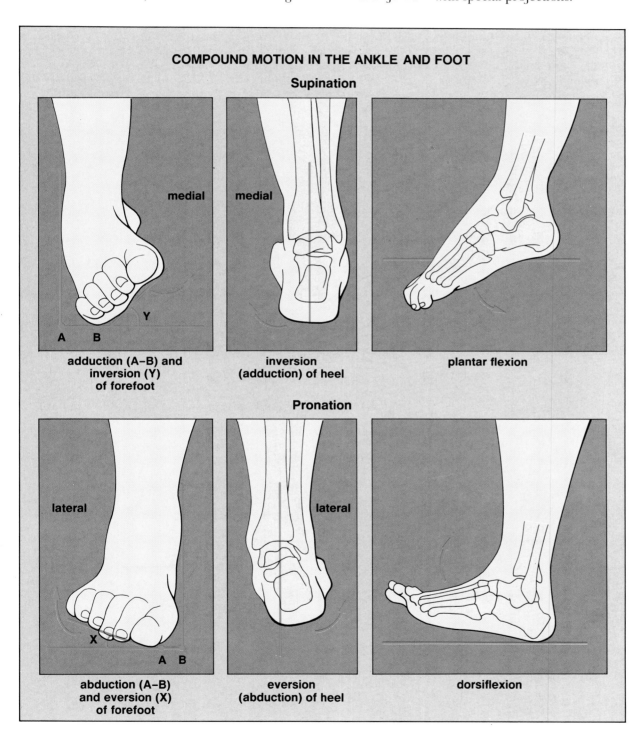

COMPOUND MOTION IN THE ANKLE AND FOOT

Supination

medial

medial

adduction (A–B) and inversion (Y) of forefoot

inversion (adduction) of heel

plantar flexion

Pronation

lateral

lateral

abduction (A–B) and eversion (X) of forefoot

eversion (abduction) of heel

dorsiflexion

Figure 9.3 Supination is a compound motion consisting of adduction and inversion of the forefoot, together with inversion of the heel and slight plantar flexion in the ankle joint. In pronation, the compound motion involves abduction and eversion of the forefoot with eversion of the heel and slight dorsiflexion in the ankle joint.

On the *anteroposterior* view, the distal tibia and fibula, including the medial and lateral malleoli, are well demonstrated (Fig. 9.4). On this projection, it is important to note that the fibular (lateral) malleolus is longer than the tibial (medial) malleolus. This anatomic feature, important for maintaining ankle stability, is crucial for reconstruction of the fractured ankle joint. Even minimal displacement or shortening of the lateral malleolus allows lateral talar shift to occur and may cause incongruity in the ankle joint, possibly leading to posttraumatic arthritis. A variant of the anteroposterior projection, in which the ankle is internally rotated 10°, is called the mortise view because the ankle mortise is well demonstrated on it (Fig. 9.5).

The *lateral* view is used to evaluate the anterior aspect of the distal tibia and the posterior lip of this bone (the so-called third malleolus) (Fig. 9.6). Some fractures oriented in the coronal plane can be better visualized on this projection.

The *oblique* view of the ankle, best obtained with the foot internally rotated about 30° to 35°, is effective in demonstrating the tibiofibular syndesmosis and the talofibular joint (Fig. 9.7). An *external oblique* view may also be required to evaluate the lateral malleolus and the anterior tibial tubercle (Fig. 9.8).

Most ankle ligament injuries require stress radiography, ankle joint arthrography, computed tomography (CT), or magnetic resonance imaging (MRI) (see below) for demonstration and sufficient evaluation. Some, however, can be deduced from the site and extension of fractures on the standard radiographic examination. A thorough knowledge of the skeletal and soft tissue topographic anatomy of the ankle, together with an understanding of the kinematics and mechanism of ankle injuries, will aid the radiologist in correctly diagnosing traumatic conditions and predicting ligament injuries. With such understanding, the radiologist can even determine the sequence of injury to the various structures.

Some ligament injuries may be diagnosed on the basis of disruption of the ankle mortise and displacement of the talus; others can be deduced from the appearance of fractured bones. For example, fibular fracture above the level of the ankle joint indicates that the distal anterior tibiofibular ligament is torn. Fracture of the fibula above its anterior tubercle strongly suggests that the tibiofibular syndesmosis is completely disrupted. Fracture of the fibula above the level of the ankle joint without accompanying fracture of the medial malleolus indicates rupture of the deltoid ligament.

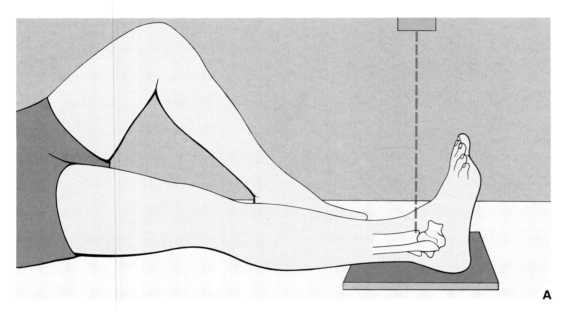 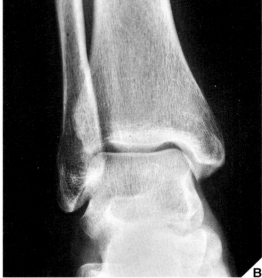

Figure 9.4 (A) For the anteroposterior view of the ankle, the patient is supine on the radiographic table with the heel resting on the film cassette. The foot is in neutral position, the sole perpendicular to the leg and the cassette. The central beam is directed vertically to the ankle joint at the midpoint between both malleoli. (B) The film in this projection demonstrates the distal tibia, particularly the medial malleolus, the body of the talus, and the tibiotalar joint. Note, however, the overlap of the distal fibula and the lateral aspect of the tibia. The tibiofibular syndesmosis is not clearly demonstrated.

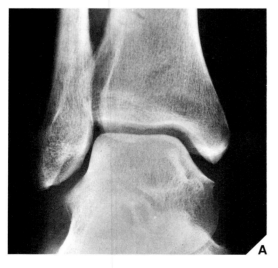 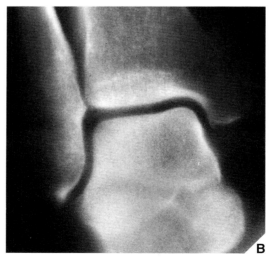 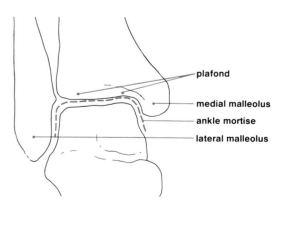

Figure 9.5 (A) The mortise view, a variant of the anteroposterior projection obtained with 10° internal rotation of the ankle, eliminates the overlap of the medial aspect of the distal fibula and the lateral aspect of the talus, so the space between these bones is well demonstrated. (B) The ankle mortise, shown here on a tomographic cut through the ankle joint, is formed by the medial malleolus, the articular surface of the distal tibia (the ceiling or plafond), and the lateral malleolus; it is shaped like an inverted U.

Transverse fracture of the medial malleolus indicates that the deltoid ligament is intact. High fracture of the fibula associated with a fracture of the medial malleolus or tear of the tibiofibular ligament, the so-called Maisonneuve fracture (see below), indicates rupture of the interosseous membrane up to the level of the fibular fracture.

When plain films of the ankle are normal, however, stress views are extremely important in evaluating ligament injuries (see Fig. 4.3).

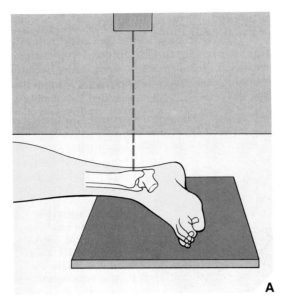 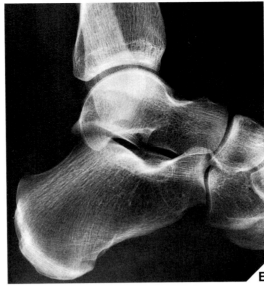

Figure 9.6 (A) For the lateral projection of the ankle, the patient is placed on his or her side with the fibula resting on the film cassette and the foot in the neutral position. The central beam is directed vertically to the medial malleolus. (The lateral view can also be obtained by placing the medial side of the ankle against the cassette.) (B) On this view, the distal tibia, talus, and calcaneus are seen in profile, and the fibula overlaps the posterior aspect of the tibia and the posterior aspect of the talus. The tibiotalar and subtalar joints are well demonstrated. Note the posterior lip of the tibia, also known as the third malleolus.

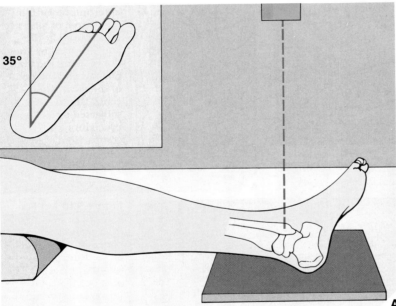 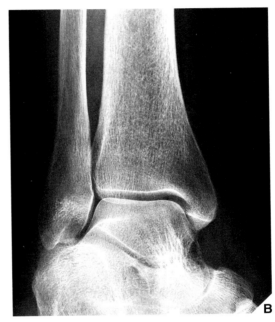

Figure 9.7 (A) For the (internal) oblique view of the ankle, the patient is supine, and the leg and foot are rotated medially about 35° *(inset)*. The foot is in the neutral position, forming a 90° angle with the distal leg. The central beam is directed perpendicular to the lateral malleolus. (B) On the radiograph, the medial and lateral malleoli, the tibial plafond, the dome of the talus, the tibiotalar joint, and the tibiofibular syndesmosis are well demonstrated.

Figure 9.8 On the external oblique view, for which the patient is positioned as for the internal oblique view but with the limb rotated laterally about 40° to 45°, the lateral malleolus and the anterior tibial tubercle are well demonstrated.

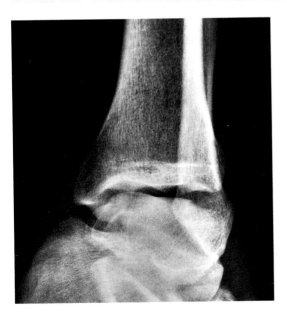 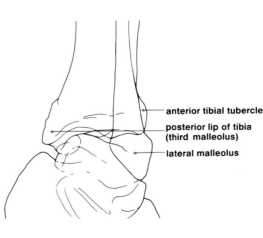

anterior tibial tubercle
posterior lip of tibia (third malleolus)
lateral malleolus

images, and inflammatory changes within or around the tendons, which again can be demonstrated by a change in the normal signal intensity.

Most injuries to the foot can be sufficiently evaluated on the standard radiographic examination of the foot, which includes the anteroposterior, lateral, and oblique projections. Only occasionally are special tangential projections required.

The *anteroposterior* view of the foot adequately demonstrates the metatarsal bones and phalanges (Fig. 9.18). This view reveals an important anatomic feature known as the first intermetatarsal angle, which normally ranges from 5° to 10° (Fig. 9.18C). This angle is an important factor in the evaluation of forefoot deformities, since it represents a way to quantify the amount of metatarsus primus varus associated with hallux valgus. On the *lateral* projec-

Figure 9.18 (A) For the anteroposterior (dorsoplantar) view of the foot, the patient is supine, with the knee flexed and the sole placed firmly on the film cassette. The central beam is directed vertically to the base of the first metatarsal bone. (B) On the film in this projection, injury to the metatarsal bones and phalanges can be adequately assessed. Note that 75% of the talar head articulates with the navicular bone. (For identification of the bones of the foot, see Figure 9.2.) (C) The first intermetatarsal angle is formed by the intersection of the lines bisecting the shafts of the first *(a)* and second *(b)* metatarsals.

A

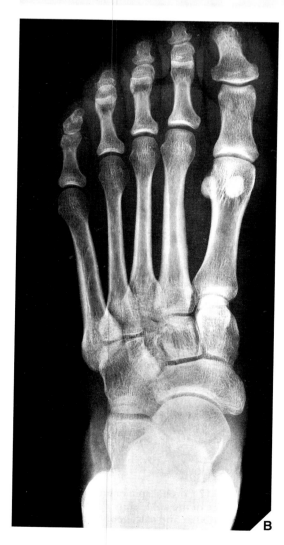

B

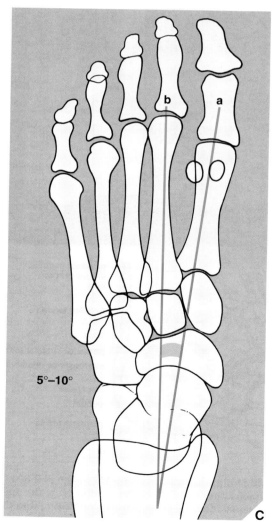

C

tion, *Boehler angle*, an important anatomic relation of the talus and the calcaneus, can be appreciated (Fig. 9.19). In fractures of the calcaneus, this angle, which normally ranges from 20° to 40°, is decreased because of compression of the superior aspect of the bone (see Fig. 9.61). This measurement also aids in evaluation of depression of the posterior facet of the subtalar joint. On anteroposterior view calcaneal pitch can also be evaluated. This measurement is an indication of the height of the foot and normally ranges from

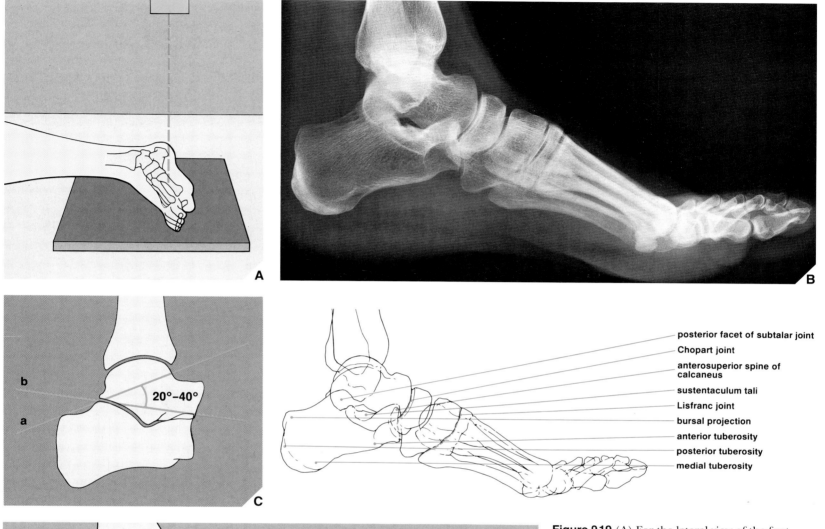

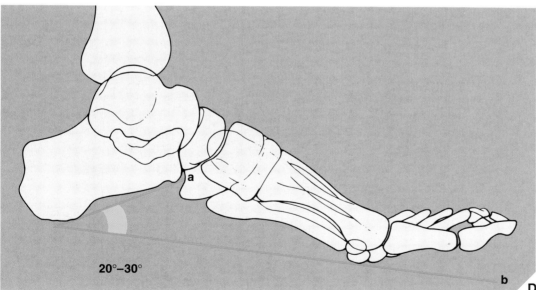

Figure 9.19 (A) For the lateral view of the foot, the patient lies on his or her side with the knee slightly flexed and the lateral aspect of the foot against the film cassette. The central beam is directed vertically to the midtarsus. (B) The lateral radiograph demonstrates the bursal projection, the most prominent feature on the posterior aspect of the calcaneus; the posterior tuberosity where the Achilles tendon inserts; the medial tuberosity on the plantar surface where the plantar fascia inserts; the anterior tuberosity; the anterosuperior spine of the calcaneus; the posterior facet of the subtalar joint; the sustentaculum tali; and the talonavicular and calcaneocuboid articulations. The Chopart and Lisfranc joints are also well visualized. (C) The lateral view also allows evaluation of the angular relationship between the talus and the calcaneus—Boehler angle. This feature is determined by the intersection of a line (*a*) drawn from the posterosuperior margin of the calcaneal tuberosity (bursal projection) through the tip of the posterior facet of the subtalar joint, and a second line (*b*) drawn from the tip of the posterior facet through the superior margin of the anterior process of the calcaneus. Normally, this angle ranges between 20° and 40°. (D) Calcaneal pitch is described by the intersection of a line drawn tangentially to the inferior surface of the calcaneus and one drawn along the plantar surface of the foot.

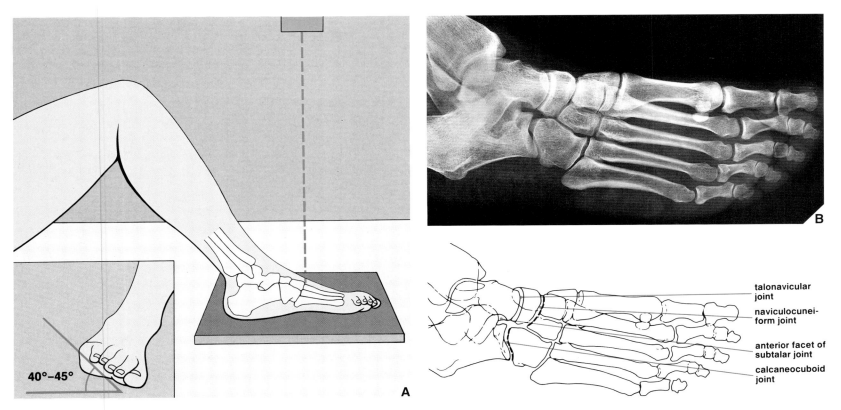

Figure 9.20 (A) For the oblique view of the foot, the patient is supine on the table with the knee flexed. The lateral border of the foot is elevated about 40° to 45° (*inset*) so that the medial border of the foot is forced against the film cassette. The central beam is directed vertically to the base of the third metatarsal. (B) On the oblique film of the foot, the phalanges and metatarsals are well demonstrated, as are the anterior part of the subtalar joint and the talonavicular, naviculocuneiform, and calcaneocuboid joints.

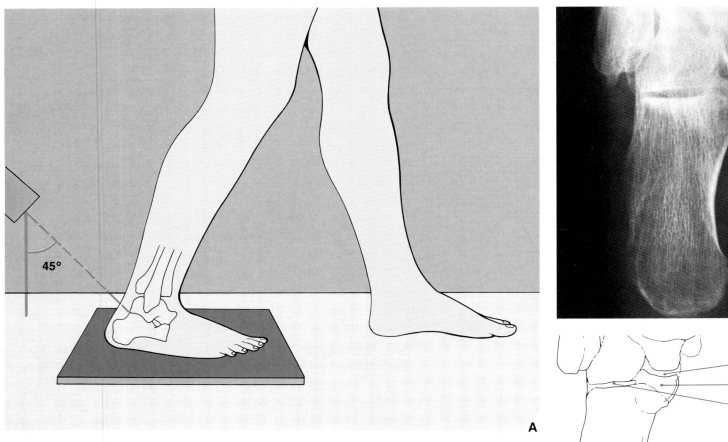

Figure 9.21 (A) For the posterior tangential (Harris-Beath) view of the foot, the patient is erect, with the sole of the foot flat on the film cassette. The central beam is usually angled 45° toward the midline of the heel, but 35° or 55° of angulation may also be used. (B) On the film in this projection, the middle facet of the subtalar joint is seen, oriented horizontally; the sustentaculum tali projects medially. The posterior facet projects laterally and is parallel to the middle facet. The body of the calcaneus is well demonstrated.

20° to 30° (Fig. 9.19D). Higher values indicate a cavus foot deformity. An *oblique* view of the foot is also obtained as part of the standard radiographic examination (Fig. 9.20). Injuries to the subtalar joint occasionally require special, tangential projections such as the posterior tangential *(Harris-Beath)* view (Fig. 9.21) or oblique tangential *(Broden)* view (Fig. 9.22). A tangential view of the sesamoid bones of the great toe (Fig. 9.23) may also be necessary.

Radiographic evaluation of foot injuries is complicated by the presence of multiple accessory ossicles, which are considered secondary centers of ossification, and the sesamoid bones, which may

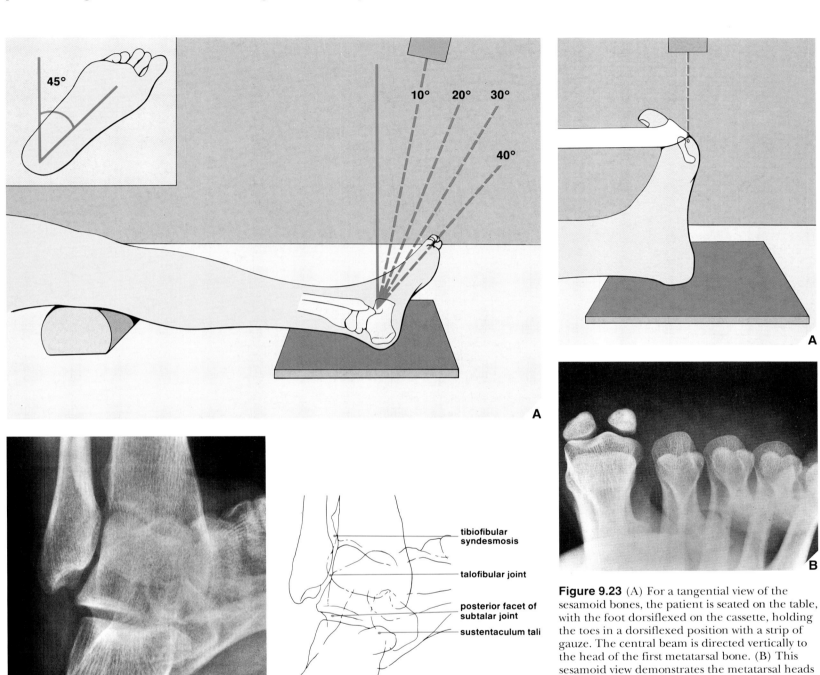

Figure 9.22 (A) For the Broden view of the foot, the patient is supine, with the knee slightly flexed and supported by a small sandbag. The foot rests on the film cassette, dorsiflexed to 90°, and, together with the leg, rotated medially about 45° (*inset*). The central beam is directed toward the lateral malleolus. Films may be obtained at 10°, 20°, 30°, and 40° of cephalad angulation of the tube. (B) A radiograph obtained at 30° cephalad angulation demonstrates the posterior facet of the subtalar joint. Note also the good demonstration of the sustentaculum tali and the excellent visualization of the talofibular joint and the tibiofibular syndesmosis.

tibiofibular syndesmosis
talofibular joint
posterior facet of subtalar joint
sustentaculum tali

Figure 9.23 (A) For a tangential view of the sesamoid bones, the patient is seated on the table, with the foot dorsiflexed on the cassette, holding the toes in a dorsiflexed position with a strip of gauze. The central beam is directed vertically to the head of the first metatarsal bone. (B) This sesamoid view demonstrates the metatarsal heads and the sesamoid bones of the first metatarsal.

mimic a fracture (Fig. 9.24A,B); conversely, a chip fracture can be misinterpreted as a mere ossicle (Fig. 9.24C,D). Thus, it is important to recognize these structures on plain radiographs.

In addition to plain-film radiography, ancillary imaging techniques may need to be employed in the evaluation of injury to the foot. Radionuclide imaging (bone scan) is a valuable means of detecting stress fractures, common foot injuries that are not always obvious on the standard radiographic examination. Likewise, tomo-graphic examination may supply useful information about occult or subtle fractures and help with evaluation of fracture healing. CT is especially effective in assessing complex fractures, particularly of the calcaneus. Tenographic examination may also be required to evaluate injury to the tendons of the foot (see above and Fig. 9.12). MRI is now frequently used to evaluate trauma to the foot.

For a tabular summary of the preceding discussion, see Figures 9.25, 9.26, and 9.27.

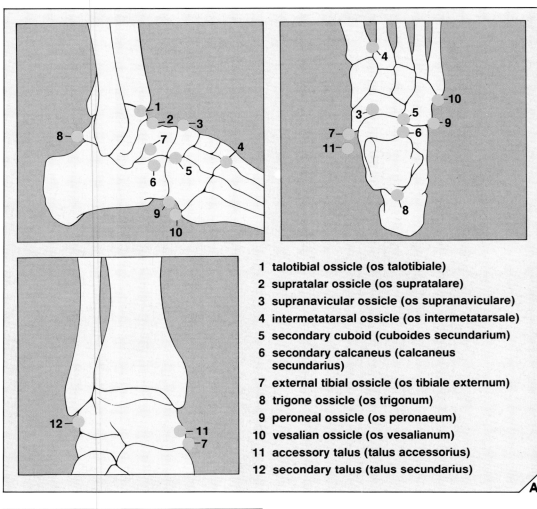

1 talotibial ossicle (os talotibiale)
2 supratalar ossicle (os supratalare)
3 supranavicular ossicle (os supranaviculare)
4 intermetatarsal ossicle (os intermetatarsale)
5 secondary cuboid (cuboides secundarium)
6 secondary calcaneus (calcaneus secundarius)
7 external tibial ossicle (os tibiale externum)
8 trigone ossicle (os trigonum)
9 peroneal ossicle (os peronaeum)
10 vesalian ossicle (os vesalianum)
11 accessory talus (talus accessorius)
12 secondary talus (talus secundarius)

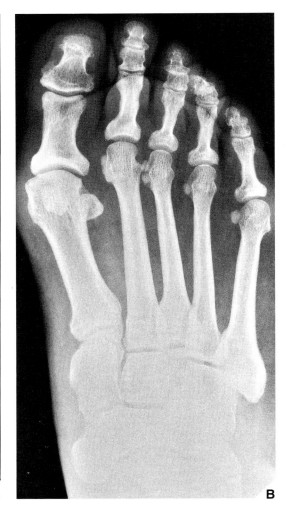

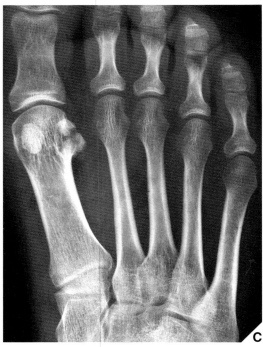

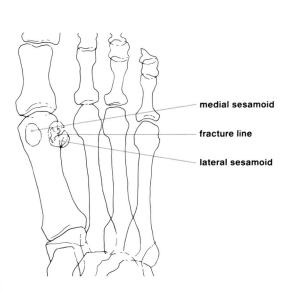

medial sesamoid

fracture line

lateral sesamoid

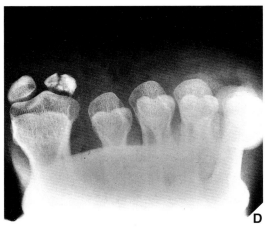

Figure 9.24 (A,B) The numerous accessory ossicles of the foot and ankle can complicate the evaluation of foot injuries by mimicking fracture. Fractures, on the other hand, may go undetected when misinterpreted as ossicles, as seen here on the anteroposterior (C) and sesamoid (D) views of the foot, which demonstrate a fracture of the lateral (fibular) sesamoid (compare with Figure 9.23B).

FIGURE 9.25 Standard and Special Radiographic Projections for Evaluating Injury to the Ankle and Foot

PROJECTION	DEMONSTRATION	PROJECTION	DEMONSTRATION

Anteroposterior (ankle)	Fractures of:
	  Distal tibia
	  Distal fibula
	  Medial malleolus
	  Lateral malleolus
	  Pilon fractures (extension into
	    tibiotalar joint)
		Lateral (ankle and foot)	Boehler angle
			Fractures of:
			  Distal tibia
			    Anterior aspect
			    Posterior lip (third malleolus)
			  Tibiotalar joint
			  Talus (particularly neck)
			  Calcaneus (particularly in
			    coronal plane)
			  Posterior facet of subtalar joint
			  Sustentaculum tali
			  Accessory ossicles
			  Cuboid bone
			Dislocations in:
			  Subtalar joint
			    Peritalar (anterior and
			      posterior types)
			  Tarsometatarsal
			    (Lisfranc) joint

(foot)	Fractures of:
	  Distal portion of talus
	  Navicular, cuboid, and
	    cuneiform bones
	  Metatarsals and phalanges
	    (including stress fractures
	    and accessory ossicles)
	Dislocations in:
	  Subtalar joint
	    Peritalar (anterior and
	      posterior types)
	    Total talar
	  Tarsometatarsal
	    (Lisfranc) joint		

With 10° internal ankle rotation (mortise view)	Same structures and
	  abnormalities as simple
	  anteroposterior but better
	  demonstration of tibial
	  plafond
		Stress (anterior-draw)	Tear of anterior talofibular
			  ligament
			Ankle instability

Stress (inversion, eversion)	Tear of lateral collateral ligament
	Ankle instability
		Oblique **Internal** **External**	Fractures of:
			  Medial malleolus
			  Talus
			  Tuberosity of calcaneus
			  Metatarsals
			  Phalanges

		Posterior Tangential **(Harris-Beath)**	Fractures involving:
			  Middle and posterior facets of
			    subtalar joint
			  Calcaneus (in axial plane)

		Oblique Tangential Broden	Fractures involving:
			  Posterior facet of subtalar joint
			  Calcaneus
			  Sustentaculum tali

		Axial **(sesamoid view)**	Fractures of sesamoid bones

FIGURE 9.26 Ancillary Imaging Techniques For Evaluating Injury to the Ankle and Foot

TECHNIQUE	DEMONSTRATION	TECHNIQUE	DEMONSTRATION

Radionuclide Imaging (scintigraphy, bone scan)	Stress fractures
	Healing process
		Tenography	Tears of:
			  Achilles tendon
			  Posterior tibialis tendon
			  Peroneal tendons
			  Digitorum longus tendon

Tomography	Position of fragments and
	  extension of fracture lines
	  in complex fractures
	Healing process and
	  complications
	  Nonunion
	  Secondary infection
		Computed Tomography	Complex fractures
			  (particularly of os calcis)
			Intraarticular extension of
			  fracture line
			Injuries to tendons (particularly
			  peroneal, tibialis, and
			  Achilles)

Arthrography (single-contrast)	Tears of ligament structures of ankle joint		

(double-contrast usually combined with tomography or CT)	Osteochondral fractures
	Osteochondritis dissecans of
	  talus
	Osteochondral bodies in joint
		Magnetic Resonance Imaging	Same as arthrography,
			  tenography, and computed
			  tomography

Injury to the Ankle

All ankle injuries can be broadly classified, according to the mechanism of injury, as resulting from inversion (Fig. 9.28) or eversion (Fig. 9.29) stress forces. Inversion injuries are much more common, as O'Donoghue has pointed out, accounting for 85% of all traumatic conditions involving the ankle. These groupings apply to both fractures and injuries to the ligament complexes of the ankle. However, it is in the latter type of injuries that they are particularly helpful in determining and evaluating the specific type of ligament injury, especially in the presence of certain fractures about the ankle.

Fractures about the Ankle Joint

In addition to being classified by mechanism of injury, fractures about the ankle joint can also be classified by the anatomic structure involved (Fig. 9.30) and designated as:

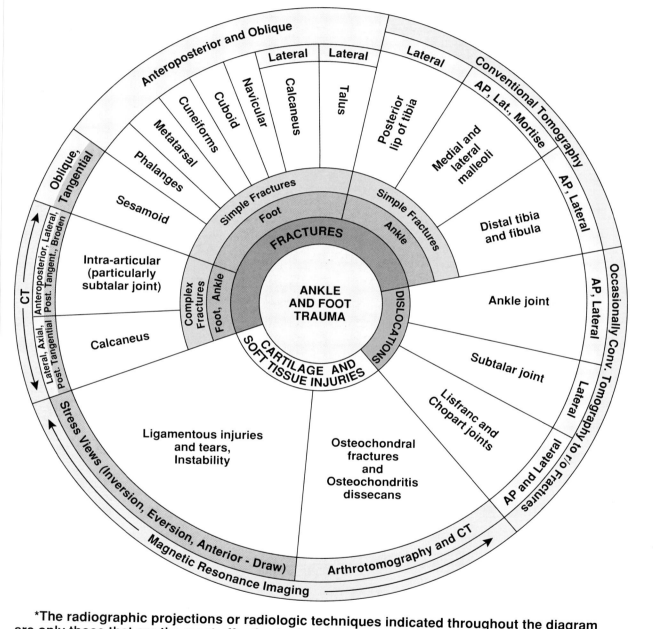

SPECTRUM OF RADIOLOGIC IMAGING TECHNIQUES FOR EVALUATING INJURY TO THE ANKLE AND FOOT*

*The radiographic projections or radiologic techniques indicated throughout the diagram are only those that are the most effective in demonstrating the respective traumatic conditions.

Figure 9.27 Spectrum of radiologic imaging techniques used to evaluate trauma to the ankle and foot.

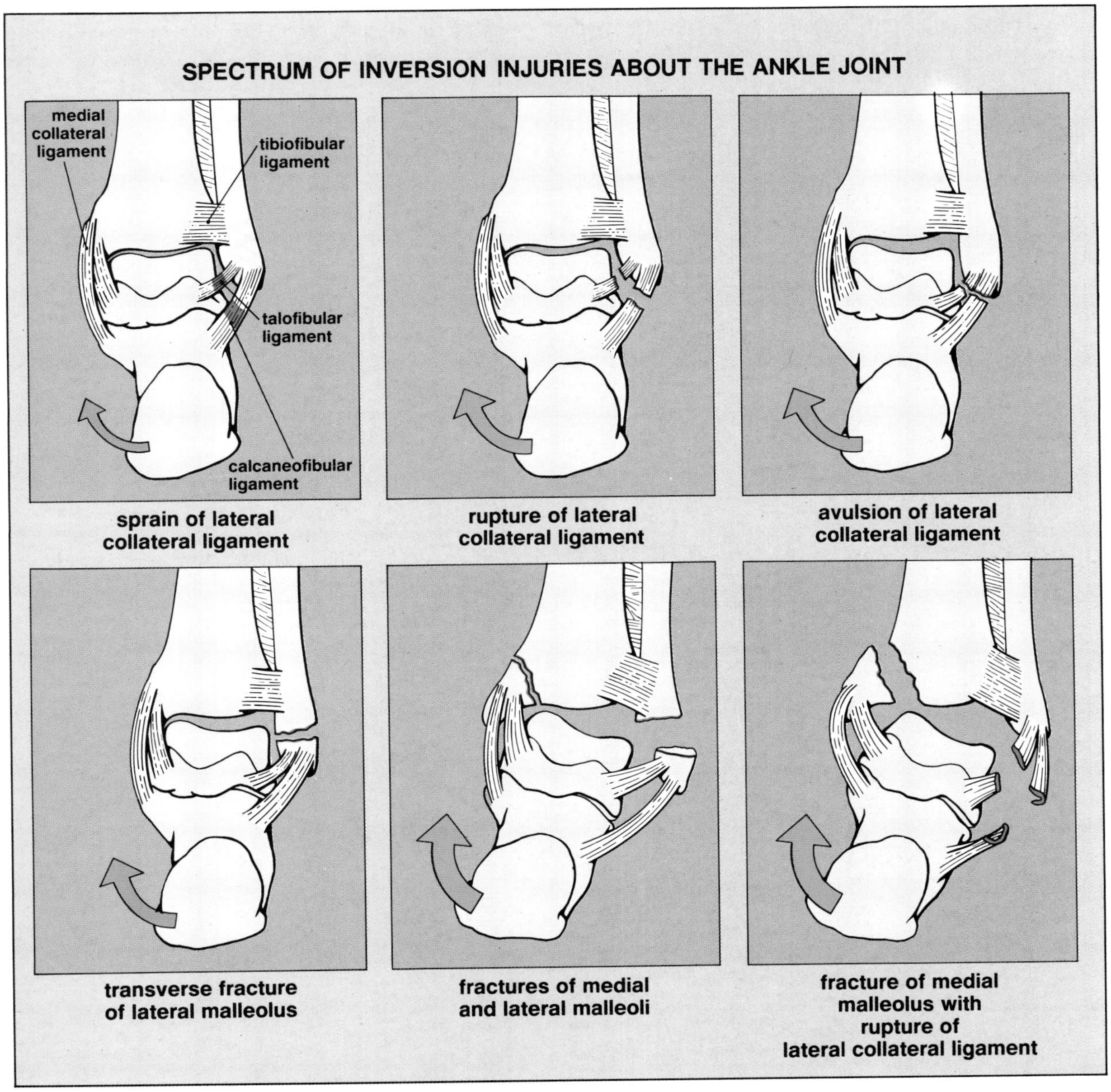

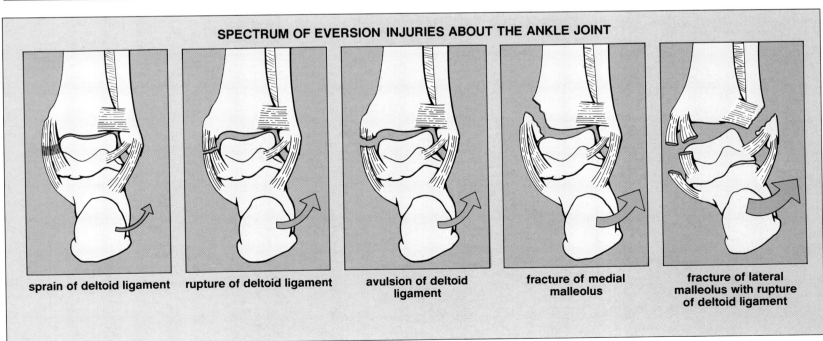

SPECTRUM OF INVERSION INJURIES ABOUT THE ANKLE JOINT

medial collateral ligament

tibiofibular ligament

talofibular ligament

calcaneofibular ligament

sprain of lateral collateral ligament

rupture of lateral collateral ligament

avulsion of lateral collateral ligament

transverse fracture of lateral malleolus

fractures of medial and lateral malleoli

fracture of medial malleolus with rupture of lateral collateral ligament

Figure 9.28 Depending on its severity, an inversion force delivered to the lateral structures of the ankle joint may manifest in a broad spectrum of injuries of the lateral collateral ligament complex, as well as the lateral and medial malleoli. Note, however, that inversion-stress forces do not affect the posterior tibiofibular or medial collateral ligaments. (Adapted from Edeiken J, 1978)

SPECTRUM OF EVERSION INJURIES ABOUT THE ANKLE JOINT

sprain of deltoid ligament

rupture of deltoid ligament

avulsion of deltoid ligament

fracture of medial malleolus

fracture of lateral malleolus with rupture of deltoid ligament

Figure 9.29 Depending on its severity, an eversion force delivered to the medial structures of the ankle joint may manifest in a broad spectrum of injuries of the medial collateral (deltoid) ligament complex, as well as the medial and lateral malleoli. Note, however, that eversion-stress forces do not affect the posterior tibiofibular or lateral collateral ligaments. (Adapted from Edeiken J, 1978)

1. *unimalleolar* when the fracture involves the medial (tibial) or lateral (fibular) malleolus (Fig. 9.31)
2. *bimalleolar* when both malleoli are fractured (Fig. 9.32)
3. *trimalleolar* when fractures involve the medial and lateral malleoli as well as the posterior lip (or tubercle) of the distal tibia (the third malleolus) (Fig. 9.33)
4. *complex fractures* when comminuted fractures of the distal tibia and fibula occur (Fig. 9.34).

These fractures, when viewed from the standpoint of pathomechanics, may be either inversion or eversion injuries or a combination of both. The various types of eversion fractures are best known by their eponyms, including the Pott, Maisonneuve, Dupuytren, and Tillaux fractures (see below).

All of the following ankle fractures involving the distal tibia and fibula can be diagnosed on the standard radiographic projections. However, conventional tomography or CT may be useful in delineating the extent of the fracture line, and either modality is particu-

larly effective in evaluating lateral displacement in the juvenile Tillaux fracture. To evaluate associated ligament injuries, stress radiography, single-contrast arthrography, or MRI are the techniques of choice.

FRACTURE OF THE DISTAL TIBIA   *PILON (PYLON) FRACTURE* Fracture of the distal tibia is called a pilon (pylon) fracture when the fracture line extends into the tibiotalar joint (see Fig. 9.34). Pilon fractures are a distinct clinical and radiologic entity and should not be confused with trimalleolar fractures. The following features distinguish pilon fractures from the trimalleolar fractures: the presence of profound comminution of the distal tibia; intra-articular extension of tibial fracture through the dome of the plafond; usual association of fracture of the talus; and usual preservation of tibiofibular syndesmosis. This fracture's significance comprises the intra-articular extension of the fracture line and its consequent potential to cause late complications of posttraumatic arthritis.

Figure 9.30 Ankle fractures can be classified according to the anatomic structure as unimalleolar, bimalleolar, trimalleolar, or complex.

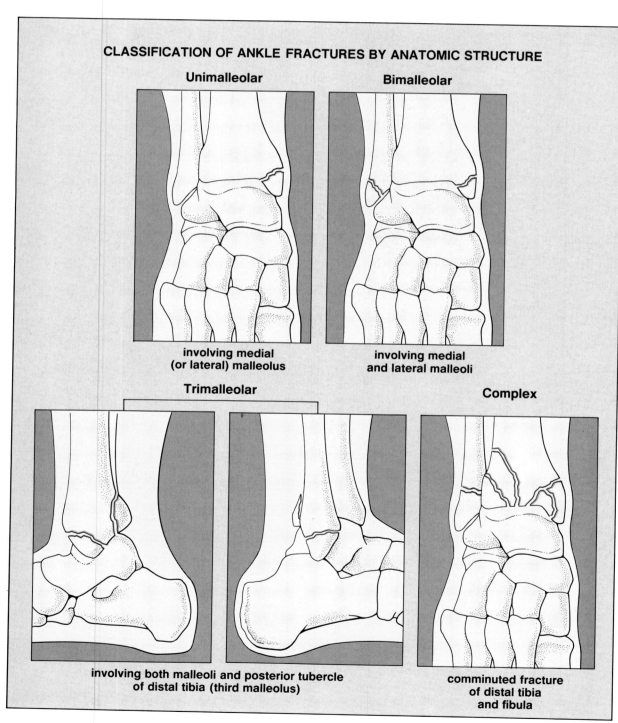

CLASSIFICATION OF ANKLE FRACTURES BY ANATOMIC STRUCTURE

Unimalleolar

involving medial
(or lateral) malleolus

Bimalleolar

involving medial
and lateral malleoli

Trimalleolar

involving both malleoli and posterior tubercle
of distal tibia (third malleolus)

Complex

comminuted fracture
of distal tibia
and fibula

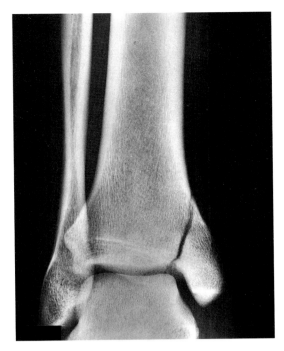

Figure 9.31 Anteroposterior view of the ankle demonstrates the typical appearance of a unimalleolar fracture involving the medial malleolus.

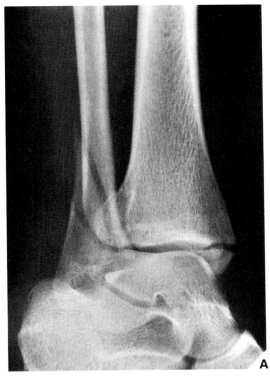

A

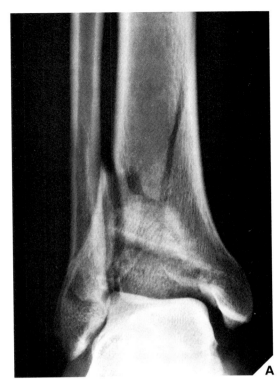

A

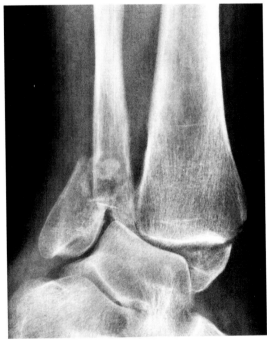

Figure 9.32 Oblique view of the ankle shows a bimalleolar fracture involving both the tibial and fibular malleoli.

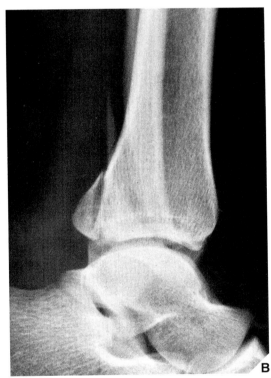

B

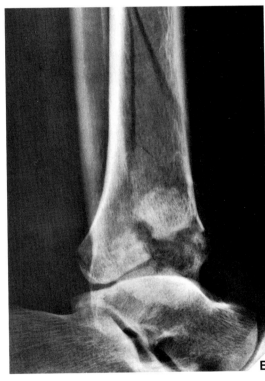

B

Figure 9.33 Oblique (A) and lateral (B) views of the ankle show a trimalleolar fracture affecting both malleoli as well as the posterior lip of the distal tibia. The latter feature is better seen on the lateral view.

Figure 9.34 Anteroposterior (A) and lateral (B) films of the ankle demonstrate a complex, comminuted fracture of the distal tibia and fibula in a 30-year-old man who fell from a third-floor window.

Müller's widely accepted classification of pilon fractures divides these injuries into three groups, depending on the displacement of the fragments and the incongruity of the joint (Fig. 9.35).

TILLAUX FRACTURE In 1872, Tillaux described an ankle fracture resulting from abduction and external-rotation injury and consist- ing of avulsion of the lateral margin of the tibia. The fracture line is vertical and extends from the distal articular surface of the tibia upward to the lateral cortex (Fig. 9.36). In children, a similar type of fracture, referred to as *juvenile Tillaux fracture*, is actually a Salter-Harris type III injury to the growth plate (Fig. 9.37; see also Fig. 4.25). This injury probably occurs because the growth plate fuses

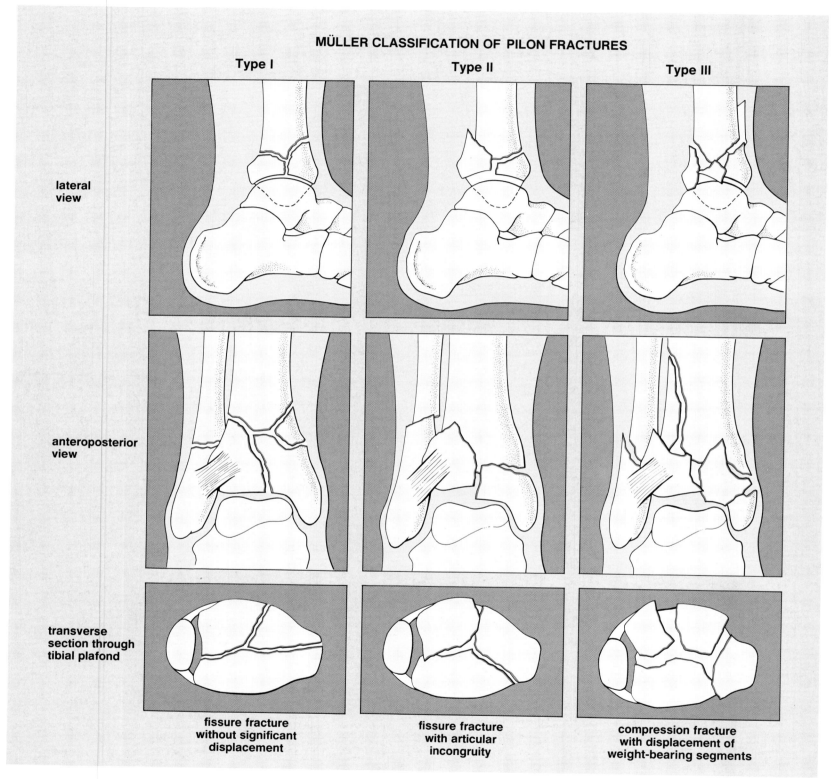

MÜLLER CLASSIFICATION OF PILON FRACTURES

Type I	Type II	Type III

lateral view

anteroposterior view

transverse section through tibial plafond

fissure fracture without significant displacement	fissure fracture with articular incongruity	compression fracture with displacement of weight-bearing segments

Figure 9.35 The Müller classification of intra-articular fractures of the distal tibia (pilon fractures) is based on the amount of displacement of the frag- ments and the consequent degree of incongruity of the joint. (Adapted from Müller ME, et al., 1979)

from medial to lateral, making the medial side stronger than the lateral.

The radiologic evaluation of a Tillaux fracture is critical for establishing whether surgery will be necessary. If the fracture fragment is laterally displaced more than 2 mm or if there is an irregularity of the articular surface of the distal tibia (a step-off), surgical rather than conservative treatment is indicated. Conventional tomography and CT are the best methods for obtaining this information (Fig. 9.38).

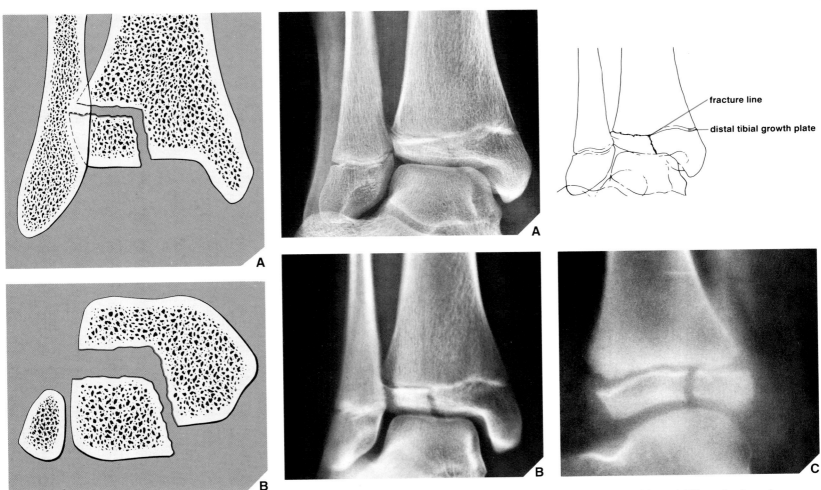

Figure 9.36 In the classic Tillaux fracture, shown here schematically in coronal (A) and transverse (B) sections through the distal tibia, the fracture line extends from the distal articular surface of the tibia upward to the lateral cortex.

Figure 9.37 A 13-year-old girl injured her right ankle during a basketball game. Oblique view of the ankle (A) and tomographic sections in the oblique (B) and lateral (C) projections demonstrate a typical Salter-Harris type III injury to the growth plate, also called juvenile Tillaux fracture.

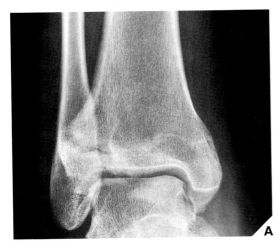

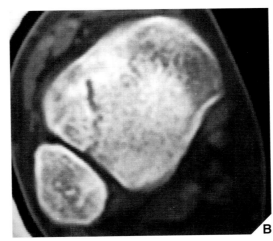

Figure 9.38 A 24-year-old woman twisted her ankle while ice skating. Anteroposterior view (A) and CT section (B) show a marginal fracture of the lateral aspect of the tibia, a characteristic Tillaux fracture. The minimal amount of displacement seen here would mandate only conservative treatment.

If, instead of avulsion of the lateral margin of the tibia, the medial portion of the fibula becomes detached and the anterior tibiofibular ligament remains intact, the fracture is called a *Wagstaffe-LeFort fracture* (Fig. 9.39).

TRIPLANAR (MARMOR-LYNN) FRACTURE Fractures involving the lateral aspect of the distal tibial epiphysis may be complicated by extension of the fracture line into two other planes, hence the term *triplanar fracture*. The mechanism of this type of injury is usually plantar flex-

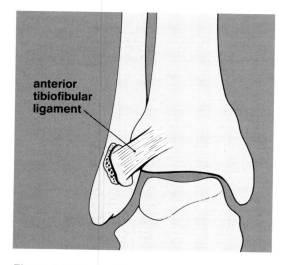

Figure 9.39 In the Wagstaffe-LeFort fracture, seen here schematically on the anteroposterior view, the medial portion of the fibula is avulsed at the insertion of the anterior tibiofibular ligament. The ligament, however, remains intact.

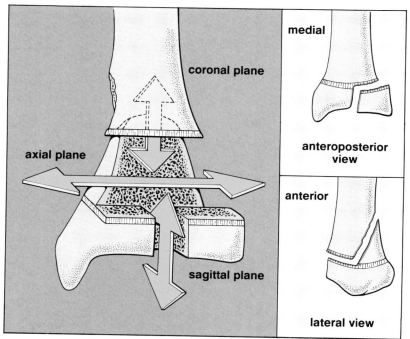

Figure 9.40 The Marmor-Lynn (or triplanar) fracture comprises a vertical fracture of the epiphysis in the sagittal plane, a horizontally oriented fracture in the axial plane through the lateral aspect of the growth plate, and an oblique fracture through the metaphysis into the diaphysis in the coronal plane, extending superiorly from the anterior aspect of the growth plate to the posterior cortex of the tibia.

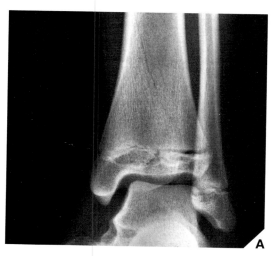

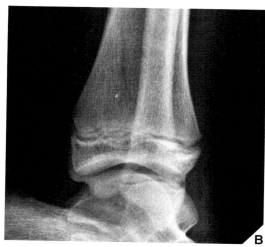

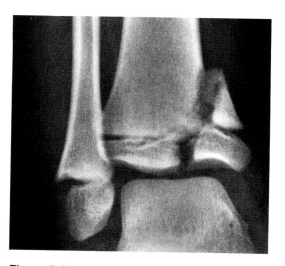

Figure 9.41 A 12-year-old girl fell on ice and sustained a typical triplanar fracture. (A) Anteroposterior view of the left ankle shows a vertical fracture of the epiphysis and horizontal extension through the lateral aspect of the growth plate. The metaphyseal and diaphyseal components of

the fracture are barely seen. (B) Lateral view clearly demonstrates the posteriorly directed fracture line in the coronal plane, the third component of a triplanar fracture (see also Figs. 9.37, 4.25).

Figure 9.42 Anteroposterior view of a Salter-Harris type IV fracture of the distal tibia in an 8-year-old boy demonstrates that the fracture line traverses the epiphysis and metaphysis, but there is no horizontal extension through the growth plate. Note the associated Salter-Harris type I fracture of the distal fibula (see Fig. 4.25).

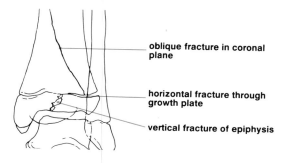

oblique fracture in coronal plane

horizontal fracture through growth plate

vertical fracture of epiphysis

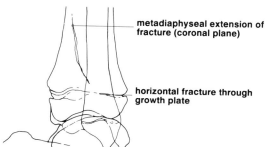

metadiaphyseal extension of fracture (coronal plane)

horizontal fracture through growth plate

ion and external rotation. The three planes involved are the *sagittal plane* in which there is a vertical fracture through the epiphysis, the *axial plane* in which a horizontally oriented fracture extends through the lateral aspect of the growth plate, and the *coronal plane* in which there is an oblique fracture through the metaphysis into the diaphysis, extending superiorly from the anterior aspect of the growth plate to the posterior cortex of the tibia (Fig. 9.40).

The epiphyseal component of this fracture is best seen on the anteroposterior view, the axial component on both the anteroposterior and lateral views, and the diaphyseal extension on the lateral view. The typical triplanar fracture thus consists of a combination of the juvenile Tillaux fracture and a Salter-Harris type II fracture (Fig. 9.41; see also Figs. 9.36, 4.25) and should not be mistaken for a Salter-Harris Type IV fracture (Fig. 9.42).

FRACTURES OF THE FIBULA *POTT FRACTURE* After suffering a fracture of his own leg, Sir Percivall Pott described in 1769 what he believed to be the most common type of ankle fracture, a fracture of the distal third of the fibula (Fig. 9.43). It is now recognized that this type of fracture usually occurs as a result of disruption of the tibiofibular syndesmosis. In fact, many authorities believe that the type of fracture Pott described does not exist as a primary fracture.

DUPUYTREN FRACTURE This is the name given to a fracture of the fibula occurring 2 cm to 7 cm above the distal tibiofibular syndesmosis and including disruption of the medial collateral ligament (Fig. 9.44). The associated tear of the syndesmosis leads to ankle instability.

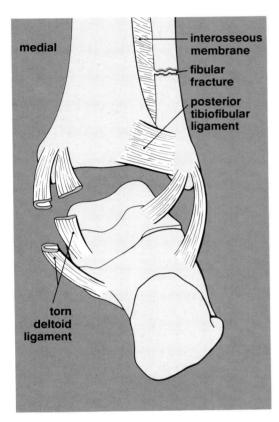

Figure 9.43 In the Pott fracture, the fibula is fractured above the intact distal tibiofibular syndesmosis, the deltoid ligament is ruptured, and the talus is subluxed laterally.

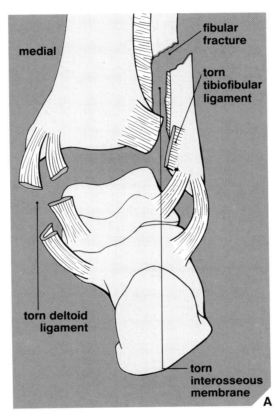

Figure 9.44 (A) The Dupuytren fracture usually occurs 2 cm to 7 cm above the distal tibiofibular syndesmosis, with disruption of the medial collateral ligament and, typically, tear of the syndesmo-

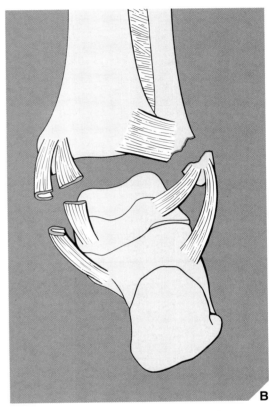

sis leading to ankle instability. (B) In the low-variant, the fracture occurs more distally and the tibiofibular ligament remains intact.

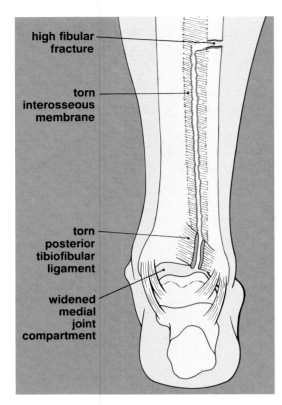

high fibular fracture

torn interosseous membrane

torn posterior tibiofibular ligament

widened medial joint compartment

Figure 9.45 The classic Maisonneuve fracture commonly occurs at the junction of the middle and distal thirds of the fibula. The tibiofibular syndesmosis is disrupted, and the interosseous membrane is torn up to the level of the fracture. The tibiotalar (medial) joint compartment is widened due to lateral subluxation of the talus.

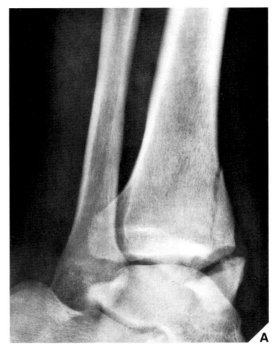

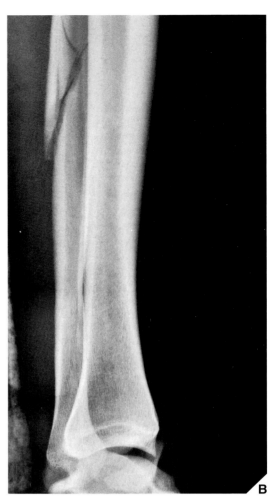

Figure 9.46 A 22-year-old man injured his right ankle in a skiing accident. (A) Oblique view of the ankle shows a comminuted fracture of the medial malleolus, with extension into the anterior lip of the tibia. (B) On the lateral view, a comminuted fracture of the fibula is apparent. This is a characteristic of a Maisonneuve-type fracture.

FIGURE 9.47 Lauge-Hansen Classification of Ankle Injuries

PRONATION-ABDUCTION INJURIES
Stage I   Rupture of the deltoid ligament or transverse fracture of the medial malleolus

Stage II   Disruption of the distal anterior and posterior tibiofibular ligaments

Stage III   Oblique fracture of the fibula at the level of the joint* (best seen on the anteroposterior projection)

PRONATION-LATERAL (EXTERNAL) ROTATION INJURIES
Stage I   Rupture of the deltoid ligament or transverse fracture of the medial malleolus

Stage II   Disruption of the anterior tibiofibular ligament and interosseous membrane

Stage III   Fracture of the fibula usually 6 cm or more above the level of the joint*

Stage IV   Chip fracture of the posterior tibia or rupture of the posterior tibiofibular ligament

SUPINATION-ADDUCTION INJURIES
Stage I   Injury to the lateral collateral ligament or transverse fracture of the lateral malleolus below the level of the joint*

Stage II   Steep oblique fracture of the medial malleolus

SUPINATION-LATERAL (EXTERNAL) ROTATION INJURIES
Stage I   Disruption of the anterior tibiofibular ligament

Stage II   Spiral fracture of the distal fibula near the joint* (best seen on the lateral projection)

Stage III   Rupture of the posterior tibiofibular ligament

Stage IV   Transverse fracture of the medial malleolus

(Adapted from Lauge-Hansen N, 1950)
*The appearance of the fibular fracture is the key to determining the mechanism of injury.

MAISONNEUVE FRACTURE Like the Dupuytren fracture, the Maisonneuve fracture is an eversion-type injury of the fibula. The fracture, however, occurs in the proximal half of the bone, commonly at the junction of the proximal and middle thirds of the shaft (Fig. 9.45). The tibiofibular syndesmosis is disrupted, and either tear of the tibiofibular ligament or fracture of the medial malleolus is also present (Fig. 9.46). The more proximal the location of the fibular fracture, the more damage to the interosseous membrane between the tibia and the fibula, which is always disrupted up to the point of the fibular fracture.

Injury to the Soft Tissues About the Ankle Joint and Foot

As mentioned earlier, all ankle injuries can be grossly classified as resulting from inversion- or eversion-stress forces (see Figs. 9.28, 9.29). However, the forces delivered to the ankle are rarely pure inversion or pure eversion. A combination of forces is usually at work to produce ligament and tendon injuries that may occur secondary to fractures or as primary injuries. Several classifications have been developed to reflect the complexity of these forces. Lauge-Hansen classified ankle injuries by combining the position of the foot (supination or pronation) with the direction of the deforming force vector (external rotation, adduction, or abduction) (Fig. 9.47). He emphasized the close relationship between bone and ligament injuries, but the complexity of his classification diminishes its value in treatment.

From the practical orthopedic point of view, the Weber classification, based on the level of fibular fracture and therefore on the type of syndesmotic ligament injury, is much more useful (Fig. 9.48):

Type A The fibular fracture may be a transverse avulsion fracture at the level of or just distal to the ankle joint. There may be an associated fracture of the medial malleolus. Alternatively, the fibula is intact, but the lateral collateral ligament is disrupted. In either case, the tibiofibular syndesmosis, the interosseous membrane, and the deltoid ligament are intact.

Type B There is a spiral fracture of the distal fibula, beginning at the level of the tibiofibular syndesmosis, with partial disruption of mainly the posterior tibiofibular ligament. It may also

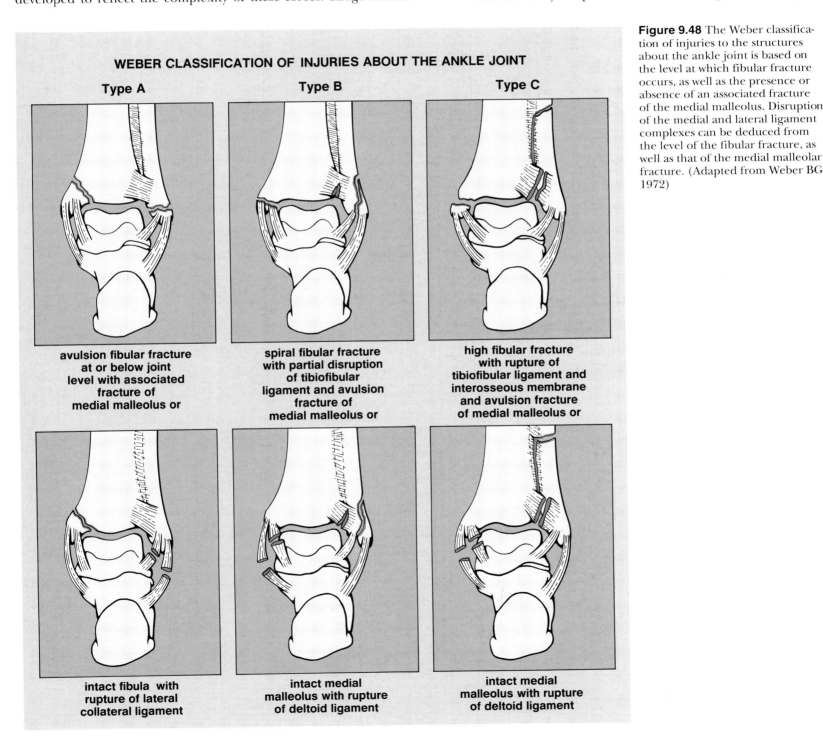

WEBER CLASSIFICATION OF INJURIES ABOUT THE ANKLE JOINT

Type A

avulsion fibular fracture at or below joint level with associated fracture of medial malleolus or

intact fibula with rupture of lateral collateral ligament

Type B

spiral fibular fracture with partial disruption of tibiofibular ligament and avulsion fracture of medial malleolus or

intact medial malleolus with rupture of deltoid ligament

Type C

high fibular fracture with rupture of tibiofibular ligament and interosseous membrane and avulsion fracture of medial malleolus or

intact medial malleolus with rupture of deltoid ligament

Figure 9.48 The Weber classification of injuries to the structures about the ankle joint is based on the level at which fibular fracture occurs, as well as the presence or absence of an associated fracture of the medial malleolus. Disruption of the medial and lateral ligament complexes can be deduced from the level of the fibular fracture, as well as that of the medial malleolar fracture. (Adapted from Weber BG, 1972)

be associated with an avulsion fracture of the medial malleolus below the level of the ankle joint (Fig. 9.49). Alternatively, the medial malleolus may be intact and the deltoid ligament may be disrupted.

Type C Fracture of the fibula occurs at a level higher than the ankle joint, with associated tear of the posterior tibiofibular ligament and resultant lateral talar instability. If the fibular fracture is high (Maisonneuve type), the interosseous membrane is torn to the level of the fracture. There is also an avulsion fracture of the medial malleolus, in which case the deltoid ligament is intact. Alternatively, the medial malleolus is intact, but the deltoid ligament is disrupted (Fig. 9.50).

The likelihood of injury to the distal tibiofibular syndesmosis can be inferred from the nature and level of the fibular fracture: The higher the fibular fracture, the more extensive the damage to the tibiofibular ligaments and, thus, the greater the risk of ankle instability. The greatest value of this classification lies in the fact that it emphasizes the lateral syndesmosis-malleolar complex as an important factor in congruence and stability in the ankle joint.

TEAR OF THE MEDIAL COLLATERAL LIGAMENT Depending on the severity of the eversion force, injury to the medial collateral ligament ranges from sprain to complete rupture (see Fig. 9.29). Tear may occur either in the body of the ligament or at its attachment to the medial malleolus. Rupture of the medial collateral ligament is typically associated with a tear of the tibiofibular ligament and lateral subluxation of the talus. On clinical examination, soft tissue swelling is prominent distal to the tip of the medial malleolus. If the standard radiographic examination of the ankle reveals lateral shift of the talus in the absence of a spiral fracture of the fibula, one must assume that both the tibiofibular and the medial collateral liga-

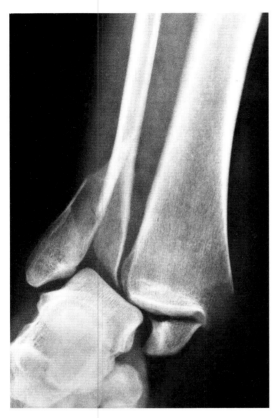

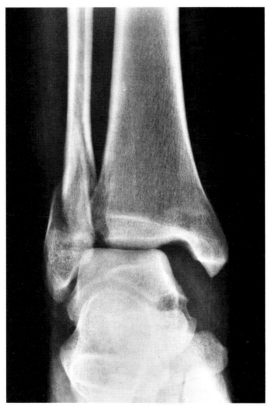

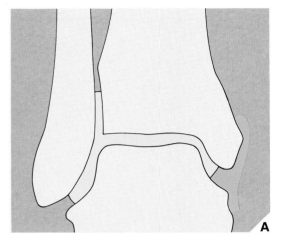

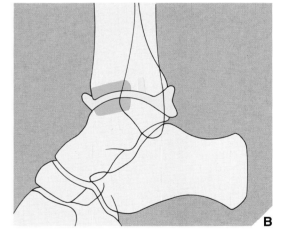

Figure 9.49 A 24-year-old woman injured her right ankle in a skiing accident. Anteroposterior view of the ankle demonstrates a spiral fracture of the fibula beginning at the level of the tibiofibular syndesmosis with consequent tear of the inferoposterior portion of the syndesmotic complex; the interosseous membrane is intact. The site of the fracture of the medial malleolus suggests that the deltoid ligament may be intact. According to the Weber classification, this is a type B fracture.

Figure 9.50 A 32-year-old woman stepped into a pothole and injured her right ankle. Anteroposterior view of the ankle demonstrates a fracture of the fibula above the level of the ankle joint, indicating disruption of the interosseous membrane. The intact medial malleolus indicates a tear of the deltoid ligament. This type of fracture is classified as a Weber type C. The risk of ankle mortise instability due to disruption of the medial and lateral ligament complexes gives this type of injury a worse prognosis than type A or B.

Figure 9.51 (A,B) Tear of the deltoid ligament in the absence of fracture is characterized on the arthrogram, represented here schematically, by leak of contrast beneath the medial malleolus (compare with Figure 9.11).

ments are torn. Arthrographic examination shows leak of contrast agent beneath the medial malleolus (Fig. 9.51).

TEAR OF THE LATERAL COLLATERAL LIGAMENT Inversion-stress forces delivered to the lateral ankle structures may cause a spectrum of injuries to the lateral collateral ligament, ranging from sprain to complete rupture (see Fig. 9.28). The body of the ligament or its attachment to the fibular malleolus may be the site of injury. In the absence of fracture of the fibular malleolus on the standard radiographic examination, disruption of the ligament complex can be recognized on the inversion-stress film of the ankle by an increase in talar tilt to 15° or more (see Figs. 9.9B, 9.52A). Arthrographic examination, however, is always diagnostic.

The component ligaments of this complex may also be injured independently. The *anterior talofibular ligament* is the most frequently injured ankle ligament. It can be diagnosed on the inversion-stress film of the ankle (see Fig. 9.9), but arthrographic examination is usually required for confirmation (Fig. 9.52). Characteristically, contrast agent is seen to leak anteriorly to the lateral malleolus and laterally alongside it (Fig. 9.53); rupture of the *posterior talofibular ligament* is better appreciated on the lateral view. Rupture of the *calcaneofibular ligament* is invariably associated with tear of the anterior

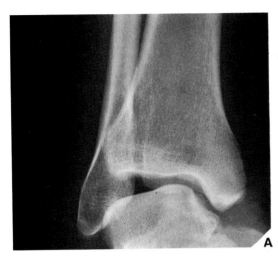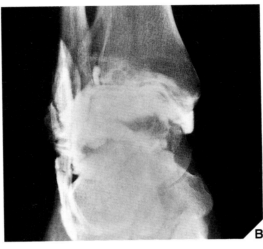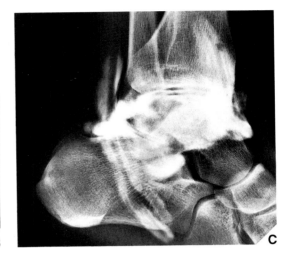

Figure 9.52 A 28-year-old woman injured her ankle in a skiing accident. (A) Inversion-stress radiograph shows a talar tilt of 22°, suggesting tear of the lateral collateral ligament complex. Single-contrast arthrograms in the anteroposterior (B) and lateral (C) projections reveal tears of several ligaments: leakage around the tip of the fibula indicates a tear of the anterior talofibular ligament, filling of the peroneal tendon sheath indicates a tear of the calcaneofibular ligament, and leak of contrast into the tibiofibular syndesmosis indicates a tear of the distal anterior tibiofibular ligament. Filling of the posterior facet of the subtalar joint indicates a tear of the posterior talofibular ligament.

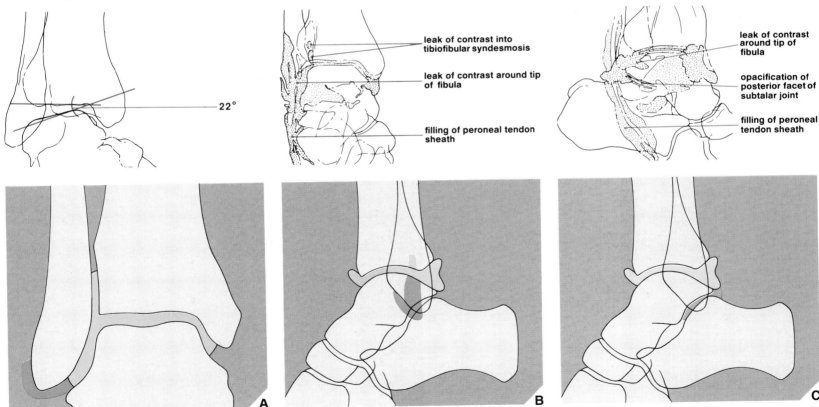

Figure 9.53 (A,B) On arthrography, leak of contrast around the tip of the lateral malleolus characterizes a tear of the anterior talofibular ligament. (C) Tear of the posterior talofibular ligament can be recognized on the lateral view by opacification of the posterior facet of the subtalar joint. In 10% of cases, however, this finding may represent a normal variant.

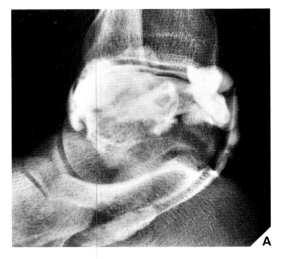

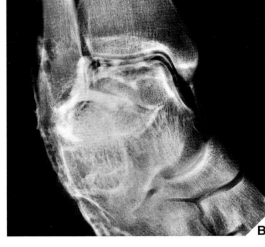

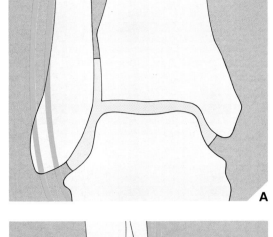

Figure 9.54 A 27-year-old man twisted his ankle during a sports activity. Plain films were normal, and stress views were equivocal. Contrast arthrograms in the lateral (A) and oblique (B) projections of the ankle show opacification of the

peroneal tendon sheath characteristic of tear of the calcaneofibular ligament. Leak of contrast agent along the fibular malleolus, seen on both views, indicates an associated tear of the anterior talofibular ligament.

leak of contrast
around tip
of fibula

filling of peroneal
tendon sheath

leak of contrast
around tip of
fibula

filling of peroneal
tendon sheath

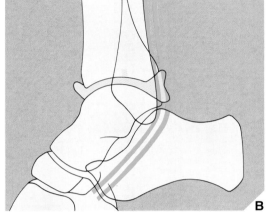

Figure 9.55 (A,B) The characteristic arthrographic finding in rupture of the calcaneofibular ligament is opacification of the peroneal tendon sheath.

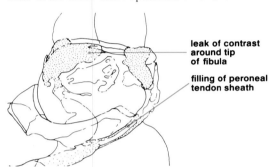

Figure 9.56 A 29-year-old man injured his ankle during a basketball game. Plain-films and stress examination revealed no abnormalities. On arthrography, however, leak of contrast into the region of the tibiofibular syndesmosis indicates a tear of the distal anterior tibiofibular ligament (compare with Figure 9.11B,D).

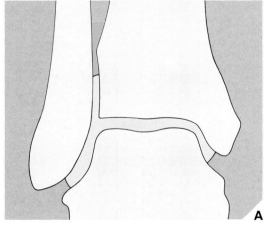

Figure 9.57
(A,B) Tear of the distal anterior tibiofibular ligament can be recognized on arthrography by leak of contrast above the syndesmotic recess. Normally, opacification of the recess does not exceed 2.5 cm.

leak of contrast into
tibiofibular
syndesmosis

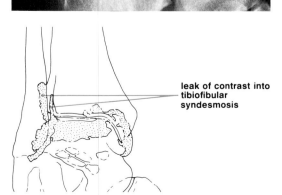

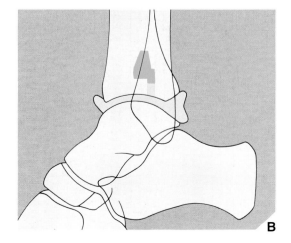

talofibular ligament (Fig. 9.54). The distinguishing arthrographic finding is opacification of the peroneal tendon sheath (Fig. 9.55).

TEAR OF THE DISTAL ANTERIOR TIBIOFIBULAR LIGAMENT Commonly associated with other ligament injuries, tear of the anterior tibiofibular ligament may also occur as an isolated injury (Fig. 9.56). Its arthrographic appearance is characterized by leak of contrast agent into the syndesmotic space (Fig. 9.57).

TENDON RUPTURES Most tendon ruptures can be diagnosed by history and clinical examination. For example, tear of the *Achilles tendon*, the most common injury to the soft tissues of the foot, is often indicated by severe tenderness at the tendon's insertion, together with limitation of plantar flexion. Ruptures of this tendon can be recognized on the lateral plain film of the foot obtained with a low-kilovoltage/soft tissue technique (Fig. 9.58), although tenography (Fig. 9.59) or MRI (see Fig. 9.16) is confirmatory. Tenography is also

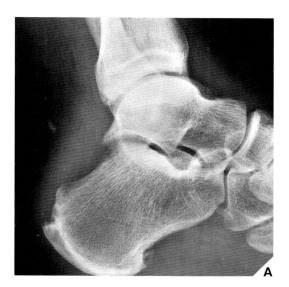
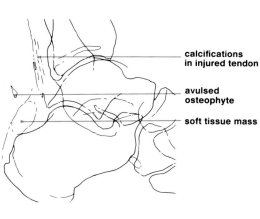
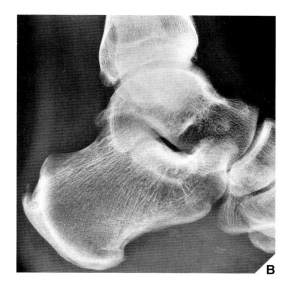

Figure 9.58 A 54-year-old man stumbled into a pothole. Physical examination revealed severe tenderness at the insertion of the Achilles tendon and marked limitation of plantar flexion. (A) Lateral view shows a lack of definition of the tendon, a lumpy soft tissue mass, and an avulsion fracture of a small osteophyte from the posterior aspect of the calcaneus at the insertion of the ruptured tendon. (B) The other, normal foot is shown for comparison.

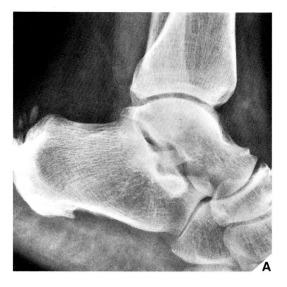
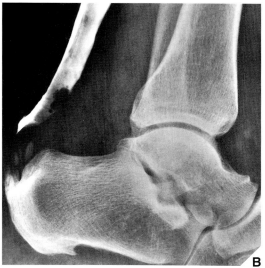
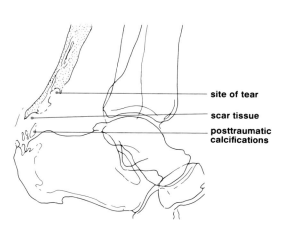

Figure 9.59 (A) Lateral plain film of the ankle shows a lack of definition of the Achilles tendon at its insertion on the posterior aspect of the os calcis and prominent soft tissue swelling. Multiple calcifications are seen at the site of the tendon's insertion. (B) The tenogram demonstrates a tear of the tendon about 5 cm proximal to the insertion by the abrupt termination of contrast filling the tendon sheath.

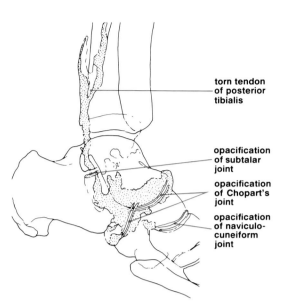

Figure 9.60 A 57-year-old man sustained an eversion injury to the left ankle while playing tennis. On clinical examination, he was diagnosed as having ruptured the tendon of the posterior tibialis muscle. Tenography confirms the clinical findings. Note the abnormal opacification of the subtalar, Chopart, and naviculocuneiform joints.

torn tendon of posterior tibialis

opacification of subtalar joint

opacification of Chopart's joint

opacification of naviculocuneiform joint

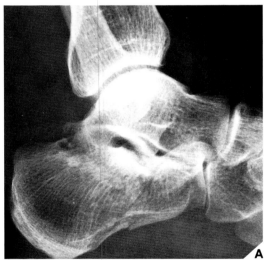

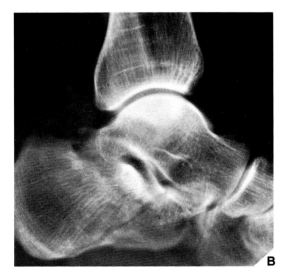

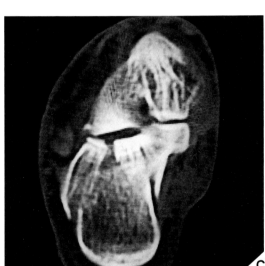

A

B

C

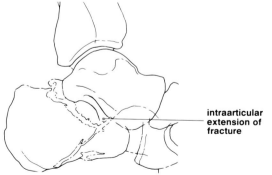

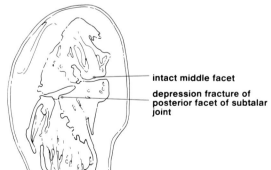

intraarticular extension of fracture

intact middle facet

depression fracture of posterior facet of subtalar joint

Figure 9.61 A 54-year-old man fell from a scaffold and sustained a fracture of the left calcaneus. (A) Lateral view shows a comminuted fracture of the calcaneus. There is a suggestion of extension of the fracture line into the subtalar joint. (B) Tomographic examination in the lateral projection confirms intra-articular extension of the fracture line. The amount of depression of the articular surface, however, cannot be definitely assessed. (C) CT section precisely demonstrates the position of the comminuted fragments and depression at the posterior facet of the subtalar joint. It also shows that the middle facet is intact, important information that the conventional and tomographic studies could not provide.

helpful in confirming rupture of the *posterior tibialis* (Fig. 9.60) and *peroneal tendons*.

Injury to the Foot
Fractures of the Foot

FRACTURES OF THE CALCANEUS Commonly sustained in falls from heights, fractures of the calcaneus are sometimes called "lover's fractures"; in 10% of cases, they are seen bilaterally. According to Cave, fractures of the calcaneus account for 60% of all major tarsal injuries.

In the evaluation of such injuries, it is critical to determine whether or not the fracture line involves the subtalar joint and, if so, to assess the degree of depression of the posterior facet. To determine the Boehler angle (see Fig. 9.19C) helps evaluate depression, but conventional tomography and CT are usually essential (Fig. 9.61). Tomographic examination may also disclose unsuspected additional fracture or fractures (Fig. 9.62). In all calcaneal fractures sustained in a fall from a height, a radiograph of the thoracolumbar spine is essential because of the commonly associ-

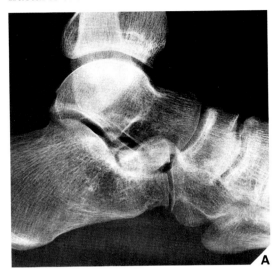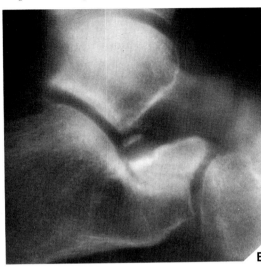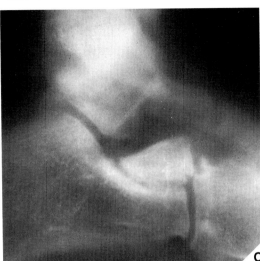

Figure 9.62 A 26-year-old man injured his ankle during a basketball game. (A) Lateral view of the ankle demonstrates an obvious fracture of the subtalar aspect of the anterior portion of the calcaneus. (B,C) Trispiral tomographic cuts demonstrate, in addition, displacement of a chip of fractured bone into the subtalar joint and a fracture of the cuboid bone.

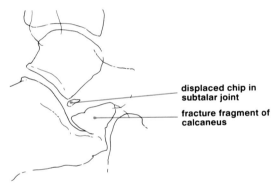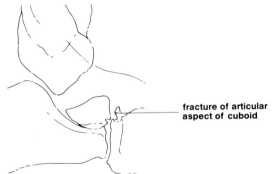

ated finding of compression fracture of one of the vertebral bodies (Fig. 9.63).

Essex-Lopresti classified calcaneal fractures into two main categories: those sparing the subtalar joint (25%) and those extending into it (75%), the latter subdivided into joint-depression fractures and tongue-type fractures. Rowe and coworkers classified calcaneal fractures into five types (Fig. 9.64):

Type I   Fractures of the tuberosity, sustentaculum tali, or anterior process (21%).
Type II   Beak fractures and avulsion fractures of the Achilles tendon insertion (3.8%).
Type III Oblique fractures not extending into the subtalar joint (19.5%).

Type IV   Fractures involving the subtalar joint (24.7%).
Type V   Fractures with central depression and varying degrees of comminution (31%).

Stress fractures of the calcaneus occur in joggers and runners but do not spare the older population when bones are weakened by osteoporosis (Fig. 9.65). Like stress fractures in long bones, these fractures are not immediately evident but typically become obvious about 10 to 14 days after the precipitating incident. They can be recognized on plain films by a band of sclerosis, representing formation of endosteal callus. The fracture line is usually oriented either vertically or parallel to the posterior contour of the bone. If stress fractures are suspected but plain films are normal, a bone scan may validate the diagnosis.

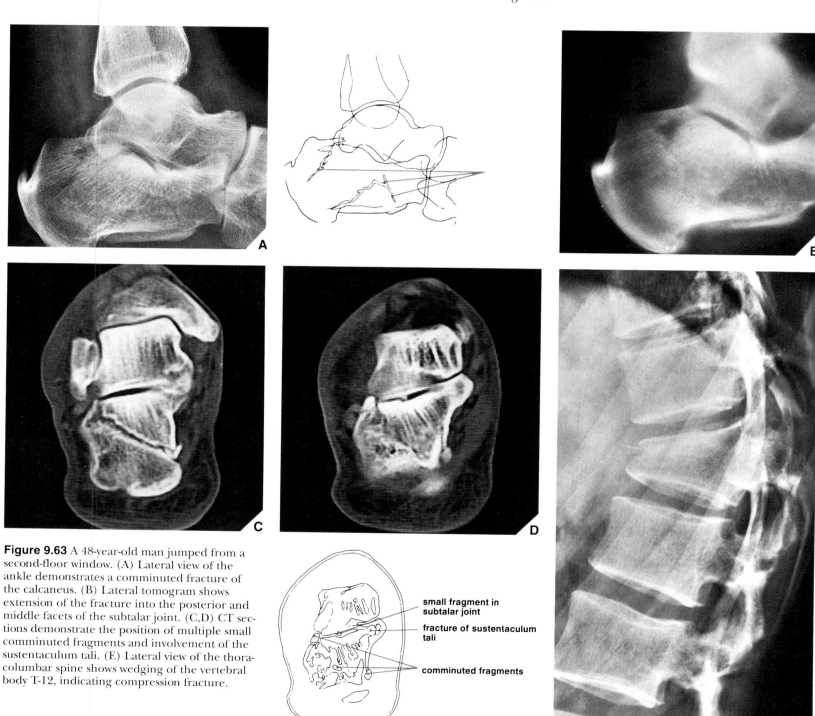

Figure 9.63 A 48-year-old man jumped from a second-floor window. (A) Lateral view of the ankle demonstrates a comminuted fracture of the calcaneus. (B) Lateral tomogram shows extension of the fracture into the posterior and middle facets of the subtalar joint. (C,D) CT sections demonstrate the position of multiple small comminuted fragments and involvement of the sustentaculum tali. (E) Lateral view of the thoracolumbar spine shows wedging of the vertebral body T-12, indicating compression fracture.

small fragment in subtalar joint

fracture of sustentaculum tali

comminuted fragments

ROWE CLASSIFICATION OF CALCANEAL FRACTURES

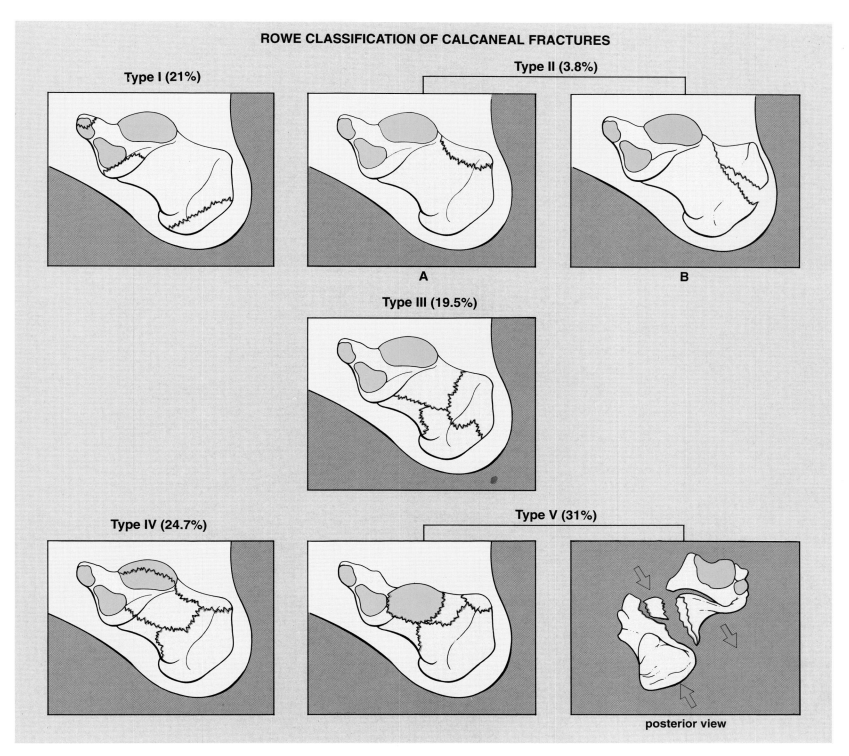

Figure 9.64 The Rowe classification of calcaneal fractures: Type I (21%)–fractures of the tuberosity, sustentaculum tali, or anterior process; type II (3.8%)–beak fractures (A) and avulsion fractures of the Achilles tendon insertion (B); type III (19.5%)–oblique fractures not extending into the subtalar joint; type IV (24.7%)–fractures involving the subtalar joint; type V (31%)–fractures with central depression and varying degrees of comminution. (Modified from Rowe CR, et al., 1963)

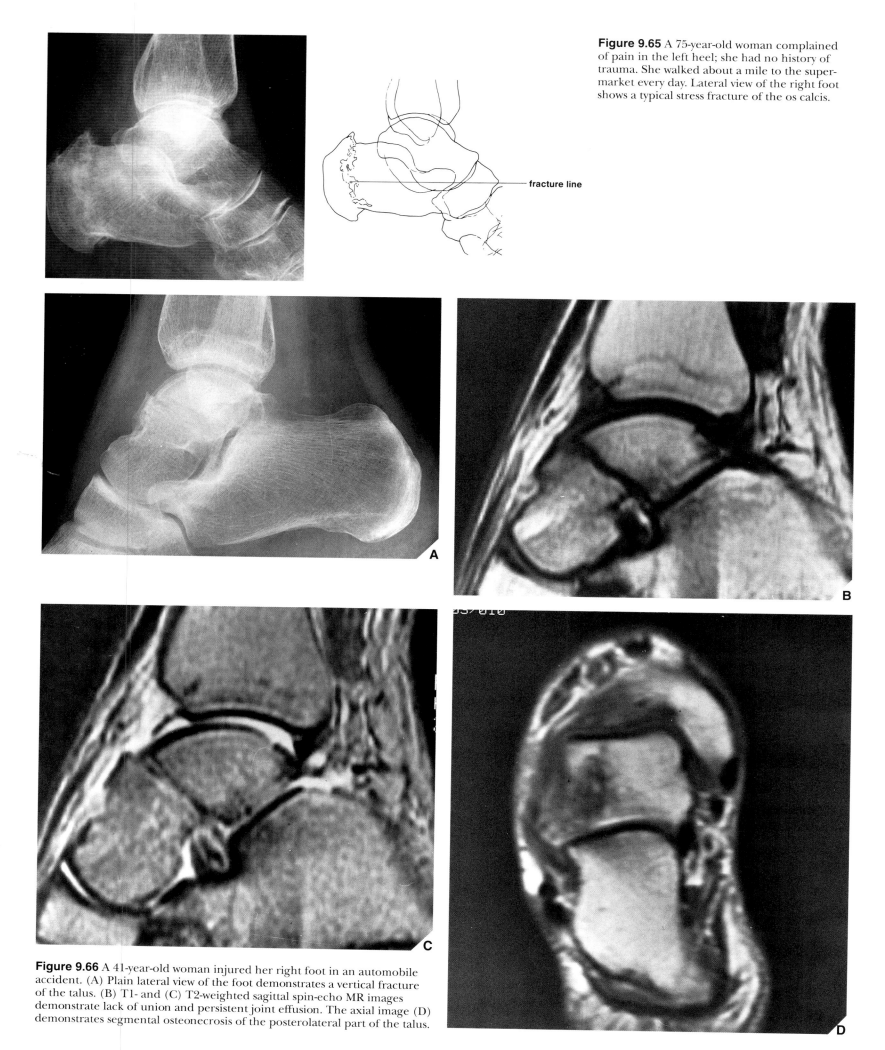

Figure 9.65 A 75-year-old woman complained of pain in the left heel; she had no history of trauma. She walked about a mile to the supermarket every day. Lateral view of the right foot shows a typical stress fracture of the os calcis.

fracture line

Figure 9.66 A 41-year-old woman injured her right foot in an automobile accident. (A) Plain lateral view of the foot demonstrates a vertical fracture of the talus. (B) T1- and (C) T2-weighted sagittal spin-echo MR images demonstrate lack of union and persistent joint effusion. The axial image (D) demonstrates segmental osteonecrosis of the posterolateral part of the talus.

FRACTURES OF THE TALUS Whether vertical (typically involving the neck of the talus) or comminuted, fractures of the talus most often result from forced dorsiflexion of the foot, as may occur in automobile accidents. Accompanying dislocation in the subtalar and talonavicular joints is common. Talar fractures are usually obvious on the standard radiographic projections. MRI may be of value for detecting various complications (Fig. 9.66).

OSTEOCHONDRITIS DISSECANS OF THE TALUS This condition should not be confused with osteochondral fracture of the dome of the talus resulting from inversion or eversion injury to the ankle. (The differ-

ential diagnosis of osteochondritis dissecans and osteochondral fracture is discussed in detail in Chapter 8.)

Osteochondritis dissecans results from chronic stress and is seen most commonly in athletes and ballet dancers. The best diagnostic procedures for demonstrating the lesion are arthrotomography (Fig. 9.67) and MRI, as is also true for osteochondritis dissecans of the femoral condyles.

JONES FRACTURE This avulsion fracture of the base of the fifth metatarsal results from inversion stress placed on the peroneus brevis tendon, which is attached to the fifth metatarsal (Fig. 9.68; see

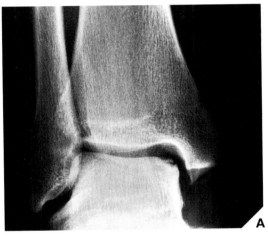 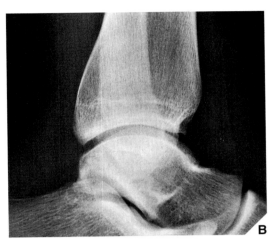 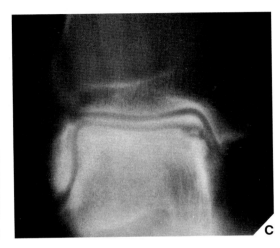

Figure 9.67 A 29-year-old man, a professional ballet dancer, complained of pain in the ankle over the preceding eight months. Anteroposterior (A) and lateral (B) radiographs demonstrate a radiolucent defect in the medial aspect of the dome of the talus and a small osteochondral body within the defect, characteristic findings in osteochondritis dissecans. (C) Arthrotomography demonstrates the intact articular cartilage over the lesion, distinguishing it as an in situ lesion.

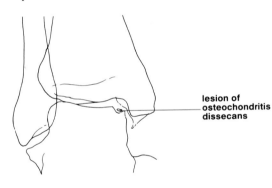 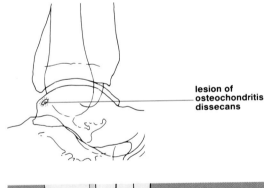

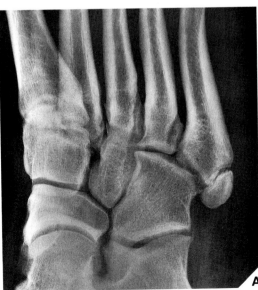 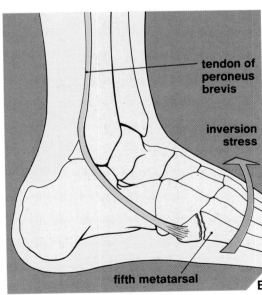

Figure 9.68 A 28-year-old man stumbled on uneven pavement and sustained an inversion injury of the right foot. (A) Oblique view demonstrates a fracture of the base of the fifth metatarsal, known as the Jones fracture. (B) Inversion-stress forces on the peroneus brevis tendon cause avulsion fracture of the base of the fifth metatarsal.

also Fig. 4.26A). From a historical point of view, however, the term "Jones fracture" is used incorrectly, since the original fracture described by Robert Jones in 1902 was one sustained about three fourths of an inch from the base of the fifth metatarsal (Fig. 9.69). The distinction between a "true" Jones fracture and an avulsion fracture of the base of the fifth metatarsal is also of prognostic value: Avulsion fractures generally heal quickly, while fractures through the proximal metatarsal shaft have a significant incidence of delayed union and fibrous union. In children, it is important not to confuse this fracture with the normal (and frequently present) secondary ossification center of the base of the fifth metatarsal (see Fig. 4.26B). The fracture line is transversely oriented, whereas the gap separating the ossification center from the fifth metatarsal is oblique.

Dislocations in the Foot

The most common dislocation in the foot occurs in the tarsometatarsal (Lisfranc) joint. In general, however, dislocations are less common than fractures of the ankle and foot. They are occasionally seen as a result of motor vehicle or aircraft accidents, as in dislocation of the talus—the so-called aviator's astragalus. According

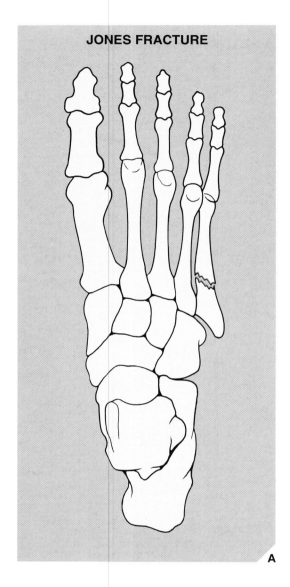

JONES FRACTURE

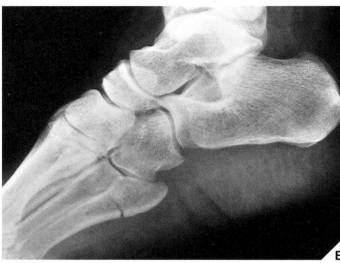

Figure 9.69 (A) A "true" Jones fracture is located about one inch distally to the base of the fifth metatarsal. (B) A 43-year-old woman, while dancing, twisted her left foot and sustained a "true" Jones fracture of the fifth metatarsal.

to Shelton and Pedowitz, aircraft accidents account for 43% of all talar injuries.

DISLOCATIONS IN THE SUBTALAR JOINT The two major types of these dislocations are peritalar dislocation of the foot and total dislocation of the talus.

PERITALAR DISLOCATION This type of abnormality involves simultaneous dislocations in the talocalcaneal and talonavicular joints with normal maintenance of the tibiotalar relationship. Often referred to as subtalar or subastragalar dislocation, peritalar dislocation, as Pennal has pointed out, accounts for about 15% of all talar injuries and about 1% of all dislocations. Patients vary in age from 10 to over 60 years, but three to ten times more men than women sustain these injuries.

Four subtypes of peritalar dislocation have been identified: medial, lateral, posterior, and anterior. *Medial dislocation* is the most common subtype, resulting from a violent inversion force acting as a fulcrum for the sustentaculum tali to cause initial dislocation of the talonavicular joint, together with rotary subluxation of the talocalcaneal joint. A greater force may cause complete dislocation. The dorsoplantar (anteroposterior) view of the foot is recommended to demonstrate this abnormality. The radiographs should carefully be scrutinized for associated fractures, particularly of both malleoli, the articular margin of the talus, and the navicular and fifth metatarsal bones.

Lateral dislocation is the next most common subtype, accounting for approximately 20% of all peritalar dislocations. At the time of injury, the foot is everted and, with the anterior calcaneal process acting as a fulcrum, the head of the talus is forced out of the talonavicular joint; the calcaneus is dislocated laterally. As in medial dislocation, the dorsoplantar view of the foot is diagnostic.

Posterior and anterior dislocations are the rarest subtypes, occurring as a result of a fall from a height onto the plantar-flexed foot (posterior dislocation) or the dorsiflexed foot (anterior dislocation). In either case, the lateral view of the foot and ankle is best for demonstrating the abnormality (Fig. 9.70).

TOTAL TALAR DISLOCATION Characterized by complete disruption of both the ankle (tibiotalar) and the subtalar joints, total talar dislocation is the most serious of all talar injuries. It is frequently complicated by osteonecrosis of the astragalus.

TARSOMETATARSAL DISLOCATION Also termed *Lisfranc fracture-dislocation,* this is the most common dislocation in the foot. It also frequently occurs in association with various types of fractures. Basically, this is a dorsal dislocation, often occurring as the result of a fall from a height or down a flight of stairs or even of stepping off a curb. There are two basic forms of injury: *homolateral*—dislocation of the first to the fifth metatarsal; and *divergent*—lateral displacement of the second to the fifth metatarsals with medial or dorsal

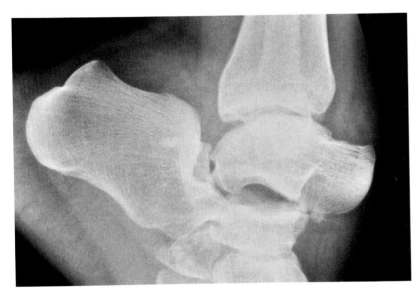

Figure 9.70 A 25-year-old man fell from a ladder and landed on his plantar-flexed left foot. Lateral view demonstrates posterior peritalar dislocation. Note that the talus articulates normally with the tibia, but there are simultaneous dislocations in the talocalcaneal and talonavicular joints. The entire foot (except for the talus) is posteriorly displaced. Associated fractures of the navicular and cuboid bones are evident.

shift of the first metatarsal (Fig. 9.71). Associated fractures most often occur at the base of the second metatarsal bone; they may also be seen in the third metatarsal, first or second cuneiform, or navicular bones. The divergent form of tarsometatarsal dislocation is most frequently associated with such fractures. These injuries are well demonstrated on the standard views of the foot (Fig. 9.72); ancillary radiographic techniques are seldom required.

Complications

The most common complications of ankle and foot fractures are nonunion and posttraumatic arthritis. Although the plain-film radiography can usually demonstrate the features of these complications, tomography is the best technique for delineating their details.

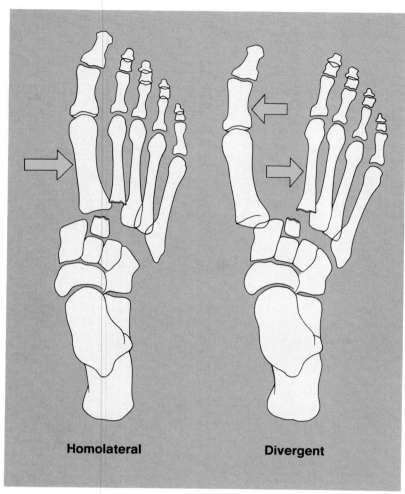

Homolateral　　　　　**Divergent**

Figure 9.71 Tarsometatarsal dislocation (Lisfranc fracture-dislocation) may be seen in two variants. In the homolateral form, the first to the fifth metatarsals are dislocated laterally. In the divergent form, the first metatarsal is medially dislocated. Both types are often associated with fracture of the base of the second metatarsal bone.

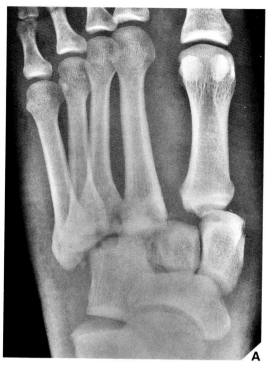

Figure 9.72 A 39-year-old man fell down a flight of stairs. Anteroposterior (A) and lateral (B) views of the right foot show the divergent type of the Lisfranc fracture-dislocation. There is lateral shift of the second to fifth metatarsals, as well as dislocation and dorsal shift in the first metatarso-cuneiform joint, which is better appreciated on the lateral film. Note the fractures at the base of the second and third metatarsals.

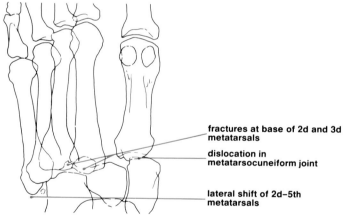

fractures at base of 2d and 3d metatarsals

dislocation in metatarsocuneiform joint

lateral shift of 2d–5th metatarsals

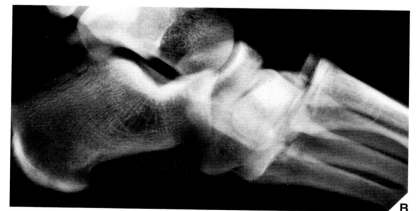

PRACTICAL POINTS TO REMEMBER

Ankle

[1] There are three principal sets of ligaments around the ankle joint:
- the medial collateral (deltoid) ligament
- the lateral collateral ligament
- the distal tibiofibular syndesmotic complex.

[2] Traumatic conditions of the ankle should be evaluated according to the mechanism that caused the injury, including:
- inversion-stress forces
- eversion-stress forces
- complex stresses combining supination or pronation with rotation, abduction, or adduction.

[3] Inversion-stress forces may manifest in a spectrum of injuries to the lateral collateral ligament, as well as in associated fractures of the distal tip of the fibula and occasionally the medial malleolus.

[4] Eversion-stress forces may manifest in a range of injuries to the medial collateral (deltoid) ligament, as well as fracture of the medial malleolus. Pott, Maisonneuve, Dupuytren, and Tillaux fractures are all eversion injuries.

[5] Pilon fracture is a comminuted fracture of the distal tibia with extension into the tibiotalar joint.

[6] Traumatic conditions of the structures about the ankle joint may not be obvious on the standard radiographic examination when only damage of soft tissue structures is present. Correct management of such injuries may be much more important to a successful orthopedic outcome than correct management of a simple fracture. For this reason, stress views, arthrographic examination and MRI are of paramount importance for full evaluation of the extent of damage to the complex structures about the joint.

[7] The ligament structure most important for congruence of the joint and ankle stability is the distal tibiofibular syndesmotic complex.

[8] The Weber classification of ankle fractures—based on the level of fibular fracture—is practical for assessing the risk of future ankle instability because of its emphasis on the lateral syndesmotic-malleolar complex as an important factor in ankle joint stability.

[9] On arthrographic examination of the ligament structures about the ankle and foot:
- leak of contrast around the tip of the fibular malleolus indicates a tear of the anterior talofibular ligament

- opacification of the peroneal tendon sheath suggests a tear of the calcaneofibular ligament
- leak of contrast more than 2.5 cm into the tibiofibular syndesmotic recess indicates a tear of the distal anterior tibiofibular ligament
- leak of contrast beneath the medial malleolus indicates a tear of the deltoid ligament.

[10] Tenography is a useful technique for evaluating tears of the tendons, such as the Achilles tendon, the posterior tibialis tendon, or the peroneal tendon.

[11] Magnetic resonance imaging is a noninvasive modality capable of demonstrating pathologic conditions of tendons and ligaments by displaying discontinuity of the anatomic structures, the presence of abnormal signal within them, and the presence of inflammatory changes.

Foot

[1] It is important to learn to recognize the multiple accessory ossicles of the foot:
- the normal appearance of these secondary ossification centers may mimic fractures
- and, conversely, an avulsion fracture may be misinterpreted as a normal ossicle.

[2] Harris-Beath and Broden views, tangential projections, are important techniques for evaluating injury to the subtalar joint.

[3] Boehler angle demonstrates an important anatomic relation of the calcaneus and subtalar joint. It is useful for evaluating compression fracture of the calcaneus, particularly with extension into the subtalar joint.

[4] In fracture of the calcaneus (so-called lover's fracture), look for an associated compression fracture of the vertebral body in the thoracic or lumbar spine.

[5] In Lisfranc fracture-dislocation in the tarsometatarsal articulation, always look for an associated fracture either:
- at the base of the metatarsals
- or in the cuneiform bones.

References

Beltran J: *MRI Musculoskeletal System.* Philadelphia, Lippincott, 1990.

Bleichrodt RP, Kingma LM, Binnendijk B, Klein J-P: Injuries of the lateral ankle ligaments: Classification with tenography and arthrography. *Radiology* 173:347, 1989.

Brostrom L, Liljedahl SO, Lindvall N: Sprained ankles. II. Arthrographic diagnosis of recent ligament ruptures. *Acta Chir Scand* 129:485, 1965.

Cave EF: Fracture of the calcis: The problem in general. *Clin Orthop* 30:64, 1963.

Cone RO III, Nguyen V, Flournoy JG, Guerra J Jr: Triplane fracture of the distal tibial epiphysis: Radiographic and CT studies. *Radiology* 153:763, 1984.

DeSmet AA, Fisher DR, Burnstein MI, Graf BK, Lange RM: Value of MR imaging in staging osteochondral lesions of the talus (osteochondritis dissecans): Result in 14 patients. *Am J Roentgenol* 154:555, 1990.

Dias LS, Giegerich CR: Fractures of the distal tibial epiphysis in adolescence. *J Bone Joint Surg* 65A:438, 1983.

Dias LS, Tachdjian MO: Physeal injuries in the ankle in children. Classification. *Clin Orthop* 136:230, 1978.

Edeiken J, Cotler JM: Ankle trauma. *Semin Roentgenol* 13:145, 1978.

Edeiken J, Cotler JM: Ankle. In: Felson B (ed): *Fractures.* New York, Grune & Stratton, 1978.

Edeiken J, Cotler JM: Ankle. In: Felson B (ed): *Roentgenology of Fractures and Dislocations.* New York, Grune & Stratton, 1978, p 151.

Eichelberger RP, Lichtenstein P, Brogdon BG: Peroneal tenography. *JAMA* 247:2587, 1982.

Erickson SJ, Quinn SF, Kneeland JB, et al: MR imaging of the tarsal tunnel and related spaces: Normal and abnormal findings with anatomic correlation. *Am J Roentgenol* 155:323, 1990.

Erickson SJ, Smith JW, Ruiz ME, et al: MR imaging of the lateral collateral ligament of the ankle. *Am J Roentgenol* 156:131, 1991.

Essex-Lopresti P: The mechanism, reduction technique and results in fracture of the os calcis. *Br J Surg* 39:395, 1982.

Feldman F, Singson RD, Rosenberg ZS, Berdon WE, Amodio J, Abramson SJ: Distal tibial triplane fractures: Diagnosis with CT. *Radiology* 164:429, 1987.

Fordyce AJW, Horn CV: Arthrography in recent injuries of the ligaments of the ankle. *J Bone Joint Surg* 54B:116, 1972.

Frost HM, Hanson CA: Technique for testing the drawer sign in the ankle. *Clin Orthop* 123:49, 1977.

Fussell ME, Godley DR: Ankle arthrography in acute sprains. *Clin Orthop* 93:278, 1973.

Gamble FO, Yale I: *Clinical Foot Roentgenology. An Illustrated Handbook.* Baltimore, Williams & Wilkins, 1966.

Giannestras NJ: *Foot Disorders. Medical and Surgical Management,* ed 2. Philadelphia, Lea & Febiger, 1973.

Giannestras NJ, Sammarco GL: Fractures and dislocations of the foot. In: Rockwood CA Jr, Green DP (eds): *Fractures,* vol 2. Philadelphia, Lippincott, 1975.

Gilula LA, Oloff LM, Caputi R, Destovet JM, Jacobs A, Solomon MA: Ankle tenography: A key to unexplained symptomatology. Part II. Diagnosis of chronic tendon disabilities. *Radiology* 151:581, 1984.

Gordon RB: Arthrography of the ankle joint. Experience in one hundred seven studies. *J Bone Joint Surg* 52A:1623, 1970.

Gould N, Seligson D, Gassman J: Early and late repair of lateral ligament of the ankle. *Foot Ankle* 1:84, 1980.

Huo Teng MM, Destovet JM, Gilula LA, Resnick D, Hembree JL, Oloff LM: Ankle tenography: A key to unexplained symptomatology. *Radiology* 151:575, 1984.

Isherwood I: A radiological approach to the subtalar joint. *J Bone Joint Surg* 43B:566, 1961.

Jahss MH: Spontaneous rupture of the tibialis posterior tendon: Clinical findings, tenographic studies, and a new technique of repair. *Foot Ankle* 3:158, 1982.

Johnson KA: Tibialis posterior tendon rupture. *Clin Orthop* 177:140, 1983.

Jones R: Fracture of the base of the fifth metatarsal by direct violence. *Ann Surg* 35:697, 1902.

Kaye JJ: The ankle. In: Freiberger RH, Kaye JJ, Spiller J (eds): *Arthrography.* New York, Appleton-Century-Crofts, 1979, pp 237-256.

Kleiger B: A review of ankle fractures due to lateral strains. *Bull Hosp Jt Dis Orthop Inst* 29:138, 1968.

Kleiger B: Mechanisms of ankle injury. *Orthop Clin North Am* 5:127, 1974.

Kleiger B, Mankin HJ: A roentgenographic study of the development of the calcaneus by means of the posterior tangential view. *J Bone Joint Surg* 43A:961, 1961.

Kleiger B, Mankin HJ: Fracture of the lateral portion of the distal tibial epiphysis. *J Bone Joint Surg* 46A:25, 1964.

Kleiger B, Greenspan A, Norman A: Radiographic examination of the normal foot and ankle. In: Jahss MH (ed): *Disorders of the Foot.* Philadelphia, Saunders, 1981.

Lauge-Hansen N: Fractures of the ankle. II. Combined experimental-surgical and experimental-roentgenologic investigations. *Arch Surg* 60:957, 1950.

Lynn MD: The triplane distal tibial epiphyseal fracture. *Clin Orthop* 86:187, 1972.

Mainwaring BL, Daffner RH, Riemer BL: Pylon fractures of the ankle: A distinct clinical and radiologic entity. *Radiology* 168:215, 1988.

Marmor L: An unusual fracture of the tibial epiphysis. *Clin Orthop* 73:132, 1970.

Meschan I: *Synopsis of Roentgen Signs.* Philadelphia, Saunders, 1962.

Müller ME, Allgower M, Willenegger H: Manual of Internal Fixation. New York, Springer Verlag, 1979.

Norman A, Kleiger B, Greenspan A, Finkel JE: Roentgenographic examination of the normal foot and ankle. In: Jahss MM (ed): *Disorders of the Foot and Ankle. Medical and Surgical Management,* vol 1. Philadelphia, WB Saunders, 1991, pp 64–90.

Olson RW: Arthrography of the ankle joint: Its use in evaluation of ankle sprains. *Radiology* 92:1439, 1969.

Olson RW: Ankle arthrography. *Radiol Clin North Am* 19:255, 1981.

Pankovich AM: Fractures of the fibula proximal to the distal tibiofibular syndesmosis. *J Bone Joint Surg* 60A:221, 1978.

Peltier LF: Guillaume Dupuytren and Dupuytren's fracture. *Surgery* 43:868, 1958.

Peltier LF: Percivall Pott and Pott's fracture. *Surgery* 51:280, 1962.

Pennal GF: Fracture of the talus. *Clin Orthop* 30:53, 1963.

Protas JM, Kornblatt BA: Fractures of the lateral margin of the distal tibia. *Radiology* 138:55, 1981.

Reckling F, McNamara G, DeSmet A: Problems in the diagnosis and treatment of ankle injuries. *J Trauma* 21:943, 1981.

Resnick D: Radiology of the talocalcaneal articulations. Anatomic considerations and arthrography. *Radiology* 111:581, 1974.

Resnick D, Georgen TG: Peroneal tenography in previous calcaneal fractures. *Radiology* 115:211, 1975.

Rijke AM, Jones B, Vierhovt PAM: Stress examination of traumatized lateral ligaments of the ankle. *Clin Orthop* 210:143, 1986.

Ritchie GW, Keim HA: Major foot deformities. Their classification and x-ray analysis. *J Can Assoc Radiol* 19:155, 1968.

Rogers LF, Campbell RE: Foot. In: Felson B (ed): *Roentgenology of Fractures and Dislocations.* New York, Grune & Stratton, 1978, p 151.

Rosenberg ZS, Feldman F, Singson RD, Kane R: Ankle tendons: Evaluation with CT. *Radiology* 166:221, 1988.

Rowe CR, Sakellarides HT, Freeman PA, Sorbie C: Fracture of the os calcis: A long-term follow-up study of 146 patients. *JAMA* 184:920, 1963.

Sauser DD, Nelson RC, Lavine MH, Wu CW: Acute injuries of the lateral ligaments of the ankle: Comparison of stress radiography and arthrography. *Radiology* 148:653, 1983.

Sclafani SJA: Ligamentous injury of the lower tibiofibular syndesmosis: Radiographic evidence. *Radiology* 156:21, 1985.

Shelton ML, Pedowitz WJ: Injuries to the talus and midfoot. In: Jahss MH (ed): *Disorders of the Foot,* vol 2. Philadelphia, Saunders, 1982, p 1463.

Shereff MJ, Johnson KA: Radiographic anatomy of the hindfoot. *Clin Orthop* 117:16, 1983.

Spiegel PK, Staples OS: Arthrography of the ankle joint: Problems in diagnosis of acute lateral ligament injuries. *Radiology* 114:587, 1975.

Staples OS: Ligamentous injuries of the ankle joint. *Clin Orthop* 42:21, 1965.

Teng MMH, Destovet JM, Gilula LA, Resnick D, Thembree JL, Oloff LM: Ankle tenography: A key to unexplained symptomatology. Part I: Normal tenographic anatomy. *Radiology* 151:575, 1984.

Watson-Jones R: *Fractures and Joint Injuries,* vols I, II. St. Louis, Mosby, 1959.

Weber BG: *Die Verletzungen des Oberen Sprunggelenkes.* Stuttgart, Verlag Hans Huber, 1972.

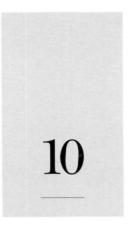

10

Spine

FRACTURES OF THE VERTEBRAL COLUMN are important not only because of the structures involved but because of the complications that may arise affecting the spinal cord. Constituting about 3% to 6% of all skeletal injuries, fractures of the vertebral column are most commonly encountered in people between the ages of 20 and 50 years, the great majority of cases (80%) being seen in males. Most spinal fractures occur at the thoracic and lumbar levels, but injury to the cervical area has a greater potential risk for spinal cord damage. Automobile accidents, sports-related activities (e.g., diving, skiing), and falls from heights are usually the circumstances in which spinal injuries are sustained.

The spine is composed of 33 vertebrae: 7 cervical, 12 thoracic, 5 lumbar, a sacrum of 5 fused segments, and a coccyx of 4 fused segments. With the exception of the first and second cervical vertebrae (C-1 and C-2), the vertebral bodies are separated from each other by intervertebral disks.

CERVICAL SPINE

Anatomic-Radiologic Considerations

Structurally, the first and second cervical vertebrae possess anatomic features distinct from those of the remaining five cervical vertebrae (Fig. 10.1). The first cervical vertebra, C-1 or atlas, is a bony ring consisting of anterior and posterior arches connected by two lateral masses. The atlas has no body; its main structures are the lateral masses, also called "articular pillars." The second vertebra, C-2 or axis, is a more complex structure whose distinguishing feature is the odontoid process, also known as the "dens" (tooth), projecting cephalad from the anterior surface of the body. The space between the odontoid process and the anterior arch of the atlas, called the "atlantal-dens interval," should not exceed 3 mm in adults whether or not the head is flexed or extended. In children under 8 years of age, this distance has been reported to be as much as 4 mm, particularly in flexion, secondary to greater ligamentous laxity.

The vertebrae C3-7 exhibit identical anatomic features and are more uniform in appearance, consisting of a vertebral body and a posterior neural arch, including the right and left pedicles and laminae, which together with the posterior aspect of the body enclose the spinal canal (Fig. 10.2). Extending caudad and cephalad from the junction of the pedicle and lamina on each side are superior and inferior articular processes, which form the apophyseal joints between the successive vertebrae. Extending laterally from the pedicle on each side is a transverse process and, in the posterior portion, a spinous process extends from the junction of the laminae in the midline. The vertebra C-7, in addition, is distinguished by its long spinous process and large transverse processes.

Radiographic examination of a patient with cervical spine trauma may be difficult and is usually limited to one or two projections, because frequently the patient is unconscious, there are associated injuries, and unnecessary movement risks damage to the cervical cord. The single most valuable projection in these instances is the lateral view, which may be obtained in the standard fashion or with the patient supine, depending on his or her condition (Fig. 10.3). This projection suffices to demonstrate most traumatic conditions of the cervical spine, including injuries involving the anterior and posterior arches of C-1; the odontoid process, which is seen in profile; and the anterior atlantal-dens interval. The bodies and spinous processes of C2-7 are fully visualized, and the intervertebral disk spaces and prevertebral soft tissues can be adequately evaluated. The lateral view may also be obtained in flexion of the neck, which is particularly effective in demonstrating suspected instability

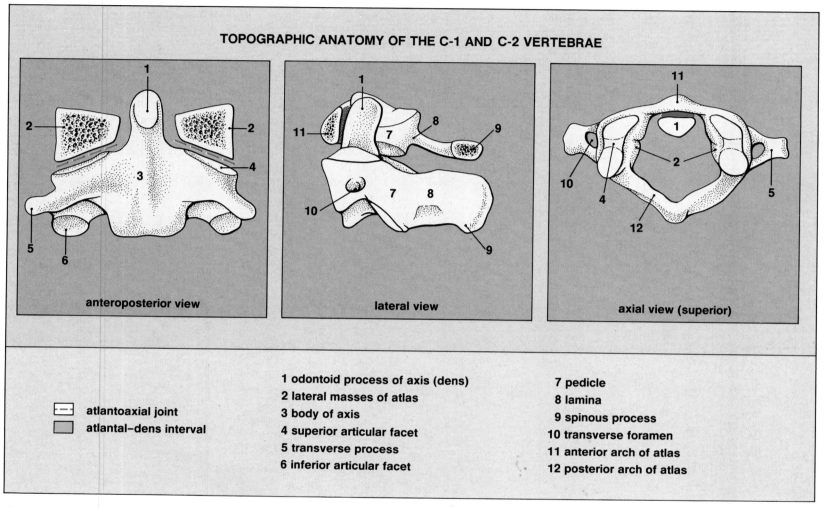

TOPOGRAPHIC ANATOMY OF THE C-1 AND C-2 VERTEBRAE

anteroposterior view

lateral view

axial view (superior)

☐ atlantoaxial joint
▨ atlantal–dens interval

1 odontoid process of axis (dens)
2 lateral masses of atlas
3 body of axis
4 superior articular facet
5 transverse process
6 inferior articular facet

7 pedicle
8 lamina
9 spinous process
10 transverse foramen
11 anterior arch of atlas
12 posterior arch of atlas

Figure 10.1 Topographic anatomy of the C-1 and C-2 vertebrae.

at C1-2 by allowing evaluation of the atlanto-odontoid distance; an increase in this distance to more than 3 mm indicates atlantoaxial subluxation. It is of the utmost importance on the lateral projection of the cervical spine that the C-7 vertebra be visualized, as this is the most commonly overlooked site of injuries.

The lateral view of the cervical spine, including the lower part of the skull, is extremely important to evaluate the vertical subluxation involving the atlantoaxial articulation and the migration of the odontoid process into the foramen magnum. Several measurements are helpful to determine atlantoaxial impaction or cranial settling resulting in superior migration of the odontoid process (Figs. 10.4–10.7).

On the anteroposterior view of the cervical spine (Fig. 10.8), the bodies of the C3-7 vertebrae (and occasionally in young persons, even the C-1 and C-2 vertebrae) are well demonstrated, as are the uncovertebral (Luschka) joints and the intervertebral disk spaces. The spinous processes are seen almost on end, casting oval shadows resembling teardrops. A variant of the anteroposterior projection

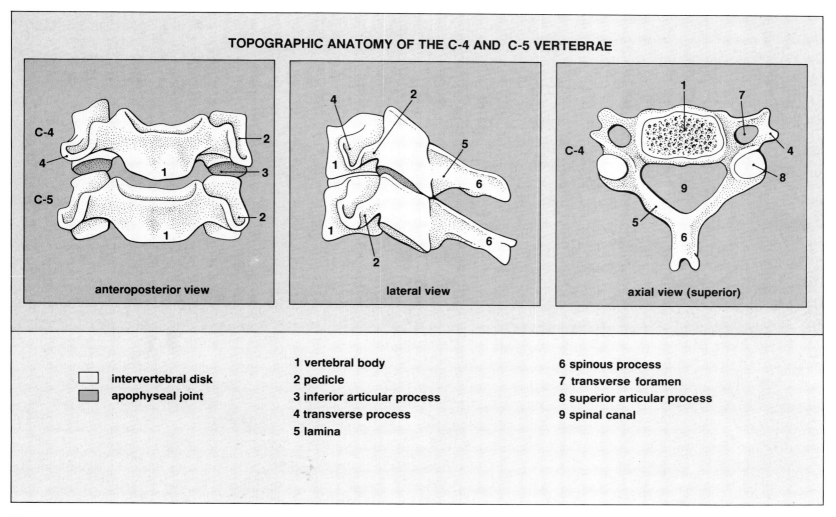

TOPOGRAPHIC ANATOMY OF THE C-4 AND C-5 VERTEBRAE

anteroposterior view   lateral view   axial view (superior)

☐ intervertebral disk
▨ apophyseal joint

1 vertebral body
2 pedicle
3 inferior articular process
4 transverse process
5 lamina

6 spinous process
7 transverse foramen
8 superior articular process
9 spinal canal

Figure 10.2 Topographic anatomy of the C-4 and C-5 vertebrae, representing the mid- and lower cervical vertebrae.

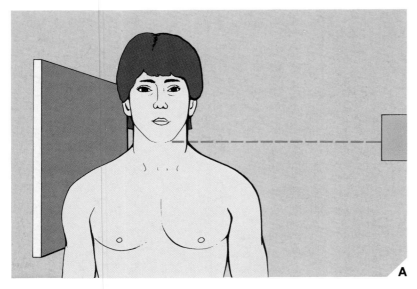

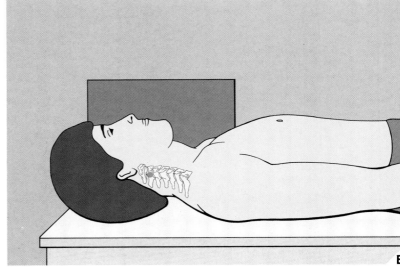

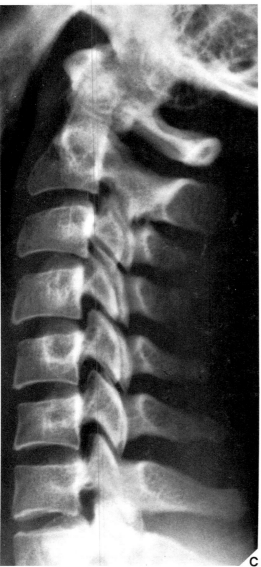

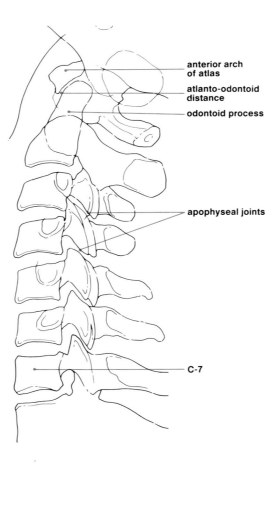

anterior arch
of atlas

atlanto-odontoid
distance

odontoid process

apophyseal joints

C-7

Figure 10.3 (A) For the erect lateral view of the cervical spine, the patient is standing or seated, with the head straight in the neutral position. The central beam is directed horizontally to the center of the C-4 vertebra (at the level of the chin). (B) For the cross-table lateral view, the patient is supine on the radiographic table. The radiographic cassette (a grid cassette to obtain a clearer image) is adjusted to the side of the neck, and the central beam is directed horizontally to a point *(red dot)* about 2.5 cm to 3 cm caudal to the mastoid tip. (C) The film in this projection clearly shows the vertebral bodies, apophyseal joints, spinous processes, and intervertebral disk spaces. It is mandatory to demonstrate the C-7 vertebra. (D) With this view the four contour lines of the normal cervical spine can be demonstrated: 1) anterior vertebral line drawn along anterior margins of the vertebral bodies; 2) posterior vertebral line (outlines anterior margin of spinal canal), drawn along posterior margins of the vertebral bodies; 3) spinolaminar line (outlines posterior margin of the spinal canal), drawn along the anterior margins of the bases of the spinous processes at the junction with lamina; 4) posterior spinous line drawn along the tips of the spinous processes from C2-7. They should be running smoothly, without angulation or interruption. The clivus-odontoid line, drawn from the dorsum sellae along the clivus to the anterior margin of the foramen magnum should point to the tip of the odontoid process at the junction of the anterior and middle thirds. The retropharyngeal space (distance from the posterior pharyngeal wall to the anteroinferior aspect of C-2) should measure about 7 mm or less; the retrotracheal space (distance from the posterior wall of the trachea to the anteroinferior aspect of C-6) should measure 22 mm in adults and 14 mm in children. (E) Low-kilovoltage technique demonstrates prevertebral soft tissues to better advantage.

LATERAL CERVICAL SPINE LANDMARKS

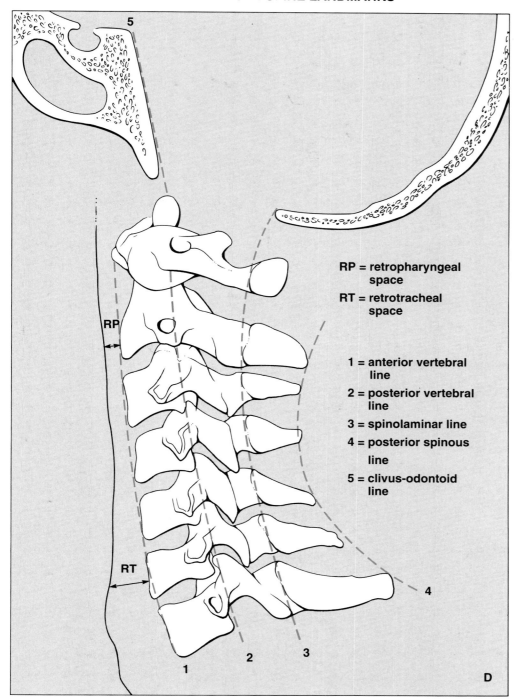

RP = retropharyngeal space

RT = retrotracheal space

1 = anterior vertebral line

2 = posterior vertebral line

3 = spinolaminar line

4 = posterior spinous line

5 = clivus-odontoid line

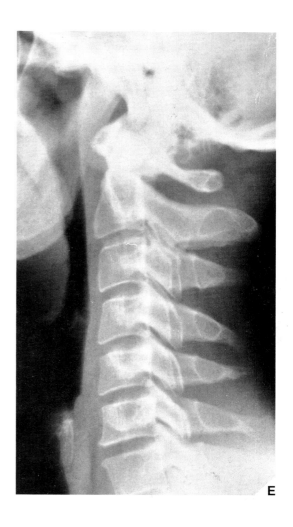

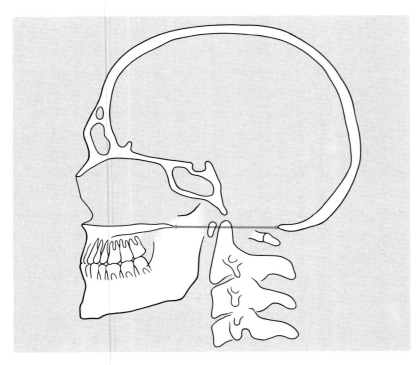

Figure 10.4 The Chamberlain line is drawn from the posterior margin of the foramen magnum (opisthion) to the dorsal (posterior) margin of the hard palate. The odontoid process should not project above this line more than 3 mm; a projection of 6.6 mm (± 2 SD) above this line strongly indicates cranial settling.

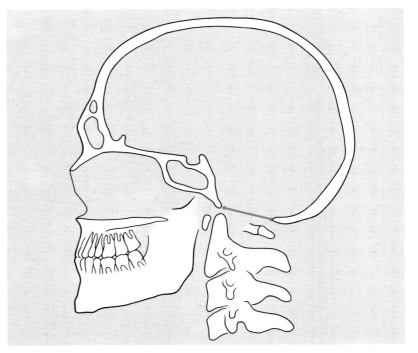

Figure 10.5 The McRae line defines the opening of the foramen magnum and connects the anterior margin (basion) with posterior margin (opisthion) of the foramen magnum. The odontoid process should be just below this line or the line may intersect only at the tip of the odontoid process. In addition, a perpendicular line drawn from the apex of the odontoid to this line should intersect it in its ventral quarter.

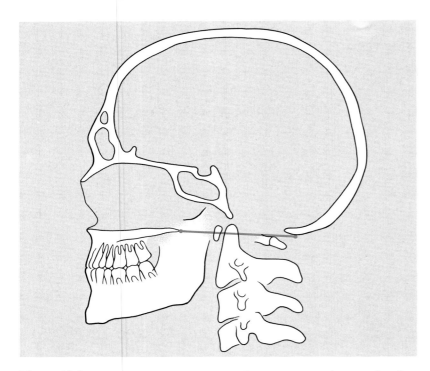

Figure 10.6 The McGregor line connects the posterosuperior margin of the hard palate to the most caudal part of the occipital curve of the skull. The tip of the odontoid normally does not extend more than 4.5 mm above the line.

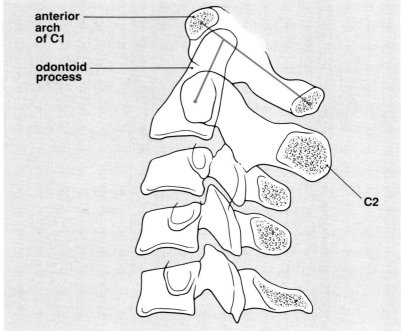

Figure 10.7 Ranawat and associates developed a method for determining the extent of the superior margin of the odontoid process, since the hard palate often is not identifiable on radiographs of the cervical spine. The coronal axis of C-1 is determined by connecting the center of the anterior arch of the first cervical vertebra with its posterior ring. The center of the sclerotic ring in C-2, representing the pedicles, is marked. The line is drawn along the axis of the odontoid process to the first line. The normal distance between C-1 and C-2 in men averages 17 mm (± 2 mm SD), and in women, 15 mm (± 2 mm). A decrease in this distance indicates cephalad migration of C-2.

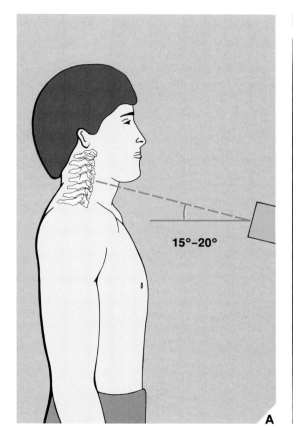

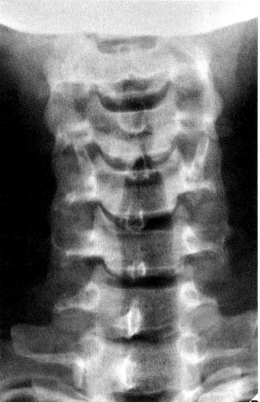

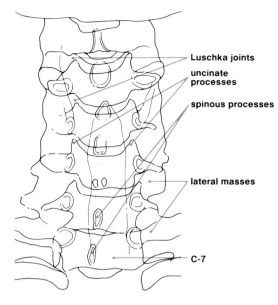

Luschka joints
uncinate processes
spinous processes

lateral masses

C-7

Figure 10.8 (A) For the anteroposterior view of the cervical spine, the patient is either erect or supine. The central beam is directed toward the C-4 vertebra (at the point of the Adam's apple) at an angle of 15° to 20° cephalad.
(B) The film in this projection demonstrates the C3-7 vertebral bodies and the intervertebral disk spaces. The spinous processes are seen superimposed on the bodies, resembling teardrops. The C-1 and C-2 vertebrae are not adequately seen. For their visualization, the patient is instructed to open and close the mouth rapidly. Motion of the mandible blurs this structure, and C-1 and C-2 become visible (C).

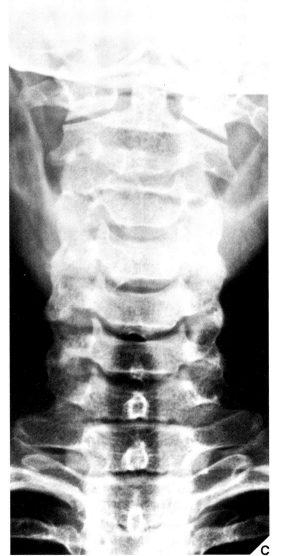

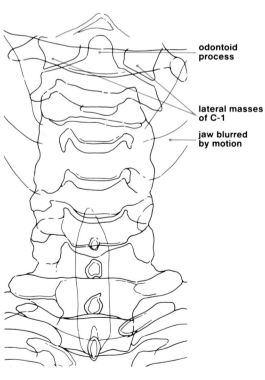

odontoid process

lateral masses of C-1

jaw blurred by motion

known as the open-mouth view (Fig. 10.9) may also be obtained as part of the standard examination. This view provides effective visualization of the structures of the first two cervical vertebrae. The body of C-2 is clearly imaged, as are the atlantoaxial joints, the odontoid process, and the lateral spaces between the odontoid process and the articular pillars of C-1. If the open-mouth view is difficult to obtain or the odontoid process is not clearly visualized, particularly its upper half, the Fuchs view may be helpful (Fig. 10.10). Oblique projections of the cervical spine (Fig. 10.11) are not routinely obtained, although at times they help visualize obscure fractures of the neural arch and abnormalities of the neural foramina and apophyseal joints. Special projections may occasionally be required for sufficient evaluation of the structures of the cervical spine. The pillar view (Fig. 10.12), which may be obtained in the anteroposte-

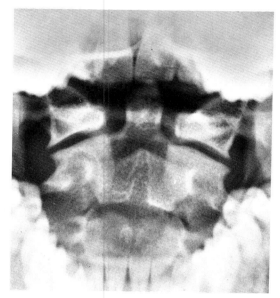
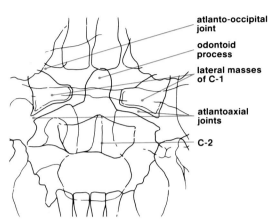

Figure 10.9 For the open-mouth view, the patient is positioned in the same manner as for the supine anteroposterior projection; the head is straight, in the neutral position. With the patient's mouth open as widely as possible, the central beam is directed perpendicular to the midpoint of the open mouth. During the exposure, the patient should softly phonate "ah" to affix the tongue to the floor of the mouth so that its shadow is not projected over C-l and C-2. On the radiograph, the odontoid process, the body of C-2, and the lateral masses of the atlas are well demonstrated; the atlantoaxial joints are seen to best advantage.

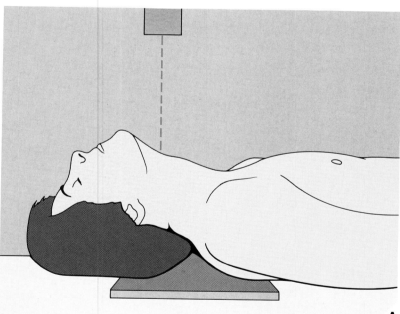
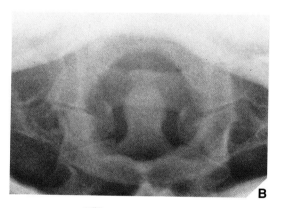
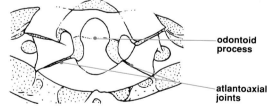

Figure 10.10 (A) For the Fuchs views of the odontoid process, the patient is supine on the table, with the neck hyperextended. The central beam is directed vertically to the neck just below the tip of the chin. (B) On the radiograph obtained in this projection, the odontoid, especially its upper half, is clearly visualized.

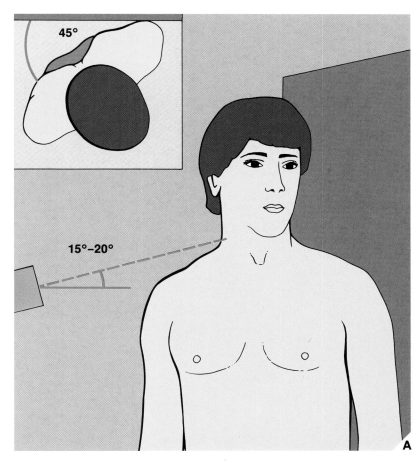

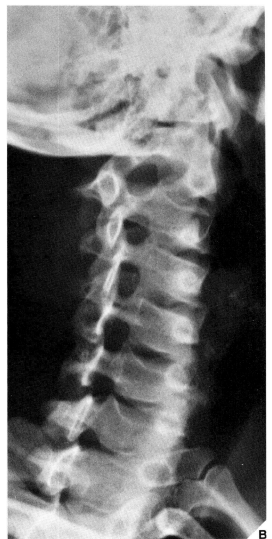

Figure 10.11 (A) An oblique view of the cervical spine may be obtained in the anteroposterior (as shown here), or posteroanterior projection. The patient may be erect or recumbent, but the erect position (seated or standing) is more comfortable. The patient is rotated 45° to one side—to the left, as shown here, to demonstrate the right-sided neural foramina and to the right to demonstrate the left-sided neural foramina. The central beam is directed to the C-4 vertebra with 15° to 20° cephalad angulation. (B) The film in this projection is effective primarily for demonstrating the intervertebral neural foramina.

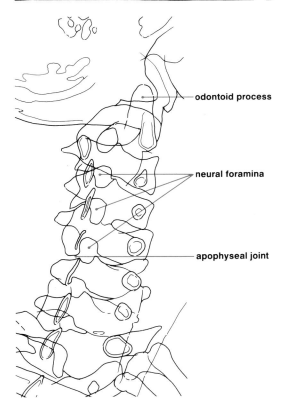

odontoid process

neural foramina

apophyseal joint

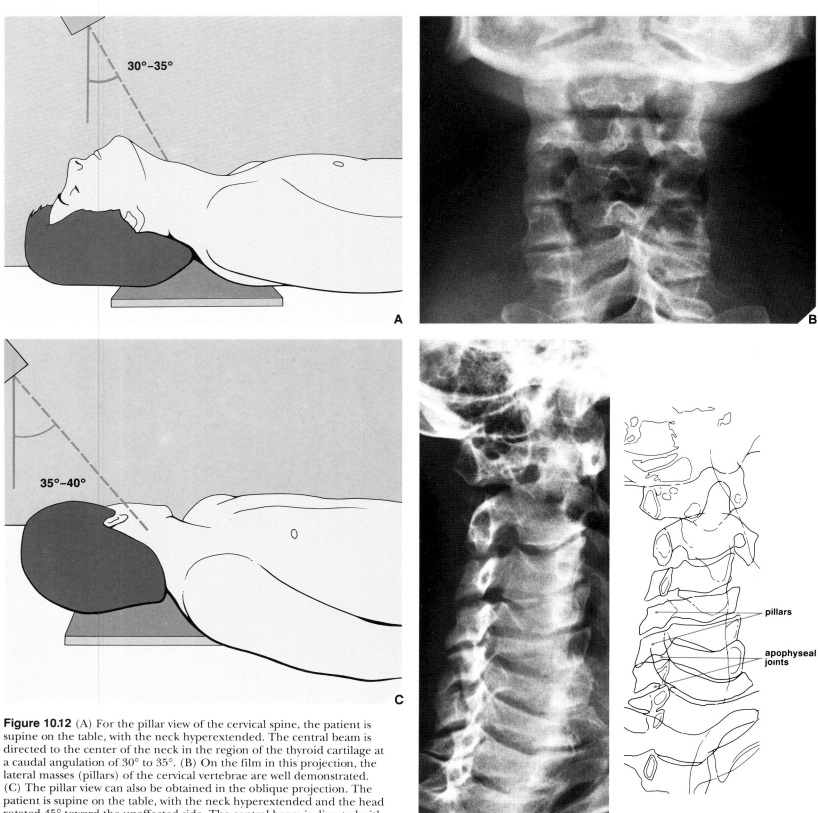

pillars

apophyseal joints

Figure 10.12 (A) For the pillar view of the cervical spine, the patient is supine on the table, with the neck hyperextended. The central beam is directed to the center of the neck in the region of the thyroid cartilage at a caudal angulation of 30° to 35°. (B) On the film in this projection, the lateral masses (pillars) of the cervical vertebrae are well demonstrated. (C) The pillar view can also be obtained in the oblique projection. The patient is supine on the table, with the neck hyperextended and the head rotated 45° toward the unaffected side. The central beam is directed with about 35° to 40° caudal angulation to the lateral side of the neck about 3 cm below the earlobe. (D) On the radiograph obtained with leftward rotation of the head, an oblique view of the right pillars is achieved.

rior or oblique projection, serves to demonstrate the lateral masses of the cervical vertebrae, and the swimmer's view (Fig. 10.13) may be employed for better demonstration of the C-7, T-1, and T-2 vertebrae, which on the standard lateral or oblique projection are obscured by the overlapping clavicle and soft tissues of the shoulder girdle. Fluoroscopy and videotaping are usually of little help in acute injuries because pain may prevent the necessary movement for positioning.

Ancillary imaging techniques play an important role in the evaluation of suspected spinal trauma. Conventional tomography and computed tomography (CT) are commonly employed techniques. In the evaluation of fractures of the odontoid process, for example,

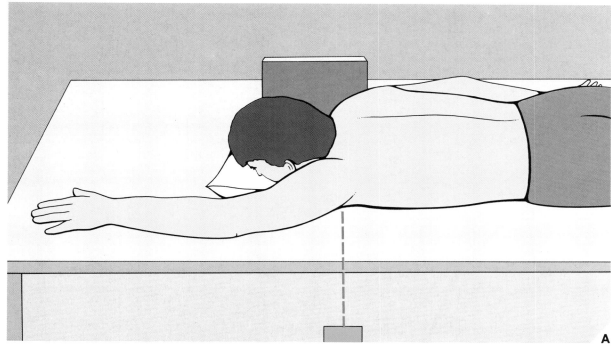

Figure 10.13 (A) For the swimmer's view of the cervical spine, the patient is placed prone on the table with the left arm abducted 180° and the right arm by the side, as if swimming the crawl. The central beam is directed horizontally toward the left axilla. The radiographic cassette is against the right side of the neck, as for the standard cross-table lateral view. (B) The film in this projection provides adequate visualization of the C-7, T-1, and T-2 vertebrae, which would otherwise be obscured by the shoulders.

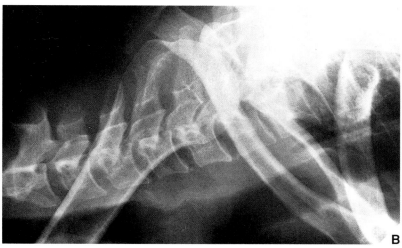

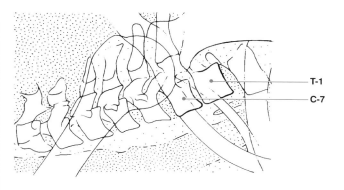

conventional tomography is particularly helpful; and in determining the extent of cervical spine injuries in general, including soft tissue trauma, CT (Fig. 10.14) provides valuable information regarding the integrity of the spinal canal and the localization of fracture fragments within the canal.

In the past several years, magnetic resonance imaging (MRI) has become the most effective modality to evaluate vertebral trauma because of the impressive quality of its images and its multiplanar capabilities, which allow examination of acutely traumatized patients without moving them. In evaluating fractures, MRI is useful not only to determine the relationship of bony fragments that may be displaced in the vertebral canal, but also to demonstrate the full extent of injury, especially to the soft tissues and the spinal cord. The effect of the trauma on the spinal cord can be directly imaged, and spinal cord compression can be diagnosed. The superior soft tissue contrast resolution of MRI can reveal minimal edema and small quantities of hemorrhage within the spinal cord. Injury to ligamentous structures and extradural pathology also may be readily identified. In the cervical spine, 3-mm-thick sagittal sections and 5-mm-thick axial sections are routinely obtained. The most effective are spin-echo T1- and T2-weighted images obtained in the sagittal plane. Sagittal MR images permit evaluation of vertebral body alignment and integrity, along with the size of the spinal canal (Fig. 10.15A). On the parasagittal section, the articular facets are well demonstrated (Fig. 10.15B). More recently, fast scans have been advocated for demonstrating injuries in the axial plane. These fast gradient-echo pulse sequences have become a popular addition to, or a replacement for, spin-echo T2-weighted sequences. Gradient-echo sequences have short acquisition times, adequate resolution, and show a satisfactory "myelographic effect" between cerebrospinal fluid and adjacent structures (Fig. 10.15C,D).

On T1-weighted sagittal images of the cervical spine, the vertebral bodies that contain yellow (or fatty) marrow are imaged as high-signal-intensity structures (see Fig. 10.15A). The intervertebral disks and the cord demonstrate intermediate signal intensity, while cerebrospinal fluid demonstrates low signal intensity.

On T2-weighted sagittal images, the vertebral bodies are imaged with low signal intensity, the intervertebral disks and cerebrospinal fluid demonstrate high signal intensity, and the cord demonstrates intermediate-to-low signal intensity.

On the axial images obtained in T1-weighting, the disk demonstrates intermediate signal intensity, the spinal fluid has low signal intensity, and the cord has high-to-intermediate signal intensity.

On the axial images obtained in T2*-weighting (MPGR), the disk is of high signal intensity and the spinal fluid is also of high signal intensity, in contrast to the spinal cord, which images as an intermediate-signal-intensity structure. The bone demonstrates low signal intensity (see Fig. 10.15C,D).

In addition to its imaging capabilities, MR also has, according to some investigators, a prognostic value when attempting to predict the degree of neurologic recovery following trauma.

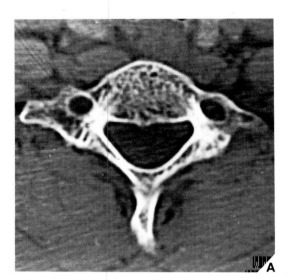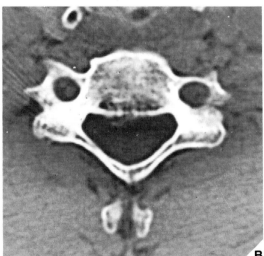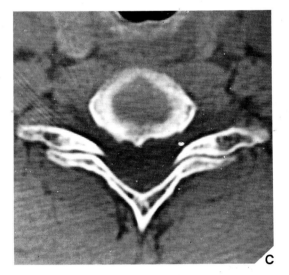

Figure 10.14 CT sections through the body of C-6 (A), C-7 (B), and the C6-7 intervertebral space (C) show the normal appearance of these structures.

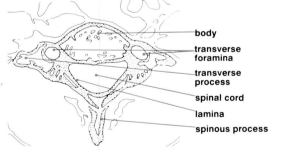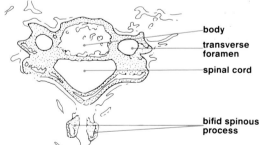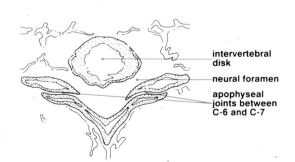

It has to be stressed, however, that CT alone or combined with myelography remains the better choice for evaluating vertebral fractures, especially when they are nondisplaced or involve the posterior elements (lateral masses, facets, laminae, spinous processes), largely because of the limitations of spatial resolution of MRI. In addition, imaging the acutely injured patient is difficult. The patient may be unstable or immobilized with either a halo or traction device unsuitable for the magnetic environment. For this reason, plain radiographs, CT, and myelography continue to play a significant role in the evaluation of the acutely traumatized spine. On the other hand, as Hyman and Gorey noted, chronic injury to the spinal cord is most accurately evaluated with MRI.

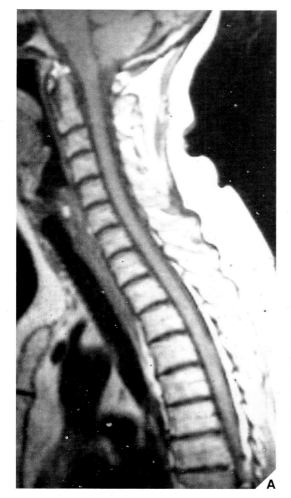
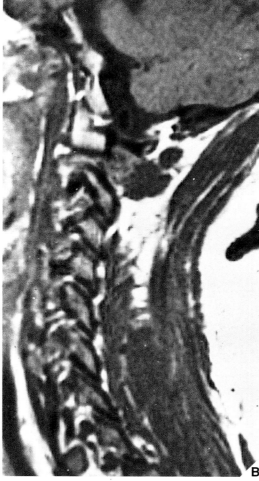
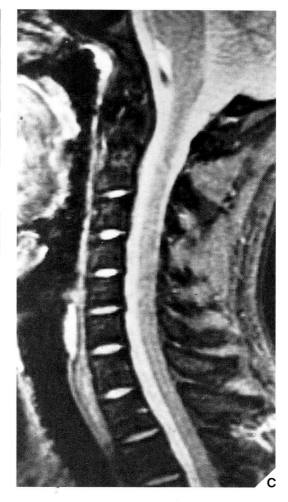

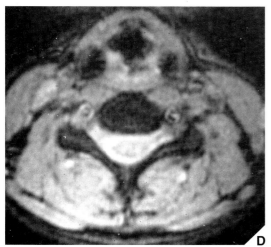

Figure 10.15 MR image of normal cervical spine. (A) T1-weighted (TR 800/TE 20) spin echo sagittal midline section demonstrates anatomic details of the bones and soft tissues. The craniocervical junction is well-outlined. The foramen magnum is defined by the fat within the occipital bone and clivus. The anterior and posterior arches of C-1 appear as small oval marrow-containing structures at the upper cervical spine. The spinal cord is of an intermediate signal intensity outlined by lower signal of CSF. The intervertebral disks are imaged with low signal intensity. (B) Parasagittal section demonstrates the apophyseal joints. (C) T2*-weighted MPGR sagittal image shows vertebral bodies and spinous processes to be of low-signal intensity. The high water content of the intervertebral disks produces a very high signal similar to that of cerebrospinal fluid. The cord is imaged as an intermediate signal intensity structure. (D) Axial section demonstrates neural foramina and nerve roots. The cervical cord is faintly outlined. (From Beltran J, 1990)

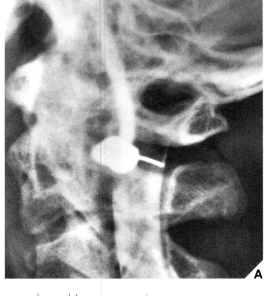

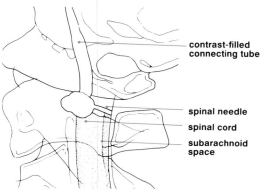

contrast-filled
connecting tube

spinal needle
spinal cord
subarachnoid
space

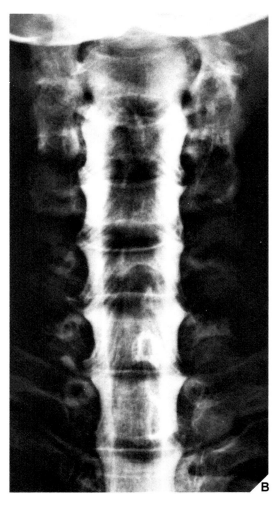

Figure 10.16 For myelographic examination of the cervical spine, the patient is recumbent on the table, lying on the left side. Using fluoroscopy, the point of entrance of the needle is marked at the C1-2 level, and a 22-gauge needle is inserted vertically, the tip being directed to the dorsal aspect of the subarachnoid space, above the lamina of C-2. Free flow of spinal fluid indicates the correct position of the needle. (A) About 10 mL of iohexol or iopamidol, water-soluble nonionic iodinated contrast agents, at a concentration of 240 mg iodine/mL, is slowly injected. Films are obtained in the posteroanterior (B), cross-table lateral (C), and oblique projections. (Oblique projections, however, are obtained not by rotating the patient but by angling the radiographic tube 45°.) If the lower segment of the cervical spine is not satisfactorily demonstrated or if the upper thoracic segment needs to be visualized, a film may also be obtained in the swimmer's position. Myelography demonstrates the thecal sac filled with contrast and the outline of the normal nerve roots and nerve root sleeves. (D) CT section at the level C3-4 obtained following myelography demonstrates the normal appearance of contrast in the subarachnoid space.

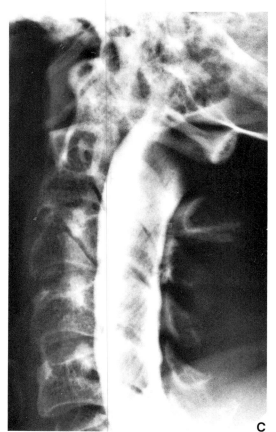

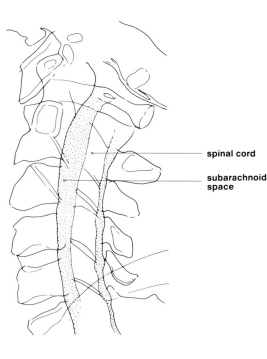

spinal cord

subarachnoid
space

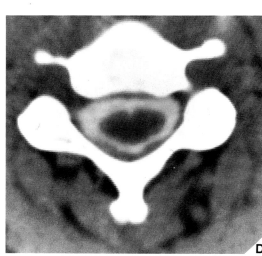

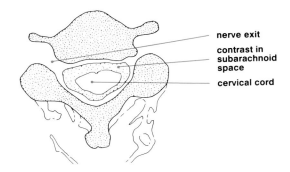

nerve exit

contrast in
subarachnoid
space

cervical cord

Since the advent of CT and MRI, myelography alone (Fig. 10.16) is nowadays rarely indicated in the evaluation of cervical injuries; if needed, this examination is usually performed in conjunction with CT (see Fig. 10.16D).

For a summary of the preceding discussion in tabular form, see Figures 10.17, 10.18, and 10.19.

Injury to the Cervical Spine

Traumatic conditions involving the cervical spine are almost always the result of indirect stress forces acting on the head and neck, the position of which at the time of impact determines the site and type of damage. As Daffner stressed, vertebral fractures occur in predictable and reproducible patterns that are related to the type of force applied to the vertebral column. The same force applied to the cervical, thoracic, or lumbar spine will result in injuries that appear quite similar, producing a pattern of recognizable signs that span the spectrum from mild soft-tissue damage to severe skeletal and ligamentous disruption. These patterns Daffner termed "fingerprints" of spinal injury; they depend on the mechanism of injury, which may be an excessive movement in any direction: flexion, extension, rotation, vertical compression, shearing, distraction—or a combination of these.

Figure 10.17 Tissue Signal Characteristics			
SIGNAL INTENSITY	T1-WEIGHTING	T2-WEIGHTING	GRADIENT ECHO (T2*)
Low signal	Cortical bone Vertebral end plates Degenerated disks Osteophytes Spinal vessels CSF	Cortical bone Vertebral end plates Ligaments Degenerated disks Osteophytes Spinal vessels Nerve roots	Bone marrow Vertebral bodies Vertebral end plates Ligaments Osteophytes
Intermediate signal	Spinal cord Paraspinal soft tissue Intervertebral disks Nerve roots Osteophytes	Paraspinal soft tissue Osteophytes Spinal cord Facet cartilage Bone marrow Vertebral bodies	Annulus fibrosus Spinal cord Nerve roots
High signal	Epidural venous plexus Hyaline cartilage Epidural and paraspinal fat Bone marrow Vertebral bodies	Intervertebral disks CSF	Intervertebral disk CSF Facet cartilage Epidural venous plexus Arteries

(Modified from: Kaiser MC, Ramos L, 1990)

Of the greatest initial importance in suspected cervical injuries, ~~is the question of stability of a fracture or dislocation. (Fig~~

ligament, and the ligamenta flava, which together with the capsule of ~~the apophyseal joints constitute the so-called posterior ligament com-~~

Several classifications of odontoid fractures have been proposed, based on the site and amount of displacement of a fracture. The system suggested by Anderson and D'Alonzo, however, is practical and has gained wide acceptance because of its emphasis on the most important feature of such fractures—their stability (Fig. 10.24):

Type I Fractures of the body of the dens distal (cephalad) to the base. They are usually obliquely oriented and are considered stable injuries. Conservative treatment usually suffices for healing.

Type II Transverse fractures through the base of the odontoid are unstable injuries. Conservative treatment has been complicated by nonunion in about 35% of cases; therefore, surgical fusion is the usual method of treatment.

Type III Fractures through the base of the odontoid extending into the body of the axis are stable injuries (Fig. 10.25). Conservative treatment is usually sufficient.

The best techniques for demonstrating fractures of the dens are the anteroposterior view, including the open-mouth variant, or Fuchs projection, and the lateral projection; thin-section trispiral tomography may also prove effective in delineating ambiguous or subtle features (Fig. 10.26).

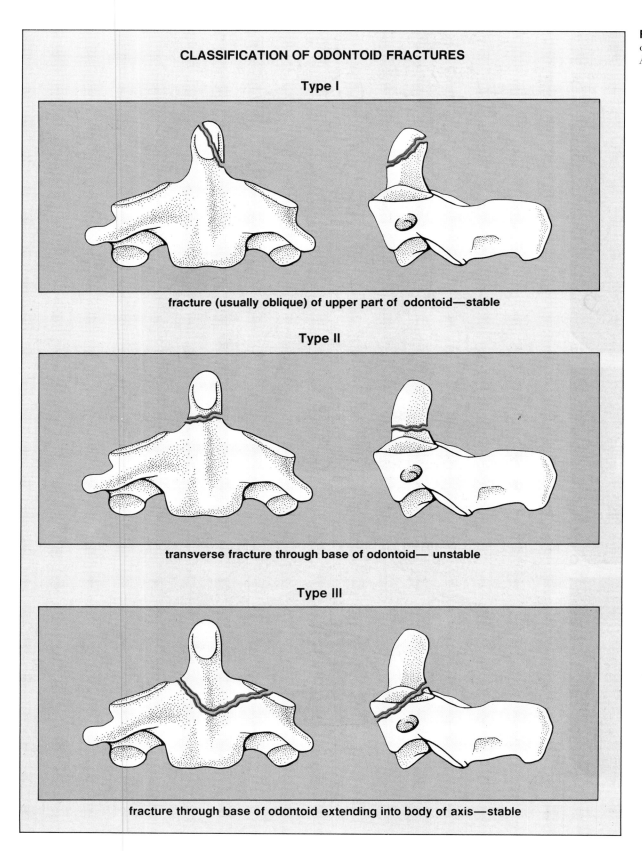

CLASSIFICATION OF ODONTOID FRACTURES

Type I

fracture (usually oblique) of upper part of odontoid—stable

Type II

transverse fracture through base of odontoid— unstable

Type III

fracture through base of odontoid extending into body of axis—stable

Figure 10.24 Classification of odontoid fractures. (Adapted from Anderson LD, D'Alonzo RT, 1974)

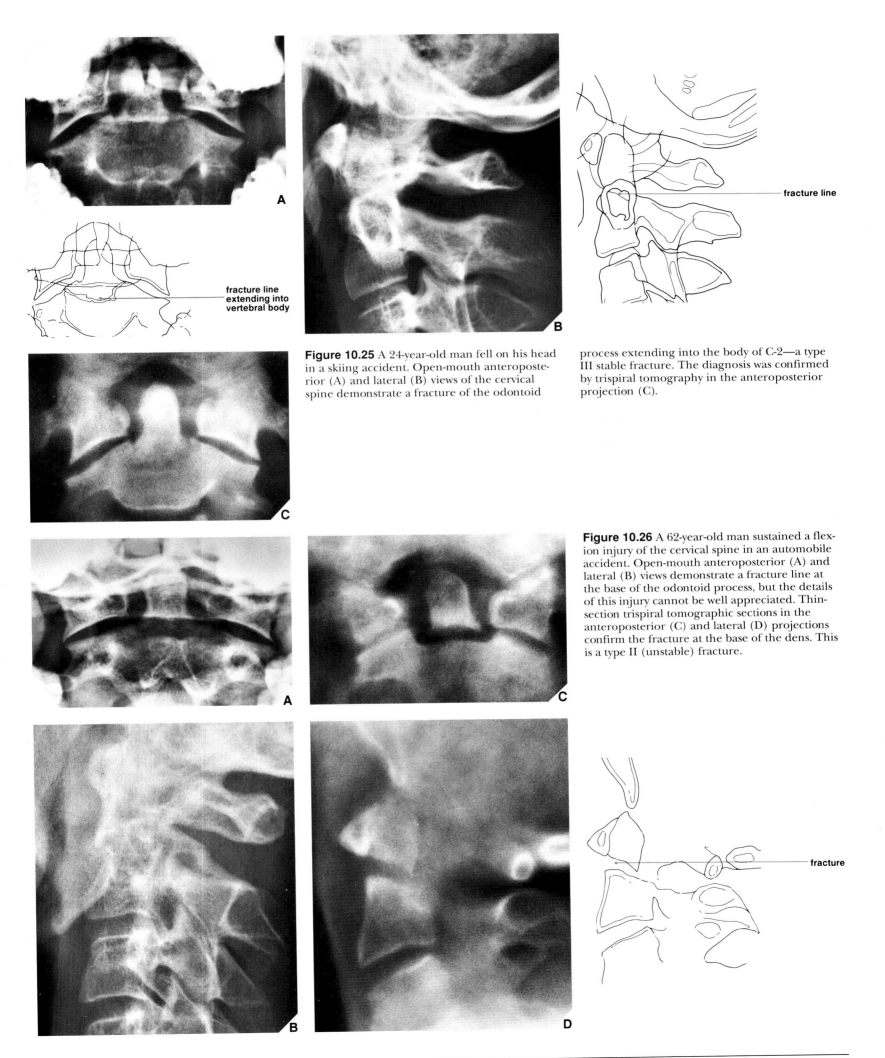

Figure 10.25 A 24-year-old man fell on his head in a skiing accident. Open-mouth anteroposterior (A) and lateral (B) views of the cervical spine demonstrate a fracture of the odontoid process extending into the body of C-2—a type III stable fracture. The diagnosis was confirmed by trispiral tomography in the anteroposterior projection (C).

Figure 10.26 A 62-year-old man sustained a flexion injury of the cervical spine in an automobile accident. Open-mouth anteroposterior (A) and lateral (B) views demonstrate a fracture line at the base of the odontoid process, but the details of this injury cannot be well appreciated. Thin-section trispiral tomographic sections in the anteroposterior (C) and lateral (D) projections confirm the fracture at the base of the dens. This is a type II (unstable) fracture.

fracture line extending into vertebral body

fracture line

fracture

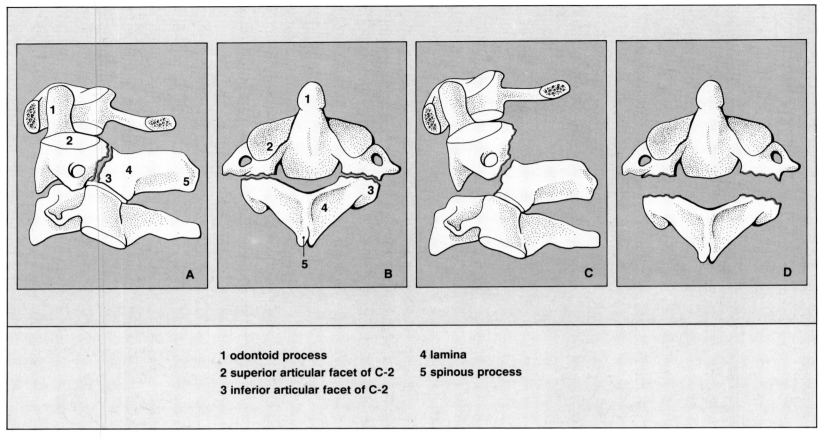

1 odontoid process
2 superior articular facet of C-2
3 inferior articular facet of C-2
4 lamina
5 spinous process

Figure 10.27 Hangman's fracture may present as nondisplaced fractures through the arches of C-2, as seen here schematically on the lateral (A) and axial (B) views, or as displaced fractures with anterior angulation (C,D) associated with disruption of ligaments, the intervertebral disk, or articular facets.

Figure 10.28 A 62-year-old man sustained a severe hyperextension injury to the cervical spine in an automobile accident. Lateral film shows a fracture through the pedicles of C-2 associated with C2-3 subluxation, a typical finding in hangman's fracture.

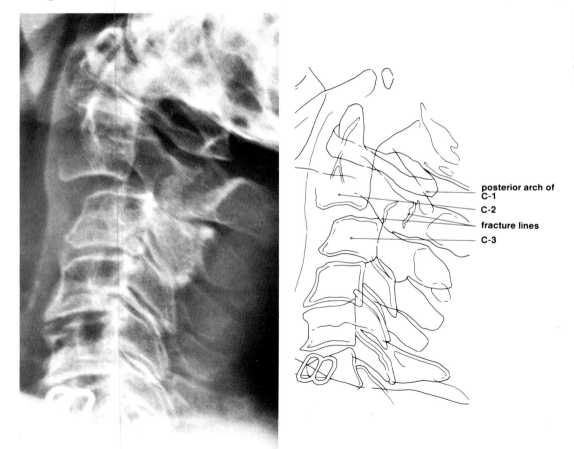

posterior arch of C-1
C-2
fracture lines
C-3

HANGMAN'S FRACTURE In 1912, Wood-Jones described the pathomechanism associated with execution by hanging. He found that hyperextension and distraction resulted in bilateral fractures through the pedicles of the axis, with anterior dislocation of the body and subsequent tearing of the spinal cord. A similar fracture, which in fact constitutes traumatic spondylolisthesis of C-2, is common in automobile accidents, when the face strikes the windshield before the vertex of the head, forcing the neck into hyperextension. This injury, which accounts for 4% to 7% of all cervical spine fractures and dislocations, may present as simple, nondisplaced fractures through the pedicles of the axis or as fractures through the arches with anterior subluxation and angulation of C-2 onto C-3 (Fig. 10.27). The fracture line usually lies anterior to the inferior articular facet of C-2 in both variants, but displaced fractures are more often associated with ligament disruption and intervertebral disk injuries. The best projection for demonstrating this injury is the lateral view (Fig. 10.28).

Fractures of the Mid- and Lower Cervical Spine

BURST FRACTURE The mechanism of this fracture is identical to that of Jefferson fractures involving C-1, but burst fractures are seen in the lower cervical vertebrae (C3-7). When the nucleus pulposus, which is normally contained within the intervertebral disk, is driven through the fractured vertebral end plate into the vertebral body, the body explodes from within, resulting in a comminuted fracture. Typically, the posterior fragment is posteriorly displaced and may cause injury to the spinal cord. If the posterior ligament complex is not disrupted, a burst fracture is stable. Occasionally, with ligamentous disruption, a burst fracture becomes unstable. Radiographically, it is characterized by a vertical split in the vertebral body, as seen on the anteroposterior view, but the plain-film lateral projection or lateral tomography better demonstrates the extent of comminution and posterior displacement (Fig. 10.29A). The most revealing modality in the case of burst fracture is, however, CT, since it demonstrates the details of fracture of the posterior part of the vertebral body in the axial plane (Fig. 10.29B).

TEARDROP FRACTURE The most severe and most unstable of injuries of the cervical spine, teardrop fracture is characterized by posterior displacement of the involved vertebra into the spinal canal, fracture of its posterior elements, and disruption of the soft tissues, including the ligamentum flavum and the spinal cord, at the level of injury. In addition, stress applied to the anterior longitudinal ligament causes it either to rupture or to avulse from the vertebral body, taking along a piece of the anterior surface of the body. This small, triangular or teardrop-shaped fragment is usually anteriorly and inferiorly displaced (Fig. 10.30). Associated spinal cord injury results in the

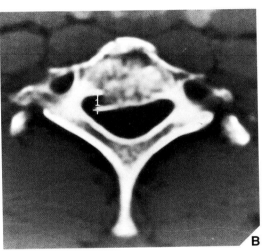

Figure 10.29 A 40-year-old man was ejected from a motorcycle and hit the pavement with the vertex of his head. (A) Lateral view of the cervical spine demonstrates a comminuted fracture of the body of C-7, involving the middle column. (B) A CT section confirms the burst fracture. The posterior part of the vertebral body is displaced into the spinal canal.

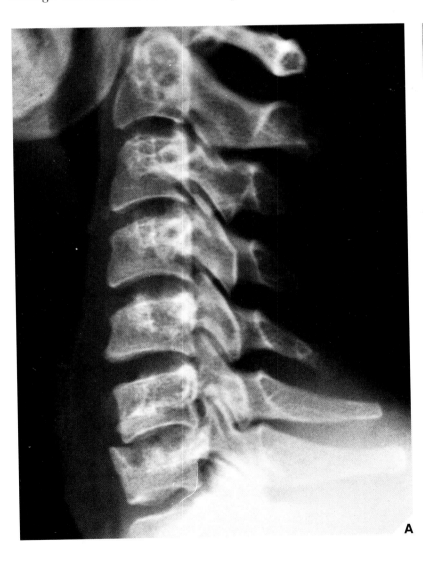

A

acute anterior cervical cord syndrome, consisting of abrupt quadriplegia and loss of pain and temperature distinction; however, posterior-column senses—position, vibration, and motion—are usually preserved.

The lateral view is the best radiographic projection for demonstrating this injury; lateral tomography may also be necessary, as well as CT (Fig. 10.31). The evaluation of spinal cord compression requires MRI.

It should be kept in mind in the evaluation of this fracture that occasionally a triangular fragment of bone similar in shape and location to that seen in the classic teardrop fracture may be noted in an extension type of injury. This "extension teardrop" fracture, however, is completely different; it is a stable fracture without the potentially dangerous complications of the flexion type of injury, and usually occurs at the level of C-2 or C-3 (Fig. 10.32).

CLAY-SHOVELER'S FRACTURE This oblique or vertical fracture of the spinous process of C-6 or C-7 is caused by an acute powerful flexion, such as that produced by shoveling. Deriving its name from its common occurrence in Australian clayminers in the 1930s, clay-shoveler's fracture was simultaneously labeled with the same name in Germany, where it was seen among workers building the Autobahn. A direct blow to the cervical spine or indirect trauma to the neck in automobile accidents can result in similar injury.

Clay-shoveler's fracture is a stable fracture, the posterior ligament complex remaining intact, and is thus not associated with neurologic damage. The best radiographic projection for demonstrating this injury is the lateral view of the cervical spine (Fig. 10.33A). If C-7 cannot be visualized despite good positioning and technique, for example, because of a short, thick neck or wide

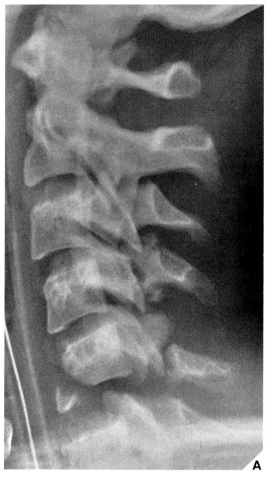

Figure 10.31 A 38-year-old man sustained an injury of the neck in a motorcycle accident. (A) Lateral view of the cervical spine demonstrates an avulsion fracture of the anteroinferior aspect of the body of C-5 and a fracture of its spinous process. The lamina of C-4 is fractured as well. There is disruption of the facets at the level of C5-6 with marked widening. There is posterior displacement of all vertebrae including and above C-5. (B) CT section demonstrates in addition a markedly comminuted fracture of the body of C-5.

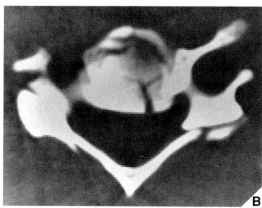

Figure 10.30 Teardrop fracture, seen here schematically in a sagittal section of the lower cervical spine, is the most serious and unstable of cervical spine injuries. Disruption of the anterior longitudinal ligament may cause avulsion of a teardrop-shaped fragment of the anterior surface of the body of C-5. This fracture is also typified by posterior displacement of the involved vertebra and fracture of its posterior elements. Depending on the severity of the injury, varying degrees of spinal cord damage may result.

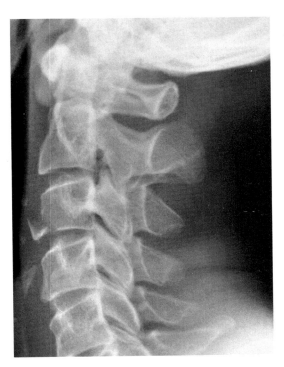

Figure 10.32 A 37-year-old man sustained an extension injury to the cervical spine in a fall. Lateral view of the spine demonstrates an extension tear-drop fracture of the vertebral body of C-3. Note that, in contrast to a flexion type injury, there is no subluxation, and the posterior, vertebral, and spinolaminar lines are not disrupted.

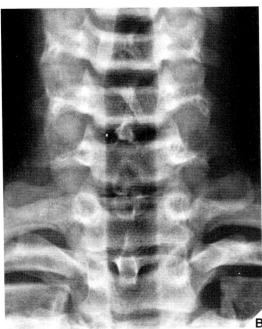

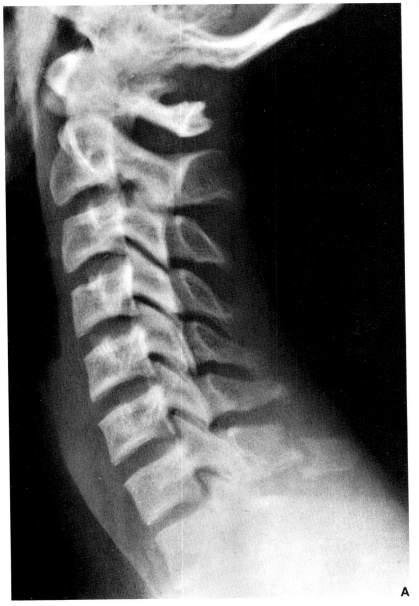

Figure 10.33 A 22-year-old man sustained a neck injury in an automobile accident. (A) Lateral view of the cervical spine shows a fracture of the spinous process of C-7, identifying this injury as a clay-shoveler's fracture. (B) On the anteroposterior view, clay-shoveler's fracture can be identified by the appearance of a double spinous process for C-7. This ghost sign is secondary to slight caudal displacement of the fractured tip of the spinous process.

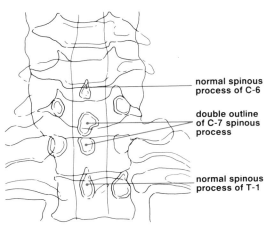

normal spinous process of C-6

double outline of C-7 spinous process

normal spinous process of T-1

shoulders, the swimmer's view should be obtained. This fracture can also be identified on the anteroposterior view by the so-called ghost sign (Fig. 10.33B) produced by displacement of the fractured spinous process.

SIMPLE WEDGE (COMPRESSION) FRACTURE Resulting from hyperflexion of the cervical spine, a simple wedge fracture generally occurs in the mid-cervical or lower cervical segment. There is anterior compression (wedging) of the vertebral body, and although the posterior ligament complex is stretched, it remains intact, making this a stable fracture. The lateral projection of the cervical spine adequately demonstrates this injury (Fig. 10.34).

Locked Facets
UNILATERAL LOCKED FACETS This type of injury is secondary to the flexion-rotation force with subsequent tearing of the joint capsule of one facet and posterior ligamentous complex. In the absence of disk space widening or subluxation, unilateral facet locking is a relatively stable injury. Frequently, however, there is about 25% anterior subluxation. These patients are at risk to sustain nerve root injury or, rarely, a Brown-Sequard type spinal cord injury.

BILATERAL LOCKED FACETS Bilateral dislocation of the cervical spine in the facet joints is the result of extreme flexion of the head and neck; it is an unstable condition due to extensive disruption of the posterior ligament complex. Interlocking of the articular facets is initiated by the forward movement of the inferior articular facet of the upper vertebra over the superior articular facet of the underlying vertebra (Fig. 10.35). This causes the lamina and spinous process of the two adjacent vertebrae to spread apart and the vertebral bodies to sublux. In the later stage of dislocation, the inferior articular facet of the upper vertebra locks in front of the superior articular facet of the lower vertebra, which results in complete anterior dislocation. The configuration of this injury leads to complete dis-

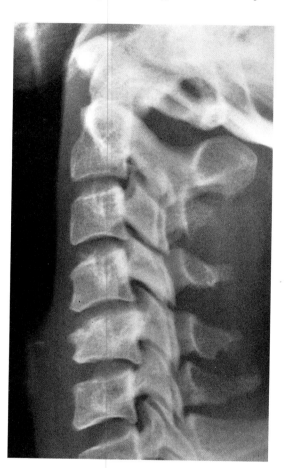

Figure 10.34 A 30-year-old woman sustained a neck injury in an automobile accident. Lateral view of the cervical spine demonstrates a simple wedge fracture of C-5.

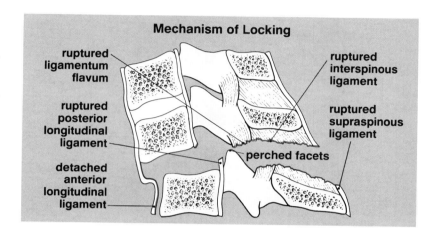

Mechanism of Locking

ruptured ligamentum flavum

ruptured posterior longitudinal ligament

detached anterior longitudinal ligament

ruptured interspinous ligament

ruptured supraspinous ligament

perched facets

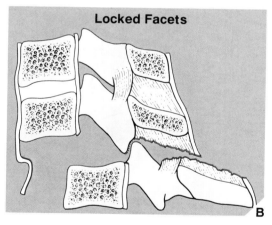

Locked Facets

B

Figure 10.35 (A,B) Bilateral locked facets is a hyperflexion injury characterized by complete anterior dislocation of the affected vertebral body. It is always associated with extensive ligament disruption and carries a great risk of cervical spinal cord damage.

ruption of the posterior ligament complex, the posterior longitudinal ligament, the annulus fibrosus, and frequently the anterior longitudinal ligament. It is also associated with a high incidence of cervical spinal cord damage.

The lateral projection of the cervical spine, preferably a cross-table lateral, is sufficient to demonstrate bilaterally locked facets. The key to the correct diagnosis is the presence of anterior displacement of the affected vertebra evident from its oblique orientation, whereas the vertebrae below are seen in true lateral projection. This results in a bowtie or bat-wing appearance of the articular pillars of the disclocated vertebra (Fig. 10.36).

THORACOLUMBAR SPINE

Anatomic–Radiologic Considerations

The standard radiographic projections for evaluating an injury to the *thoracic spine* are the anteroposterior (Fig. 10.37) and lateral (Fig. 10.38) views. The lateral projection is obtained using a technique called autotomography, which requires shallow breathing by the patient to blur the structures involved in respiratory motion and give a clear view of the thoracic vertebral column.

As in cervical spine injuries, conventional tomography, CT, and MRI play leading roles in the evaluation of fractures of the thoracic

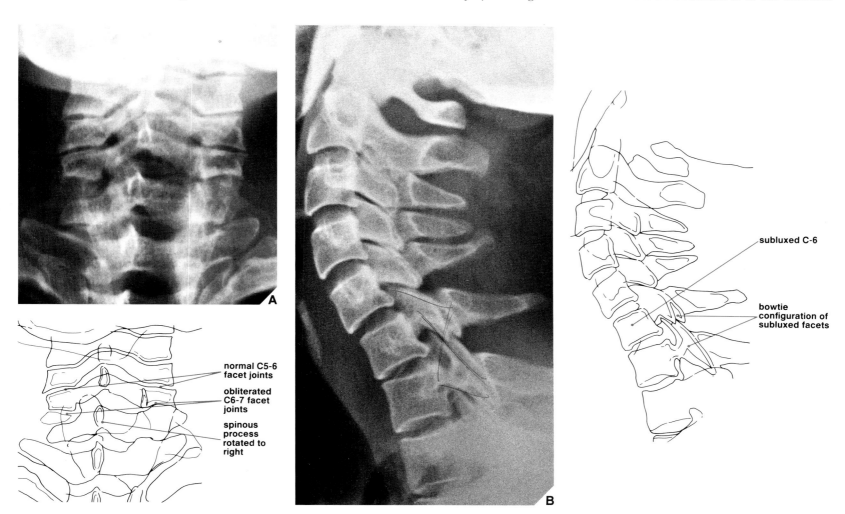

Figure 10.36 A 34-year-old woman injured her neck in a skiing accident. (A) Pillar view of the cervical spine demonstrates bilateral obliteration of the facet joints at the C6-7 level. The joints above appear normal. Displacement of the spinous process to the right is the result of rotation. (B) Lateral view shows subluxation of C-6 onto C-7, as well as rotation, yielding the typical bowtie appearance of this injury.

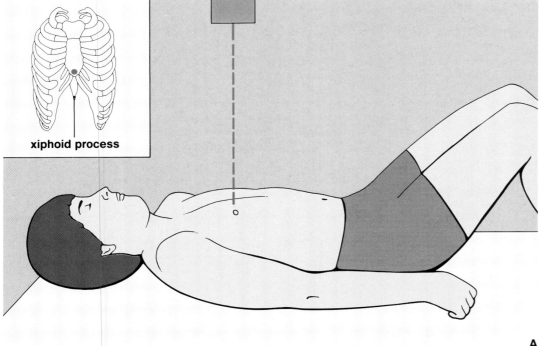

xiphoid process

A

Figure 10.37 (A) For the anteroposterior view of the thoracic spine, the patient is supine on the table, with the knees flexed to correct the normal thoracic kyphosis. The central beam is directed vertically about 3 cm above the xiphoid process. (B) On the film in this projection, the vertebral end plates and pedicles and the intervertebral disk spaces are seen. The height of the vertebrae can be determined, and changes in the paraspinal line can be evaluated.

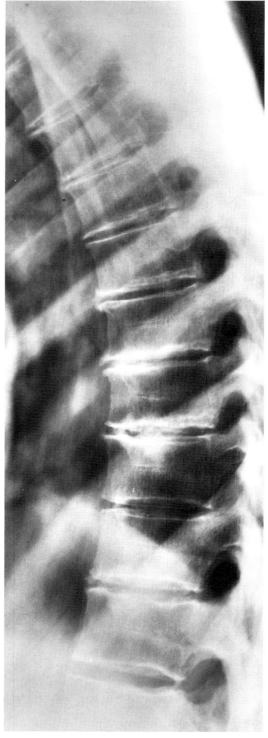

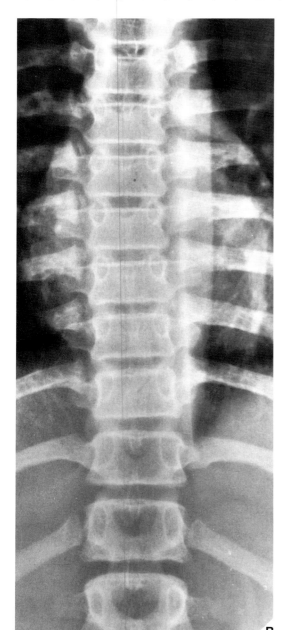

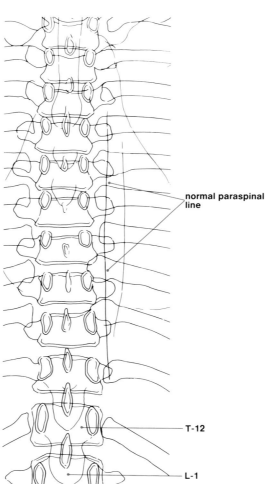

normal paraspinal line

T-12

L-1

B

Figure 10.38 For the lateral view of the thoracic spine, the patient is erect with the arms elevated. To eliminate structures that would obscure the bony elements of the thoracic spine, the patient is instructed to breathe shallowly during the exposure. The central beam is directed horizontally to the level of the T-6 vertebra with about 10° cephalad angulation. The film in this projection demonstrates a lateral image of the vertebral bodies and intervertebral disk spaces.

spine, particularly in defining the extent of injury. Conventional tomography offers the possibility of obtaining direct coronal and sagittal sections of spine, but it has the disadvantages of not being able to obtain axial sections and exposing the patient to a relatively high dose of radiation. Axial images can be obtained on CT, which provides in addition an excellent means of evaluating soft tissue injuries and exposes the patient to a relatively low dose of radiation. Unless reformation images are obtained, however, axially oriented fracture lines can be missed on axial CT sections. MR images are ideal for evaluating concomitant soft-tissue injury, particularly to the spinal cord and thecal sac.

The standard radiographic examination for evaluating injuries of the *lumbar spine* includes the anteroposterior, lateral, and oblique projections, supplemented by coned-down lateral spot films of the lumbosacral junction (L5-S1). The anteroposterior view is usually sufficient for evaluating traumatic conditions involving the vertebral bodies and transverse processes; the intervertebral disk spaces are also well demonstrated, except for the lowest (L5-S1) (Fig. 10.39).

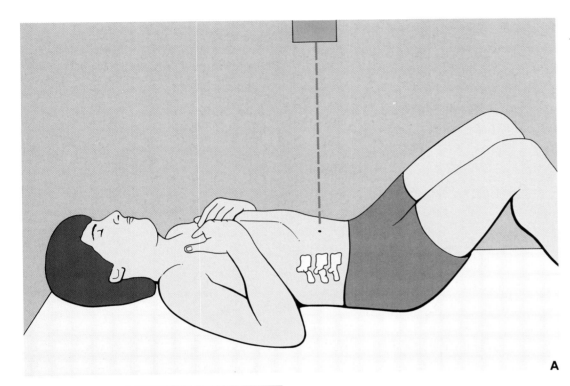

Figure 10.39 (A) For the anteroposterior projection of the lumbar spine, the patient is supine on the table, with the knees flexed to eliminate the normal physiologic lumbar lordosis. The cen-tral beam is directed vertically to the center of the abdomen at the level of the iliac crests. (B) The radiograph in this projection demonstrates the vertebral bodies, vertebral end plates, and the transverse processes; the intervertebral disk spaces are also well delineated. The spinous processes are seen en face, appearing as teardrops; the pedicles, also visualized en face, project as oval densities on either side of the bodies.

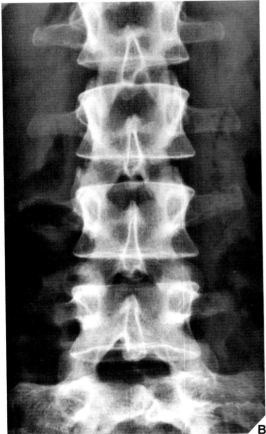

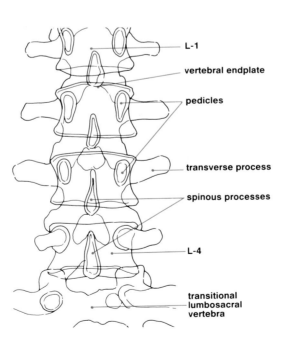

L-1

vertebral endplate

pedicles

transverse process

spinous processes

L-4

transitional lumbosacral vertebra

The spinous processes, seen as teardrops, and the articular facets, however, are not well demonstrated on this projection. A characteristic configuration of the end plates of the L3-5 vertebral bodies can be observed on the anteroposterior projection. Normally, the inferior aspects of these vertebrae form what is called a "Cupid's-bow" contour (Fig. 10.40), which is lost in cases of compression fractures affecting this part of the column.

On the lateral projection of the lumbar spine, the vertebral bodies are seen in profile, and the superior and inferior end plates are well demonstrated (Fig. 10.41). Fractures of the spinous processes

can be adequately evaluated on this projection, as can abnormalities involving the intervertebral disk spaces, including L5-S1. As in the cervical spine, an oblique projection of the lumbar spine can be obtained from either the patient's anterior or posterior aspect, although the posteroanterior oblique projection is preferable (Fig. 10.42). This view is particularly effective in demonstrating the facet joints (articular facets) and reveals a configuration of the elements of adjoining vertebrae, known as the "Scotty-dog" formation (Fig. 10.42C), which was first identified by Lachapele.

Ancillary imaging techniques are frequently used in the evalua-

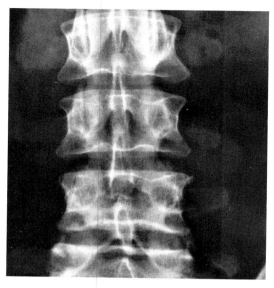

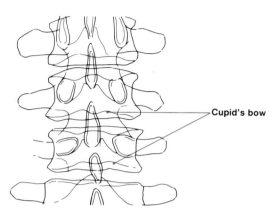

Cupid's bow

Figure 10.40 Anteroposterior coned-down view of the lumbar spine demonstrates a characteristic configuration of the lower aspects of L-3 and L-4. This "Cupid's-bow" contour is lost in cases of compression fracture.

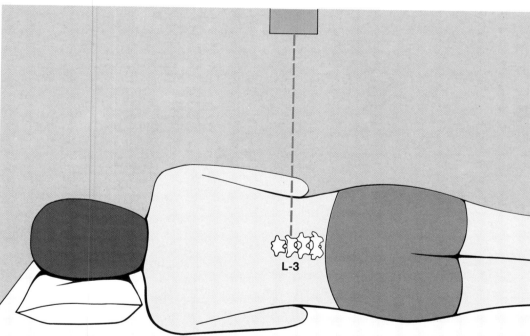

L-3

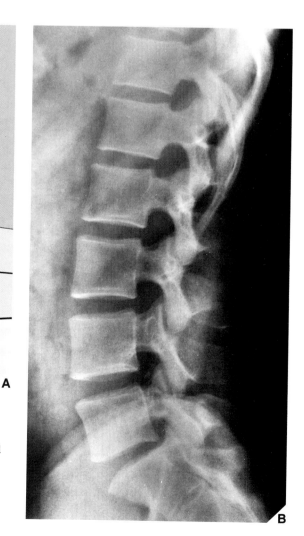

A

B

Figure 10.41 (A) For the lateral projection of the lumbar spine, the patient is recumbent on the radiographic table on either the left or right side; the knees and hips are flexed to eliminate the lordotic curve. The central beam is directed vertically to the center of the body of L-3, at the level of the patient's waist. (B) The lateral film of the lumbar spine allows adequate demonstration of the vertebral bodies, pedicles, and spinous processes, as well as the intervertebral foramina and disk spaces.

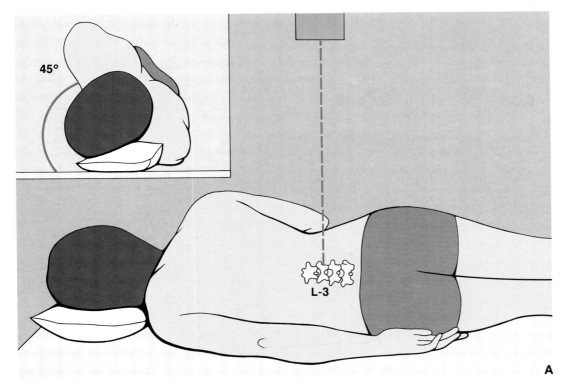

45°

L-3

A

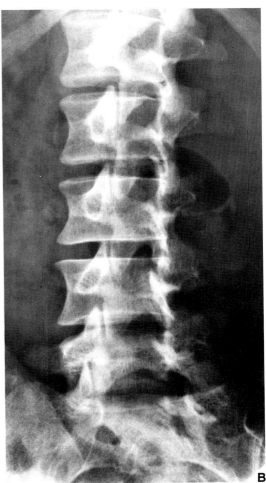

B

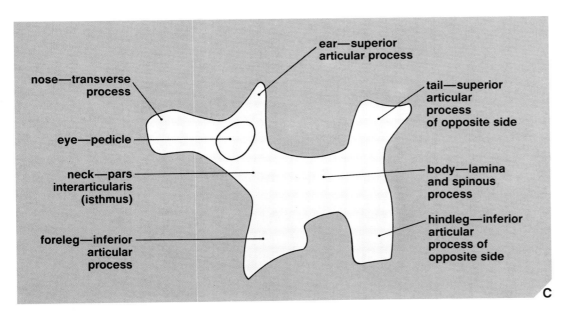

ear—superior
articular process

nose—transverse
process

tail—superior
articular
process
of opposite side

eye—pedicle

neck—pars
interarticularis
(isthmus)

body—lamina
and spinous
process

foreleg—inferior
articular
process

hindleg—inferior
articular
process of
opposite side

C

Figure 10.42 (A) For the posteroanterior oblique projection of the lumbar spine, the patient is recumbent on the table, with the right side rotated 45° to demonstrate the right-sided articular facets. (Elevation of the left side allows demonstration of the left-sided articular facets.) The central beam is directed vertically toward the center of L-3. (B) The posteroanterior oblique film demonstrates the facet joints, the superior and inferior articular process, the pedicles, and the pars interarticularis. (C) The oblique film also demonstrates a characteristic configuration of the elements of adjacent lumbar vertebrae known as the "Scotty dog."

tion of traumatic conditions of the lumbar spine. As in cervical and thoracic injuries, conventional tomography and CT provide useful information; CT is frequently used to assess the extent of damage in vertebral body fractures and abnormalities involving the intervertebral disks (Fig. 10.43). Moreover, myelography (Fig. 10.44) and diskography (Fig. 10.45) are often required, and they are frequently performed in conjunction with CT examination (Fig. 10.46).

MRI is now frequently used in the evaluation of injury to the thoracic and lumbar spine. In general, the images are obtained using a planar surface coil with its long axis oriented parallel to the spine. The slice thickness used to image the thoracic and lumbar spine in both sagittal and axial planes is usually 5.0 mm, with a 1-mm gap between slices to reduce the artifactual signal from adjacent slices. Sagittal images of the thoracic and lumbar spine are obtained with

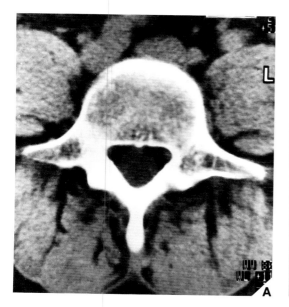
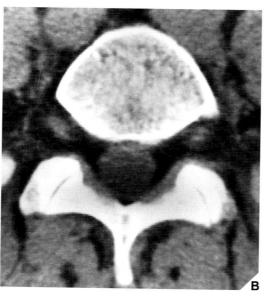
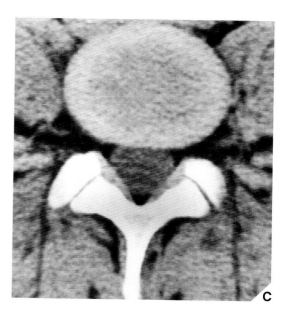

Figure 10.43 (A) CT section through the body of L-3 demonstrates an axial view of the pedicles, transverse processes, and laminae, as well as a cross-section of the thecal sac and the superior part of the spinous process. (B) In a section through the base of the intervertebral foramina, the caudal part of the body and spinous process are seen. Note the L3-4 facet joints. (C) At the L3-4 disk space, the facet joints are shown in full view, and the spinous process and laminae of L-4 can now be seen. Note the appearance of the ligamentum flavum.

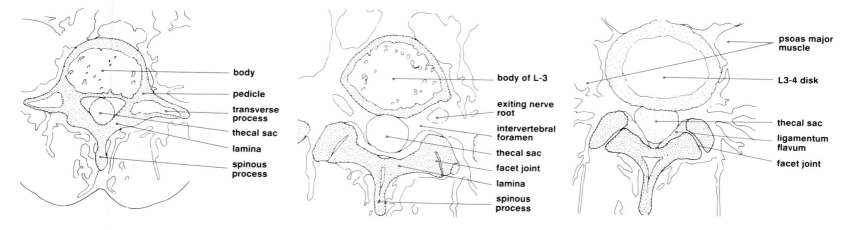

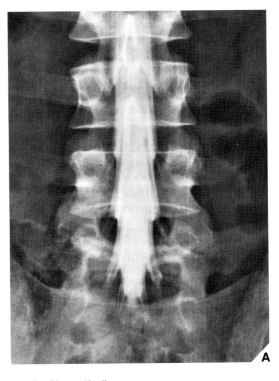

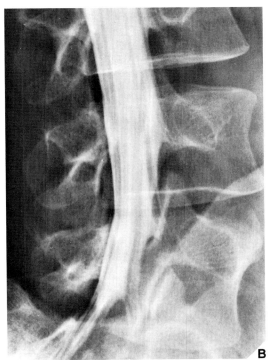

Figure 10.44 For myelographic examination of the lumbar spine, the patient is prone on the table. The puncture site, usually at the L3-4 or L2-3 level, is marked under fluoroscopic control. A 22-gauge needle is inserted into the subarachnoid space, and free flow of spinal fluid indicates proper placement. Fifteen mL of iohexol or iopamidol, in a concentration of 180 mg iodine/mL is slowly injected, and films are obtained in the posteroanterior (A), left and right oblique (B), and cross-table lateral (C) projections. In these normal studies, contrast is seen outlining the subarachnoid spaces of the thecal sac, as well as the cul-de-sac or most caudal part of the subarachnoid space. The nerve roots appear symmetric on both sides of the contrast column. A linear filling defect represents a nerve root in its contrast-filled sleeve. The length of the root pocket may vary from one patient to another, but in each patient, all roots are approximately equal in length. It is imperative during myelographic examination of the lumbar segment to obtain one spot film of the thoracic segment at the level T10-12 (D), since tumors localized in the conus medullaris may mimic the clinical symptoms of a herniated lumbar disk.

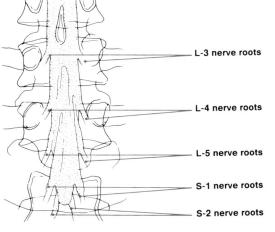

- L-3 nerve roots
- L-4 nerve roots
- L-5 nerve roots
- S-1 nerve roots
- S-2 nerve roots

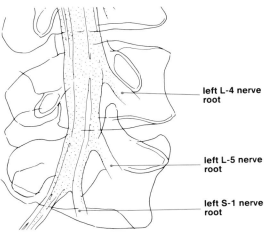

- left L-4 nerve root
- left L-5 nerve root
- left S-1 nerve root

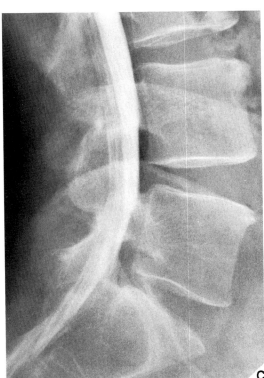

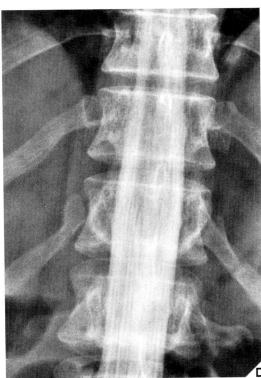

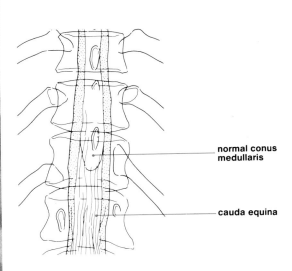

- normal conus medullaris
- cauda equina

T1- and T2-weighting. In the axial plane, T1- and T2*-gradient re-called echo pulse sequences (MPGR or GRASS) are usually obtained. Similarly to the imaging of the cervical spine, cerebrospinal fluid is visualized with low signal intensity on the sagittal images in T1-weighting, in contrast to the intermediate signal intensity of the spinal cord. The marrow within the vertebral bodies is seen as a high signal intensity in contrast to the intermediate signal intensity of the intervertebral disks (Fig. 10.47A).

On T2-weighted images, the thoracic cord is visualized as a low to intermediate signal intensity in contrast to the high signal intensity of the cerebrospinal fluid. The intervertebral disks demonstrate high signal intensity on both T2- and T2-* (MPGR) weighted images. The vertebral body marrow is imaged as an intermediate signal intensity on T2-weighted images and a low signal intensity on T2*-weighted MPGR and GRASS images (Fig. 10.47B).

The axial images effectively demonstrate the relation of the intervertebral disk spaces to the thecal sac. On axial T1-weighted images, the vertebral body, pedicles, laminae, transverse, and spinous processes demonstrate high signal intensity, while the nucleus pulposus yields intermediate signal intensity in contrast to the low signal intensity peripherally of the annulus fibrosus. The nerve roots demonstrate low to intermediate signal intensity and are in contrast with the high signal intensity of the surrounding fat (Fig. 10.47C). On T2-weighted images, the nucleus pulposus demonstrates high signal intensity, in contrast to the low signal intensity of the annulus fibrosus. The nerve roots are imaged as low-signal-intensity structures (Fig. 10.47D).

For a summary of the preceding discussion in tabular form, see Figures 10.19, 10.48, and 10.49.

Injury to the Thoracolumbar Spine
Fractures of the Thoracolumbar Spine

CLASSIFICATION Fractures of the thoracolumbar segment of the spine may involve the vertebral body and arch, as well as the transverse, spinous, and articular processes. They can generally be grouped by mechanism of injury as compression fractures, burst fractures, distraction fractures (Chance and other seat-belt injuries), and fracture-dislocations.

Because different classifications of thoracolumbar spine fractures have been used in the past by numerous authors, reports concerning the stability or lack of stability of a particular fracture pattern have varied. In 1983, Denis introduced the concept of the three-column spine classification of acute injuries to the thoracic and lumbar segments (Fig. 10.50). The significance of this system is its usefulness in determining the stability of various fractures, based on the site of injury in one or more of the spinal columns or elements:

The *anterior column* comprises the anterior two thirds of the annulus fibrosus and vertebral body and the anterior longitudinal ligament. The *middle column* includes the posterior longitudinal ligament and the posterior third of the vertebral body and annulus fibrosus. The *posterior column* consists of the posterior ligament complex, which has been defined by Holdsworth to include the supraspinous and infraspinous ligaments, the capsule of the intervertebral joints, and the ligamentum flavum (or interlaminar ligament), as well as the posterior portion of the neural arch. Generally, one-column fractures are stable, and three-column unstable; two-column fractures may be stable or unstable, depending on the extent of injury.

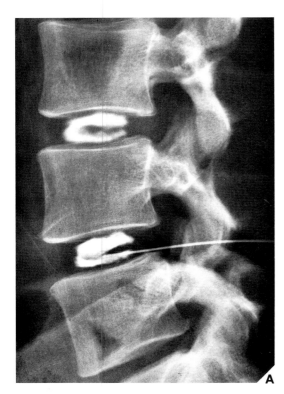

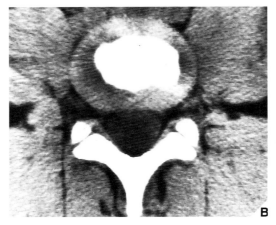

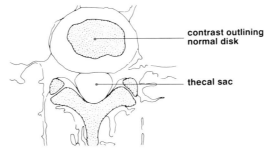

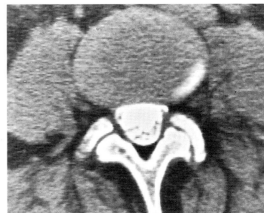

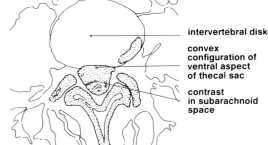

Figure 10.45 For diskographic examination of the lumbar spine, the patient is prone on the table, and the level of the injection, depending on the indication, is marked. The needle is inserted into the center of the nucleus pulposus, and about 2 mL to 3 mL of metrizamide is injected. (A) Lateral view of a normal diskogram shows a concentration of contrast medium in the nucleus pulposus outlining the disk; there should be no leak of contrast while the needle is in place. (B) CT section through the L3-4 disk space following diskography shows the normal appearance of this structure.

Figure 10.46 CT section obtained following myelography shows the normal appearance of contrast medium in the subarachnoid space. Note that the disk does not encroach on the ventral aspect of the thecal sac.

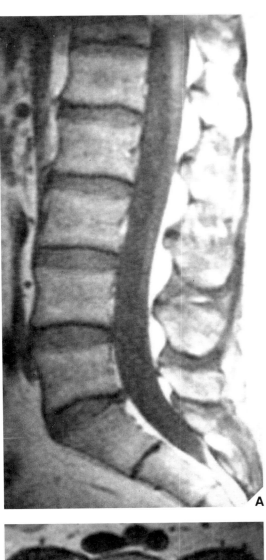

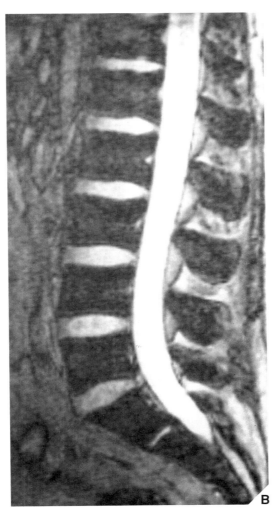

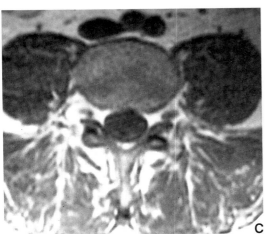

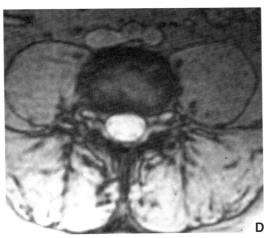

Figure 10.47 MRI appearance of a normal lumbar spine. (A) On this spin echo T1-weighted sagittal midline section (TR 800/TE 20) the tip of the conus medullaris is identified at T12-L1 level, surrounded by low-signal intensity cerebrospinal fluid. Epidural fat is of a very high-signal intensity. It is most clearly seen posteriorly but also some fat is present anteriorly at the lumbosacral junction. Intervertebral disks are of a somewhat low-signal intensity due to their high water content. The low-signal intensity lines along the ventral and dorsal aspects of the vertebral body are related to the anterior and posterior longitudinal ligaments and cortical bone of the vertebral bodies. These ligaments also span and cover the anterior and posterior portions of the disks. The thin black line along the inferior end plate and the bright line at the superior portion of each vertebral body are due to a chemical shift artifact. (B) Gradient echo T2-weighted sagittal midline section (TR 1000/TE 12, flip angle 22.5°) provides an image with a similar appearance to that of the myelographic technique, due to its very high gray-scale contrast. There is clear delineation of the thecal sac filled with high-signal-intensity cerebrospinal fluid. The posterior longitudinal ligament and dura are silhouetted against the high water signal of the cerebrospinal fluid and the intervertebral disks. The epidural fat is of intermediate-to-low signal intensity and the vertebral bodies are of a very low signal intensity. A high signal intensity of the midposterior cleft in the vertebral bodies is related to the basivertebral veins. (C) On the spin echo T1-weighted axial section (TR 800/TE 20), the nerve roots are surrounded by high signal intensity fat in the neural foramen. The ventral margin of the thecal sac at the disk level is convex outward and the canal is ample in size. The facet joints are well seen as the two low-signal intensity arcs of the cortical bone. (D) Gradient echo T2-weighted axial section (TR 1000/TE 12, flip angle 22.5 °) demonstrates low-signal nerve roots of the cauda equina surrounded by high signal intensity cerebrospinal fluid. The anterior margin of the thecal sac is well delineated. The individual nerve-root sheaths in the foramen also appear at a somewhat higher signal intensity. Some signal is visible from the disk interspace. (From Beltran J, 1990)

COMPRESSION FRACTURES Usually resulting from anterior or lateral flexion, compression fracture is a failure of the anterior column under compression forces; the middle column remains intact, acting as a hinge, even in severe cases where there may also be partial failure of the posterior column. The standard radiographic examination of the thoracic and lumbar segments is usually sufficient to demonstrate this injury, although conventional tomography or CT may be required to delineate the extent of the fracture or demonstrate obscure features. The anteroposterior view reveals buckling of the lateral cortices of the body close to the involved end plate, together with a decrease in the height of the body. In lateral-flexion injuries, compression forces may result in a wedge-shaped deformity of the body. In subtle cases, a clue to the diagnosis may be seen in a localized bulge of the paraspinal line secondary to hemorrhage and edema. However, it should be kept in mind that this finding may also be seen in pathologic fractures secondary to skeletal metastases to the spine. On the lateral projection, a simple vertebral compression fracture can be identified by a decrease in the height of the anterior part of the body, while the height of the posterior part and posterior cortex is maintained (Fig. 10.51).

SPECTRUM OF RADIOLOGIC IMAGING TECHNIQUES FOR EVALUATING INJURY TO THE SPINE*

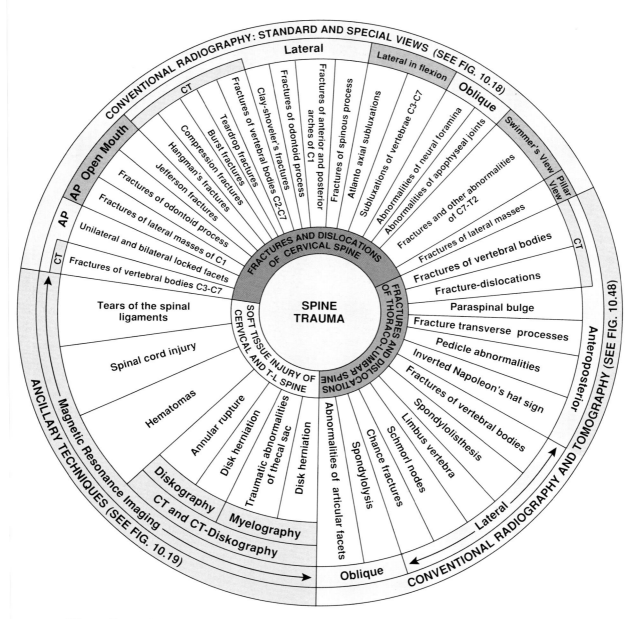

*The radiographic projections or radiologic techniques indicated throughout the diagram are only those that are the most effective in demonstrating the respective traumatic conditions.

Figure 10.48 Spectrum of radiologic imaging techniques for evaluating injury to the spine.

Figure 10.49 Standard and Special Radiographic Projections for Evaluating Injury to the Thoracic and Lumbar Spine*

PROJECTION	DEMONSTRATION
Anteroposterior	Fractures of:
	Vertebral bodies
	Vertebral end plates
	Pedicles
	Transverse processes
	Fracture-dislocations
	Abnormalities of intervertebral
	disk spaces
	Paraspinal bulge
	Inverted Napoleon's-hat sign
Lateral	Fractures of:
	Vertebral bodies
	Vertebral end plates
	Pedicles
	Spinous processes
	Chance fracture (seat-belt fractures)
	Abnormalities of:
	Intervertebral foramina
	Intervertebral disk spaces
	Limbus vertebra
	Schmorl node
	Spondylolisthesis
	Spinous-process sign
Oblique	Abnormalities of:
	Articular facets
	Pars interarticularis
	Spondylolysis
	"Scotty-dog" configuration

*For the ancillary imaging techniques, see Figure 10.19.

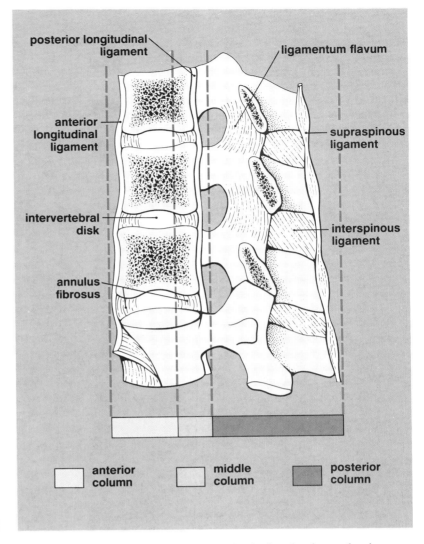

Figure 10.50 The three-column concept in viewing the thoracolumbar spine is helpful in determining the stability of various injuries. Fractures involving all three columns are unstable and those affecting one column are stable. (Adapted from Denis F, 1983)

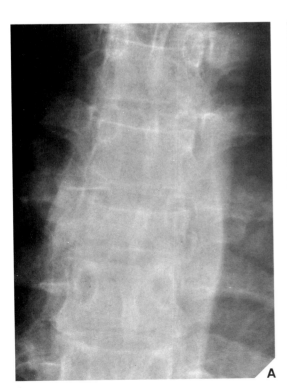

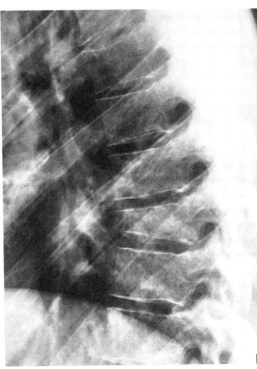

Figure 10.51 A 48-year-old woman fell from a ladder and hurt her back. (A) Anteroposterior view of the thoracic spine demonstrates a decrease in the height of the vertebral body of T-8, secondary to compression fracture. Note the localized widening of the paraspinal line secondary to hemorrhage and edema. (B) The lateral view demonstrates anterior wedging. Note the intact posterior vertebral body line. These are the features of simple compression fracture affecting only the anterior column.

BURST FRACTURES A burst fracture results from a failure of the anterior and middle columns secondary to axial-compression forces or a combination of axial compression with rotation or anterior or lateral flexion. The anteroposterior and lateral projections of the thoracic and lumbar spine are usually adequate to demonstrate these fractures. The anteroposterior view characteristically reveals a vertical fracture of the lamina, together with an increase in the interpedicular distance and splaying of the posterior facet joints. On the lateral view, fracture of the posterior part of the vertebral body results in a decrease in the height of this portion of the bone.

Comminution is often present, and fragments are retropulsed into the spinal canal, leading to compression of the thecal sac. For this reason, CT is an essential technique in the evaluation of burst fractures (Fig. 10.52A-C), and MRI (Fig. 10.52D) or myelography (Fig. 10.53) or may be required to localize the site and demonstrate the degree of compression on the thecal sac.

CHANCE FRACTURE Originally described by G. Q. Chance, this type of distraction injury of the lumbar spine has also come to be called a "seat-belt" fracture, because of the frequency of its occurrence in

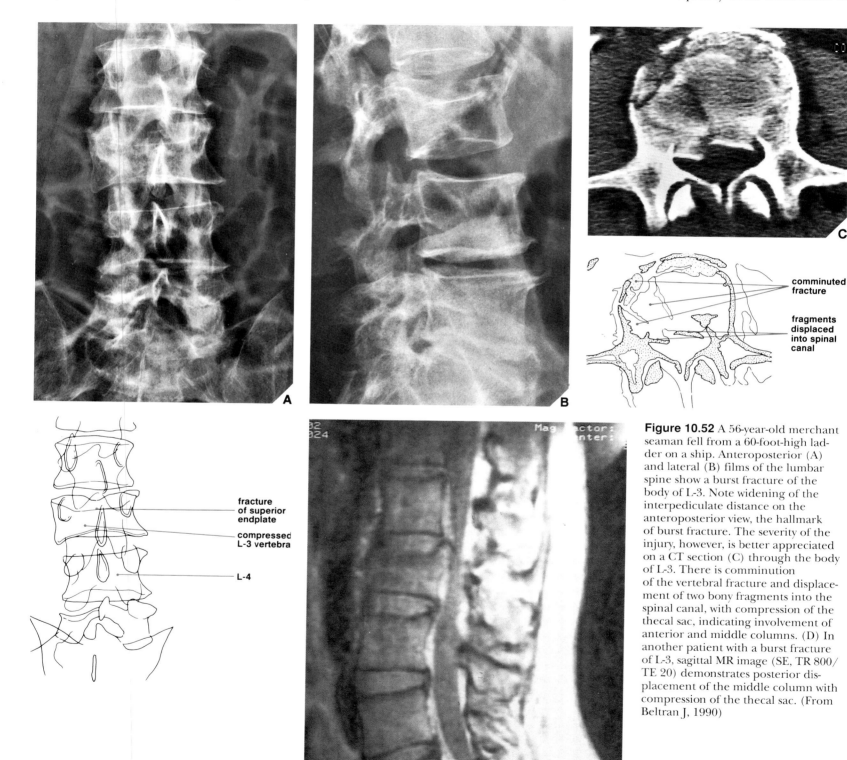

comminuted fracture

fragments displaced into spinal canal

fracture of superior endplate

compressed L-3 vertebra

L-4

Figure 10.52 A 56-year-old merchant seaman fell from a 60-foot-high ladder on a ship. Anteroposterior (A) and lateral (B) films of the lumbar spine show a burst fracture of the body of L-3. Note widening of the interpediculate distance on the anteroposterior view, the hallmark of burst fracture. The severity of the injury, however, is better appreciated on a CT section (C) through the body of L-3. There is comminution of the vertebral fracture and displacement of two bony fragments into the spinal canal, with compression of the thecal sac, indicating involvement of anterior and middle columns. (D) In another patient with a burst fracture of L-3, sagittal MR image (SE, TR 800/TE 20) demonstrates posterior displacement of the middle column with compression of the thecal sac. (From Beltran J, 1990)

automobile accidents in individuals wearing only lap seat belts. Acute forward flexion of the spine across a restraining lap seat belt during sudden deceleration causes the spine above the belt to be pushed forward and distracted from the lower, fixed part of the spine. The classic Chance fracture involves a horizontal splitting of the vertebra, beginning in the spinous process or lamina and extending through the pedicles and the vertebral body without dam-

age to ligament structures. Its constant feature is a transverse fracture without dislocation or subluxation (Fig. 10.54). The transverse process may be horizontally fractured as well, and at times there is compression of the anterior aspect of the vertebral body. Chance fracture tends to be stable, because the upper half of the neural arch remains firmly attached to the vertebra above and the lower half to the vertebra below. Since the original description of this frac-

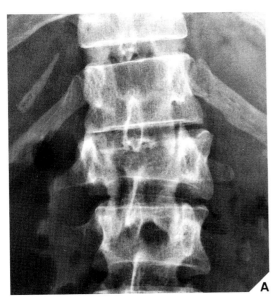
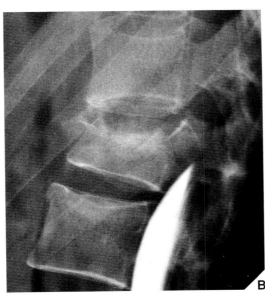
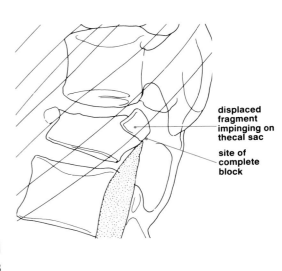

Figure 10.53 A 28-year-old woman made a parachute jump and landed on her back. She developed hemiplegia and became incontinent. (A) Anteroposterior projection of the lumbar spine shows a burst fracture of L-1.

(B) Lateral view as part of a myelogram shows complete obstruction of the flow of contrast medium at the level of fracture due to a small bony fragment impinging on the thecal sac.

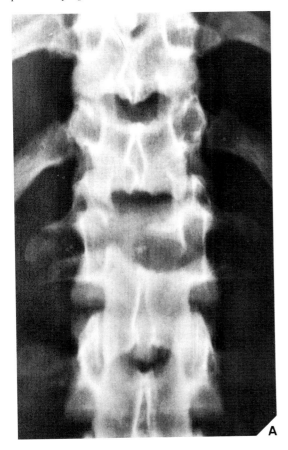
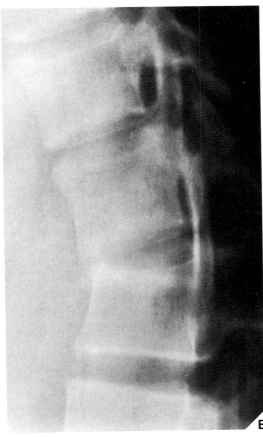
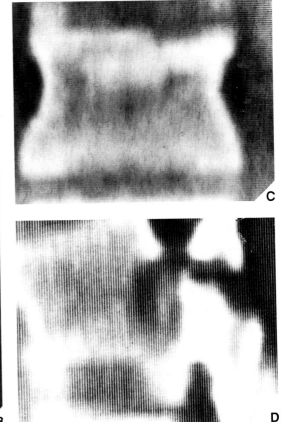

Figure 10.54 A 30-year-old woman sustained an injury to the lower back in a car collision; she had been wearing a lap seat belt. Anteroposterior (A) and lateral (B) tomograms of the lumbar spine show a fracture of the verte-

bral body of L-1 extending into the lamina and spinous process. Frontal (C) and sagittal (D) CT reformation images confirm the conventional tomographic findings. (Courtesy of Dr. D. Faegenburg, Mineola NY)

ture, three more types of seat-belt fractures have been reported, which involve varying degrees of ligament and intervertebral disk disruption (Figs. 10.55, 10.56). According to the Denis three-column concept of thoracolumbar spine injuries, these latter types of fractures are essentially the result of failure of the posterior and middle columns, with the intact anterior element acting as a hinge. These injuries may be stable or unstable, depending on their extent and severity.

FRACTURE-DISLOCATIONS Resulting from various forces—flexion, rotation, distraction, or anteroposterior or posteroanterior shear—acting on the thoracolumbar segment either alone or in combination, fracture-dislocations result in failure of all three columns of the spine, and hence such injuries are unstable.

In the *flexion-rotation type* of injury, the posterior and middle columns are completely disrupted, and the anterior column may show anterior wedging of the vertebral body. The lateral film also demonstrates subluxation or dislocation, together with an increase in the interspinous distance. The posterior wall of the vertebral body may be intact if the dislocation occurs at the level of the intervertebral disk. The anteroposterior projection may not be diagnostic, but it occasionally reveals a displaced fracture of the superior articular process on one side, representing failure of the posterior column secondary to rotational forces.

In the *shear types* of fracture-dislocation, all three columns are disrupted, including the anterior longitudinal ligament. The *posteroanterior shear variant* is characterized by forward displacement of the spinal segment onto the vertebra below at the point of shear; the vertebral bodies are intact without any decrease in their anterior or posterior height. However, the posterior elements of the dislocated vertebral segment, including the laminae, articular facets, and the spinous processes, are usually fractured at several levels. In *anteroposterior shear*, the spinal segment above the point of shear is dislocated posterior to the segment below. It may be accompanied by a fracture of the spinous process.

Fracture-dislocation of the *flexion-distraction type* resembles seat-belt injuries involving failure of the posterior and middle columns (see Fig. 10.55). However, unlike seat-belt injuries, the entire annu-

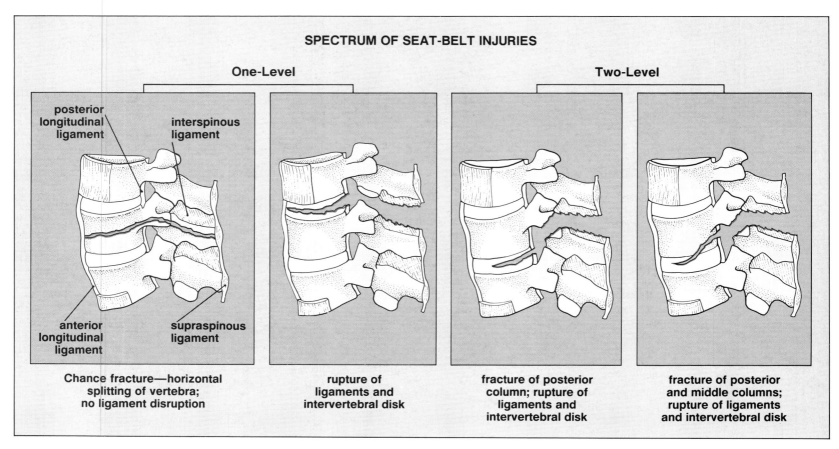

SPECTRUM OF SEAT-BELT INJURIES

One-Level   Two-Level

posterior longitudinal ligament

interspinous ligament

anterior longitudinal ligament

supraspinous ligament

Chance fracture—horizontal splitting of vertebra; no ligament disruption

rupture of ligaments and intervertebral disk

fracture of posterior column; rupture of ligaments and intervertebral disk

fracture of posterior and middle columns; rupture of ligaments and intervertebral disk

Figure 10.55 The spectrum of seat-belt injuries involving the lumbar spine.

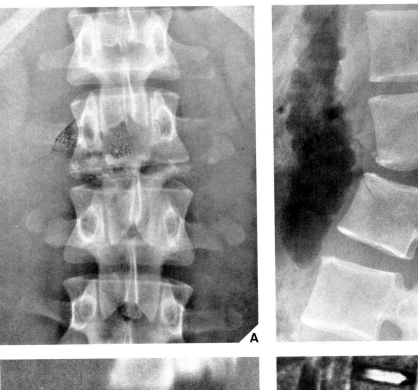

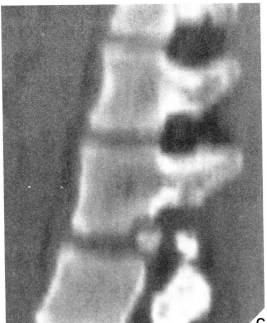

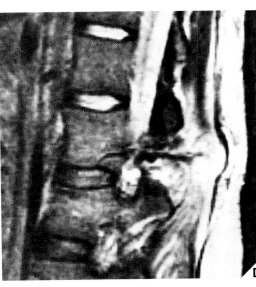

Figure 10.56 A 21-year-old woman sustained an injury to the lower back in a car accident. (A) Anteroposterior view of the lumbar spine demonstrates a horizontal cleft in the L-2 vertebral body. Note increased distance between the pedicles of L-2 and L-3 and fractures of several transverse processes. (B) Lateral view shows posterior angulation at the L2-3 level and an oblique fracture extending from the inferoposterior part of the L-2 vertebral body to the lamina and posterior elements. (C) Sagittal CT reformation demonstrates the fracture of posterior elements to better advantage. (D) Parasagittal MR image demonstrates disruption of the posterior ligaments and a large soft tissue hematoma. The findings are typical of a two-level seat-belt injury.

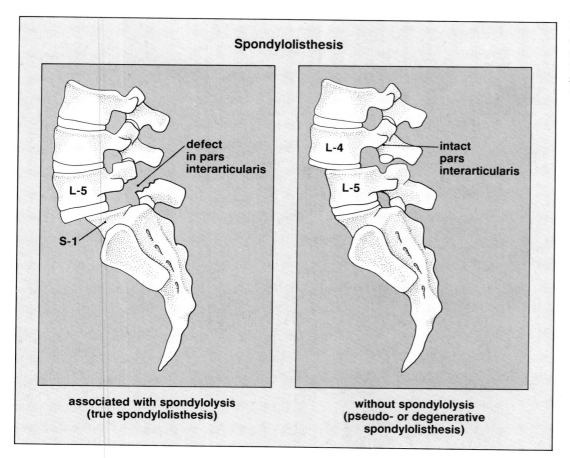

Figure 10.57 Spondylolisthesis may occur in association with spondylolysis resulting from a defect in the pars interarticularis, or secondary to degenerative disk disease and degeneration and subluxation of the apophyseal joints (pseudospondylolisthesis).

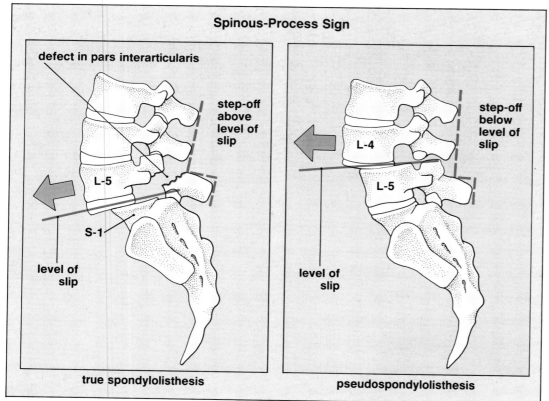

Figure 10.58 The spinous-process sign can help differentiate true spondylolisthesis from pseudospondylolisthesis by the appearance of a step-off in the spinous processes above the level of vertebral slip in the former and below that level in the latter.

lus fibrosus is torn, which allows the vertebra above to dislocate or sublux onto the vertebra below.

Spondylolysis and Spondylolisthesis

Spondylolysis, a defect in the pars interarticularis (neck of the "Scotty dog") of a vertebra, may be an acquired abnormality, secondary to an acute fracture; or as is more commonly the case, it may result from chronic stress (stress fracture). Rarely is it seen as a result of a congenital defect in the isthmus. Spondylolisthesis, a term introduced by Killian in 1854, is defined as ventral slipping or gliding of all or part of one vertebra on a stationary vertebra beneath it. These abnormalities are seen predominantly in the lumbar spine (90% of cases) and most commonly at the L4-5 and L5-S1 levels.

It is important to distinguish spondylolisthesis associated with spondylolysis from spondylolisthesis occurring without an associated defect in the pars interarticularis (Fig. 10.57). As a rule, this latter form, designated "pseudospondylolisthesis" by Junghanns in 1931, is associated with degenerative disk disease and degeneration and subluxation in the apophyseal joints, and it is often referred to as degenerative spondylolisthesis (see Chapter 12). Although the defect in the pars interarticularis cannot always be demonstrated on conventional radiographs, true spondylolisthesis can be differentiated from pseudospondylolisthesis by the spinous-process sign introduced by Bryk and Rosenkranz (Fig. 10.58). The sign is a logical outgrowth of the different processes at work in the two conditions. In true spondylolisthesis, a bilateral defect in the pars interarticularis leads to forward (ventral) slippage of the body, pedicles, and superior articular process of the involved vertebra, while the spinous process, laminae, and inferior articular process remain in normal position. Therefore, study of the most dorsal aspects of the spinous processes reveals a step-off at the interspace above the level of the slip (Fig. 10.59A). In pseudospondylolisthesis, on the other hand, the entire vertebra, including the spinous process, moves forward; in this situation, the most dorsal

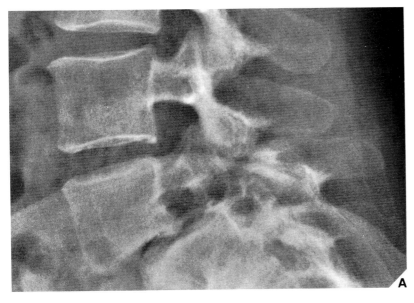
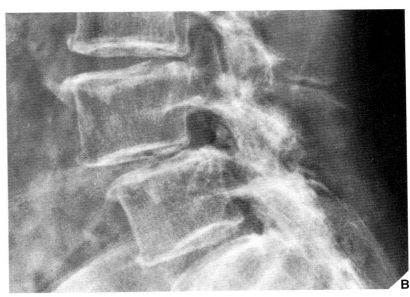

Figure 10.59 (A) Lateral view of the lumbar spine demonstrates the typical appearance of spondylolisthesis secondary to a defect in the pars interarticularis. Note that the most dorsal aspect of the spinous process of L-5 forms a step with that of L-4 above the level of slippage of L-5. (B) In spondylolisthesis without spondylolysis (degenerative spondylolisthesis), a step-off in the spinous processes below the level of vertebral slippage is an identifying feature.

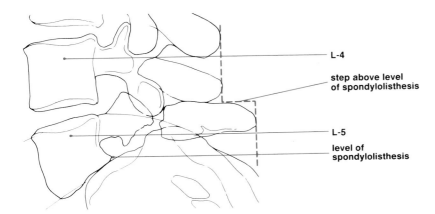
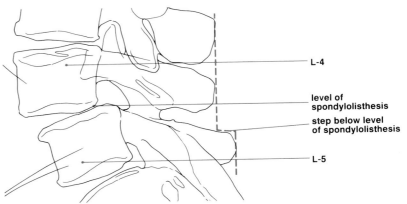

aspects of the spinous processes exhibit a step-off at the interspace below the level of the slipped vertebra (Fig. 10.59B). Application of this sign allows a correct diagnosis to be made on a single lateral film; oblique projections are not necessary. In obtaining the films, however, it is important to avoid overexposure, which may obscure the posterior margins of the spinous processes.

The defect in the pars interarticularis precipitating spondylolisthesis can be demonstrated on the standard oblique projection of the lumbar spine, which may need to be supplemented by conventional tomography or CT (Fig. 10.60 A-C); myelography on the lateral view may show an extradural defect on the ventral aspect of the thecal sac, similar to that created by disk herniation (Fig. 10.60D). A severe degree of spondylolisthesis at the L5-S1 level can be identified on the anteroposterior view by the ventrocaudal displacement of L-5 over the sacrum. This configuration creates curvilinear densities forming what is called the "inverted Napoleon's hat" sign (Fig. 10.61). The simple grading of spondylolisthesis proposed by Meyerding is based on the amount of forward slipping (Fig. 10.62).

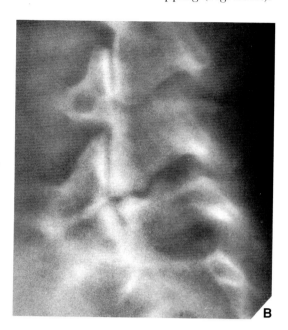

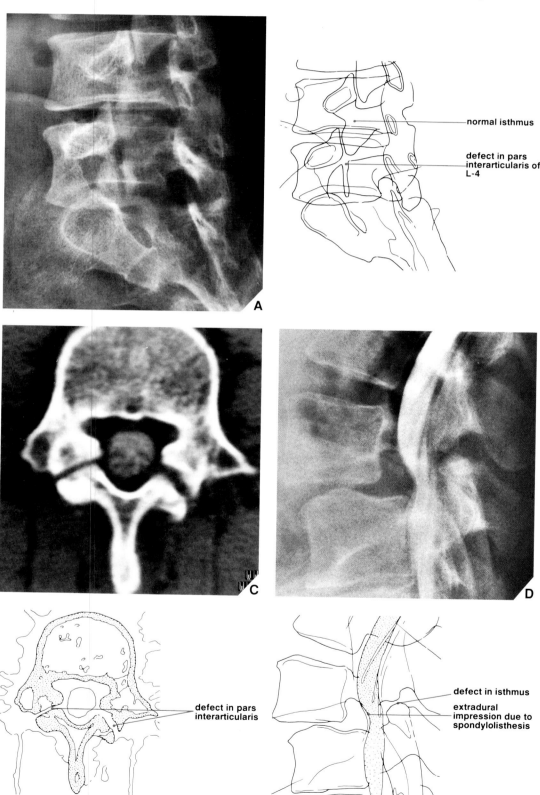

Figure 10.60 Oblique plain film (A) and trispiral tomogram (B) of the lumbar spine in a 28-year-old man show a defect in the pars interarticularis (neck of the "Scotty dog") of L-4 typical of spondylolysis. (C) CT section through the body clearly demonstrates defects in the left and right pars interarticularis. (D) Lateral spot film obtained during myelography shows an extradural defect, similar to that of disk herniation, on the ventral aspect of the thecal sac due to grade-2 spondylolisthesis at L4-5 (see Fig. 10.61). The defect in the pars interarticularis is also clearly seen.

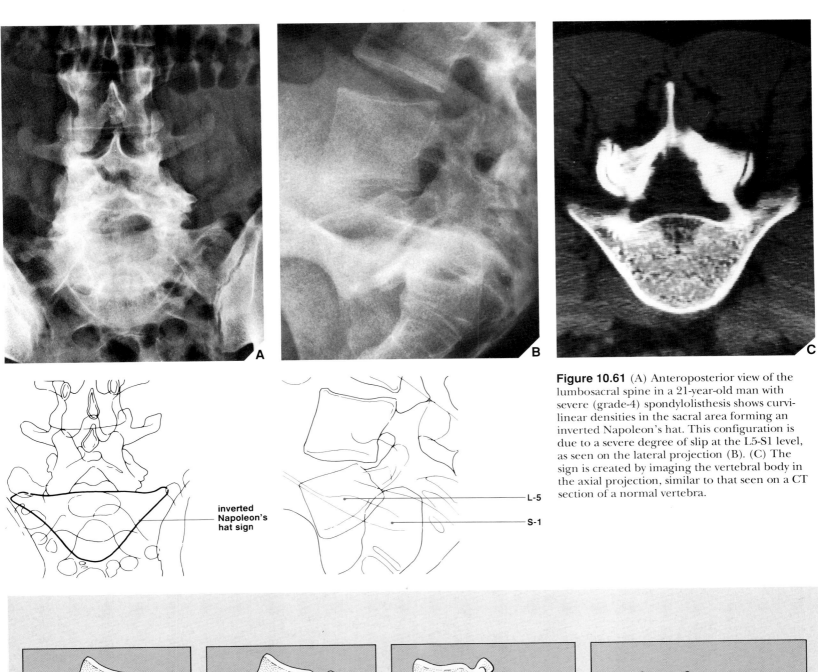

Figure 10.61 (A) Anteroposterior view of the lumbosacral spine in a 21-year-old man with severe (grade-4) spondylolisthesis shows curvilinear densities in the sacral area forming an inverted Napoleon's hat. This configuration is due to a severe degree of slip at the L5-S1 level, as seen on the lateral projection (B). (C) The sign is created by imaging the vertebral body in the axial projection, similar to that seen on a CT section of a normal vertebra.

inverted Napoleon's hat sign

L-5

S-1

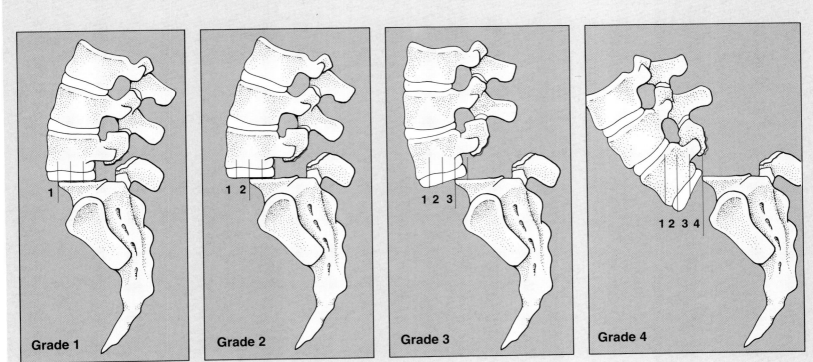

Grade 1 Grade 2 Grade 3 Grade 4

Figure 10.62 The grading of spondylolisthesis, as proposed by Meyerding, is based on the amount of forward displacement of L-5 on S-1.

Injury to the Diskovertebral Junction

One of the most frequent conditions affecting the diskovertebral junction is herniation of an intervertebral disk. The chief structural unit between adjacent vertebral bodies, the intervertebral disk comprises a soft central portion, the nucleus pulposus, composed of collagen fibrils and mucoprotein gel, lying eccentrically and somewhat posteriorly; and a firm fibrocartilaginous ring, the annulus fibrosus, surrounding the nucleus pulposus and reinforced by the anterior and posterior longitudinal ligaments. Injury to the intervertebral disk and the diskovertebral junction can result from acute trauma or from subtle subclinical, often endogenous injury. Depending on the direction of herniation of disk material, a spectrum of injuries of the intervertebral disk and adjacent vertebrae may be seen (Fig. 10.63).

ANTERIOR DISK HERNIATION When the normal attachments of the annulus fibrosus to the vertebral rim by Sharpey fibers and to the anterior longitudinal ligament loosen, disk material (nucleus pulposus) herniates anteriorly. Elevation of the anterior longitudinal ligament by herniating material stimulates the formation of peripheral osteophytes, leading to a degenerative condition known as spondylosis deformans (see Chapter 12 on arthritides), which can be demon-

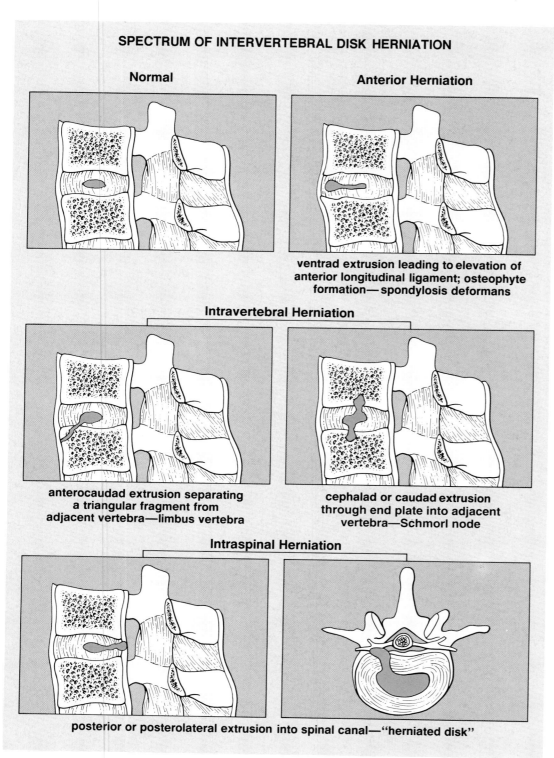

SPECTRUM OF INTERVERTEBRAL DISK HERNIATION

Normal

Anterior Herniation

ventrad extrusion leading to elevation of anterior longitudinal ligament; osteophyte formation— spondylosis deformans

Intravertebral Herniation

anterocaudad extrusion separating a triangular fragment from adjacent vertebra—limbus vertebra

cephalad or caudad extrusion through end plate into adjacent vertebra—Schmorl node

Intraspinal Herniation

posterior or posterolateral extrusion into spinal canal—"herniated disk"

Figure 10.63 The spectrum of intervertebral disk herniation.

strated on the lateral view of the lumbar spine (Fig 10.64A; see also Fig. 12.25). Anterior herniation can also be demonstrated on diskography (Fig. 10.64B).

INTRAVERTEBRAL DISK HERNIATION Ventrocaudal disk herniation, as well as ventrocephalad herniation, which is much less commonly seen, produces an abnormality known as limbus vertebra. Herniation of disk material into a vertebral body at the site of attachment of the annulus fibrosus to the body's rim separates a small, triangu-

lar fragment of bone, which is commonly mistaken for an acute fracture or infectious spondylitis. Reactive bone sclerosis adjacent to the defect, however, indicates a chronic process. The adjacent disk space is invariably narrowed, and a radiolucent cleft known as the vacuum phenomenon may be seen in the disk space, representing degeneration of the disk (Fig. 10.65). This abnormality is invariably asymptomatic due to the fact that it is the product of chronic, endogenous trauma. The characteristic radiographic changes are best seen on the lateral projection of the lumbar spine (see Fig. 10.65); only rarely

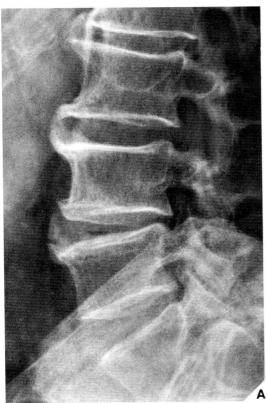

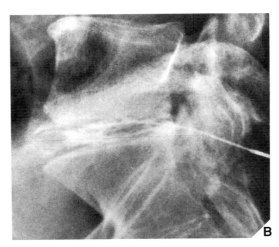

contrast outlining
anterior disk
herniation

spinal needle
in intervertebral
disk

Figure 10.64 (A) Lateral view of the lumbar spine shows a late stage of spondylosis deformans at the L2-3, L3-4, and L4-5 levels characterized by large osteophytes on the anterior aspects of adjacent vertebral bodies as a result of anterior disk herniation. (B) Anterior disk herniation can also be identified on diskography by contrast medium outlining the extruded material, as seen here at the L5-S1 level.

Figure 10.65 Lateral view of the lumbar spine in a 55-year-old woman with breast cancer who underwent radiographic examination to exclude bone metastases shows anterior disk herniation into the body of L-2 (limbus vertebra). Note the vacuum phenomenon, indicating disk degeneration.

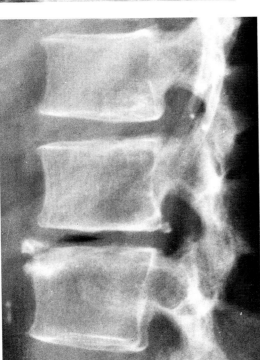

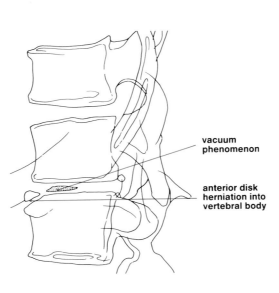

vacuum
phenomenon

anterior disk
herniation into
vertebral body

is conventional tomography or CT indicated to exclude a true vertebral fracture (Fig. 10.66). Occasionally, more than one vertebra is affected and although limbus vertebra is usually seen in the lumbar spine, it may also be present in a thoracic vertebra.

Limbus vertebra should not be confused with the secondary ossification centers of the vertebral ring apophysis, which are commonly seen in the growing skeleton (Fig. 10.67); at skeletal maturity, these centers become fully united with the vertebral body.

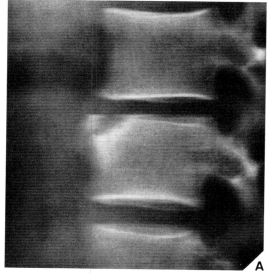

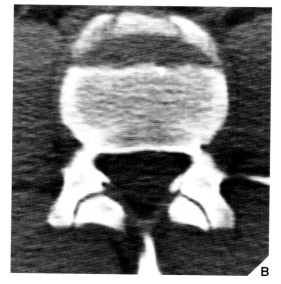

Figure 10.66 An 18-year-old male injured his lumbar spine in an automobile accident. The standard radiographic examination was equivocal regarding fracture. (A) Lateral tomogram shows the typical appearance of a limbus vertebra secondary to anterior herniation of the nucleus pulposus. The small triangular segment is separated from the body of L-4 by a rim of reactive sclerosis, indicating a chronic process. Note the characteristic disk space narrowing. (B) CT examination was performed to investigate the possibility of concomitant posterior disk herniation into the spinal canal. The examination was negative for posterior herniation but confirmed the anterior herniation into the vertebral body, as seen in this more proximal section.

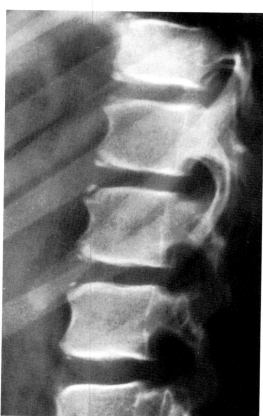

Figure 10.67 The secondary ossification centers of the vertebral ring apophysis in the growing skeleton, as seen here in a 5-year-old girl, should not be mistaken for limbus vertebrae.

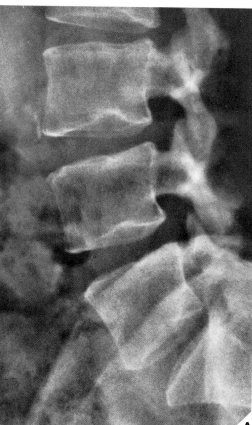

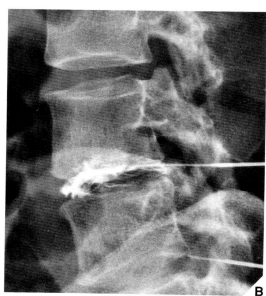

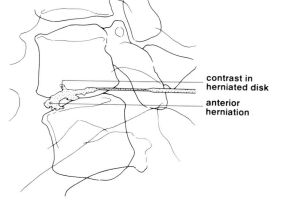

contrast in herniated disk

anterior herniation

Figure 10.68 (A) Lateral radiograph of the lumbar spine in an asymptomatic 77-year-old woman with osteoporosis of the spine shows multiple indentations particularly of the inferior end plates. representing the Schmorl nodes, secondary to intravertebral disk herniation due to weakening of the vertebral end plates. (B) In another patient, a small Schmorl node is demonstrated on diskography by opacification of extruded disk material in the body of L-4. Some anterior herniation is also evident.

Intravertebral disk herniation may also occur when the nucleus pulposus breaks through the vertebral end plate, extruding into a vertebra. This abnormality may be the result of acute trauma, as in a burst fracture, but it is much more commonly encountered secondary to weakening of the vertebral body, as in osteoporosis. In the latter condition the lesion is known as a Schmorl node. It may be small and localized, or large and diffuse, in which case it is often referred to as "ballooned disk" (Fig. 10.68).

Involvement of more than three consecutive thoracic vertebrae by Schmorl nodes is known as Scheuermann disease. This condition, which usually affects adolescent boys and young adults, is characterized by anterior wedging of the vertebral bodies and a kyphotic curve of the thoracic spine ("juvenile thoracic kyphosis"), in addition to a wavy outline of the vertebral end plates (Fig. 10.69).

POSTERIOR OR POSTEROLATERAL DISK HERNIATION Intraspinal herniation or "herniated disk" is the most serious of the three variants of diskovertebral junction injury. It is most commonly seen in the lumbar spine, particularly L4-5 and L5-S1, although it may be seen in the cervical region. It is commonly associated with clinical symptoms such as sciatic pain and weakening of the lower extremity, especially when herniation in the lumbar segment causes compression on an exiting nerve root or the thecal sac. A predisposing factor in some patients may be the loss of elasticity of the annulus fibrosus due to degenerative changes, with subsequent rupture of the annulus or even the posterior longitudinal ligament and retropulsion of the nucleus pulposus into the spinal canal. Typically, the patient, usually a young adult man, gives a history of straining his back by lifting a heavy object. The subsequent pain in the lumbar region radiates to the posterior aspect of the thigh and buttock and the lateral aspect of the leg, and is aggravated by coughing and sneezing; sometimes, there is associated paresthesia or numbness in the foot. Physical examination reveals muscular spasm, limitation of forward bending, and restriction of straight-leg raising on the affected side. Various other symptoms and physical findings may be present depending on the level and degree of injury.

The standard radiographic examination in herniated disks is usually normal, and ancillary radiologic techniques including myelography and CT, either alone or in conjunction with one another, as well as diskography, and nowadays MRI, are required to make a diagnosis. The myelographic findings in disk herniation may be very subtle, such as absent opacification of a nerve sheath (Fig. 10.70); or more

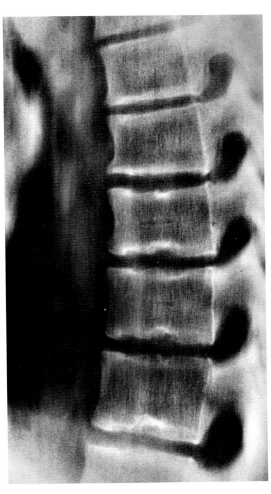

Figure 10.69 Lateral tomogram of the thoracic spine in a 23-year-old man demonstrates several Schmorl nodes in T5-8 and slight anterior wedging of the vertebral bodies. Involvement of multiple thoracic vertebrae by Schmorl nodes is known as Scheuermann disease. Note the wavy outline of the superior and inferior end plates and the mild kyphotic curve of the thoracic spine in this patient, an abnormality also called juvenile thoracic kyphosis.

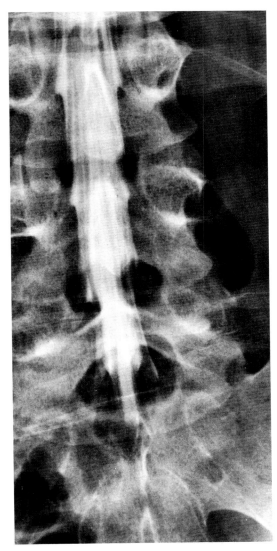

Figure 10.70 In lifting a heavy object, a 27-year-old man felt sudden, sharp pain in the lower back radiating to the left lower extremity. The standard radiographs of the lumbosacral spine were normal. Anteroposterior view of a myelo-

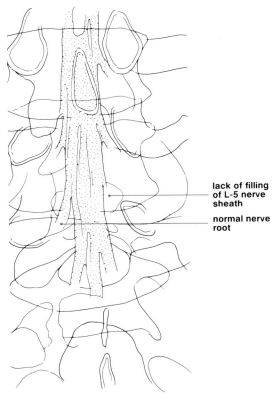

lack of filling of L-5 nerve sheath

normal nerve root

gram demonstrates a subtle lack of filling of the left L-5 nerve sheath, which at surgery was found to be compressed by a lateral herniation of the L4-5 disk.

obvious, such as an extradural pressure defect in the contrast-filled thecal sac (Fig. 10.71). Disk herniation can also be diagnosed on plain CT examination (Fig. 10.72) or on CT sections obtained following myelography or diskography (Figs. 10.73, 10.74), or on MRI (Fig. 10.75).

The latter imaging modality is being used increasingly for the diagnosis of conditions causing acute low back pain and sciatica. The sensitivity of MRI for the diagnosis of herniated disk and spinal stenosis is equivalent to or better than that of computed tomography, even in combination with myelography and diskography.

Radicular symptoms represent one of the most common reasons patients are referred for MRI of the spine. MRI is particularly sensitive and is used to detect and characterize disk herniation because it allows for direct evaluation of the internal morphology of the disk. The sagittal imaging plane is more sensitive for defining disk impingement on the thecal sac, or for demonstrating extruded frag-

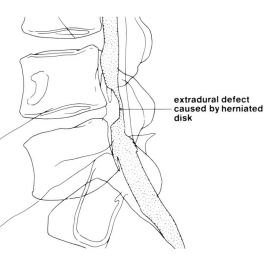

Figure 10.71 Lateral spot film obtained during myelography in a 38-year-old man demonstrates a large posterior herniation of the intervertebral disk at L4-5.

extradural defect caused by herniated disk

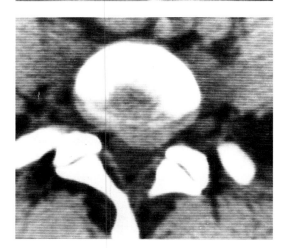

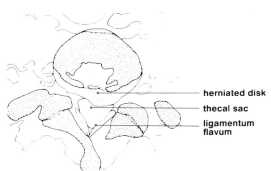

Figure 10.72 CT section of the lumbar spine at the L5-S1 level demonstrates a large centrolateral disk herniation encroaching on the left intervertebral foramen.

herniated disk

thecal sac

ligamentum flavum

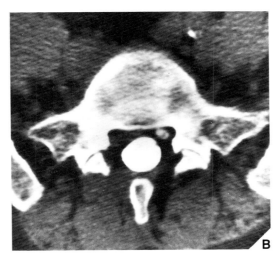

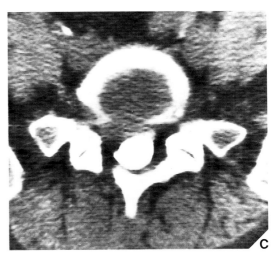

Figure 10.73 A 47-year-old man presented with severe back pain radiating to the right buttock and leg. (A) Spot film in the oblique projection obtained during myelography shows an extradural defect on the right side of the thecal sac at the L5-S1 disk space involving the right S-1 nerve root. The L-5 and S-2 nerve roots are normally outlined. CT sections (B,C) also obtained during myelography, demonstrate the lack of opacification of the S-1 nerve root on the right side and a large herniation of the L5-S1 disk compressing the thecal sac from the right.

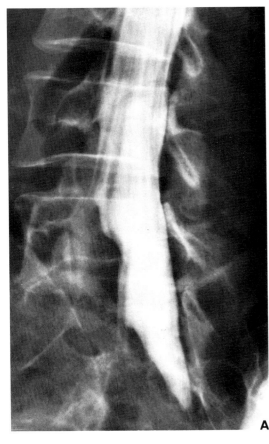

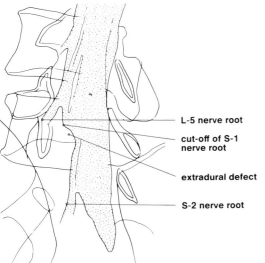

L-5 nerve root

cut-off of S-1 nerve root

extradural defect

S-2 nerve root

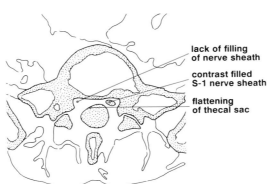

lack of filling of nerve sheath

contrast filled S-1 nerve sheath

flattening of thecal sac

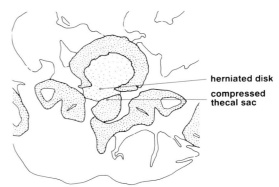

herniated disk

compressed thecal sac

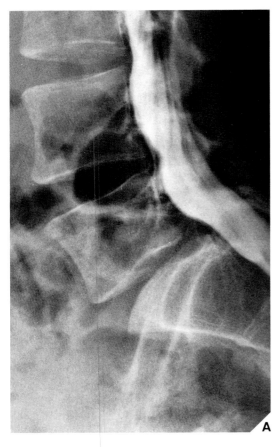

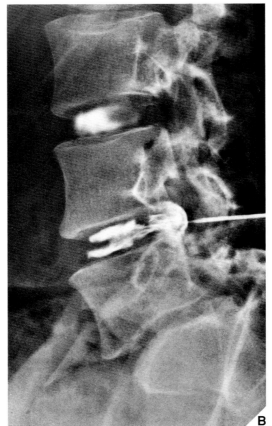

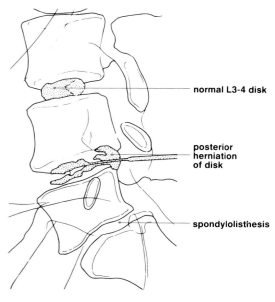

normal L3-4 disk

posterior
herniation
of disk

spondylolisthesis

Figure 10.74 A 30-year-old male construction
worker strained his lower back at work and
was admitted to the hospital with severe sciatica.
(A) Lateral view of the lumbar spine during myelographic examination reveals a slight separation
of the ventral aspect of the dural sac from the
dorsal aspect of L-5 due to grade-1 spondylolisthesis. In addition, there is an extradural pressure
defect on the ventral aspect of the dural sac at
the L4-5 level and a much smaller defect at the
L3-4 disk space. (B) A diskogram using metrizamide was performed at the L3-4 and L4-5 levels,
the latter demonstrating posterior herniation.
(C) CT at the L4-5 level following diskography
shows posterior protrusion of the opacified disk
material.

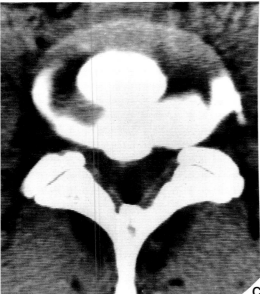

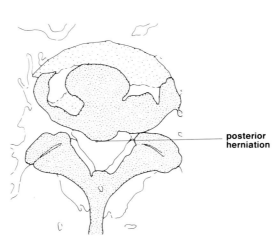

posterior
herniation

ments and showing the relationship to the vertebral bodies and intervertebral disk spaces (Fig. 10.75A). The axial imaging plane can demonstrate the effect of the herniated disk on the exiting nerve roots and thecal sac (Fig. 10.75B). Axial images are also important in evaluating neural foramina and nerve root effacement in cases of lateral and posterolateral disk herniation. Free disk fragments can be easily identified.

The use of T1-weighted images in the axial plane provides excellent contrast between high-signal fat and low-signal thecal sac, nerve roots, and disk fragments. Fast-scan techniques provide increased cerebrospinal fluid signal and allow enhanced contrast between herniated fragments and CSF. Some advantages of MRI in comparison with myelography and CT of lumbar disk disease are evident. MRI is sensitive to the water content of the nucleus pulposus. As the water content of this structure decreases with aging or degeneration,

decreased signal appears, particularly on T2-weighted images. In addition, the myelographic effect provided with heavily T2-weighted images and fast-scan techniques allows the visualization of nerve roots within the thecal sac. Anomalies such as conjoint nerve roots, which may simulate a herniated nucleus pulposus on CT studies, can be visualized directly with MRI. It has to be stressed, however, that evaluating patients with radiculopathy and herniated disk is an area in which both MRI and CT can be complementary. In cases where an extradural defect is identified with MRI, it may be difficult to ascertain whether the lesion represents a herniated nucleus pulposus or an osteophyte; in these situations, CT can make the distinction easily, by identifying the increased mineralization within the osteophyte. When the herniated fragment is clearly in continuity with the intervertebral disk and is of the same signal intensity, the diagnosis is suggested by MRI alone.

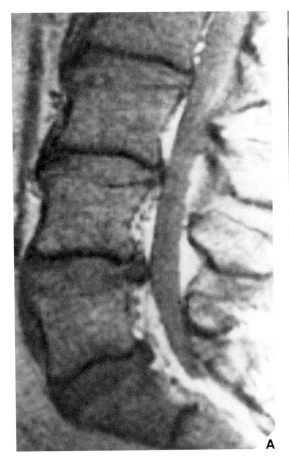

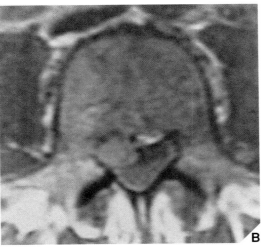

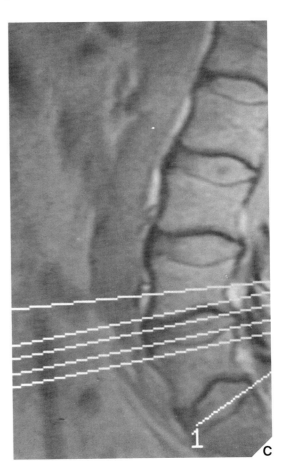

Figure 10.75 A 44-year-old man presented with sciatic pain radiating to the right buttock and thigh. (A) Sagittal MRI (SE, TR 1500/TE 20) demonstrates a posterior herniation of the disk L4-5 and a bulging disk at L5-S1. (B) Axial MRI (SE, TR 1500/TE 30) clearly shows posterolateral disk herniation with marked compression of the thecal sac. (C) The levels of the several axial sections obtained at the L4-5 disk space are indicated.

PRACTICAL POINTS TO REMEMBER

Cervical Spine

[1] The single most important projection in the radiographic examination of the cervical spine is the lateral view—either the erect or cross-table lateral.

[2] In the evaluation of injury to the cervical spine, it is mandatory to visualize the C-7 vertebra, the site of the most commonly missed fractures. If this cannot be accomplished on the lateral projection, the swimmer's view should be attempted.

[3] CT examination and MRI are useful techniques for evaluating vertebral-column trauma and associated soft-tissue and spinal cord injuries.

[4] Stability of a cervical spine fracture is the most important practical factor in evaluation of injuries to this region.

[5] Jefferson fracture—a symmetrical fracture of the anterior and posterior arches of C-1—can be diagnosed on the anteroposterior open-mouth view by the lateral displacement of the lateral masses.

[6] In the evaluation of fractures of the odontoid process (dens), note that:
- type I (an oblique fracture distal [cephalad] to the base) and type III (a fracture through the base extending into the body) are stable
- type II (a transverse fracture through the base) is unstable.

[7] Teardrop fracture, a flexion injury, is the most severe and unstable of cervical spine fractures; it is frequently associated with spinal cord damage.

[8] Clay-shoveler's fracture, involving the spinous processes of C-6 or C-7, can be recognized on the anteroposterior projection of the cervical spine by the ghost sign produced by caudal displacement of the fractured spinous process.

[9] In the radiographic evaluation of bilateral locked facets, a bow-tie or bat-wing appearance of the dislocated articular pillars on the lateral projection is characteristic.

Thoracolumbar Spine

[1] The three-column spine classification of acute injuries to the thoracic and lumbar segments is a practical approach to defining the stability of various fractures.

[2] Subtle fractures of the thoracic vertebrae can be recognized by a localized bulge in the paraspinal line secondary to edema and hemorrhage.

[3] Chance fracture, known also as a seat-belt fracture, is a horizontal fracture through a lumbar vertebral body with extension into the lamina and spinous process.

[4] Spondylolysis, a defect in the pars interarticularis (neck of the "Scotty dog"), leads to ventral slipping of one vertebra on the vertebra beneath it—spondylolisthesis.

[5] Spondylolisthesis
- may be associated with a defect in the pars interarticularis, so-called true spondylolisthesis
- or exist without an isthmic defect, so-called pseudospondylolisthesis or degenerative spondylolisthesis (associated with degenerative changes in the intervertebral disk and apophyseal joints).

[6] A simple test to distinguish between the two types of spondylolisthesis is the spinous-process sign.

[7] A severe degree of spondylolisthesis at the L5-S1 level can be recognized on the anteroposterior projection by the phenomenon known as the "inverted Napoleon's hat" sign.

[8] An intervertebral disk can herniate anteriorly or anterolaterally, as well as posteriorly, or posterolaterally. Intraosseous herniation into a vertebral body may occur caudad or ventrocaudad, cephalad, or ventrocephalad.

[9] Intravertebral ventrocaudad or ventrocephalad herniation results in separation of a small, triangular segment of a vertebra. This limbus vertebra should not be mistaken for a fracture.

[10] Posterior disk herniation can be documented by:
- CT
- myelography
- diskography
- MRI
- or a combination of these.

[11] As a rule, diskography is performed if the results of CT, myelography, and MRI are equivocal.

References

Amato M, Totty WG, Gilula LA: Spondylolysis of the lumbar spine: Demonstration of defects and laminal fragmentation. *Radiology* 153:627, 1984.

Amundsen P, Skalpe IO: Cervical myelography with a water soluble contrast medium (Metrizamide). *Neuroradiology* 8:209,1975.

Anand AK, Lee BCP: Plain and metrizamide CT of lumbar disk disease: Comparison with myelography. *AJNR* 3:567, 1982.

Anderson LD, D'Alonzo RT: Fractures of the odontoid process of the axis. *J Bone Joint Surg* 56A:1663, 1974.

Beltran J: *MRI: Musculoskeletal System.* Philadelphia, Lippincott, 1990.

Boden SD, Davis DO, Dina TS, et al: Abnormal magnetic-resonance scans of the lumbar spine in asymptomatic subjects. *J Bone Joint Surg* 72A:403, 1990.

Boyd WR, Gardiner A Jr: Metrizamide myelography. *Am J Roentgenol* 129:481, 1977.

Brant-Zawadzki M, Miller EM, Federle MP: CT in the evaluation of spine trauma. *Am J Roentgenol* 136:369, 1981.

Brashear HR Jr, Venters GC, Preston ET: Fractures of the neural arch of the axis: A report of twenty-nine cases. *J Bone Joint Surg* 57A:879, 1975.

Brodsky AE, Binder WF: Lumbar discography. Its value in diagnosis and treatment of lumbar disc lesions. *Spine* 4:110, 1979.

Brown RC, Evans ET: What causes the "eye in the Scotty dog" in the oblique projection of the lumbar spine? *Am J Roentgenol* 118:435, 1973.

Bryk D, Rosenkranz W: True spondylolisthesis and pseudospondylolisthesis—the spinous process sign. *J Can Assoc Radiol* 20:53, 1969.

Bucholz RW: Unstable hangman's fractures. *Clin Orthop* 154:119, 1981.

Burke JT, Harris JH: Acute injuries of the axis vertebra. *Skel Radiol* 18:335, 1989.

Cancelmo JJ: Clay shoveler's fracture: A helpful diagnostic sign. *Am J Roentgenol* 115:540, 1972.

Chance CQ: Note on a type of flexion fracture of the spine. *Br J Radiol* 21:452, 1948.

Christenson PC: The radiologic study of the normal spine: Cervical, thoracic, lumbar, and sacral. *Radiol Clin North Am* 15:133, 1977.

Clark WM, Gehweiler JA Jr, Laib R: Twelve significant signs of cervical spine trauma. *Skeletal Radiol* 3:201, 1979.

Collins JS Jr, Gardner WJ: Lumbar discography: An analysis of one thousand cases. *J Neurosurg* 19:452, 1962.

Daffner RH: Injuries of the thoracolumbar vertebral column. In: Dalinka MK, Kaye JJ (eds): *Radiology in Emergency Room Medicine.* New York, Churchill Livingstone, 1984, pp 317-341.

Daffner RH: "Fingerprints" of vertebral trauma—a unifying concept based on mechanism. *Skeletal Radiol* 15:518, 1986.

Daffner RH: *Imaging of Vertebral Trauma.* Rockville, Aspen Publishers, 1988.

Denis F: The three column spine and its significance in the classification of acute thoracolumbar spine injuries. *Spine* 8:817, 1983.

Denis F: Spinal instability as defined by the three-column spine concept in acute spinal trauma. *Clin Orthop* 189:65, 1984.

Dietz GW, Christensen EE: Normal "Cupid's bow" contour of the lower lumbar vertebrae. *Radiology* 121:577, 1976.

Dolan KD: Cervical spine injuries below the axis. *Radiol Clin North Am* 15:247, 1977.

Dortwart RH, DeGroot J, Sauerland EK, Helms CA, Vogler JB: Computed tomography of the lumbosacral spine: Normal anatomy, anatomic variants and pathologic anatomy. *RadioGraphics* 2:459, 1982.

Dublin AB, McGahan JP, Reid MH: The value of computed tomographic metrizamide myelography in the neuroradiological evaluation of the spine. *Radiology* 146:79, 1983.

Epstein BS, Epstein JA, Jones MD: Lumbar spondylolisthesis with isthmic defect. *Radiol Clin North Am* 15:261, 1977.

Ferguson RL, Allen BL Jr: A mechanistic classification of thoracolumbar spine fractures. *Clin Orthop* 189:77, 1984.

Firooznia H, Benjamin V, Kricheff II, Rafii M, Golimbu C: CT of lumbar spine disc herniation: Correlation with surgical findings. *Am J Roentgenol* 142:587, 1984.

Fuchs, AW: Cervical vertebrae (Part I). *Radiogr Clin Photogr* 16:2,1940.

Gerlock AJ Jr, Kirchner SG, Heller RM, Kaye JJ: *The Cervical Spine in Trauma.* Philadelphia, Saunders, 1978.

Gerlock AJ Jr , Mirfakhraee M: Computed tomography and hangman's fractures. *South Med J* 76:727, 1983.

Geweiler JA, Osborn RL, Becker FG: *The Radiology of Vertebral Trauma.* Saunders, Philadelphia, 1980.

Glickstein MF, Burke DL, Kessel HY: Magnetic resonance demonstration of hyperintense herniated discs and extruded disc fragments. *Skeletal Radiol* 18:527, 1989.

Guerra J Jr, Garfin SR, Resnick D: Vertebral burst fractures: CT analysis of the retropulsed fragment. *Radiology* 153:769, 1984.

Gumley G, Taylor TKF, Ryan MD: Distraction fractures of the lumbar spine. *J Bone Joint Surg* 64B:520, 1982.

Hadley MN, Browner C, Sonntag VKH: Axis fractures: A comprehensive review of management and treatment in 107 cases. *Neurosurgery* 17:281, 1985.

Han SY, Witten DM, Mussleman JP: Jefferson fracture of the atlas: Report of six cases. *J Neurosurg* 44:368, 1976.

Harrington PR, Tullos HS: Spondylolisthesis in children: Observations and surgical treatment. *Clin Orthop* 79:75, 1971.

Hartman JT, Kendrick I, Lorman P: Discography as an aid in evaluation for lumbar and lumbosacral fusion. *Clin Orthop* 81:77, 1971.

Haughton VM: MR imaging of the spine. *Radiology* 166:297, 1988.

Haughton VM, Eldevik OP, Magnaes B, Amundsen P: A prospective comparison of computed tomography and myelography in the diagnosis of herniated lumbar disks. *Radiology* 142:103, 1982.

Hayes CW, Conway WF, Walsh JW, Coppage L, Gervin AS: Seat belt injuries: Radiologic findings and clinical correlation. *RadioGraphics* 11:23, 1991.

Holdsworth F, Chir M: Fractures, dislocations, and fracture-dislocations of the spine. *J Bone Joint Surg* 52A:1534, 1970.

Holt EP Jr: The question of lumbar discography. *J Bone Joint Surg* 50A:720, 1968.

Hyman RA, Gorey MT: Imaging strategies for MR of the spine. *Radiol Clin North Am* 26:505, 1988.

Irstan L: Lumbar myelography with Amipaque. *Spine* 3:70, 1978.

Johansen JG, Orrison WW, Amundsen P: Lateral C1-2 puncture for cervical myelography. Part I: Report of a complication. *Radiology* 146:391, 1983.

Kaiser MC, Ramos L: *MRI of the Spine. A Guide to Clinical Applications.* Stuttgart, Thieme Verlag, 1990.

Kassel EE, Cooper PW, Rubenstein JD: Radiology of spinal trauma: Practice experience in a trauma unit. *J Can Assoc Radiol* 34:189, 1983.

Keene JS, Goletz TH, Lilleas F, Alter AJ, Sackett JF: Diagnosis of vertebral fractures: A comparison of conventional radiography, conventional tomography, and computed axial tomography. *J Bone Joint Surg* 64A:585, 1982.

Kim KS, Chen HH, Russell EJ, Rogers LF: Flexion teardrop fracture of the cervical spine: radiographic characteristics. *Am J Roentgenol* 152:319, 1989.

Kornberg M: Discography and magnetic resonance imaging of the diagnosis of lumbar disc disruption. *Spine* 14:1368, 1989.

Martel W, Seeger JF, Wicks JD, Washburn RL: Traumatic lesions of the discovertebral junction in the lumbar spine. *Am J Roentgenol* 127:457, 1976.

McKim TH: Atlantoaxial injuries. *Semin Orthop* 2:110, 1987.

Meyer GA, Haughton VM, Williams AL: Diagnosis of herniated lumbar disk with computed tomography. *N Engl J Med* 301:1166, 1979.

Mirvis SE, Young JWR, Lim C, Greenberg J: Hangman's fracture: Radiologic assessment in 27 cases. *Radiology* 163:713, 1987.

Mirvis SE, Geisler FH, Jelinek JJ, Joslyn JN, Gellad F: Acute cervical spine trauma: evaluation with 1.5T MR imaging. *Radiol* 166: 807, 1988.

Myerding HW: Spondylolisthesis. *Surg Gynecol Obstet* 34:371, 1932.

Newman PH: The etiology of spondylolisthesis. *J Bone Joint Surg* 45B:39, 1963.

Orrison WW, Eldevik OP, Sackett JF: Lateral C1-2 puncture for cervical myelography. Part III: Historical, anatomic and technical considerations. *Radiology* 146:401, 1983.

Pech P, Kilgore DP, Pojunas KW, Haughton VM: Cervical spinal fractures: CT detection. *Radiology* 157:117, 1985.

Raskin SP, Keating JW: Recognition of lumbar disk disease: Comparison of myelography and computed tomography. *AJNR* 3:215, 1982.

Rogers LF: The roentgenographic appearance of transverse or Chance fractures of the spine: The seat belt fracture. *Am J Roentgenol* 111:844, 1971.

Rogers LF, Lee C: Cervical spine trauma. In: Dalinka MK, Kaye JJ (eds): *Radiology in Emergency Room Medicine.* New York, Churchill Livingstone, 1984.

Russell EJ, D'Angelo CM, Zimmerman RD, Czervionke LF, Huckman MS: Cervical disk herniation: CT demonstration after contrast enhancement. *Radiology* 152:703, 1984.

Scher AT: Unilateral locked facet in cervical spine injuries. *Am J Roentgenol* 129:45, 1977.

Scher AT: "Tear-drop" fractures of the cervical spine: Radiologic features. *S Afr Med J* 61:355, 1982.

Schneider RC, Livingston KE, Cave AJE, Hamilton G: "Hangman's fracture" of the cervical spine. *J Neurosurg* 22:141, 1965.

Smith GR, Northrop CH, Loop JW: Jumper's fractures: Patterns of thora-columbar spine injuries associated with vertical plunges. A review of 38 cases. *Radiology* 122:657, 1977.

Turski PA, Sackett JF: Applications of computed tomography in spinal trauma. *Appl Radiol* Sept-Oct:87, 1982.

Whittley JE, Forsythe HF: Classification of cervical spine injuries. *Am J Roentgenol* 83:633, 1958.

Wiltse LL: Spondylolisthesis: Classification and etiology. In: *Symposium on the Spine.* American Academy of Orthopedic Surgery, St. Louis, Mosby, 1969, p 143.

Wiltse LL, Winter RB: Terminology and measurement of spondylolisthesis. *J Bone Joint Surg* 65A:768, 1983.

Wiltse LL, Newman PH, McNab I: Classification of spondylolysis and spondy-lolisthesis. *Clin Orthop* 117:23, 1976.

Yu S, Sether IA, Ho PSP, Wagner M, Haughton VM: Tears of the annulus fibrosus: Correlation between MR and pathologic findings in cadavers. *AJNR* 9:367, 1988.

Zanca P, Lodmell EA: Fracture of spinous process: New sign for recognition of fractures of cervical and upper dorsal spinous processes. *Radiology* 56:427, 1951.

PART III

Arthritides

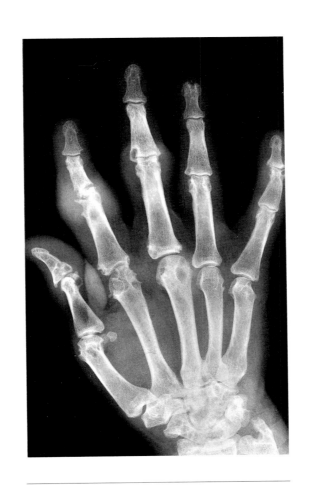

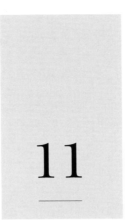

11

Radiologic Evaluation of the Arthritides

IN ITS GENERAL MEANING, the term *arthritis* indicates an abnormality of the joint as the result of a degenerative, inflammatory, infectious, or metabolic process (Fig. 11.1). Also included among the arthritides are connective tissue arthropathies, such as those associated with systemic lupus erythematosus and scleroderma.

RADIOLOGIC IMAGING MODALITIES

PLAIN-FILM RADIOGRAPHY The radiologic modalities used to evaluate arthritis are very similar to those employed in traumatic conditions involving the bones and joints (see Chapter 4), although there are some modifications. The most important modality for the evaluation of arthritis is plain-film radiography. As in the radiographic examination of traumatic conditions, standard films of the involved joint should be obtained in at least two projections at 90° to each other (Fig. 11.2; see also Fig. 4.1). A weight-bearing view may be of value, particularly for a dynamic evaluation of any decre-

ment in the joint space under the weight of the body (Fig. 11.3). Special projections may at times be required to demonstrate destructive changes in the joint to better advantages. The radial head-capitellum view (see Chapter 5), by eliminating overlap of the radial head and coronoid process and by more clearly demonstrating the humeroradial and humeroulnar joints, shows the inflammatory changes in the elbow joint to better advantage (Fig. 11.4). The semisupinated oblique view of the hand and wrist (the so-called Allstate or ball-catcher's view), introduced by Norgaard in 1965, effectively demonstrates the radial aspects of the metacarpal heads and of the base of the proximal phalanges in the hand and the triquetrum and pisiform in the wrist (Fig. 11.5). Since the earliest erosive changes of some inflammatory arthritides begin in these areas, the Norgaard view may provide important information at the early stages of arthritides (Fig. 11.6). It may also demonstrate subtle subluxations in metacarpophalangeal joints frequently seen in systemic lupus erythematosus.

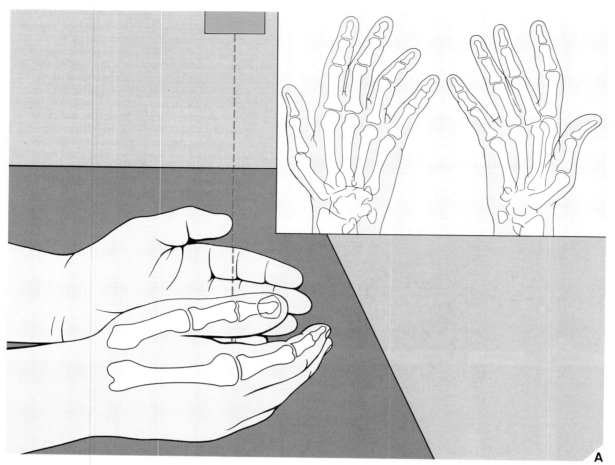

Figure 11.5 (A) For the "Allstate" Norgaard view of the hands and wrists, the patient's arm is fully extended and resting on its ulnar side. Fingers are extended. The hands are in slight pronation, as when catching a ball. The central beam is directed toward the metacarpal heads. (B) On the film in this projection, the radial aspects of the base of the proximal phalanges, the triquetrum, and pisiform bones are well demonstrated.

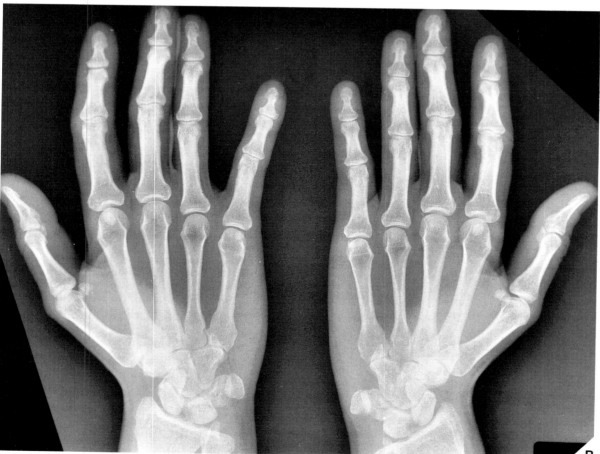

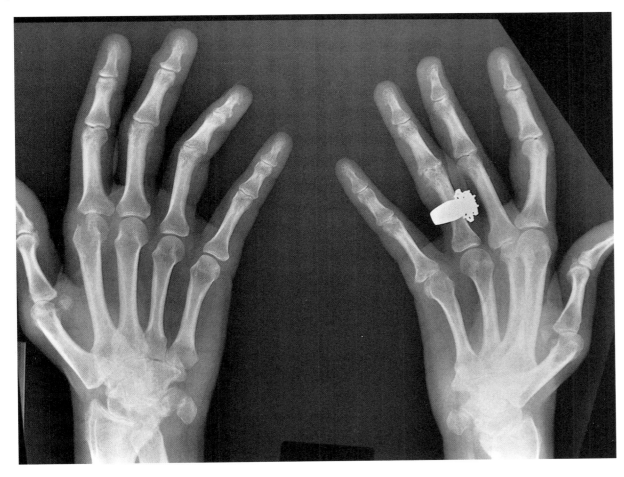

Figure 11.6 The "Allstate" view of the hands and the wrists of this 62-year-old woman with rheumatoid arthritis demonstrates erosions in the radiocarpal and intercarpal articulations as well as the carpometacarpal joint, bilaterally. Note, in addition, subtle erosions of the head of the first, third, fourth, and fifth metacarpals of the left hand, and of the head of the second metacarpal of the right hand. A small erosion at the base of the middle phalanx of the ring finger of the left hand is also well seen.

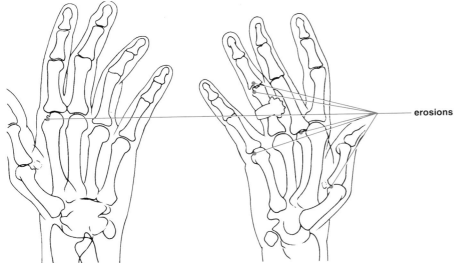

erosions

MAGNIFICATION RADIOGRAPHY This technique is used to diagnose the very early articular changes of arthritis, which are not well appreciated on standard projections (Fig. 11.7). This technique involves a special screen-film system and geometric enlargement that yields magnified images of the bones and joints with greater sharpness and bony detail.

TOMOGRAPHY, CT, AND ARTHROGRAPHY Among the ancillary imaging techniques used to evaluate the arthritides, conventional tomography is rarely employed for the purpose of making a specific diagnosis, its major purpose being rather demonstration to better advantage of the degree of joint destruction (Fig. 11.8).

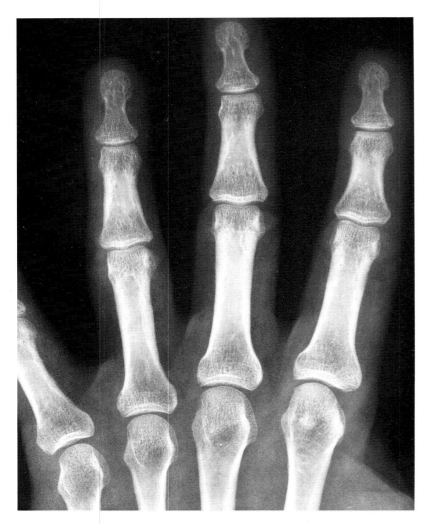

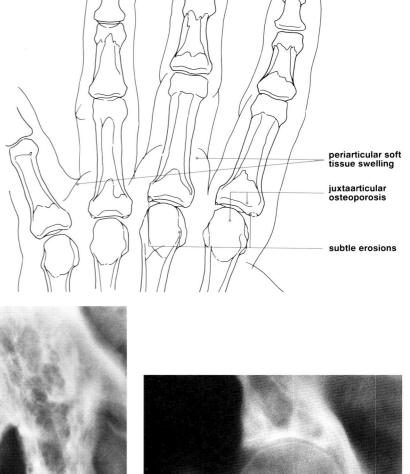

Figure 11.7 Dorsovolar view of the fingers obtained with the magnification technique demonstrates the early changes of rheumatoid arthritis: juxtaarticular osteoporosis, periarticular soft tissue swelling representing intracapsular fluid, and subtle erosions at the bases of the proximal phalanges and heads of the metacarpals—a finding not appreciated on the standard radiographs of this patient.

periarticular soft tissue swelling

juxtaarticular osteoporosis

subtle erosions

Figure 11.8 A 74-year-old woman with Paget disease and secondary degenerative changes in the hip joint was evaluated for a possible total hip arthroplasty. (A) Standard anteroposterior view of the right hip shows extensive Paget disease evident in the thickening of the cortex of the pelvic bones, particularly the ischium, and a coarse trabecular pattern. Note the narrowing of the radiographic joint space indicative of degenerative changes in the hip joint. Conventional tomograms show predominant involvement of the acetabulum (B) with preservation of the femoral head (C).

Except for its use in evaluating degenerative changes in the spine, particularly spinal stenosis, computed tomography (CT) is less commonly used than it is in trauma (Fig. 11.9). In the assessment of spinal stenosis secondary to degenerative changes, CT examination may also be performed following myelography (Fig. 11.10), although myelography alone is often sufficient (Fig. 11.11).

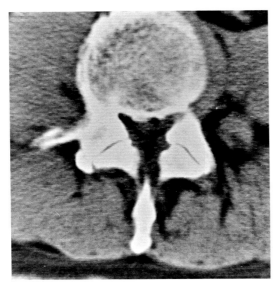

Figure 11.9 CT scan in a 66-year-old patient with advanced osteoarthritis of the facet joints shows marked narrowing of the spinal canal secondary to degenerative changes. At 8 mm, the transverse diameter is well below normal.

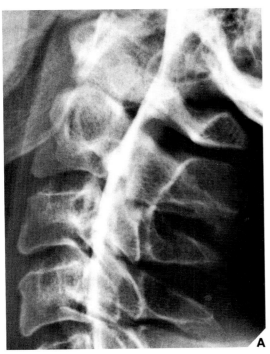

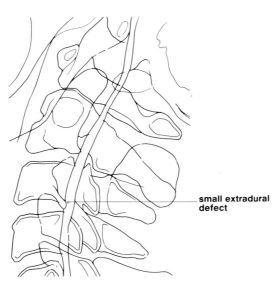

small extradural defect

A

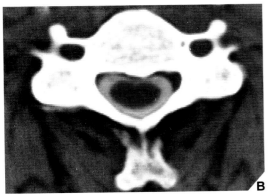

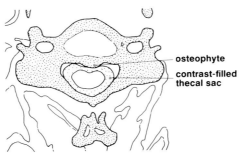

osteophyte

contrast-filled thecal sac

B

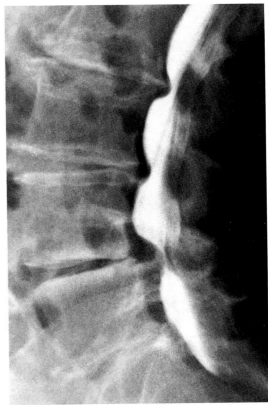

Figure 11.11 Lateral film of the lumbosacral spine obtained after injection of metrizamide into the subarachnoid space shows an "hourglass" configuration of the contrast medium in the thecal sac, a feature characteristic of spinal stenosis. This appearance results from concomitant hypertrophy of the facet joints and posterior bulging of the intervertebral disks.

Figure 11.10 A 56-year-old man complained of constant pain in the neck radiating to the left arm; there was also associated weakness and numbness in the left hand. (A) Cervical myelogram in the lateral projection shows a small extradural defect on the ventral aspect of the thecal sac at C3-4. (B) CT section obtained following myelography shows impingement of a posterior osteophyte on the thecal sac at the corresponding level.

Arthrography has some limited application in the evaluation of degenerative (Fig. 11.12), inflammatory, and infectious (see Fig. 19.17B) conditions of the joint.

SCINTIGRAPHY Radionuclide bone scan is much more commonly used than these other techniques, mainly for evaluating the distribution of arthritis in different joints (see Chapter 2). The radiopharmaceuticals currently in use in bone scan include organic diphosphonates—ethylene diphosphonate (HEPD) and methylene diphosphonate (MDP)—labeled with technetium-99m, a gamma emitter with a six hour half-life; MDP is more commonly used, typically in a dose that provides 15 mCi (555 MBq) of technetium-99m.

After intravenous injection of the radiopharmaceutical, approximately 50% of the dose localizes in bone, the remainder circulating freely in the body and eventually excreted by the kidneys. A gamma camera can then be used in a procedure known as a three-phase radionuclide bone scan. Scintigraphy can determine the distribution of arthritic changes in large and small joints (Fig. 11.13). It can also distinguish an infected joint from infected periarticular soft tissues (see Fig. 18.9).

SONOGRAPHY This technique is rarely used in evaluation of joint abnormalities. Occasionally it helps to differentiate popliteal fossa masses in patients with rheumatoid arthritis, in whom complications of

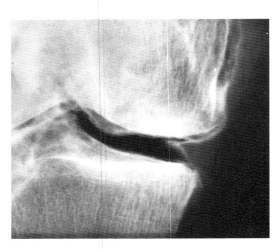

Figure 11.12 Double-contrast arthrogram in a 62-year-old man with progressive pain localized to the medial femorotibial joint compartment demonstrates advanced degeneration of the articular cartilage.

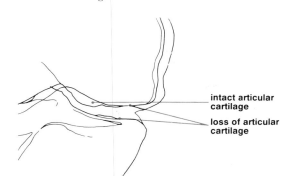

intact articular cartilage

loss of articular cartilage

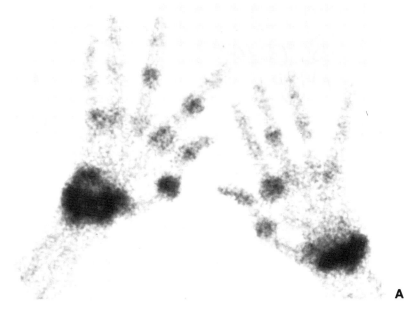

Figure 11.13 Radionuclide bone scan (A) obtained two hours after the intravenous injection of 15 mCi (555 MBq) of technetium-99m-labeled MDP shows an increased uptake of radiopharmaceutical in several joints of the hand and wrist. A plain radiograph (B) of the same patient shows advanced psoriatic arthritis.

A

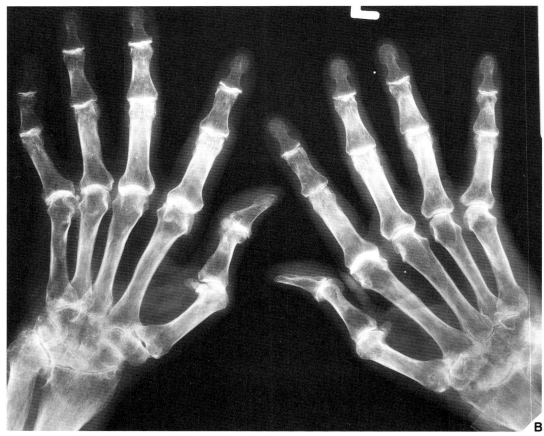

B

an arthritic process (such as popliteal cyst or hypertrophied synovium) may be distinguished from conditions not related to arthritis (such as popliteal artery aneurysm). It may also effectively diagnose deep vein thrombosis, occasionally seen in patients with rheumatoid arthritis.

MAGNETIC RESONANCE IMAGING. MRI of the joints provides excellent contrast between soft tissues and bone. Articular cartilage, fibrocartilage, cortex, and spongy bone can be distinguished from each other by their specific signal intensities. It is an excellent modality for demonstrating the rheumatoid nodules and synovial abnormalities

in patients with rheumatoid arthritis. MRI's ability to contrast the synovial-covered joint from other soft tissue structures allows for noninvasive delineation of the degree of synovial hypertrophy that accompanies synovitis, previously demonstrable only by means of arthrography or arthroscopy. Since synovitis is often accompanied by joint effusion, this too can be effectively demonstrated by MRI (Fig. 11.14). Joint fluid normally gives an intermediate signal intensity on T1-weighted images and a high signal intensity on T2-weighted images. This has proved to be helpful in diagnosing Baker cysts (Fig. 11.15). Although MRI is quite sensitive in detecting joint effusion, it

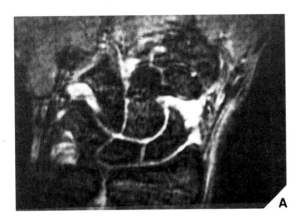
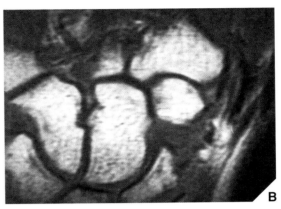

Figure 11.14 Plain film examination was normal in this patient with known rheumatoid arthritis of the wrist. MRI in the coronal plane using gradient echo technique (A) and spin echo sequence (B) demonstrates marginal scaphoid erosions with adjacent

fluid and inflammatory panus. Inflammatory fluid is also seen in the radioulnar, midcarpal, radio-carpal, and carpometacarpal joints. (From Beltran J, 1990)

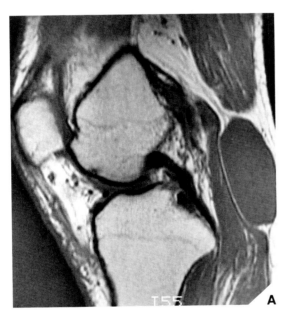
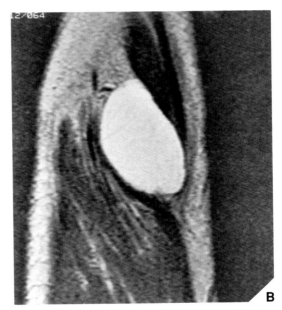

Figure 11.15 A 68-year-old woman with rheumatoid arthritis complained of pain in the region of the popliteal fossa. The presumptive diagnosis of thrombophlebitis was made. (A) Sagittal MRI (TR 900/ TE 20) demonstrates an oval structure in the popliteal fossa displaying intermediate signal inten-

sity. Also note a small subchondral erosion of the anterior aspect of the medial femoral condyle. (B) Coronal MRI (TR 1800/TE 80) at the level of the popliteal fossa demonstrates a large Baker cyst that displays a high signal intensity due to fluid content.

cannot yet distinguish between inflammatory and noninflammatory fluid. Occasionally, MRI may provide some additional information in hemophilic arthropathy (Fig. 11.16).

The most promising role of MRI, however, is in the evaluation of the spine. MR images in the sagittal plane are useful for demonstrating hypertrophy of the ligamentum flavum or the vertebral facets, grading the degree of foramina stenosis, and measuring the sagittal diameter of the spinal cord. MR images in the axial plane facilitate detailed analysis of the facet joints and more accurate measurement of the thickness of the ligamentum flavum and the diameter of the spinal canal. The quality of evaluation of spinal cord abnormalities by MRI in the cervical area in patients with rheumatoid arthritis and of spinal stenosis in patients with advanced degenerative changes of the spine surpasses that obtained with other modalities. MRI is particularly useful in examination of patients with pain related to disk disease since it can differentiate normal, degenerated, and herniated disks noninvasively (see also

Chapter 10). In fact, the changes of disk degeneration can be identified by MRI long before they can be detected by conventional radiography or CT.

THE ARTHRITIDES

Diagnosis

Clinical Information

The clinical manifestations and laboratory data, in conjunction with the radiographic findings, are of significant help in making the diagnosis of a specific arthritic process. The various arthritides, for example, have different frequencies of occurrence between the sexes. Rheumatoid arthritis is much more common in females, and erosive osteoarthritis is seen almost exclusively in middle-aged women. Psoriatic arthritis, Reiter syndrome, and gouty arthritis, on the other hand, are more common in males. Clinical symptoms are

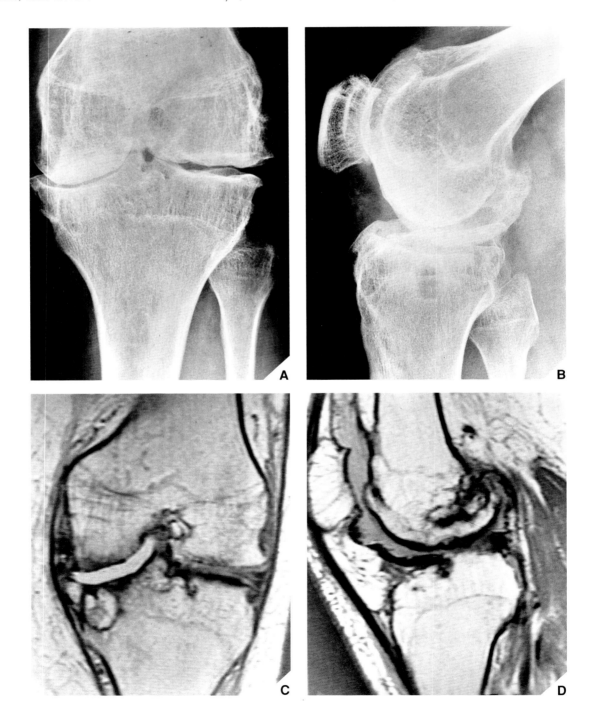

of further assistance. Patients with Reiter syndrome, for example, usually present with urethritis, conjunctivitis, and mucocutaneous lesions, and those with psoriatic arthritis may present with swelling of a single finger, the so-called "sausage digit," as well as changes in the skin and fingernails. Patients with gouty arthritis may exhibit soft tissue masses, representing chronic tophi, on the dorsal aspect of the hands or feet.

Laboratory data are also essential. Gouty arthritis, for instance, is associated with elevated serum uric acid concentrations, and a synovial fluid examination reveals monosodium urate crystals in leukocytes in the fluid. The synovial fluid of patients with pseudogout (CPPD), on the other hand, contains calcium pyrophosphate crystals. The detection of autoantibodies is another important aid in the diagnostic workup. Rheumatoid factor (RF) is a typical finding in rheumatoid arthritis. Patients lacking the specific antibodies represented by rheumatoid factor are said to have "seronegative" arthritis. Patients with lupus arthritis have a positive lupus erythematosus

(LE) cell test. Lastly, identification of the antigens of the major histocompatibility complex, particularly human leukocyte-associated antigens HLA-B27 and HLA-DR4, has in recent years become a crucial test in the diagnosis of arthritic disease. It has been reported that 95% of patients with ankylosing spondylitis, 86% of patients with Reiter syndrome, and 60% of patients with psoriatic arthropathy test positively for antigen HLA-B27, while a great majority of those with rheumatoid arthritis exhibit the HLA-DR4 antigen. This is helpful in differentiating certain types of arthritides, as well as distinguishing psoriatic arthritis from rheumatoid arthritis in cases in which the radiographic presentation of these conditions may be very similar.

Radiographic Features of the Arthritides

The true or diarthrodial joint consists of cartilage covering the articular ends of the bones forming the joint; the articular capsule, which is reinforced by ligamentous structures; and the joint space,

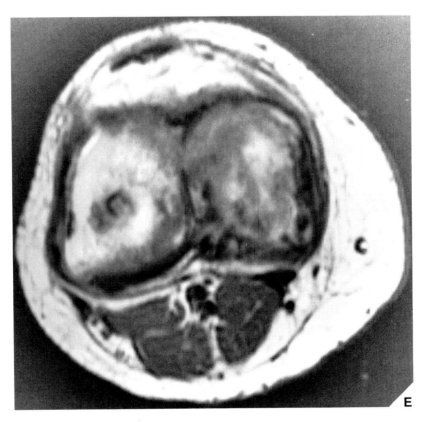

Figure 11.16 A 29-year-old male with hemophilia and multiple episodes of intra-articular bleeding. (A,B) Anteroposterior and lateral views of the knee demonstrate an advanced stage of hemophilia. Abnormalities include periarticular osteoporosis, irregularity of subchondral bone at the tibial plateau and femoral condyles, narrowing of the radiographic joint space, and erosion of the subchondral bone. (C) Coronal MRI (TR 1900/TE 20) demonstrates, in addition, complete destruction of articular cartilage at the medial joint compartment, and a large, subchondral cyst in the proximal tibia, not well appreciated on the plain films. (D) Sagittal MRI (TR 800/TE 20) demonstrates to better advantage the intra-articular blood in the suprapatellar and infrapatellar bursae, displaying intermediate signal intensity. (E) Axial MRI (TR 400/TE 20) shows erosive changes of the articular cartilage of the femoral condyles.

which is lined with synovial membrane and filled with synovial fluid (Fig. 11.17). Because of its physicochemical constitution, articular cartilage absorbs only a minimal amount of x-rays, thus appearing radiolucent on a radiographic film. The radiolucent articular cartilage, together with the joint cavity filled with synovial fluid, creates the so-called radiographic joint space.

The abnormality of the joint in arthritis usually consists of destruction of the articular cartilage, which appears on a film as a narrowing of the radiographic joint space, usually accompanied by subchondral erosion; narrowing of the joint is the cardinal sign of arthritis (Fig. 11.18). It should be kept in mind, however, that in some arthritic processes the joint space may not become narrow, appearing instead slightly expanded. This happens, for example, in the early stages of some arthritides, when joint effusion and ligamentous laxity cause distention of the joint with fluid, but the articular cartilage has not yet been destroyed. It may also be seen in rare instances when granulation pannus erodes the subchondral bone without destroying the articular cartilage (Fig. 11.19).

Other radiographic signs specific to different types of arthritis include periarticular soft tissue swelling, periarticular osteoporosis, and, in the more advanced stages of some arthritides, complete destruction of the joint with subluxation or dislocation and ankylosis (joint fusion) (Fig. 11.20).

The radiographic presentation of arthritis depends on the type and stage of the disease, as well as the site of the original insult characteristic for the various forms of arthritis (Fig. 11.21)—whether it is the articular cartilage, as in osteoarthritis (see Figs. 11.2, 11.25); the synovial membrane, as in inflammatory arthritis (Fig. 11.22A); the synovial membrane, subchondral bone, and periarticular soft tissues, as in infectious arthritis (see Fig. 19.17); or the synovial membrane, articular cartilage, subchondral bone, and periarticular soft tissues as in some metabolic arthritides (Fig. 11.22 B,C).

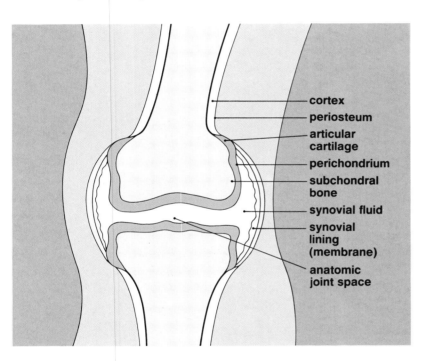

Figure 11.17 The constituent structures of a true or diarthrodial joint.

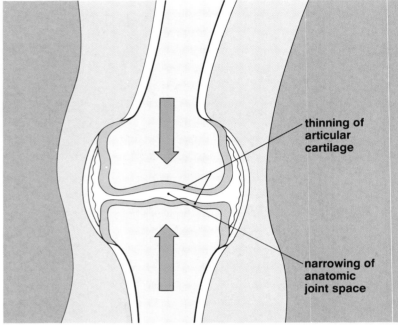

Figure 11.18 The cardinal sign of an arthritic process is narrowing of the radiographic joint space. Thinning of the articular cartilage reduces the space mechanically.

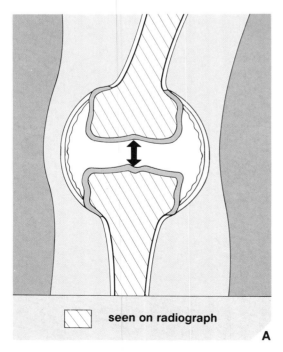

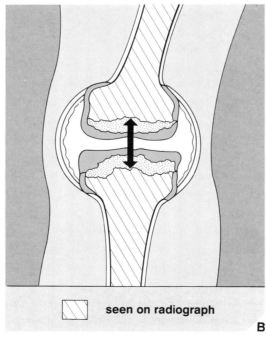

Figure 11.19 In the early stage of some arthritides, widening rather than narrowing of the joint space may be seen radiographically. This may be due to distention of the joint with fluid (A) or erosion of the subchondral bone by granulation pannus with some preservation of the articular cartilage (B).

The radiographic diagnosis of arthritis, as Resnick observed, is based on the evaluation of two fundamental parameters: the *morphology* of the articular lesion and its *distribution* in the skeleton. If these findings are combined with the history, physical examination, and relevant laboratory data in a given case, the accuracy of the diagnosis is markedly improved.

MORPHOLOGY OF THE ARTICULAR LESION The various arthritides exhibit morphologically distinct features, as observed radiographically in the large (Fig. 11.23) and small (Fig. 11.24) joints. In the degenerative form of the disease known as osteoarthritis, thinning of the articular cartilage results in localized narrowing of the joint space; there is also subchondral sclerosis and osteophyte and cyst formation, but generally osteoporosis is absent (Fig. 11.25). Inflammatory arthritides, such as rheumatoid arthritis, are characterized by a diffuse, usually multicompartmental narrowing of the joint space associated with marginal or central erosions, periarticu-

lar osteoporosis, and symmetric periarticular soft tissue swelling; subchondral sclerosis is minimal or absent and formation of osteophytes is lacking (Fig. 11.26). In a metabolic arthritis such as gout, well defined bony erosions displaying a so-called overhanging edge are usually associated with preservation of part of the joint space and a localized, asymmetric soft tissue mass; osteophyte formation and osteoporosis are absent (Fig. 11.27). Infectious arthritis is characterized by the complete destruction of both articular ends of the bones forming the joint; all communicating joint compartments are invariably involved, with diffuse osteoporosis, joint effusion, and periarticular soft tissue swelling (see Fig. 19.16). Neuropathic arthritis is marked by destruction of the articular surfaces, which leaves bony debris, and a substantial joint effusion; osteoporosis is usually lacking. Depending on the amount of destruction, varying degrees of joint instability are present (Fig. 11.28).

Analysis of the morphologic features of an arthritic lesion at certain sites other than the diarthrodial joints may be of further

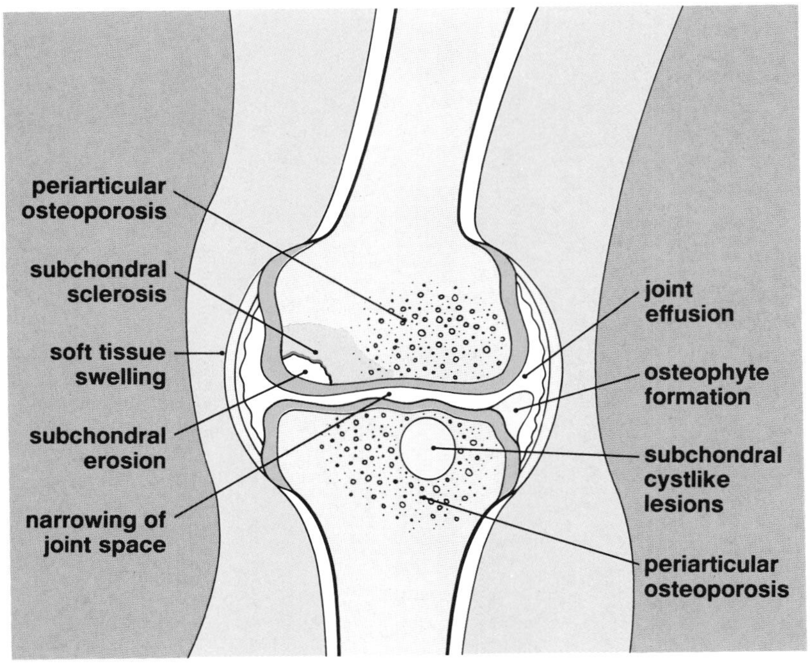

Figure 11.20 Summary representation of radiographic features seen in the arthritides. Not all of these features are seen in every type of arthritis.

Figure 11.21 Target sites of various arthritides in a joint.

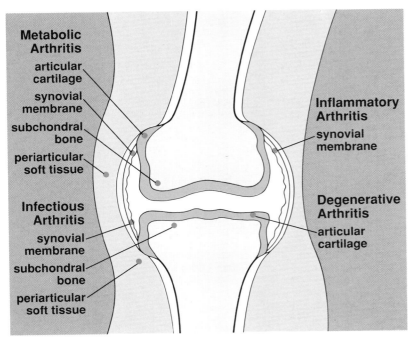

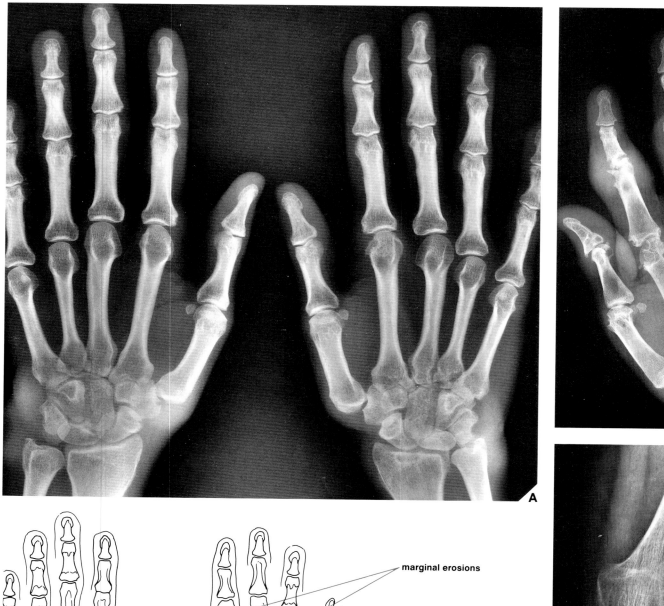

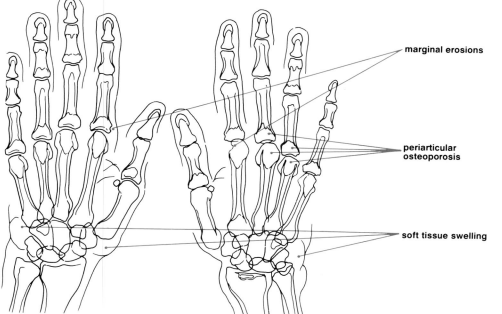

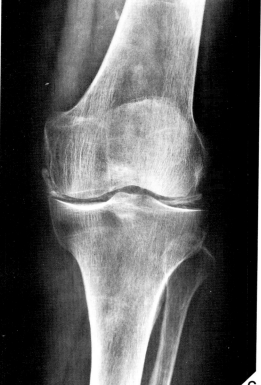

Figure 11.22 (A) Early changes of rheumatoid arthritis, as seen in the hands of a 40-year-old woman, present as marginal erosions in so-called bare areas at the locus of attachment of the capsular synovial lining. Also note the periarticular osteoporosis and soft tissue swelling, particularly in both wrists. (B) The asymmetric marginal erosions affecting various articulations in the hand of a 38-year-old man with tophaceous gout are characteristic of a metabolic process involving the subchondral bone. Note the preservation of part of the joint and the location of several erosions at some distance from the joint space. (C) In CPPD crystal deposition arthropathy, seen here in the knee of a 70-year-old woman, there is calcification of the fibrocartilage (semilunar cartilage or menisci) and hyaline cartilage (articular cartilage) in association with narrowing of the medial femorotibial joint compartment. Aspirated fluid from the knee joint yielded calcium pyrophosphate dihydrate crystals.

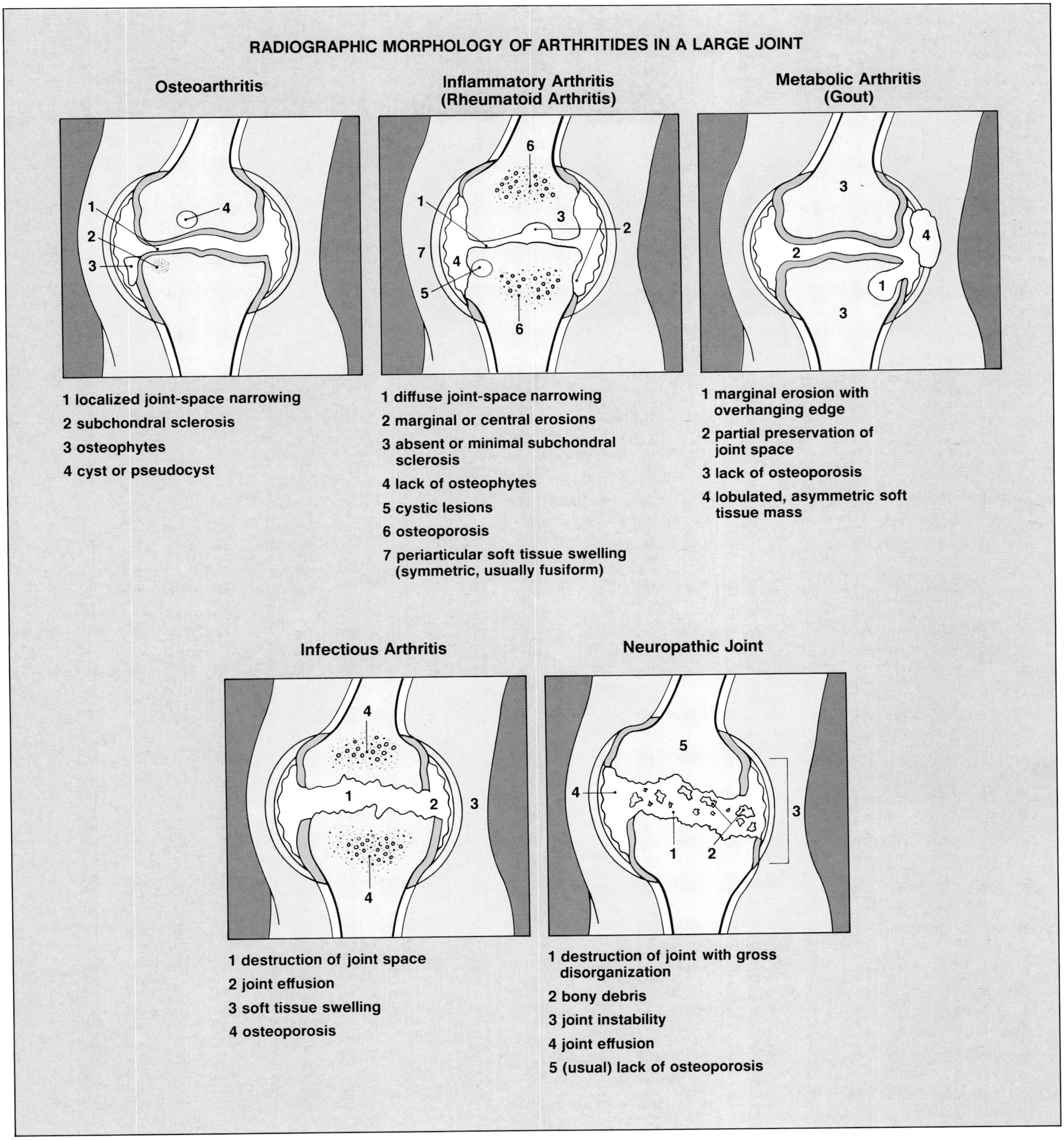

RADIOGRAPHIC MORPHOLOGY OF ARTHRITIDES IN A LARGE JOINT

Osteoarthritis

1 localized joint-space narrowing

2 subchondral sclerosis

3 osteophytes

4 cyst or pseudocyst

Inflammatory Arthritis (Rheumatoid Arthritis)

1 diffuse joint-space narrowing

2 marginal or central erosions

3 absent or minimal subchondral sclerosis

4 lack of osteophytes

5 cystic lesions

6 osteoporosis

7 periarticular soft tissue swelling (symmetric, usually fusiform)

Metabolic Arthritis (Gout)

1 marginal erosion with overhanging edge

2 partial preservation of joint space

3 lack of osteoporosis

4 lobulated, asymmetric soft tissue mass

Infectious Arthritis

1 destruction of joint space

2 joint effusion

3 soft tissue swelling

4 osteoporosis

Neuropathic Joint

1 destruction of joint with gross disorganization

2 bony debris

3 joint instability

4 joint effusion

5 (usual) lack of osteoporosis

Figure 11.23 Morphologic features distinguishing the various arthritides in a large joint.

RADIOGRAPHIC MORPHOLOGY OF ARTHRITIDES IN THE HAND

Osteoarthritis

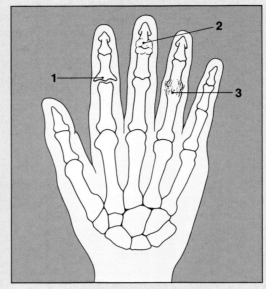

1 Heberden nodes
2 Bouchard nodes
3 joint space narrowing
4 subchondral sclerosis

Erosive Osteoarthritis

1 gull-wing erosion
2 Heberden nodes (occasionally)
3 interphalangeal ankylosis

Rheumatoid Arthritis

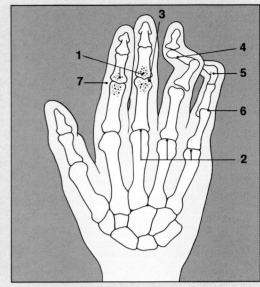

1 periarticular osteoporosis
2 joint space narrowing
3 marginal erosions
4 boutonniére deformity
5 swan-neck deformity
6 subluxations and dislocations
7 soft tissue swelling (symmetric, fusiform)

Gouty Arthritis

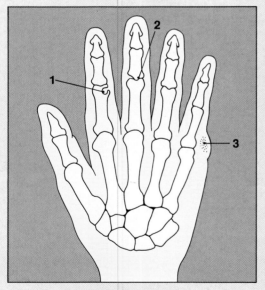

1 asymmetric erosion with
  overhanging edge
2 partial preservation of joint space
3 asymmetric soft tissue swelling with
  or without calcifications (tophus)
  (usually at dorsal aspect)

Psoriatic Arthritis

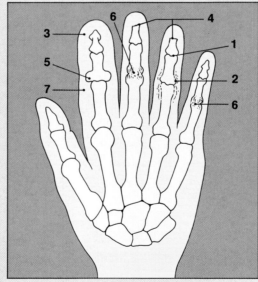

1 joint space narrowing
2 fluffy periostitis
3 "sausage digit" (soft tissue
  swelling of single digit)
4 erosion of terminal tufts
5 "mouse-ear" type of articular erosion
6 interphalangeal ankylosis
7 soft tissue swelling

Lupus Arthritis

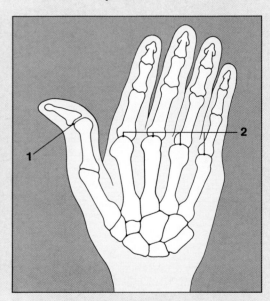

1 hitchhiker's thumb deformity
2 flexible deformities
  (subluxations)

Figure 11.24 Morphologic features distinguishing the various arthritides in the small joints of the hand.

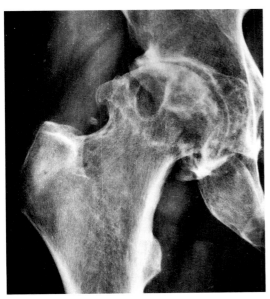

Figure 11.25 Plain radiograph of the hip demonstrates the typical morphologic changes seen in degenerative joint disease: segmented narrowing of the joint space (here at the weight-bearing segment), subchondral sclerosis, cyst-like lesions, and marginal osteophytes. Note the lack of osteoporosis.

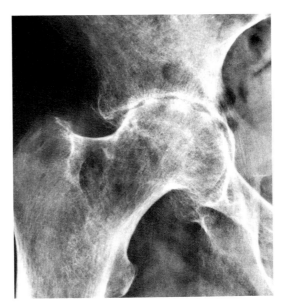

Figure 11.26 Inflammatory arthritis, seen here in the hip, is marked by diffuse, uniform narrowing of the joint space, marginal and central subchondral erosions, and severe periarticular osteoporosis. Note the almost total absence of reactive subchondral sclerosis and the lack of osteophyte formation.

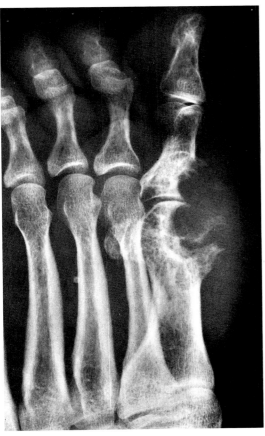

Figure 11.27 Asymmetric periarticular erosions that spare part of the joint are typical of gouty arthritis, seen here involving the first metatarsophalangeal joint of the right foot. Note the characteristic overhanging edge at the site of erosion and the soft tissue mass representing a tophus; osteophytes and osteoporosis are absent.

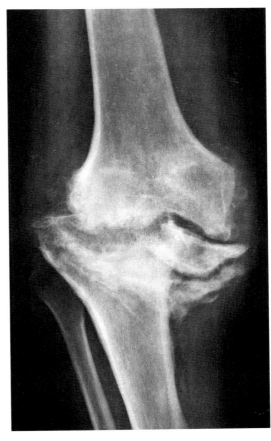

Figure 11.28 The neuropathic joint is morphologically identified by gross articular disorganization, multiple bony debris, and joint effusion, as seen here in the knee. Note the lack of osteoporosis. The amount of destruction evident in this case results in severe joint instability.

assistance in differentiating the various arthritides and reaching a correct diagnosis. Two such sites that are frequently affected are the heel (Fig. 11.29) and the spine (see Fig. 11.31). In the heel, degenerative changes are usually manifested by a traction osteophyte at the posterior and plantar aspects of the os calcis (Fig. 11.30A). Rheumatoid arthritis produces erosive changes in the area of the retrocalcaneal bursa sec-

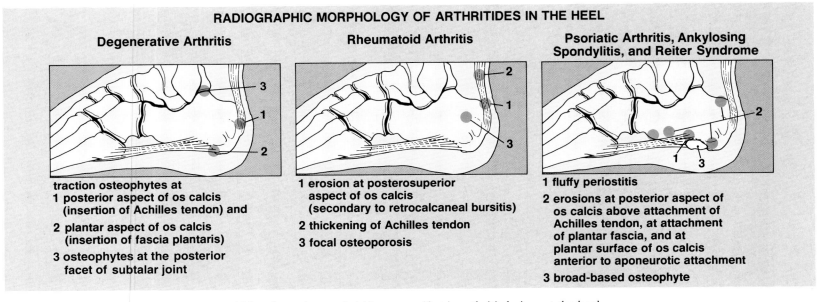

RADIOGRAPHIC MORPHOLOGY OF ARTHRITIDES IN THE HEEL

Degenerative Arthritis

traction osteophytes at
1 posterior aspect of os calcis (insertion of Achilles tendon) and
2 plantar aspect of os calcis (insertion of fascia plantaris)
3 osteophytes at the posterior facet of subtalar joint

Rheumatoid Arthritis

1 erosion at posterosuperior aspect of os calcis (secondary to retrocalcaneal bursitis)
2 thickening of Achilles tendon
3 focal osteoporosis

Psoriatic Arthritis, Ankylosing Spondylitis, and Reiter Syndrome

1 fluffy periostitis
2 erosions at posterior aspect of os calcis above attachment of Achilles tendon, at attachment of plantar fascia, and at plantar surface of os calcis anterior to aponeurotic attachment
3 broad-based osteophyte

Figure 11.29 Morphologic features distinguishing the various arthritides as manifest in arthritic lesions at the heel.

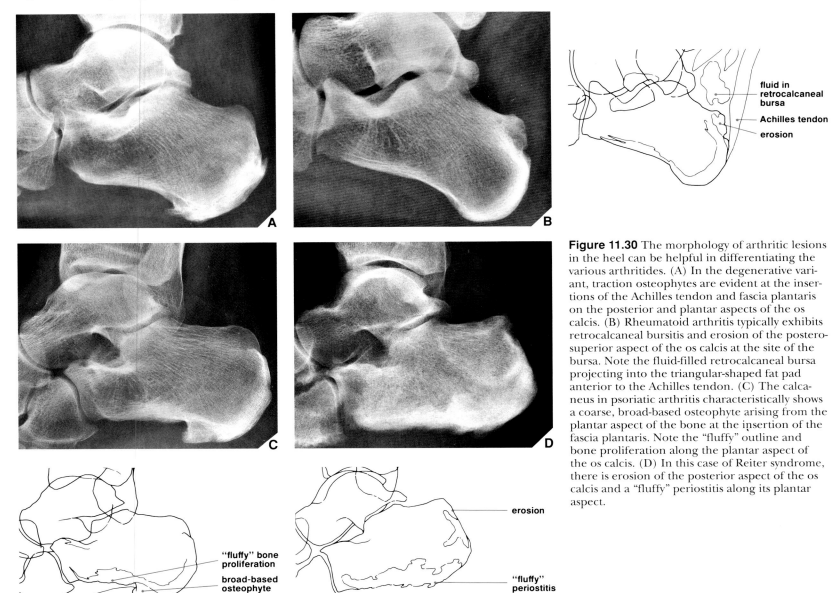

Figure 11.30 The morphology of arthritic lesions in the heel can be helpful in differentiating the various arthritides. (A) In the degenerative variant, traction osteophytes are evident at the insertions of the Achilles tendon and fascia plantaris on the posterior and plantar aspects of the os calcis. (B) Rheumatoid arthritis typically exhibits retrocalcaneal bursitis and erosion of the posterosuperior aspect of the os calcis at the site of the bursa. Note the fluid-filled retrocalcaneal bursa projecting into the triangular-shaped fat pad anterior to the Achilles tendon. (C) The calcaneus in psoriatic arthritis characteristically shows a coarse, broad-based osteophyte arising from the plantar aspect of the bone at the insertion of the fascia plantaris. Note the "fluffy" outline and bone proliferation along the plantar aspect of the os calcis. (D) In this case of Reiter syndrome, there is erosion of the posterior aspect of the os calcis and a "fluffy" periostitis along its plantar aspect.

ondary to inflammatory rheumatoid bursitis (Fig. 11.30B). Psoriatic arthritis (Fig. 11.30C), Reiter syndrome (Fig. 11.30D), and ankylosing spondylitis all produce a characteristic "fluffy" periostitis that results in a broad-based osteophyte at the site of attachment of the fascia plantaris on the plantar aspect of the os calcis, associated with erosions of the plantar surface and the posterior aspect of the calcaneus.

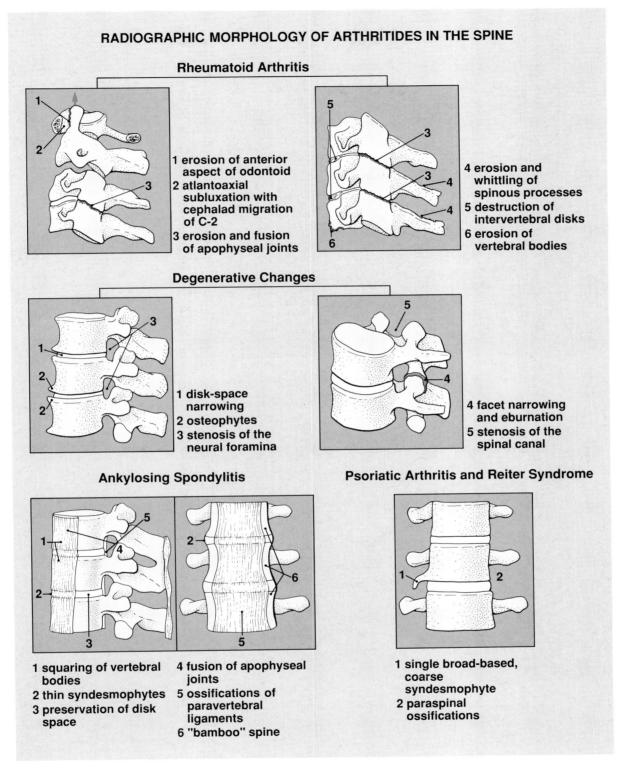

Figure 11.31 Morphologic features distinguishing the various arthritides as manifested in the spine.

Similarly, the morphology of arthritic lesions in the spine offers important indications of the disease process at work (Fig. 11.31). Among the inflammatory arthritides, for instance, rheumatoid arthritis causes a characteristic erosion of the odontoid process (Fig. 11.32). Moreover, as a result of inflammatory pannus and erosion of the transverse ligament between the anterior arch of the atlas and C-2, there may be subluxation in the atlantoaxial joint. This is usually manifested by an increase to more than 3 mm in the distance between the arch of the atlas and the dens, as demonstrated on a lateral view of the cervical spine in flexion (Fig. 11.33). Erosion of the apophyseal joints of the cervical spine, sometimes leading to fusion, is frequently seen in juvenile rheumatoid arthritis (Fig. 11.34).

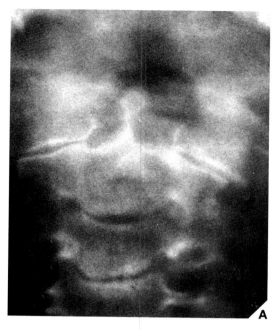
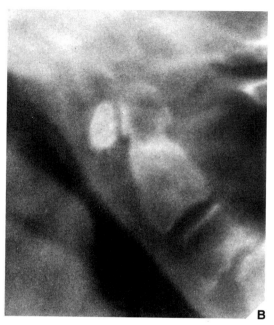

Figure 11.32 Anteroposterior (A) and lateral (B) trispiral tomograms of the cervical spine in a 55-year-old woman with a 15-year history of rheumatoid arthritis show erosion of the odontoid process typical for this condition.

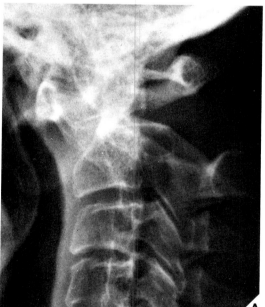
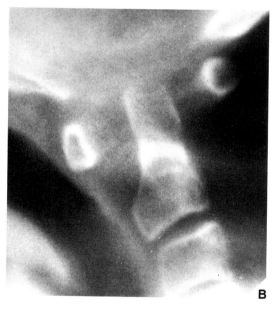

Figure 11.33 (A) Lateral film of the cervical spine in flexion in a 68-year-old woman with a long history of rheumatoid arthritis shows a marked increase in the distance between the anterior arch of the atlas and the odontoid process, measuring 12 mm; normally, it should not exceed 3 mm. (B) Trispiral tomogram demonstrates the atlantoaxial subluxation in detail.

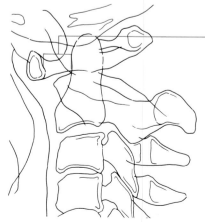

increased
distance
between
anterior
arch of atlas
and odontoid

Arthritic lesions involving other segments of the spine also exhibit distinguishing features that help in differentiating the disease process. Degenerative changes may manifest in the cervical, thoracic, or lumbar (Fig. 11.35) spine by the appearance of marginal osteophytes, narrowing and sclerosis of the apophyseal joints, and narrowing of the disk spaces. In ankylosing spondylitis, there is a characteristic "squaring" of the vertebral bodies, with the formation of delicate syndesmophytes, which differ morphologically from degenerative osteophytes, arising from the anterior aspects of the vertebral bodies. In the later stages of this condition, inflammation and fusion of the apophyseal joints lead to the appearance of what has been called "bamboo" spine; the sacroiliac joints are also

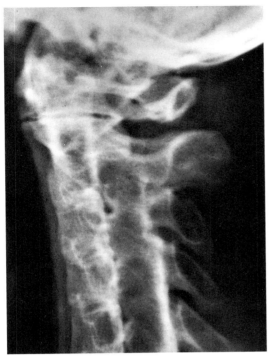

Figure 11.34 Lateral view of the cervical spine in a 34-year-old woman with juvenile rheumatoid arthritis since age 20 shows the typical involvement of the apophyseal joints. In this case, there is complete fusion of the joints.

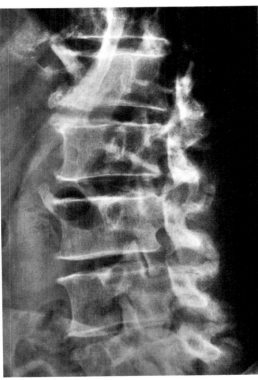

Figure 11.35 Oblique view of the lumbar spine in a 72-year-old woman shows narrowing and eburnation of the articular margins of the facet joints, osteophytosis, and narrowing of the intervertebral disk spaces—a combination of the effects of true facet joint arthritis, spondylosis deformans, and degenerative disk disease.

invariably affected (Fig. 11.36). In psoriasis and Reiter syndrome, one can occasionally see a single, coarse osteophyte in the lumbar spine, frequently bridging adjacent vertebral bodies, as well as paravertebral ossifications; there are also associated inflammatory changes in the sacroiliac joints (Fig. 11.37).

DISTRIBUTION OF THE ARTICULAR LESION Osteoarthritis tends to have a characteristic distribution in the skeletal system. Typically, the large joints such as the hip and knee and the small joints of the hand and wrist are involved, while the shoulder, elbow, and ankle are spared (Fig. 11.38). Inflammatory arthritides, on the other hand, have

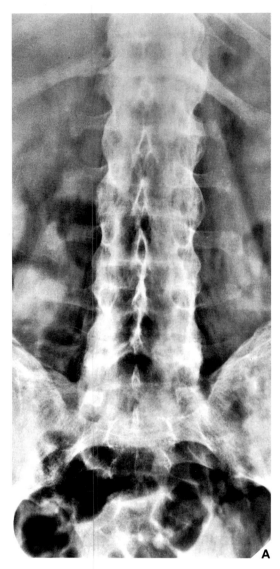
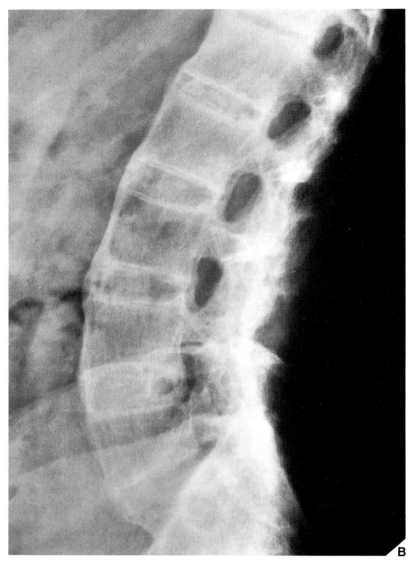

Figure 11.36 Antero-posterior (A) and lateral (B) radiographs of the lumbar spine in a 31-year-old man with advanced ankylosing spondylitis demonstrate the typical appearance of "bamboo spine" secondary to inflammation, ossification, and fusion of the apophyseal joints associated with ossification of the anterior and posterior longitudinal ligaments, as well as the supraspinous and interspinous ligaments. Note also the fusion of the sacroiliac joints.

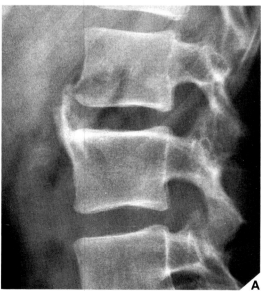
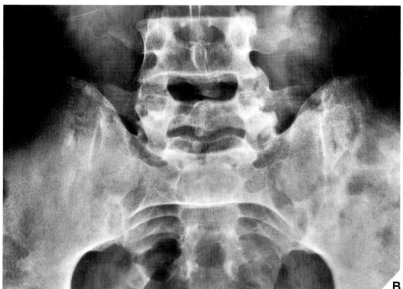

Figure 11.37 Lateral view (A) of the lumbar spine in a 27-year-old man shows a single, coarse osteophyte bridging the bodies of L-1 and L-2. Antero-posterior view (B) of the lumbosacral segment shows the effects of the inflammatory process on the sacroiliac joints.

different sites of predilection in the skeleton, depending on the specific variant of the disease. Rheumatoid arthritis, for example, involves most of the large joints such as the hip, knee, elbows, and shoulders. In the hand, it has a characteristic distribution that spares the distal interphalangeal joints (see Fig. 11.38), and in the cervical spine, the C1-2 articulation and the apophyseal joints are frequently affected. Juvenile rheumatoid arthritis has a similar pattern of distribution, except that the distal interphalangeal joints of the hand may also be affected. Psoriatic arthritis, in contrast to rheumatoid arthritis, has a predilection for the distal interphalangeal joints, as well as the sacroiliac joints, resembling Reiter syndrome in this respect (see Fig. 11.38). Erosive osteoarthritis, which some investigators consider a variant of osteoarthritis, others a variant of rheumatoid arthritis, and still others a distinct form of arthritis, has a tendency to affect the proximal and distal interphalangeal joints of the hand (see Fig. 11.24).

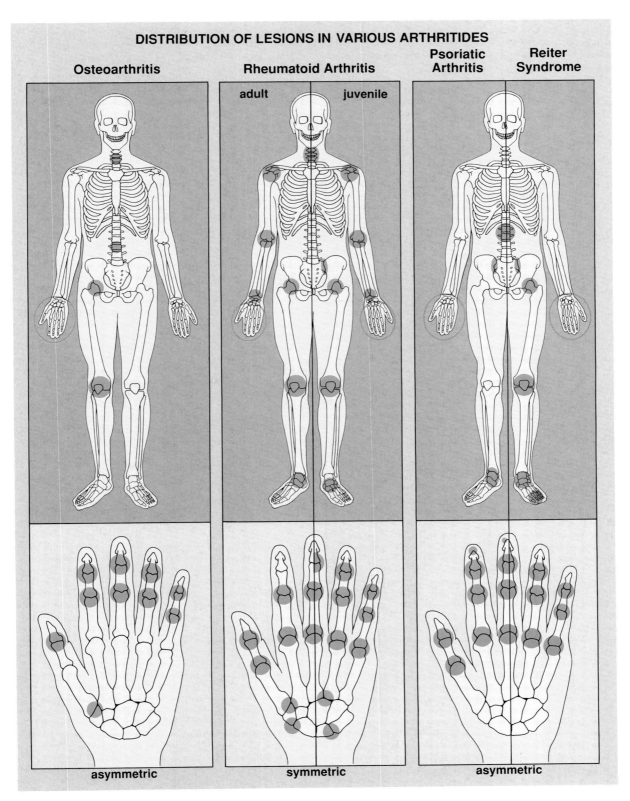

Figure 11.38 Distribution of arthritic lesions in the skeleton in various arthritides.

Management

Monitoring the Results of Treatment

Similar modalities are used for monitoring the results of medical and surgical treatment of arthritis. Since the most effective treatment, particularly when large joints are involved, entails corrective and reconstructive procedures such as femoral or tibial osteotomy or total joint replacement of the hip or knee, the surgeon follows the postsurgical progress of the patient with sequential radiographic examinations. In osteoarthritis of the hip, the corrective procedures most often performed are varus or valgus osteotomies of the proximal femur, to improve the congruence of the articular surfaces and redistribute the stress forces over different areas of the joint. Similarly, a high tibial osteotomy is done to correct severe varus or valgus deformities in osteoarthritis of the knee, particularly in cases of unicompartmental involvement. The radiographic techniques used in monitoring the outcome of these procedures, which in fact represent iatrogenic surgical fractures, are similar to those used in evaluating traumatic fractures. And as in traumatic fractures, the radiologist also pays attention to similar features, such as bone union, nonunion, or delayed union (see Chapter 4). In elderly patients, in whom total hip or total knee arthroplasties are common, radiographic scrutiny is also essential. After total hip replacement, for instance, it is important to evaluate the position of the prosthesis, with particular reference to the degree of inclination of the acetabular component, the position of the stem of the prosthesis (whether it is in valgus, varus, or the neutral position), and the status of the separated and rejoined greater trochanter, among other features (Fig. 11.39). After a total knee arthroplasty with a condylar type of prosthesis, it is important to evaluate the position of the tibial component relative to the tibial shaft, as well as the axial alignment and the status of the methylmethacrylate fixation of the components (Fig. 11.40).

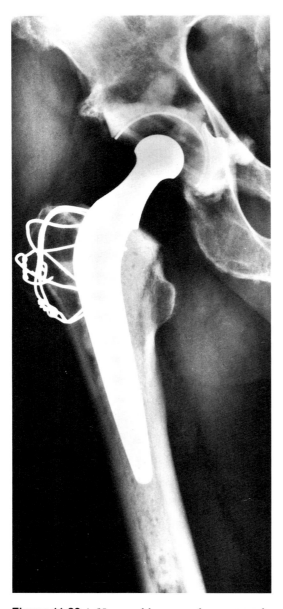

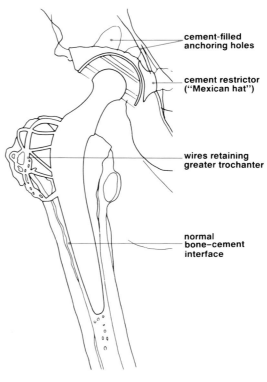

cement-filled anchoring holes

cement restrictor ("Mexican hat")

wires retaining greater trochanter

normal bone–cement interface

Figure 11.39 A 69-year-old man underwent total hip replacement because of advanced degenerative joint disease; a Charnley low-friction arthroplasty was performed. On the anteroposterior view of the right hip, one can evaluate all of the parts of the prosthesis. Note that the acetabular component is oriented about 45° to the horizontal plane and is cemented to the bone with methylmethacrylate previously impregnated with barium sulfate to make it visible radiographically. A wire-mesh cement restrictor ("Mexican hat") prevents significant leakage of methylmethacrylate into the pelvis. The stem of the prosthesis is in the neutral position in the medullary canal of the femur. Note the extent of cement below the distal end of the prosthesis, for secure anchoring. The greater trochanter, which was osteotomized to facilitate exposure of the joint, has been reattached by metallic wires slightly distal and lateral for improved stability. Note the normal appearance of the bone-cement interface.

Complications of Surgical Treatment

As important as evaluating the outcome of the surgical treatment of arthritic disease is monitoring the complications that may arise from such treatment, especially those following osteotomies and joint-replacement procedures. These complications include thrombophlebitis, hematomas, heterotopic bone formation, the intrapelvic leakage of acrylic cement, infection, loosening, subluxation or dislocation of a prosthesis, and fracture of a prosthesis.

THROMBOPHLEBITIS A rather frequent complication in the immediate postoperative period, particularly in patients with previous circulatory problems, thrombophlebitis is related to venous stasis and the lack of movement of the surgically treated extremity; sudden pain and swelling of the leg are common clinical findings. The venous soleal plexus in the calf is the most common site of thrombus forma-tion. Radiologically, this complication can be detected by venography, radionuclide scanning, or sonography. On radionuclide scan, an increased gamma-count rate in an area of the lower extremities following intravenous administration of ^{125}I-labeled fibrinogen suggests adherence of the tracer to a developing clot. Sonography can detect venous thrombosis using "compression ultrasound." Lack of compressibility of a vein is thought to be the single most reliable finding in differentiating between thrombosed and normal veins. Other criteria useful in detection of vein thrombosis are the presence of echogenic intraluminal material and enlargement of the vein.

HEMATOMA The formation of a hematoma is a common complication of surgery for arthritic disease. However, it usually subsides within a short time, unless it is associated with infection. This complication can be easily detected with MRI.

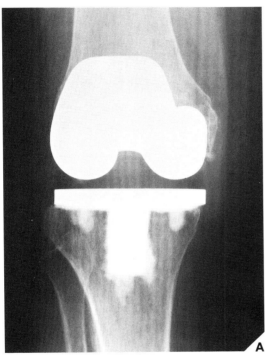

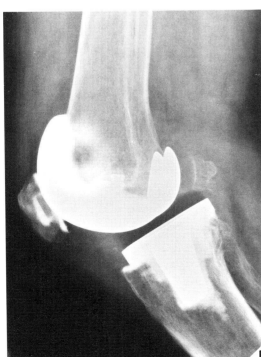

Figure 11.40 A 62-year-old woman underwent total knee arthroplasty using a semiconstrained, cemented condylar prosthesis. (A) Anteroposterior view demonstrates that the tibial component is aligned with the surface of the bone, forming a 90° angle with the long axis of the tibia. There is no evidence of a radiolucent line at the cement-bone interface. The slight valgus configuration at the knee (about 7°) is acceptable. On the lateral projection (B), note the tight adherence of the femoral component of the prosthesis to the bone.

LEAKAGE OF ACRYLIC CEMENT Intrapelvic leakage of methylmethacrylate may lead to vascular and neurologic damage, visceral necrosis, and urinary tract disorders, as a result of the heat of polymerization of the acrylic cement. To prevent an accidental leak, a wire mesh restrictor ("Mexican hat") is applied around the acetabular anchoring holes of the prosthesis (see Fig. 11.39).

HETEROTOPIC BONE FORMATION This is a relatively frequent complication of surgery for arthritic disease in the hip. The amount of new bone that forms in the adjacent soft tissues varies; if extensive, it may interfere with function of the hip joint. Plain film radiography and occasionally CT is sufficient to evaluate this complication.

INFECTION Although infection may occur at any time postoperatively, it is usually observed shortly after the joint-replacement procedure. Clinically, it is manifested by pain, elevation of temperature, and discharge from the wound. The radiographic findings in cases of infection include soft tissue swelling, rarefaction of bone, and, occasionally, a periosteal reaction. Scintigraphy using indium-111-oxine-labeled white blood cells has been reported to be very useful in these circumstances.

LOOSENING OF A PROSTHESIS Infection following a joint-replacement procedure may result in loosening of a prosthesis, but loosening may also be seen as a late complication resulting from mechanical factors. The standard radiographic projections are usually sufficient to reveal this development (Fig. 11.41). The most effective technique for demonstrating loosening of a prosthesis, however, is arthrography. The subtraction technique is commonly used to demonstrate the cardinal sign of loosening—the extension of contrast medium into the gap that develops at the interface of the bone and acrylic cement (Fig. 11.42). At times, when even arthrography is inconclusive, traction applied on the examined hip by pulling on the leg can be helpful in demonstrating occult loosening of a prosthesis. A radionuclide bone scan may

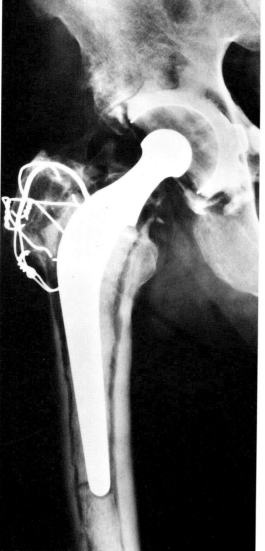

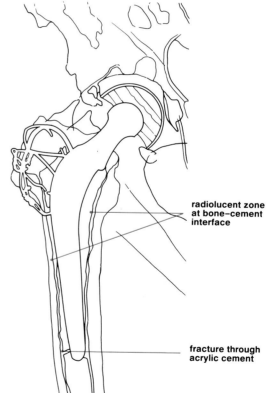

Figure 11.41 Anteroposterior view of the right hip of a 69-year-old woman shows a wide radiolucent zone at the bone-cement interface characteristic of loosening of a Charnley prosthesis. Note the fracture through the acrylic cement at the distal segment of the prosthetic stem.

radiolucent zone
at bone–cement
interface

fracture through
acrylic cement

occasionally be helpful in differentiating mechanical loosening from infectious loosening. Foci of increased activity, representing accumulation of radioisotope, are consistent with mechanical loosening, while diffuse increased activity indicates infection.

DISLOCATION OF A PROSTHESIS This complication is easily diagnosed on the lateral view of the knee or anteroposterior view of the hip. Tomography may occasionally be required, particularly if there are difficulties in reducing a dislocation (Fig. 11.43).

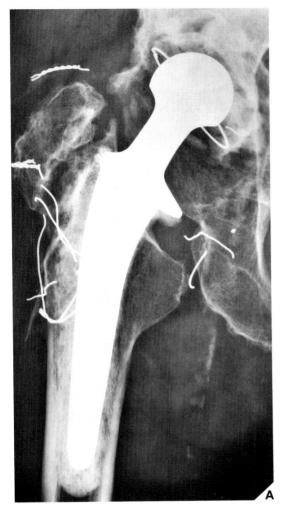

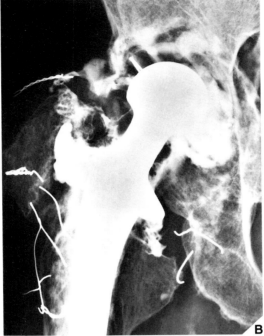

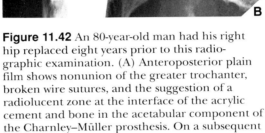

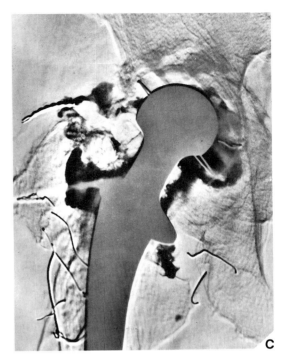

Figure 11.42 An 80-year-old man had his right hip replaced eight years prior to this radiographic examination. (A) Anteroposterior plain film shows nonunion of the greater trochanter, broken wire sutures, and the suggestion of a radiolucent zone at the interface of the acrylic cement and bone in the acetabular component of the Charnley–Müller prosthesis. On a subsequent arthrogram (B) and a subtraction-enhanced film (C), loosening of the prosthesis is clearly evident from the contrast medium seen entering the bone–cement gap and leaking medial and lateral to the neck of the prosthesis; the gap between the femur and separated greater trochanter is also opacified.

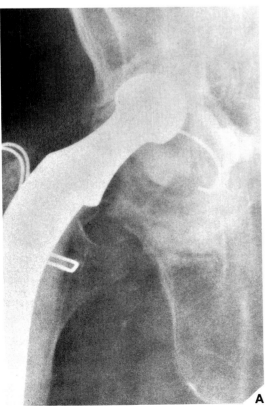

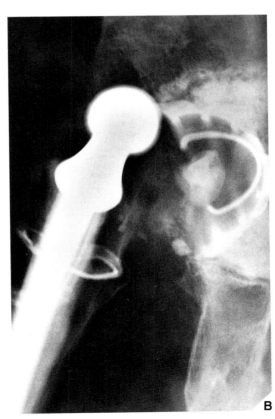

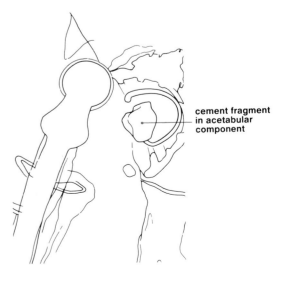

cement fragment in acetabular component

Figure 11.43 A 77-year-old man had had a Charnley low-friction arthroplasty ten years previously for osteoarthritis of the right hip. Recently, he fell and dislocated the prosthesis, as shown on this anteroposterior view (A). Several attempts to reduce the dislocation, even under anesthesia, failed. (B) Tomographic cut demonstrates a small fragment of cement in the acetabular component of the prosthesis, which blocked reduction of the dislocation.

PRACTICAL POINTS TO REMEMBER

[1] The radiographic hallmarks of an arthritic process regardless of etiology are:
- narrowing of the joint space
- bony erosion of various forms depending on the specific type of arthritis.

[2] The most important radiologic imaging modality for evaluating arthritis is plain-film radiography. Ancillary techniques, in order of their frequency of use, include:
- radionuclide bone scan
- magnification radiography
- magnetic resonance imaging
- arthrography
- computed tomography.

[3] Radionuclide imaging is an effective technique for:
- determining the skeletal distribution of arthritic changes
- differentiating arthritis from periarticular soft tissue infection
- monitoring the various complications of joint-replacement surgery.

[4] The radiographic diagnosis of arthritis is based on:
- the morphology of an articular lesion
- its distribution in the skeleton.

[5] The morphologic changes characteristic of different arthritides can be effectively analyzed in several important anatomic sites, including the hand, heel, and spine. These changes, together with the characteristic distribution of lesions in the skeleton and the clinical and laboratory data in a given case, facilitate arriving at a specific diagnosis.

[6] In the hand, the various arthritides have predilections for specific sites:
- in osteoarthritis and erosive osteoarthritis—the proximal and distal interphalangeal joints
- in psoriatic arthritis—the distal interphalangeal joints
- in rheumatoid arthritis—the metacarpophalangeal and proximal interphalangeal joints.

[7] In the spine, the various arthritides exhibit characteristic morphologic features in:
- degenerative disease—marginal osteophytes and narrowing of the apophyseal joints and disk spaces
- rheumatoid arthritis—atlantoaxial subluxation and erosion of the odontoid process
- juvenile rheumatoid arthritis—fusion of the apophyseal joints of the cervical spine
- psoriatic arthritis and Reiter syndrome—coarse, asymmetric paraspinal ossifications
- ankylosing spondylitis—a delicate syndesmophyte.

[8] Sacroiliitis is commonly seen in ankylosing spondylitis, Reiter syndrome, and psoriatic arthritis.

[9] Monitoring the results of treatment of the arthritides involves detecting possible complications of various osteotomies and joint-replacement procedures. These complications include:
- thrombophlebitis
- intrapelvic leakage of methylmethacrylate cement
- heterotopic bone formation
- infection
- loosening, dislocation, and fracture of a prosthesis.

[10] Contrast arthrography utilizing the subtraction technique is useful in detecting loosening of a prosthesis.

References

Aisen AM, Martel W, Ellis JE, McCune WJ: Cervical spine involvement in rheumatoid arthritis: MR imaging. *Radiology* 165:159, 1987.

Alazraki NP, Fierer J, Resnick D: The role of gallium and bone scanning in monitoring response to therapy in chronic osteomyelitis. *J Nucl Med* 19:696, 1978.

Anderson LS, Staple TW: Arthrography of total hip replacement using subtraction technique. *Radiology* 109:470, 1973.

Beabout JW: Radiology of total hip arthroplasty. *Radiol Clin North Am* 13:2, 1975.

Beltran J: *MRI: Musculoskeletal System.* Philadelphia, Lippincott, 1990.

Beltran J, Caudill JL, Herman LA, et al: Rheumatoid arthritis: MR imaging manifestations. *Radiology* 165:153, 1987.

Breedveld FC, Algra PR, Vielvoye CJ, Cats A: Magnetic resonance imaging in the evaluation of patients with rheumatoid arthritis and subluxations of the cervical spine. *Arthritis Rheum* 30:624, 1987.

Brower AC: *Arthritis in Black and White.* Philadelphia, Saunders, 1988.

Charkes MD: Skeletal blood flow: Implication for bone-scan interpretation. *J Nucl Med* 21:91, 1980.

Forrester DM, Brown JC: *The Radiology of Joint Diseases*, ed 3. Philadelphia, Saunders, 1987.

Freiberger RH: Evaluation of hip prostheses by imaging methods. *Semin Roentgenol* 21:20, 1986.

Gelman MI, Coleman RE, Steven PM, Davey BW: Radiography, radionuclide imaging, and arthrography in the evaluation of total hip and knee replacement. *Radiology* 128:677, 1978.

Genant HK, Doi K, Mall JC, Sickles EA: Direct radiographic magnification for skeletal radiology. *Radiology* 123:47, 1977.

Greenspan A, Norman A: Gross hematuria: A complication of intrapelvic cement intrusion in total hip replacement. *Am J Roentgenol* 130:327, 1978.

Greenspan A, Norman A: Letter to the Editor (reply). *Am J Roentgenol* 140:1273, 1983.

Greenspan A, Norman A: Radial head-capitellum view: An expanded imaging approach to elbow injury. *Radiology* 164:272, 1987.

Gristina AG, Kolkin J: Current concepts review. Total joint replacement and sepsis. *J Bone Joint Surg* 65A:128, 1983.

Habermann ET: Total joint replacement: An overview. *Semin Roentgenol* 21:7, 1986.

Hendrix RW, Wixson RL, Rana NA, Rogers LF: Arthrography after total hip arthroplasty: A modified technique used in the diagnosis of pain. *Radiology* 148:647, 1983.

Insall J, Tria AJ, Scott WN: The total condylar knee prosthesis: The first five years. *Clin Orthop* 145:68, 1979.

Jones MM, Moore WH, Brewer EJ, Sonnemaker RE, Long SE: Radionuclide bone/joint imaging in children with rheumatic complaints. *Skeletal Radiol* 17:1, 1988.

Kattan KR, Marsch JT: Some extra-articular manifestations of arthritis and complications of therapy. A pictorial essay. *Radiol Clin North Am* 26:1277, 1988.

Kursunoglu-Brahme S, Riccio T, Weissman MH, et al: Rheumatoid knee: Role of gadopentetate-enhanced MR imaging. *Radiology* 176:831, 1990.

Larsson EM, Holtas S, Zygmunt S: Pre- and postoperative MR imaging of the craniocervical junction in rheumatoid arthritis. *Am J Roentgenol* 152:561, 1989.

McAfee JG: Update on radiopharmaceuticals for medical imaging. *Radiology* 171:593, 1989.

Perri JA, Rodman P, Mankin HJ: Giant synovial cysts of the calf in patients with rheumatoid arthritis. *J Bone Joint Surg* 50A:709, 1968.

Rupani HD, Holder LE, Espinola DA, Engin SI: Three-phase radionuclide bone imaging in sports medicine. *Radiology* 156:187, 1985.

Salvati EA, Ghelman B, McLaren T, Wilson PD Jr: Subtraction technique in arthrography for loosening of total hip replacement fixed with radiopaque cement. *Clin Orthop* 101:105, 1974.

Schneider R, Hood RW, Ranawat CS: Radiologic evaluation of knee arthroplasty. *Orthop Clin North Am* 13:225, 1982.

Schneider R, Abenavoli AM, Soundry M, Insall J: Failure of total condylar knee replacement. *Radiology* 152:309, 1984.

Schneider R, Goldman AB, Insall JN: Knee prosthesis. *Semin Roentgenol* 21:29, 1986.

Schumacher TM, Genant HK, Kellet MJ, Mall JC, Fye KM: HLA-B27 associated arthropathies. *Radiology* 126:289, 1978.

Sebes JI, Nasrallah NS, Rabinowitz JG, Masi AT: The relationship between HLA-B27 positive peripheral arthritis and sacroiliitis. *Radiology* 126:299, 1978.

Seltzer SE, Weissman BN, Finberg HJ: Improved diagnostic imaging in joint diseases. *Semin Arthritis Rheum* 11:315, 1982.

Steinbach L, Hellman D, Petri M, Sims R, Gillespy T, Genant H: Magnetic resonance imaging: A review of rheumatologic applications. *Semin Arthritis Rheum* 16:79, 1986.

Subramanian G, McAfee JG: A new complex of 99m-Tc for skeletal imaging. *Radiology* 99:192, 1971.

Subramanian G, McAfee JG, Blair RJ, Kallfelz FA, Thomas FD: Technetium-99m methylene diphosphonate—a superior agent for skeletal imaging. Comparison with other technetium complexes. *J Nucl Med* 16:744, 1975.

Weissman BN: Spondyloarthropathies. *Radiol Clin North Am* 25:1235, 1987.

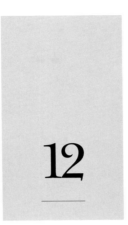

12

Degenerative Joint Disease

OSTEOARTHRITIS

DEGENERATIVE JOINT DISEASE (osteoarthritis, osteoarthrosis) is the most common form of arthritis. In its primary (idiopathic) form, it affects individuals in their fifth decade and above; in its secondary form, however, osteoarthritis may be seen in a much younger age group. Patients in the latter group have clearly defined underlying conditions leading to the development of degenerative joint disease (see Fig. 11.1).

Some authorities postulate that there are two types of primary degenerative joint disease. The first form is apparently closely related to the aging process ("wear and tear") and represents not a true arthritis but a senescent process of the joint. It characteristically shows limited destruction of the cartilage, slow progression, lack of significant joint deformity, and no restriction of joint function. This process is not affected by sex or race. The second type, a true

osteoarthritis, is unrelated to the aging process, although it shows an increased prevalence with age. Marked by progressive destruction of the articular cartilage and reparative processes such as osteophyte formation and subchondral sclerosis, true osteoarthritis progresses rapidly, leading to significant joint deformity. This form may be related to genetic factors, as well as to sex, race, and obesity. It has been shown that osteoarthritis tends to affect women more commonly than men, particularly in the proximal and distal interphalangeal joints and the first carpometacarpal joints. In the population over age 65, osteoarthritis affects whites more frequently than blacks. Obesity is associated with a higher incidence of osteoarthritis in the knees, which may be related to an excessive weight-bearing load on these joints.

Generally, in osteoarthritis the large diarthrodial joints such as the hip or knee and the small joints such as the interphalangeal joints of the hand are most often affected; the spine, however, is just as frequently involved in the degenerative process (Fig. 12.1). The shoulder, elbow, wrist, and ankle are unusual sites for primary osteoarthritis, and if degenerative changes are encountered in these locations, secondary arthritis should be considered. It should be kept in mind, however, that evidence exists for an association between degenerative arthritis in unusual sites and certain occupations. Even primary osteoarthritic changes may develop more rapidly, for example, in the lumbar spine, knees, and elbows of coal miners and in the wrists, elbows, and shoulders of pneumatic drill operators. Degenerative changes are also commonly seen in the ankles and feet of ballet dancers and in the femoropatellar joints of bicyclists.

An overview of the clinical and radiographic hallmarks of degenerative joint disease is presented in Figure 12.2.

OSTEOARTHRITIS OF THE LARGE JOINTS

The hip and knee joints are the most common sites of osteoarthritis. The severity of radiographic changes does not always correlate with the clinical symptoms, which may vary from stiffness and pain to severe deformities and limitation of joint function.

Osteoarthritis of the Hip

There are four cardinal radiographic features of degenerative joint disease in the hip:

1. Narrowing of the joint space as a result of thinning of the articular cartilage
2. Subchondral sclerosis (eburnation) due to reparative processes (remodeling)
3. Osteophyte formation (osteophytosis) as a result of reparative processes in sites not subjected to stress (so-called low-stress areas), which are usually marginal (peripheral) in distribution
4. Cyst or pseudocyst formation resulting from bone contusions that lead to microfractures and intrusion of synovial fluid into the altered spongy bone; in the acetabulum, these subchondral cyst-like lesions are referred to as *Eggers cysts*.

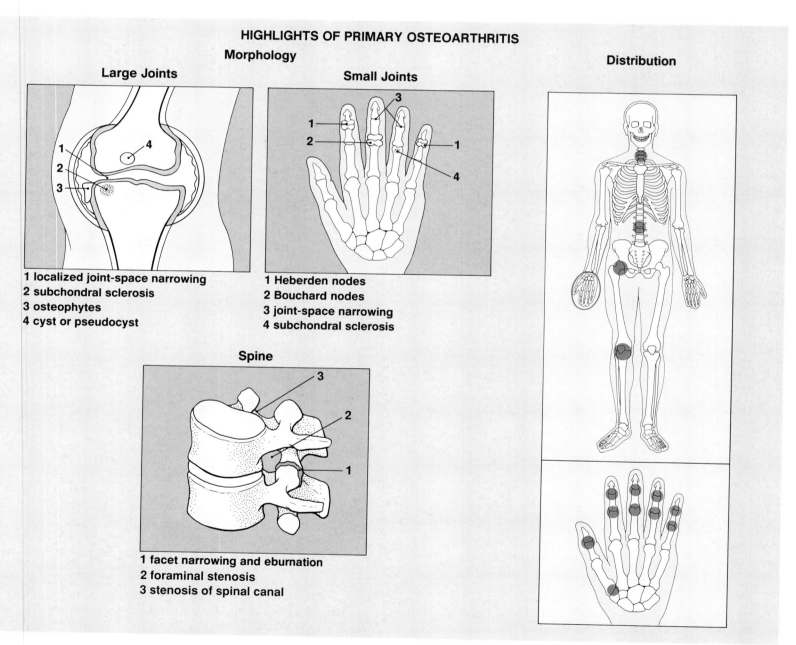

Figure 12.1 Highlights of the morphology and distribution of arthritic lesions in primary osteoarthritis.

Figure 12.2 Clinical and Radiographic Hallmarks of Degenerative Joint Disease

TYPE OF ARTHRITIS	SITE	CRUCIAL ABNORMALITIES	TECHNIQUE*/PROJECTION
Primary Osteoarthritis (F > M; >50 years)	Hand	Degenerative changes in: Proximal interphalangeal joints (Bouchard nodes) Distal interphalangeal joints (Heberden nodes)	Dorsovolar view
	Hip	Narrowing of joint space Subchondral sclerosis Marginal osteophytes Cysts and pseudocysts Superolateral subluxation	Anteroposterior view
	Knee	Same changes as in hip Varus or valgus deformity Degenerative changes in: Femoropatellar compartment Patella (tooth sign)	Anteroposterior view Weight-bearing anteroposterior view Lateral view Axial view of patella
	Spine	Degenerative disk disease: Narrowing of disk space Degenerative spondylolisthesis Osteophytosis Spondylosis deformans Degenerative changes in apophyseal joints Foraminal stenosis Spinal stenosis	Lateral view Lateral flexion/extension views Anteroposterior and lateral views Anteroposterior and lateral views Oblique views (cervical, lumbar) CT, myelogram, MRI
Secondary Osteoarthritis Posttraumatic	Hip Knee Shoulder, elbow, wrist, ankle (unusual sites)	Similar changes to those in primary osteoarthritis History of previous trauma Younger age	Standard views Tomography
Slipped Capital Femoral Epiphysis	Hips	Herndon hump Narrowing of joint space Osteophytosis	Anteroposterior and frog-lateral views
Congenital Hip Dislocation (F > M)	Hips	Signs of acetabular hypoplasia	Anteroposterior and frog-lateral views
Perthes Disease (M > F)	Hip	Unilateral or bilateral Osteonecrosis of femoral head Coxa magna Lateral subluxation	Anteroposterior and frog-lateral views
Inflammatory Arthritis	Hip Knee	Medial and axial migration of femoral head Periarticular osteoporosis Limited osteophytosis	Standard views
Osteonecrosis	Hip Shoulder	Increased bone density Joint space usually preserved or only slightly narrowed Crescent sign (hip, shoulder) Coarse trabeculations Thickening of cortex	Anteroposterior views (hip, shoulder) Grashey view (shoulder) Frog-lateral view (hip) Standard views of affected joints Radionuclide bone scan
Paget Disease (>40 years)	Hips, knees, shoulders	Dysplastic changes Narrowing of joint space Osteophytes	Standard views of affected joints
Multiple Epiphyseal Dysplasia	Epiphyses of long bones		
Hemochromatosis	Hands	Degenerative changes in second and third metacarpophaleangeal joints with beak-like osteophytes Chondrocalcinosis	Dorsovolar view Standard views of affected joint
Acromegaly	Large joints Hands	Joints spaces widened or only slightly narrowed Enlargement of terminal tufts Beak-like osteophytes in heads of metacarpals	Dorsovolar view

*Radionuclide bone scan is used to determine the distribution of arthritic lesions in the skeleton.

These hallmarks of degenerative joint disease can be readily demonstrated on the standard projections of the hip (Figs. 12.3, 12.4). Occasionally, tomography is used to demonstrate the details of the degenerative process; it is not used to make a specific diagnosis but rather to confirm or exclude possible complications (see Fig. 11.8).

As articular cartilage is destroyed and reparative changes develop, evidence emerges of a change in the relation of the femoral head with respect to the acetabulum, known as "migration." Generally, three patterns of femoral-head migration can be observed: superior, which may be either superolateral or superomedial; medial; and axial (Fig. 12.4). The most common pattern is superolateral migration; the medial pattern is uncommon, while axial migration is exceptionally seen. It should be kept in mind, however, that in inflammatory arthritis of the hip, such as rheumatoid arthritis,

where a prior axial or medial migration of the femoral head is commonly associated with acetabular protrusio, degenerative changes may develop as a complication of the inflammatory process. Thus, one may see secondary osteoarthritis with medial or axial migration (Fig. 12.5).

Occasionally, the degenerative process in the hip may run a more rapid course. This destructive arthrosis of the hip joint is known as *Postel coxarthropathy*, a condition that may quickly lead to complete destruction of the hip joint. Because of the rapidity of the process, the radiographic presentation of this condition is marked by very little, if any, reparative changes, mimicking infectious or neuropathic arthritis (Charcot joint) (Fig. 12.6).

Secondary osteoarthritis is often seen in the hip joint in patients with predisposing conditions such as previous trauma, slipped capital femoral epiphysis, congenital hip dislocation, Perthes disease,

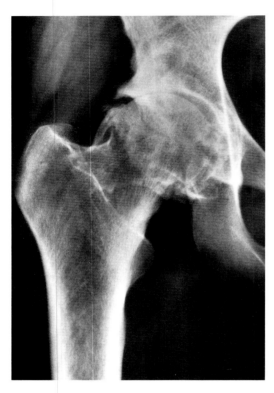

Figure 12.3 A 51-year-old woman presented with a history of right hip pain for the past ten years and no previous history suggesting predisposing factors for osteoarthritis. Anteroposterior view of the hip demonstrates the radiographic hallmarks of osteoarthritis: narrowing of the joint space, particularly at the weight-bearing segment; formation of marginal osteophytes; and subchondral sclerosis. Note the lack of osteoporosis.

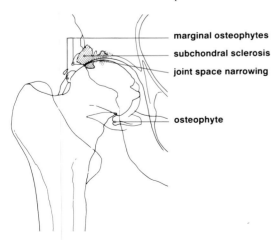

marginal osteophytes

subchondral sclerosis

joint space narrowing

osteophyte

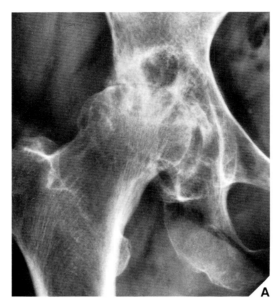

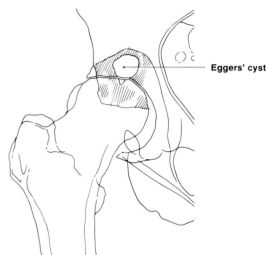

Eggers' cyst

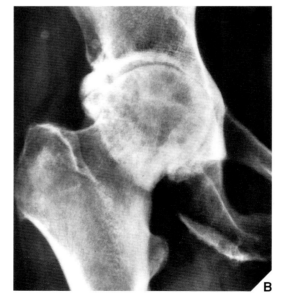

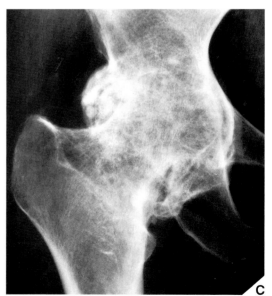

Figure 12.4 (A) Anteroposterior view of the right hip of a 65-year-old woman with long-standing degenerative joint disease in both hips demonstrates superolateral migration of the femoral head, the most common pattern seen in osteoarthritis of the hip joint. Note the typical Eggers cyst in the acetabulum. (B) Medial migration of the femoral head is apparent in this 48-year-old woman. Note also the minimal degree of acetabular protrusio. (C) Axial migration of the femoral head is evident in this 57-year-old woman who was suspected of having inflammatory arthritis. Clinical and laboratory investigations, however, led to a diagnosis of idiopathic osteoarthritis, which was confirmed on histopathologic examination after total hip replacement.

osteonecrosis, Paget disease, and inflammatory arthritides. The radiographic findings are the same as those described for primary osteoarthritis, but the features of the underlying process also can often be detected. Although the standard radiographic views are usually sufficient for demonstrating these changes, arthrography, or magnetic resonance imaging may at times be needed for a more accurate assessment of the status of the articular cartilage.

TREATMENT Advanced osteoarthritis, whether primary or secondary, is usually treated surgically by total hip arthroplasty using, among the various types available, either a cemented or a noncemented prosthesis. The reader is referred to Chapter 11 for further discussion of management.

Osteoarthritis of the Knee

The knee is a complex joint comprising three major compartments—the medial femorotibial, the lateral femorotibial and the femoropatellar—each of which may be affected by degenerative changes. The radiographic features of these changes are similar to those seen in osteoarthritis of the hip, including narrowing of the joint space (usually one or two compartments), subchondral sclerosis, osteophytosis, and subchondral cyst (or pseudocyst) formation. The standard anteroposterior and lateral projections of the knee are sufficient to demonstrate these processes (Fig. 12.7). If the medial joint compartment is affected, the knee may assume a varus configuration, which is best demonstrated on the weight-bearing anteroposterior view (Fig. 12.8A); involvement of the lateral compartment may lead to a

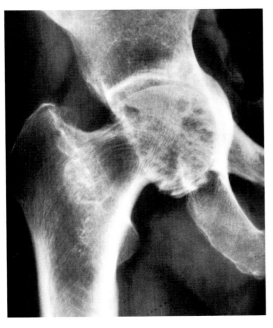

Figure 12.5
Anteroposterior view of the right hip of a 42-year-old woman with a known history of long-standing rheumatoid arthritis shows the typical changes of inflammatory arthritis, including medial migration of the femoral head and acetabular protrusio. Superimposition of secondary osteoarthritis is evident in subchondral sclerosis and marginal osteophytes.

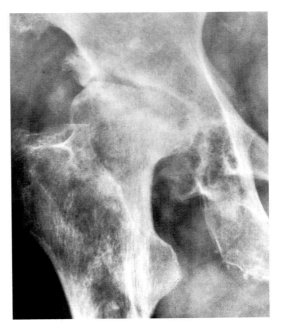

Figure 12.6
Anteroposterior radiograph of the right hip of a 72-year-old man who had pain in the hip for four months shows the typical appearance of Postel coxarthropathy, which often mimics Charcot joint or infectious arthritis. Note the destruction of the articular portion of the femoral head, which is laterally subluxed. The same destructive process has led to widening of the acetabulum.

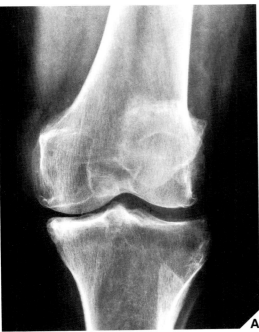

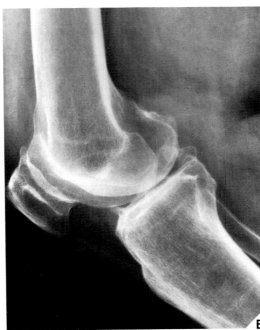

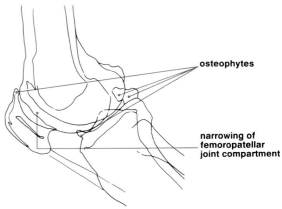

osteophytes

narrowing of femoropatellar joint compartment

Figure 12.7 Anteroposterior (A) and lateral (B) projections of the knee of a 57-year-old woman demonstrate narrowing of the medial femorotibial and femoropatellar compartments, subchondral sclerosis, and osteophytosis, the typical features of osteoarthritis. Note that osteophytes that were not obvious on the frontal projection are much better demonstrated on the lateral view.

valgus configuration (Fig. 12.8B). A frequent complication of osteoarthritis of the knee is the formation of osteochondral bodies, which can be demonstrated on the standard projections of the knee (Fig. 12.9) but may occasionally require arthrography. The femoropatellar joint compartment is also commonly involved in primary osteoarthritis. The lateral view of the knee and axial views of the patella are the most effective means of visualizing the degenerative changes (Fig. 12.10).

Often, particularly in individuals past their fifth decade, degenerative changes unrelated to femoropatellar osteoarthritis are seen at the insertion of the quadriceps tendon into the base of the patella. These changes are manifest as vertical ridges resembling teeth on an axial view of the patella and have been designated by Greenspan and colleagues as the "tooth" sign (Fig. 12.11A). The dentate structures represent an enthesopathy probably related to stress at the attachment of the quadriceps apparatus, and their nature is clearly

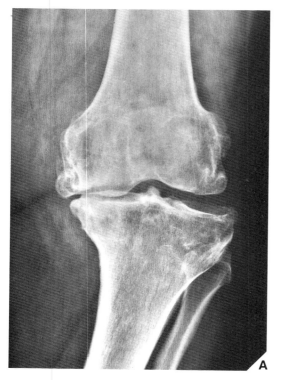

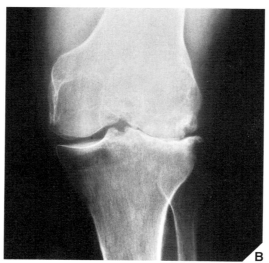

Figure 12.8 (A) Weight-bearing anteroposterior view of the knee of a 58-year-old woman demonstrates advanced osteoarthritis of the medial femorotibial joint compartment, which has led to a varus configuration of the joint. (B) Involve-ment of the lateral femorotibial joint compartment in advanced osteoarthritis, as seen on this weight-bearing anteroposterior view of another patient, has resulted in a valgus configuration.

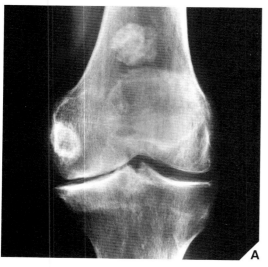

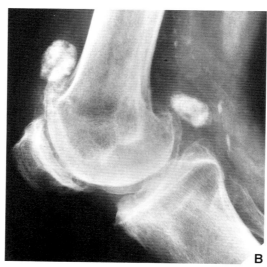

Figure 12.9 Anteroposterior (A) and lateral (B) views of the knee of a 66-year-old man with advanced osteoarthritis demonstrate predominant involvement of the medial femorotibial and femoropatellar joint compartments, with formation of two large osteochondral bodies.

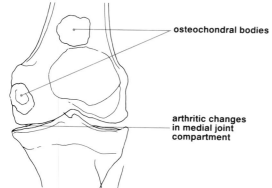

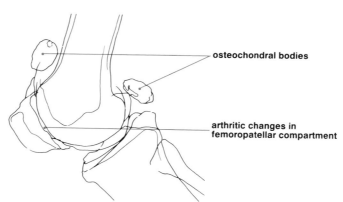

demonstrated on the lateral projection (Fig. 12.11B). At times they can be recognized on the anteroposterior view as well (Fig. 12.11C).

As in the hip joint, one may encounter secondary osteoarthritis in the knee. One of the most common predisposing factors is previous trauma or surgery.

Osteoarthritis of Other Large Joints

Other large joints such as the shoulder and ankle can be affected by osteoarthritis (Fig. 12.12), but involvement of these sites in the idiopathic form of the disease is much less common than involvement of the hip or knee. In fact, with evidence of degenerative changes in

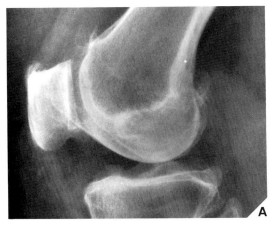
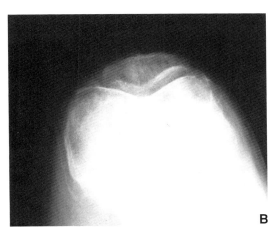

Figure 12.10 Lateral view of the knee (A) and axial view of the patella (B) of a 72-year-old woman demonstrate narrowing of the medial femoropatellar joint compartment and osteophyte formation on the medial aspect of the joint.

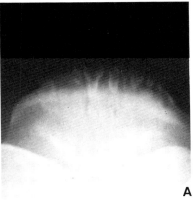
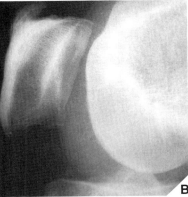
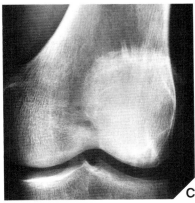

Figure 12.11 (A) Axial view of the patella demonstrates dentate structures (the "tooth" sign), which represent degenerative ossifications (enthesopathy) at the insertion of the quadriceps tendon into the base of patella, as seen on the lateral view (B) in this 55-year-old man. (C) Occasionally, the tooth sign can also be demonstrated on the anteroposterior projection of the knee, seen here in a 54-year-old woman. (A, B: Reprinted with permission from Greenspan A, et al., 1977)

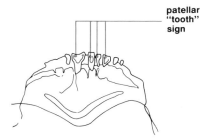
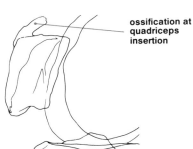
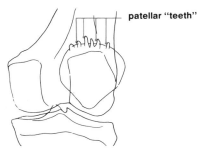

patellar "tooth" sign

ossification at quadriceps insertion

patellar "teeth"

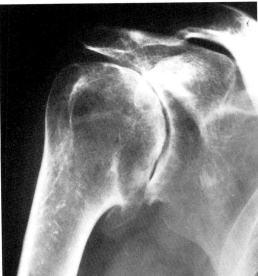

Figure 12.12 Anteroposterior view of the right shoulder of a 58-year-old man shows the typical features of osteoarthritis; both shoulders were affected. The patient had no history of trauma or other underlying condition to suggest the possibility of secondary arthritis.

such sites, one must consider the possibility of secondary rather than idiopathic arthritis (see Fig. 12.2).

OSTEOARTHRITIS OF THE SMALL JOINTS

Primary Osteoarthritis of the Hand

The most commonly affected small joints are those of the hand, particularly the proximal and distal interphalangeal and the first carpometacarpal articulations (see Figs. 11.24, 12.1). In the distal interphalangeal joints, if hypertrophic phenomena supervene and osteophytes are prominent, degenerative changes are accompanied by *Heberden nodes*. Similar deformities in the proximal interphalangeal joints are called *Bouchard nodes* (Fig. 12.13). If the degenerative changes involve the first carpometacarpal joint, they may result in an odd deformation of the thumb (Fig. 12.14). The midcarpal articulations may also be affected, particularly the scaphotrapeziotrapezoid joint.

Secondary Osteoarthritis of the Hand

ACROMEGALY   The most characteristic secondary osteoarthritic changes in the small joints may be observed in acromegalic patients. Although the degenerative process in acromegaly also affects large joints such as the hip, knee, and shoulder, as well as the spine, the hand displays the most typical features of this condition. These include soft tissue prominence and enlargement of the terminal tufts and the bases of the terminal phalanges; there may also be widening of some articular spaces and narrowing of others; beak-like osteophytes at the heads of the metacarpals are a prominent feature (Fig. 12.15). Degenerative changes in acromegaly are the result of hypertrophy of articular cartilage, which is not properly nourished by synovial fluid because of its abnormal thickness. (The reader is also referred to the discussion of acromegaly in Chapters 14 and 25.)

HEMOCHROMATOSIS   Commonly associated with the development of secondary osteoarthritis in the small joints, hemochromatosis (iron storage disease) is a rare disorder characterized by iron deposition in internal organs, articular cartilage, and synovium. Some investiga-

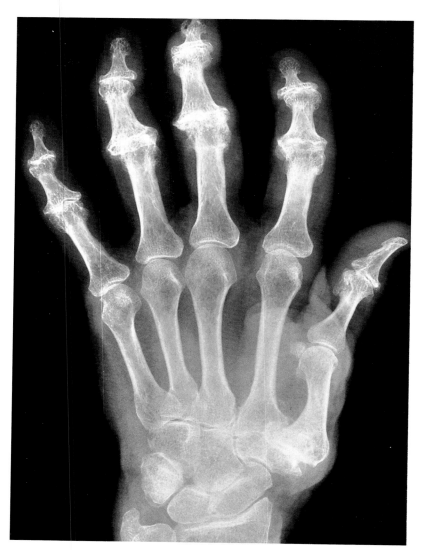

Figure 12.13 Dorsovolar view of right hand of a 74-year-old woman shows degenerative changes in the distal interphalangeal joints, manifested by Heberden nodes, and in the proximal interphalangeal joints, manifested by Bouchard nodes. Note also degenerative changes in the first carpometacarpal joint.

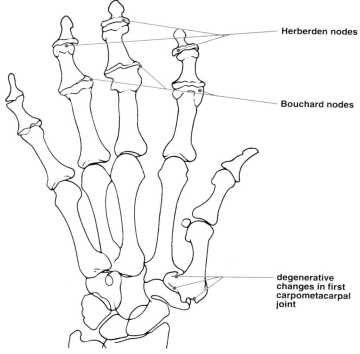

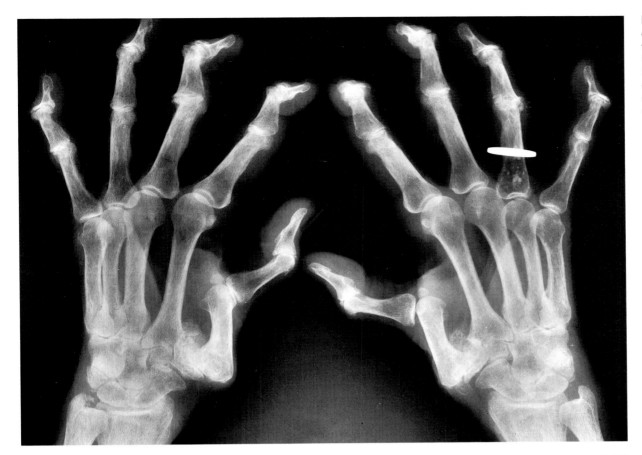

Figure 12.14 Dorsovolar view of both hands of a 52-year-old woman with osteoarthritis in addition to the typical Herberden and Bouchard nodes shows deformative changes at the first carpometacarpal articulations, resulting in an odd configuration of both thumbs.

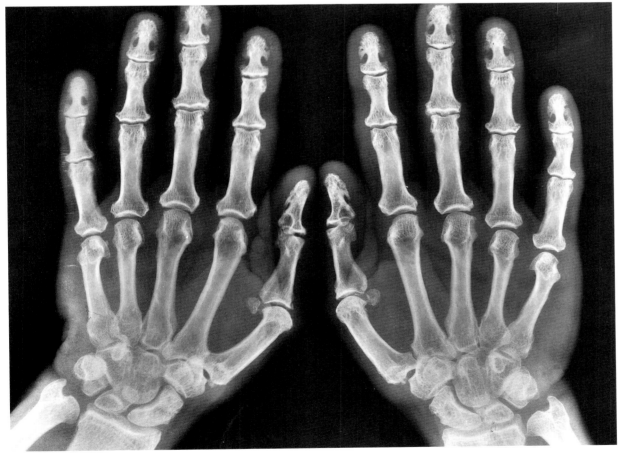

Figure 12.15 Dorsovolar view of both hands of a 42-year-old man with acromegaly shows widening of some and narrowing of other joint spaces, enlargement of the distal tufts and the bases of terminal phalanges, and beak-like osteophytes affecting particularly the heads of metacarpals. Note the soft tissue prominence and the large sesamoid bones at the first metacarpophalangeal joints. The sesamoid index (derived by multiplying the vertical and horizontal diameters of the sesamoid bone) is 48 in this patient; normally it should not exceed 20 to 25.

tors believe that the arthropathy seen in this condition differs from typical degenerative joint disease and warrants classification in the group of metabolic arthritides (see Chapter 14).

In the hand, the second and third metacarpophalangeal joints are characteristically affected (Fig. 12.16), although other small joints such as the interphalangeal and carpal articulations may be involved. Degenerative changes may also be seen at the shoulders, knees, hips, and ankles. Loss of the articular space, eburnation, subchondral cyst formation, and osteophytosis are the most prominent radiographic features of hemochromatosis. The changes may occasionally mimic those seen in calcium pyrophosphate dihydrate deposition disease (CPPD) and rheumatoid arthritis.

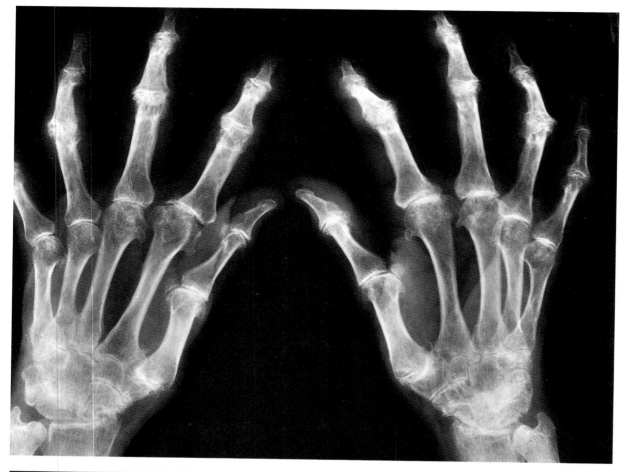

Figure 12.16 Oblique view of both hands of a 53-year-old woman with hemochromatosis arthropathy shows beak-like osteophytes arising from the heads of the second and third metacarpals on the radial aspect. The interphalangeal, metacarpophalangeal, and carpal articulations are also affected.

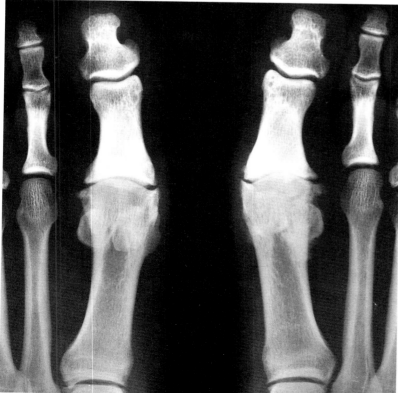

Figure 12.17 Dorsoplantar view of the first and second phalanges of the feet of a 33-year-old man shows degenerative changes bilaterally involving the first metatarsophalangeal joints, known as hallux rigidus. Note the narrowing of the joint space, subchondral sclerosis, and marginal osteophytes.

Osteoarthritis of the Foot

In the foot, the most commonly affected articulation is the metatarsophalangeal joint of the great toe. This condition is known as *hallux rigidus* (Fig. 12.17).

DEGENERATIVE DISEASES OF THE SPINE

Degenerative changes may involve the spine at the following sites:

1. The synovial joints—atlantoaxial, apophyseal, costovertebral, and sacroiliac—leading to *osteoarthritis* of these structures
2. The intervertebral disks, leading to the condition known as *degenerative disk disease*
3. The vertebral bodies and annulus fibrosus, leading to the condition known as *spondylosis deformans*, and

4. The fibrous articulations, ligaments, or sites of ligament attachment to the bone (entheses), leading to the condition known as *diffuse idiopathic skeletal hyperostosis* (DISH).

Frequently, all four conditions coexist in the same patient.

Osteoarthritis of the Synovial Joints

Degenerative changes of the vertebral facet joints are very common, particularly in the mid- and lower cervical and the lower lumbar segments. As in the other synovial joints, the characteristic radiographic features include diminution of the joint space, eburnation of subchondral bone, and osteophyte formation, all of which are most easily demonstrated on the oblique projection of the spine (Fig. 12.18). In the cervical spine, osteophytes on the posterior aspect of a vertebral body may encroach on the neural

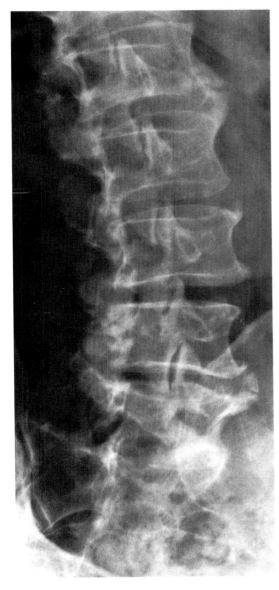
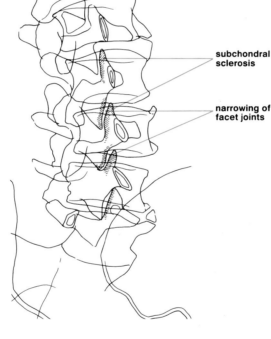

subchondral sclerosis

narrowing of facet joints

Figure 12.18 Oblique view of the lumbar spine in a 68-year-old man demonstrates advanced osteoarthritis of the facet joints. Narrowing of the joint spaces, eburnation of the articular margins, and small osteophytes are similar to the changes seen in osteoarthritis of the large synovial joints.

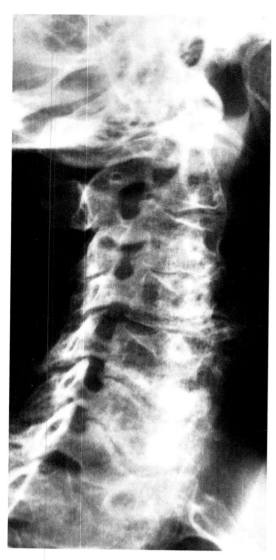

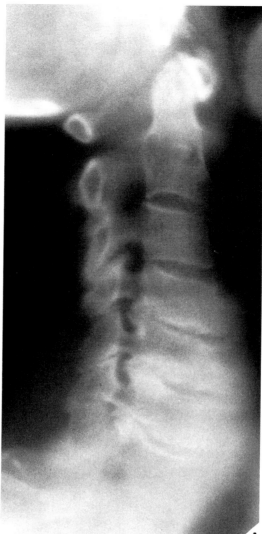

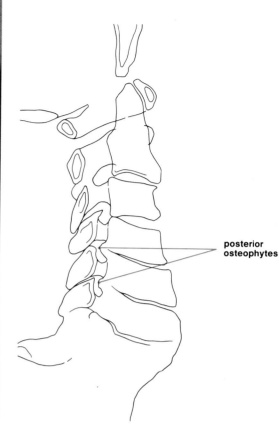

posterior
osteophytes

Figure 12.19 Oblique view of the cervical spine in a 72-year-old woman who complained of neck pain radiating to both shoulders reveals multiple posterior osteophytes encroaching on numerous neural foramina.

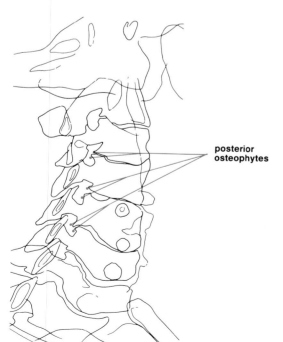

posterior
osteophytes

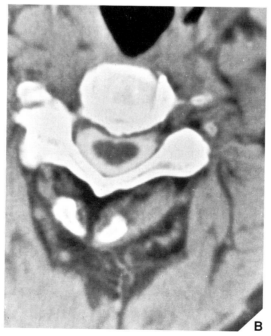

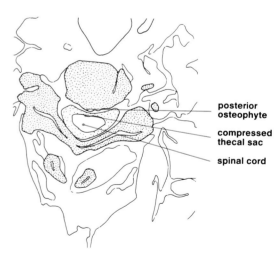

posterior
osteophyte

compressed
thecal sac

spinal cord

Figure 12.20 (A) Conventional lateral tomogram of the cervical spine in a 56-year-old man demonstrates encroachment of the neural foramina by posterior osteophytes. (B) CT section at the level of C-3 obtained during myelography demonstrates a large posterior osteophyte impinging on the thecal sac and compressing the subarachnoid space filled with contrast medium.

foramina or the thecal sac, causing various neurologic symptoms. In addition to the standard oblique views (Fig. 12.19), conventional tomography or computed tomography (CT) is usually required to demonstrate these changes (Fig. 12.20). Anterior osteophytes, on the other hand, are as a rule asymptomatic unless they are unusually prominent. Involvement of the apophyseal joints may exhibit a "vacuum phenomenon" (Fig. 12.21), which in fact represents gas in the joint. This finding is almost pathognomonic for a degenerative process.

As in other diarthrodial joints, degenerative changes of the sacroiliac joints are manifested by narrowing of the joint space, sub-chondral sclerosis, and osteophytosis (Fig. 12.22). It is important to note in the evaluation of the sacroiliac joints that only the lower half of the radiographic sacroiliac joint space is lined by synovium; the upper portion is a syndesmotic joint (Fig. 12.23).

Degenerative Disk Disease

The vacuum phenomenon may also be seen in the intervertebral disk secondary to degenerative disk disease. These radiolucent collections of gas, principally nitrogen, are related to the negative pressure created by abnormally altered joint or disk spaces.

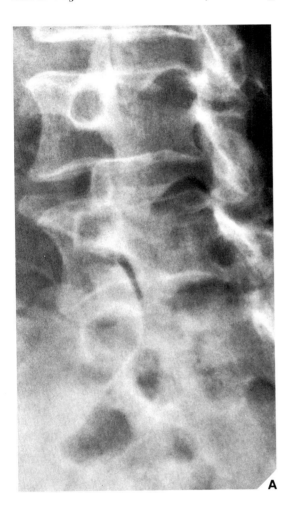

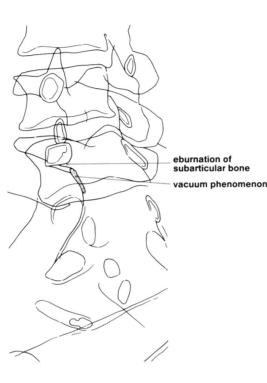

eburnation of
subarticular bone

vacuum phenomenon

A

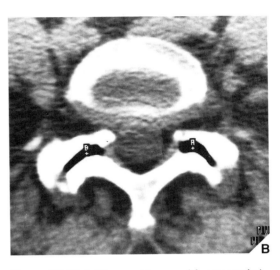

B

Figure 12.21 A 56-year-old man with osteoarthritis affecting the apophyseal joints of the lumbar spine. (A) Oblique view of the lumbosacral spine demonstrates a vacuum phenomenon of the facet joint L5-S1 and eburnation of the subarticular bone. (B) CT section through both facets clearly demonstrates the presence of gas, as confirmed by the Hounsfield values. These units are related to the attenuation coefficient for various tissues in the body and represent absorption values directly related to tissue density. Note also the hypertrophic spur arising from the right facet and encroaching on the spinal canal.

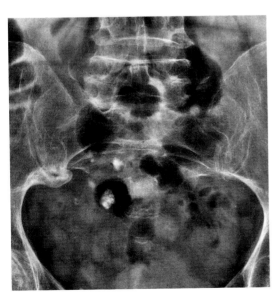

Figure 12.22 Degenerative changes in the sacroiliac joints, seen here affecting predominantly the right sacroiliac joint in an 82-year-old woman, are manifested by narrowing of the joint space and osteophytosis.

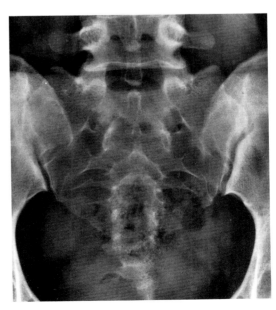

Figure 12.23 The true diarthrodial portion of the sacroiliac joint comprises only about 50% of the radiographic joint space. The upper part is a syndesmotic joint.

Other radiographic findings of degenerative disk disease include disk space narrowing and osteophytosis at the marginal borders of the adjacent vertebral bodies (Fig. 12.24). Degenerative disk disease, in combination with degenerative changes in the apophyseal joints, may lead to degenerative spondylolisthesis (see Figs. 10.58, 12.24).

Spondylosis Deformans

Spondylosis deformans is a degenerative condition marked by the formation of anterior and lateral osteophytes as a result of anterior and anterolateral disk herniation (see Figs. 10.62, 10.63). As Schmorl and other investigators have pointed out, the initiating factors in the development of this condition are abnormalities in the peripheral fibers of the annulus fibrosus that result in weakening the anchorage of the intervertebral disk to the vertebral body at the site where Sharpey fibers attach to the vertebral rim. Unlike degenerative disk disease, the intervertebral spaces in spondylosis deformans are relatively well preserved, the primary radiographic feature being extensive osteophytosis (Fig. 12.25). These osteophytes must be differentiated from the delicate syndesmophytes of ankylosing spondylitis, from the large, characteristically asymmetric bone excrescences that are seen in psoriatic arthritis and Reiter syndrome involving the lateral aspect of vertebral bodies, and from the flowing, usually anterior, hyperostosis of the DISH syndrome.

Diffuse Idiopathic Skeletal Hyperostosis

DISH, originally described by Forestier and popularized by Resnick, is characterized by flowing ossification along the anterior aspect of the vertebral bodies extending across the disk spaces. It is also associated with hyperostosis at the sites of tendon and ligament attachments to the bone, ligament ossification, and osteophytosis involving the axial and appendicular skeleton. A lateral radiograph of the spine best demonstrates these changes. As in spondylosis deformans, the disk spaces are usually well preserved (Fig. 12.26). It is important to distinguish this condition from the apparently similar "bamboo spine" seen in ankylosing spondylitis (see Fig. 13.26).

Complications of Degenerative Disease of the Spine

DEGENERATIVE SPONDYLOLISTHESIS One of the most common complications of degenerative disease of the spine, degenerative spondylolisthesis, results from degenerative changes in the disk and apophyseal joints. In this condition, there is anterior displacement of a vertebra onto the one below, which usually is easily recognized on the lateral view of the spine by the spinous-process sign (Fig. 12.27; see also Fig. 10.57). However, on occasion the displacement may not be obvious on the standard lateral film, and radiographs must be obtained while the patient maximally extends and

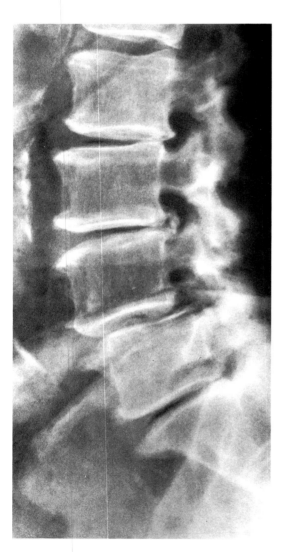

Figure 12.24 Lateral view of the lumbosacral spine in a 66-year-old woman demonstrates advanced degenerative disk disease at multiple levels. Note the radiolucent collections of gas in several disks (the vacuum phenomenon) as well as the narrowing of the disk spaces and marginal osteophytes. Grade 1 degenerative spondylolisthesis is seen at the L4-5 level.

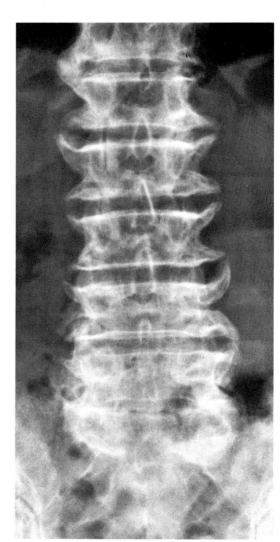

Fig.12.25 Anteroposterior projection of the lumbosacral spine in a 68-year-old woman exhibits the typical changes of spondylosis deformans. Note the extensive osteophytosis and relatively well preserved intervertebral disk spaces.

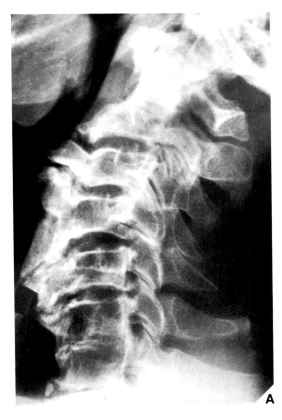

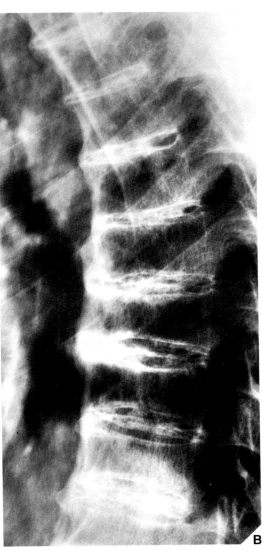

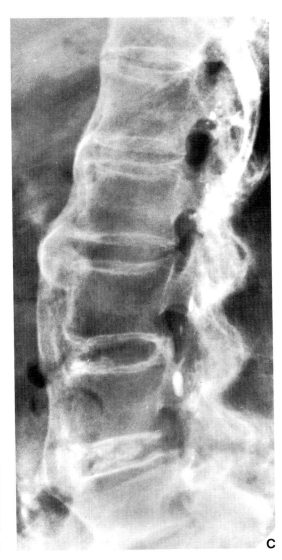

Figure 12.26 Lateral views of the cervical (A), thoracic (B), and lumbar (C) spine in a 72-year-old man with Forestier disease (DISH) show the characteristic flowing hyperostosis extending across the vertebral disk spaces, which are relatively well preserved.

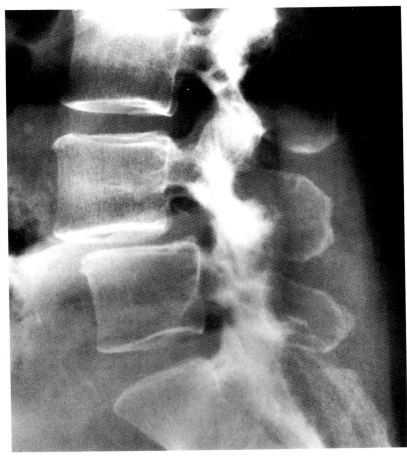

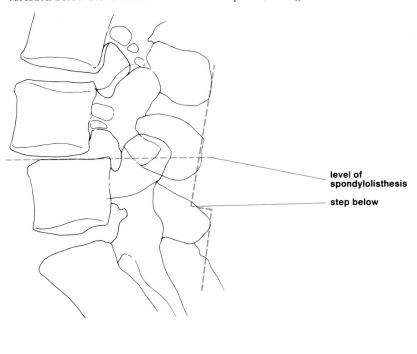

Figure 12.27 A 55-year-old woman with degenerative disk disease at L4-5 and degenerative facet arthritis developed spondylolisthesis, a common complication of this condition. Lateral view of the lumbosacral spine is sufficient to differentiate this condition from spondylolisthesis associated with spondylolysis by the appearance of a step-off of the spinous process at the vertebra below the involved intervertebral space (see Fig. 10.57).

level of spondylolisthesis

step below

flexes the spine (Fig. 12.28). As Milgram pointed out, the stress applied by forward and backward motion of the spine discloses instability (spondylolisthesis), which may be overlooked on other projections.

Degenerative spondylolisthesis occurs in approximately 4% of patients with degenerative disk disease and affects females more frequently than males. It has a predilection for the L4-5 spinal level. This predilection has been attributed to developmental or acquired alterations in the neural arch that lead to instability and abnormal stress. The stress applied to the vertebra may result in decompensation of the ligaments, hypermobility, instability, and osteoarthritis of adjacent apophyseal joints.

Clinical symptoms associated with degenerative spondylolisthesis include low back pain with or without radiation into the leg, sciatic pain with signs of nerve root compression, and intermittent claudication of the cauda equina. It should be noted, however, that many patients with degenerative spondylolisthesis are asymptomatic.

Radiographic findings of degenerative spondylolisthesis include osteoarthritic changes of the facet joints (joint narrowing, marginal eburnation, and osteophyte formation), anterior slippage of the superior vertebra on the inferior vertebra, and, in many instances, intervertebral vacuum phenomenon. Invariably the affected intervertebal disk space is narrowed.

SPINAL STENOSIS Spinal stenosis is a much more severe complication of degenerative disease of the spine. In its acquired form, it results from hypertrophy of the structures surrounding the spinal canal, such as the pedicles, laminae, articular processes, and poste-rior aspect of the vertebral bodies, as well as the ligamentum flavum. These alternations usually are apparent on plain film radiography; however, spinal stenosis can be better demonstrated by ancillary techniques. Spinal stenosis can be demonstrated by myelography, which can show the impingement of the thecal sac by hypertrophic changes of the posterior parts of the vertebral body and bulging disks, but CT best delineates its details (Fig. 12.29). Magnetic resonance imaging is also an effective modality in this respect.

Spinal stenosis in the lumbar segment can be divided into three groups on the basis of its anatomic location: stenosis of the spinal canal, stenosis of the subarticular or lateral recesses, and stenosis of the neural foramina.

The causes of stenosis of the central canal are related to hypertrophic changes of osteoarthritis of the apophyseal joints, thickening of the ligamentum flavum, and osteophytes arising from the vertebral bodies. Bone hypertrophy at the site of the facet joints is a major cause of stenosis of the subarticular or lateral recesses, leading to encroachment on the neural elements in this region. Clinical manifestations of lateral recess syndrome include unilateral or bilateral leg pain, which is initiated or aggravated by long periods of standing or walking. These symptoms are usually relieved entirely by sitting or squatting.

The stenosis of the neural foramina is caused by hypertrophic changes and osteophytosis involving the vertebral body and articular process. Moreover, degenerative spondylolisthesis may be associated with distortion of the intervertebral foramen and may lead to compromise of the exiting nerve.

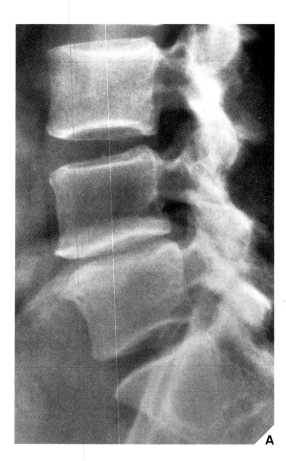
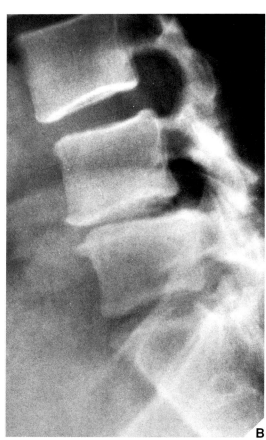

Figure 12.28 A 50-year-old man presented with chronic low back pain. (A) Standard lateral view of the lumbosacral spine in the neutral position shows narrowing of the L4-5 disk space, indicating degenerative disk disease. There is no evidence of vertebral list. (B) Lateral view in flexion, however, demonstrates grade 1 spondylolisthesis at L4-5.

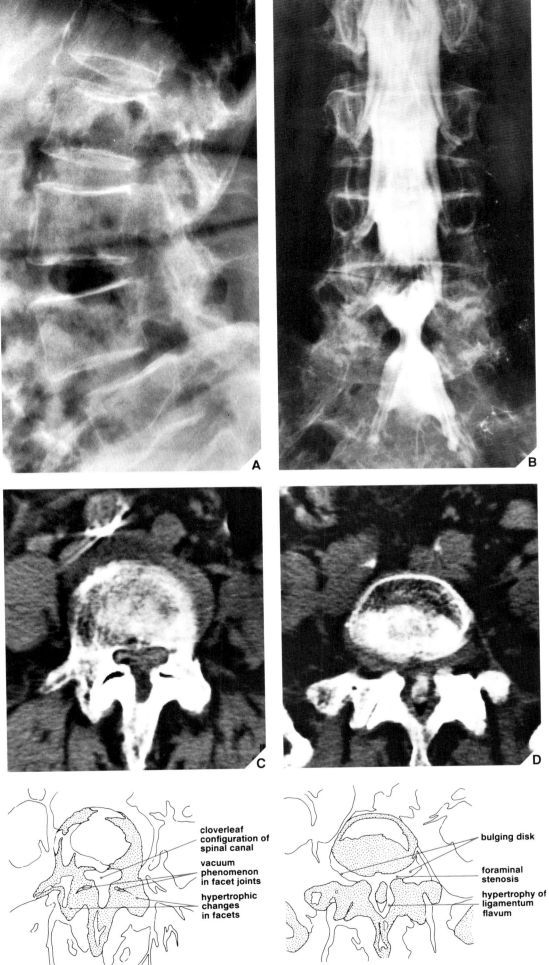

Figure 12.29 A 71-year-old woman was evaluated for severe low back pain. (A) Standard lateral view of the lumbar spine shows degenerative spondylolisthesis at the L4-5 interspace. Note the short appearance of the pedicles. (B) A myelogram in the anteroposterior projection also discloses segmental narrowing of the thecal sac; the upper defect is related to spondylolisthesis, the lower to spinal stenosis. CT sections (C, D) demonstrate the details of the abnormalities—severe spinal and foraminal stenosis, hypertrophy of the ligamenta flava, and posterior bulging of the intervertebral disk. Note the cloverleaf configuration of the spinal canal secondary to marked hypertrophy of the facet joints. The vacuum phenomenon in the apophyseal joints is well demonstrated.

cloverleaf
configuration of
spinal canal

vacuum
phenomenon
in facet joints

hypertrophic
changes
in facets

bulging disk

foraminal
stenosis

hypertrophy of
ligamentum
flavum

NEUROPATHIC ARTHROPATHY

This acute or chronic destructive arthritis, also known as Charcot joint, is grouped with other degenerative joint diseases because it exhibits manifestations similar to those seen in other forms of osteoarthritis—destruction of articular cartilage, subchondral sclerosis, and marginal osteophytosis—but in their most severe form. Pathognomonic for neuropathic joints are fragmentation of the bone and cartilage, which are discharged as debris into the joint; chronic synovitis with accumulation of varying amounts of fluid in the joint; and joint instability manifested by subluxation and dislocation (Fig. 12.30). Underlying conditions leading to neuropathic joint include diabetes mellitus, syphilis, leprosy, syringomyelia, congenital indifference to pain, and spina bifida with meningomyelocele. In diabetic patients, the condition has a greater predilection for the joints of the foot and ankle; in patients with syringomyelia, joints of the upper extremities are more commonly affected (Fig. 12.31). The eponym *Charcot joint* was originally reserved for neuropathic joint in syphilitic patients with tabes dorsalis. Currently, this term applies to any joint displaying features of neuropathic arthropathy, regardless of the etiologic factor.

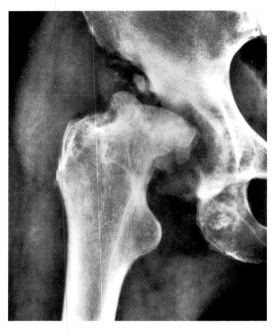

Figure 12.30
Anteroposterior view of the right hip of a 57-year-old woman with neurosyphilis (tabes dorsalis) shows the typical features of neuropathic (Charcot) joint. There is complete disorganization of the joint, fragmentation, and subluxation. The absence of osteoporosis is a characteristic feature of the neuropathic joint. This condition represents the most severe manifestation of degenerative joint disease.

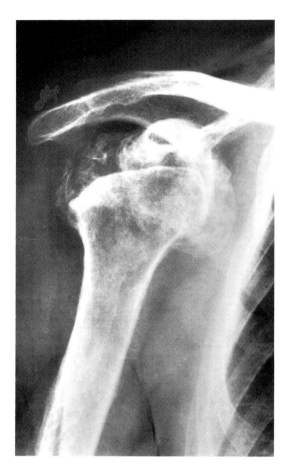

Figure 12.31
A 59-year-old woman with syringomyelia developed a neuropathic shoulder joint. Anteroposterior radiograph shows destruction of the joint, bony debris, and subluxation of the humeral head.

PRACTICAL POINTS TO REMEMBER

Osteoarthritis

[1] Degenerative joint disease (osteoarthritis, degenerative arthritis) is classified as primary (idiopathic) or secondary; in the latter there is an underlying, predisposing disorder.

[2] The radiographic hallmarks of osteoarthritis are:
- diminution (narrowing) of the joint space
- subchondral sclerosis
- osteophytosis
- cyst or pseudocyst formation
- lack of pronounced osteoporosis.

Osteoarthritis of the Large Joints

[1] In the hip joint, the degenerative process results in migration of the femoral head, most commonly in a superolateral direction.

[2] Postel coxarthropathy is a rapidly destructive arthrosis of the hip joint, which radiographically can mimic infection or neuropathic joint.

[3] The medial femorotibial and femoropateller compartments of the knee joint are commonly involved in osteoarthritis. Weight-bearing examination may reveal a varus configuration of the knee.

[4] The "tooth" sign of the patella, recognized on an axial view by vertical ridges at the insertion of the quadriceps tendon into the base of the patella, represents a type of degenerative change (enthesopathy) unrelated to femoropatellar osteoarthritis. It is commonly seen after the fifth decade of life.

[5] If the shoulder, elbow, or ankle joints are affected by degenerative joint disease, a diagnosis of secondary rather than primary osteoarthritis should be considered.

Osteoarthritis of the Small Joints

[1] In the hand, the hallmarks of primary degenerative joint disease are:
- Heberden nodes affecting the distal interphalangeal joints
- Bouchard nodes affecting the proximal interphalangeal joints.

[2] The first carpometacarpal articulation is frequently involved in primary degenerative joint disease.

Degenerative Disease of the Spine

[1] In the spine, degenerative changes may be present in four major forms:
- as osteoarthritis of the synovial joints, including the atlantoaxial, apophyseal, costovertebral, and sacroiliac
- as spondylosis deformans, a condition manifested by formation of anterior and lateral marginal osteophytes with preservation of the disk spaces (at least in the early stages)
- as degenerative disk disease, a condition primarily involving the intervertebral disks and manifested by destruction of these structures, the vacuum phenomenon, and narrowing of the disk spaces
- as diffuse idiopathic skeletal hyperostosis (DISH syndrome or Forestier disease), characterized by flowing ossifications along the anterior aspects of vertebral bodies extending across the disk spaces, relative preservation of the intervertebral disks, and hyperostosis at the sites of tendon and ligament attachment to the bone (enthesopathy).

[2] Two common conditions can complicate degenerative spine disease:
- degenerative spondylolisthesis
- spinal stenosis.

[3] Degenerative spondylolisthesis is marked by anterior (ventral) displacement of a vertebra onto the one below and recognized on the lateral view of the spine by the spinous-process sign.

[4] Spinal stenosis can readily be diagnosed using computed tomography or magnetic resonance imaging.

Neuropathic Arthropathy

[1] Neuropathic (Charcot) joint manifests with the same degenerative changes as osteoarthritis, but they are seen in their most severe form. This condition is also marked by:
- fragmentation of the bone and cartilage, filling the joint with debris
- chronic synovitis with joint effusion
- joint instability with subluxation or dislocation.

[2] The underlying conditions leading to neuropathic joint include diabetes mellitus, syphilis, leprosy, syringomyelia, and congenital indifference to pain.

References

Adamson TC III, Resnik CS, Guerra Jr J, Vint VC, Weisman MH, Resnick D: Hand and wrist arthropathies of hemochromatosis and calcium pyrophosphate deposition disease: Distinct radiographic features. *Radiology* 147:377, 1983.

Beggs I: Radiological assessment of degenerative diseases of the cervical spine. *Semin Orthop* 2:63, 1987.

Bennett GL, Leeson MC, Michael A: Extensive hemosiderin deposition in the medial meniscus of a knee. Its possible relationship to degenerative joint disease. *Clin Orthop* 230:182, 1988.

Bora FW Jr, Miller G: Joint physiology, cartilage metabolism, and the etiology of osteoarthritis. *Hand Clin* 3:325, 1987.

Brandt KD: Osteoarthritis. *Clin Geriatr Med* 4:279, 1988.

Bullough PG, Bansal M: The differential diagnosis of geodes. *Radiol Clin North Am* 26:1165, 1988.

Cone RO, Resnick D: Degenerative disease of the shoulder. *Australas Radiol* 28:232, 1984.

Danielsson L: Incidence and osteoarthritis of the hip (coxarthrosis). *Clin Orthop* 45:67, 1966.

Davis MA: Epidemiology of osteoarthritis. *Clin Geriatr Med* 4:241, 1988.

Fairbank TJ: Knee joint changes after meniscectomy. *J Bone Joint Surg* 30B:664, 1948.

Forestier J, Rotes Querol J: Senile ankylosing hyperostosis of the spine. *Ann Rheum Dis* 9:321, 1950.

Freeman MAR: Total replacement of the knee. *Orthop Rev* 3:21, 1974.

Greenspan A, Norman A, Tchang FKM: "Tooth" sign in patellar degenerative disease. *J Bone Joint Surg* 59A:483, 1977.

Harrison MHM, Schajowicz F, Trueta J: Osteoarthritis of the hip: A study of the nature and evolution of the disease. *J Bone Joint Surg* 35B:598, 1953.

Hayward I, Bjorkengren AG, Pathria MN, Zlatkin MB, Sartoris DJ, Resnick D: Patterns of femoral head migration in osteoarthritis of the hip: A reappraisal with CT and pathologic correlation. *Radiology* 166:857, 1988.

Kellgren JH, Moore R: Generalized osteoarthritis and Heberden's nodes. *Br Med J* 1:181, 1952.

Kerr R, Resnick D, Pineda C, Haghighi P: Osteoarthritis of the glenohumeral joint: A radiologic-pathologic study. *Am J Roentgenol* 144:967, 1985.

Kirkaldy-Willis WH, Farfan HF: Instability of the lumbar spine. *Clin Orthop* 165:110, 1982.

Knutsson F: The vacuum phenomenon in the intervertebral discs. *Acta Radiol* 23:173, 1942.

Kumpan W, Salomonowitz E, Seidl G, Wittich GR: The intervertebral vacuum phenomenon. *Skeletal Radiol* 15:444, 1986.

Leach RE, Gregg T, Siber FJ: Weight-bearing radiography in osteoarthritis of the knee. *Radiology* 97:265, 1970.

Lefkowitz DM, Quencer RM: Vacuum facet phenomenon: A computed tomographic sign of degenerative spondylolisthesis. *Radiology* 144:562, 1982.

Maldague BE, Noel HM, Malghem JJ: The intervertebral vacuum cleft: A sign of ischemic vertebral collapse. *Radiology* 129:23, 1978.

McAfee PC, Ullrich CG, Levinsohn EM, Yuan HA, Cacayorill ED, Lockwood RC: Computed tomography in degenerative lumbar spinal stenosis: The value of multiplanar reconstruction. *RadioGraphics* 2:529, 1982.

Milgram JE: Recurrent articular spondylolisthesis: Common cause of vertebral instabilities, root pain, sciatica, and ultimately spinal stenosis. Early detection and blocking of specific dislocations. *Bull Hosp Jt Dis Orthop Inst* 46:47, 1986.

Norman A, Robbins H, Milgram JE: The acute neuropathic arthropathy—a rapid severely disorganizing form of arthritis. *Radiology* 90:1159, 1968.

O'Donoghue DM: *Treatment of Injuries to Athletes*, ed 2. Philadelphia, Saunders, 1970.

Pathria M, Sartoris DJ, Resnick D: Osteoarthritis of the facet joints: Accuracy of oblique radiographic assessment. *Radiology* 164:227, 1987.

Pepper HW, Noonan CD: Radiographic evaluation of total hip arthroplasty. *Radiology* 108:23, 1973.

Peyron JG: Epidemiologic and etiologic approach of osteoarthritis. *Semin Arthritis Rheum* 8:288, 1979.

Postachinni F, Pezzeri G, Montanaro A, Natali G: Computerized tomography in lumbar stenosis. *J Bone Joint Surg* 62B:78, 1980.

Postel M, Kerboull M: Total prosthetic replacement in rapidly destructive arthrosis of the hip joint. *Clin Orthop* 72:138, 1970.

Pritzker KPH: Aging and degeneration in the lumbar intervertebral disc. *Orthop Clin North Am* 8:65, 1977.

Resnick D: Patterns of migration of the femoral head in osteoarthritis of the hip. Roentgenographic-pathologic correlation and comparison with rheumatoid arthritis. *Am J Roentgenol* 124:62, 1975.

Resnick D: Degenerative diseases of the vertebral column. *Radiology* 156:3, 1985.

Resnick D, Niwayama G: Entheses and enthesopathy. Anatomical, pathological and radiological correlation. *Radiology* 146:1, 1983.

Resnick D, Niwayama G, Goergen TG: Degenerative disease of the sacroiliac joint. *Investig Radiol* 10:608, 1975.

Resnick D, Shaul SR, Robins JM: Diffuse idiopathic skeletal hyperostosis (DISH): Forestier's disease with extraspinal manifestations. *Radiology* 115:513, 1975.

Resnick D, Niwayama G, Coutts RD: Subchondral cysts (geodes) in arthritic disorders: Pathologic and radiographic appearance of the hip joint. *Am J Roentgenol* 128:799, 1977.

Schmorl G, Junghanns H: *The Human Spine in Health and Disease*, ed 2 (Tr, Besemann EF). New York, Grune & Stratton, 1971.

Schumacher HR: Articular cartilage in the degenerative arthropathy of hemochromatosis. *Arthritis Rheum* 25:1460, 1982.

Sokoloff L: Pathology and pathogenesis of osteoarthritis. In: Hollander JL, McCarty DJ (eds): *Arthritis and Allied Conditions*, ed 8. Philadelphia, Lea & Febiger, 1972, pp 1009-1031.

Watt I, Dieppe P: Osteoarthritis revisited. *Skeletal Radiol* 19:1, 1990.

Weber BG: Total hip replacement: Rotating versus fixed and metal versus ceramic heads. In: *Proceedings of the Ninth Open Scientific Meeting of the Hip Society, 1981*. St. Louis, Mosby, 1981, pp 264-275.

Weisz GM: Value of computerized tomography in diagnosis of diseases of the lumbar spine. *Med J Aust* 1:216, 1982.

Weisz GM, Lee P: Spinal canal stenosis. *Clin Orthop* 179:134, 1983.

Weisz GM, Lee P: Spinal reserve capacity. A radiologic concept of lumbar canal stenosis. *Orthop Rev* 13:579, 1984.

Yazici H, Saville PD, Salvati EA, Bohne WHO, Wilson PD Jr: Primary osteoarthrosis of the knee or hip. Prevalence of Heberden nodes in relation to age and sex. *JAMA* 231:1256, 1975.

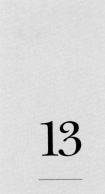

Inflammatory Arthritides

INFLAMMATORY ARTHRITIDES

THE INFLAMMATORY ARTHRITIDES comprise a group of different and for the most part systemic disorders (see Fig. 11.1) that have in common one important feature: inflammatory pannus eroding articular cartilage and bone (Fig. 13.1). An overview of the clinical and radiographic hallmarks of the various inflammatory arthritides is shown in Figure 13.2.

EROSIVE OSTEOARTHRITIS

Erosive osteoarthritis, which tends to be hereditary, is an inflammatory arthritis seen predominantly in middle-aged women. This condition combines certain clinical manifestations of rheumatoid arthritis with certain radiographic features of degenerative joint disease. Involvement is limited to the hands, with the proximal and distal interphalangeal joints being the most frequently affected.

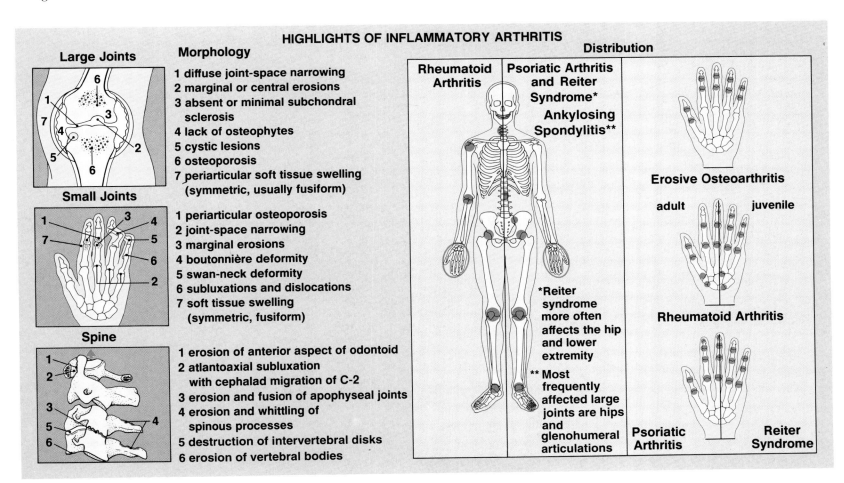

Figure 13.1 Highlights of the morphology and distribution of arthritic lesions in the inflammatory arthritides.

Figure 13.2 Clinical and Radiographic Hallmarks of Inflammatory Arthritides

TYPE OF ARTHRITIS	SITE	CRUCIAL ABNORMALITIES	TECHNIQUE*/PROJECTION

Erosive Osteoarthritis **(F; middle age)**	Hands	Involvement of:
		  Proximal interphalangeal joints
		  Distal interphalangeal joints
		Gull-wing deformities associated with erosions
		Heberden nodes
		Joint ankylosis
			Dorsovolar view

Rheumatoid Arthritis **(F > M; presence of rheumatoid factor and DRW4)**	Hands and wrists	Involvement of:
		  Metacarpophalangeal joints
		  Proximal interphalangeal joints
		Central and marginal erosions
		Periarticular osteoporosis
		Joint deformities: swan-neck, boutonnèire, main en lorgnette, hitchhiker's thumb
			Dorsovolar view
			
			Dorsovolar and lateral views

	Hip	Narrowing of joint space Erosions Acetabular protrusio	Anteroposterior and lateral views
	Knee	Narrowing of joint space Synovial cysts Erosions	Anteroposterior and lateral views
	Ankle and foot	Involvement of subtalar joint Erosions of calcaneus	Anteroposterior and lateral views Lateral and Broden views Lateral view (heel)
Juvenile Rheumatoid Arthritis	Hands	Joint ankylosis Periosteal reaction Growth abnormalities	Dorsovolar view (wrist and hand)
	Knees	Growth abnormalities	Anteroposterior and lateral views
	Cervical spine	Fusion of apophyseal joints C1-2 subluxation	Anteroposterior, lateral, and oblique views Lateral view in flexion
Rheumatoid Variants			
Ankylosing Spondylitis (M > F; young adult; 95% positive for HLA-B27)	Spine	Squaring of vertebral bodies Syndesmophytes "Bamboo" spine Paravertebral ossifications	Anteroposterior and lateral views
	Sacroiliac joints	Inflammatory changes Fusion	Posteroanterior and Ferguson views
	Pelvis	Whiskering of iliac crests and ischial tuberosity	Anteroposterior view
Reiter Syndrome (M > F)	Foot	Involvement of great toe articulations Erosions of calcaneus	Anteroposterior and lateral views
	Spine	Single, coarse syndesmophyte	Anteroposterior and lateral views
	Sacroiliac joints	Unilateral or bilateral but asymmetric involvement	Posteroanterior and Ferguson views
Psoriatic Arthritis (M ≥ F; skin changes; HLA-B27 positive)	Hands	Involvement of distal interphalangeal joints Erosion of terminal tufts Mouse-ear erosions Pencil-in-cup deformities Sausage digit Joint ankylosis Fluffy periosteal reaction	Dorsovolar view
	Foot	Involvement of distal interphalangeal joints Erosions of terminal tufts and calcaneus	Anteroposterior and lateral views (ankle and foot)
	Spine	Single, coarse syndesmophyte	Anteroposterior and lateral views
	Sacroiliac joints	Unilateral or bilateral but asymmetric involvement	Posteroanterior and Ferguson views
Enteropathic Arthropathies	Sacroiliac joints	Symmetric involvement	Posteroanterior and Ferguson views

*Radionuclide bone scan is used to determine the distribution of arthritic lesions in the skeleton.

In the early stage of the disease, the main feature is symmetric synovitis of the interphalangeal joints. Later this is followed by articular erosions, which exhibit a characteristic radiographic feature named the "gull-wing" deformity by Martel. This configuration is seen as a result of central erosion and marginal proliferation of bone (Fig. 13.3); Heberden nodes may also be present. Later in the disease process, bone ankylosis of the phalanges may develop. About 15% of patients with erosive osteoarthritis may develop clinical, laboratory, and radiographic manifestations of rheumatoid arthritis (Fig. 13.4). The exact relationship between these two conditions is still unclear. Some investigators believe that erosive osteoarthritis is actually rheumatoid arthritis originating in unusual sites but subsequently progressing to the articulations that are more typically involved. Others suggest that each is a distinct entity, citing as evidence the fact that the synovial fluid of patients with rheumatoid arthritis does not resemble that of patients with erosive osteoarthritis, that the immunologic abnormalities commonly seen in rheumatoid arthritis are absent in the latter condition, and that the serologic test for rheumatoid factor is negative.

Occasionally, a variant of erosive osteoarthritis may be seen as one of the features of Cronkhite-Canada syndrome. This rare systemic disorder also manifests with generalized gastrointestinal polyposis, hyperpigmentation of the skin, and nail atrophy.

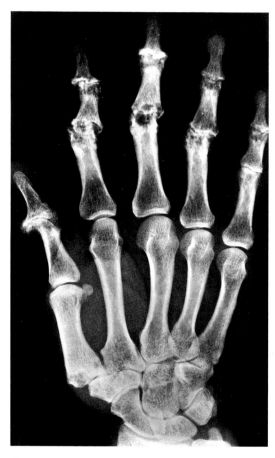

Figure 13.3 Dorsovolar film of the left hand of a 48-year-old woman with erosive osteoarthritis shows the typical involvement of the proximal and distal interphalangeal joints. Note the "gull-wing" pattern of articular erosion, a configuration resulting from peripheral bone erosion in the distal side of the joint and central erosion in the proximal side of the joint associated with marginal bone proliferation.

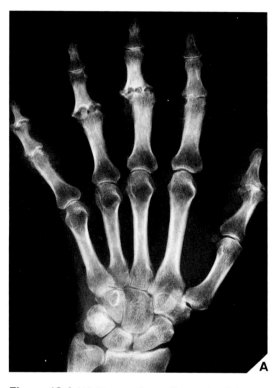

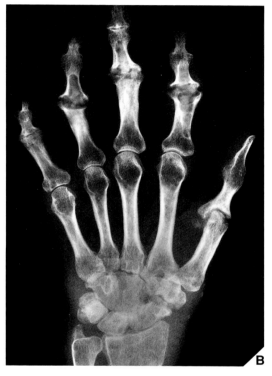

Figure 13.4 (A) Dorsovolar radiograph of the hand of a 58-year-old woman demonstrates the gull-wing configuration of erosive changes in the proximal interphalangeal joints and the distal interphalangeal joint of the small finger. Because of protracted pain and lack of response to conservative treatment, she underwent joint resection followed by implantation of silicone-rubber prostheses in the proximal interphalangeal joints of the index, middle, and ring fingers, together with fusion of the interphalangeal joint of the thumb and the distal interphalangeal joint of the small finger. Five years after surgery she developed the classic radiographic features of rheumatoid arthritis involving the wrists (B), elbows, shoulders, hips, and cervical spine. Note the surgical fusion of interphalangeal joints of the thumb and fifth finger, as well as the spontaneous fusion of the distal interphalangeal joints of the index and ring fingers.

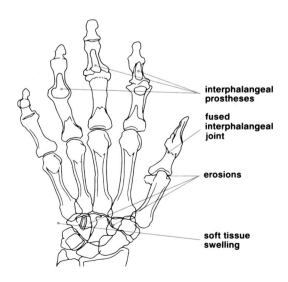

interphalangeal prostheses

fused interphalangeal joint

erosions

soft tissue swelling

TREATMENT The main objective of therapy in patients with inflammatory erosive osteoarthritis is relief of pain and restoration of joint function. Surgical intervention is often necessary for the relief of persistent pain and the correction of severe deformities. One of the most effective procedures is joint replacement by means of silicone-rubber arthroplasties (see Fig. 13.4B). The indications for this type of surgery are loss of the joint space, synovial proliferation with joint destruction, loss of normal alignment, and uncontrolled pain.

RHEUMATOID ARTHRITIS

Adult Rheumatoid Arthritis

Rheumatoid arthritis is a progressive, chronic, systemic inflammatory disease affecting primarily the synovial joints; women are affected three times more often than men. The course of the disease varies from patient to patient, and there is a striking tendency toward spontaneous remissions and exacerbations. The detection of rheumatoid factor, representing specific antibodies in the patient's serum, is an important diagnostic finding. Although it is still debatable, some investigators also include under this rubric a condition called *seronegative rheumatoid arthritis* (see below), in which patients present without rheumatoid factor but with the clinical and radiographic picture of rheumatoid arthritis.

Rheumatoid Factors

Rheumatoid factors, so widely used by clinicians, are antigammaglobulin antibodies that are elaborated in part by rheumatoid synovium. Rheumatoid factors in synovial fluid are either of the IgG or IgM variety. They combine with their antigens (immunoglobulin G [IgG]) to form immune complexes. These complexes activate the complement system, which releases mediators responsive for producing inflammation within the joint structures. Since rheumatoid factors can be found in the joint fluids of patients with nonrheumatoid disorders, their presence alone is not diagnostic of rheumatoid arthritis. However, finding high titers of these factors in a joint effusion strongly suggests the diagnosis of rheumatoid arthritis. Early in the course of disease, rheumatoid factors may be demonstrated in the synovial fluid before they are positive in the serum, allowing early diagnosis.

Rheumatoid factors participate in the pathogenesis of rheumatoid arthritis through the formation of local and circulating antigen-antibody complexes. In synovial fluid, both IgM and IgG rheumatoid factors can combine with antigen (IgG) to form immune complexes. The complement system is activated, resulting in the attraction of polymorphonuclear leukocytes into the joint space. Discharge of their hydrolytic enzymes causes destruction of joint tissues. The process initiating these events is as yet unknown.

Radiographic Features

Rheumatoid arthritis is characterized by a diffuse, usually multicompartmental symmetric narrowing of the joint space associated with marginal or central erosions, periarticular osteoporosis, and periarticular soft tissue swelling; subchondral sclerosis is minimal or absent and formation of osteophytes is lacking.

Large Joint Involvement

Any of the large weight-bearing and nonweight-bearing joints can be affected by rheumatoid arthritis. Regardless of the size of the joint

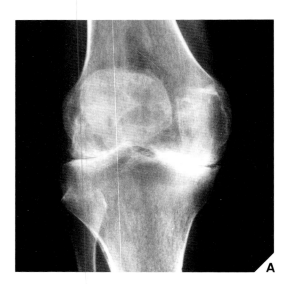
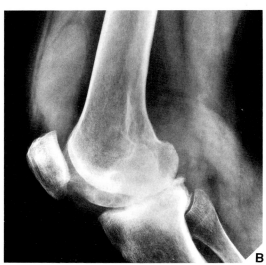

Figure 13.5 Anteroposterior (A) and lateral (B) radiographs of the knee of a 52-year-old woman with rheumatoid arthritis affecting several joints show tricompartmental involvement. Note the periarticular osteoporosis and joint effusion.

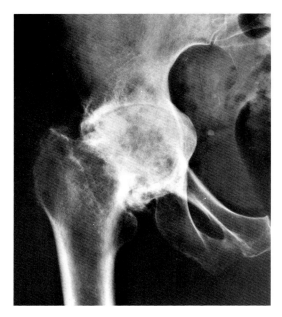

Figure 13.6 Anteroposterior view of the right hip of a 60-year-old woman with advanced rheumatoid arthritis shows concentric joint space narrowing, with axial migration of the femoral head leading to acetabular protrusio.

and the site of involvement, certain radiographic features can be identified that are characteristic of this inflammatory process.

OSTEOPOROSIS In rheumatoid arthritis, unlike osteoarthritis, osteoporosis is a striking feature. In the early stage of the disease, osteoporosis is localized to periarticular areas, but with progression of the condition a generalized osteoporosis can be observed.

JOINT SPACE NARROWING This is usually a symmetric process with concentric narrowing of the joint. In the knee, all three joint compartments are involved (Fig. 13.5). Narrowing in the hip joint leads to axial or, less commonly, medial migration of the femoral head, which in more advanced stages may result in acetabular protrusio (Fig. 13.6). Cephalad migration of the humeral head may also be seen secondary to destructive changes in the shoulder joint and rupture of the rotator cuff (Fig. 13.7); resorption of the distal end of the clavicle, which assumes a pencil-like appearance, may also be observed. Tear of the rotator cuff in this condition must be differentiated from the chronic traumatic form of this abnormality (see Figs. 5.32-5.34).

ARTICULAR EROSIONS Erosive destruction of a joint may be central or peripheral in location. As a rule, reparative processes are absent or very minimal, thus there is no evidence of subchondral sclerosis or osteophytosis (Fig. 13.8), which may be present only if secondary degenerative changes are superimposed on the underlying inflammatory process (see Fig. 12.5).

SYNOVIAL CYSTS AND PSEUDOCYSTS These radiolucent defects are usually seen in close proximity to the joint (Fig. 13.9). They may or may not communicate with the joint space.

JOINT EFFUSION Fluid can be best demonstrated in the knee joint on the lateral projection (see Fig. 13.5B). Fluid in the other large joints such as the shoulder, elbow, and hip can be best demonstrated by magnetic resonance imaging.

Small Joint Involvement

Rheumatoid arthritis characteristically affects the small joints of the wrist, as well as the metacarpophalangeal and proximal interphalangeal joints of the hands and feet. As a rule, the distal interphalangeal joints in the hand are spared, although in advanced stages of the disease even these may be affected. This latter point, however, is controversial, since some investigators believe that if the distal interphalangeal joints are involved, the condition may represent juvenil-rheumatoid arthritis or another form of polyarthritis, not classic rheumatoid arthritis.

In addition to the characteristic changes exhibited in large joint involvement, the small joints may also show radiographic features specific for these sites.

SOFT TISSUE SWELLING This earliest sign of rheumatoid arthritis usually has a fusiform, symmetric shape. It is periarticular in location and represents a combination of joint effusion, edema, and tenosynovitis.

JOINT DEFORMITIES Although not pathognomonic for rheumatoid arthritis, certain deformations such as the *swan-neck deformity* and the *boutonnière deformity* are more often seen in this form of arthritis than in other inflammatory arthritides. The first of these represents hyperextension in the proximal interphalangeal joint and flexion in the distal interphalangeal joint, a configuration resembling a swan's neck (Fig. 13.10). In the boutonnière deformity, the

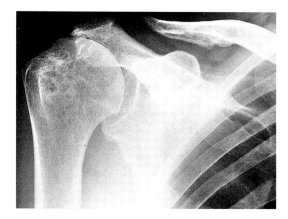

Figure 13.7 Anteroposterior view of the right shoulder of a 72-year-old man with advanced rheumatoid arthritis shows upward migration of the humeral head secondary to rotator cuff tear, a common complication of rheumatoid changes in the shoulder joint. Note the characteristic tapered erosion of the distal end of the clavicle, erosions of the humeral head, and the substantial degree of periarticular osteoporosis.

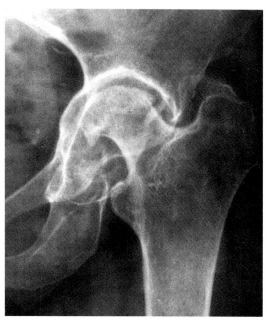

Figure 13.8 Anteroposterior view of the left hip of a 59-year-old woman with advanced rheumatoid polyarthritis demonstrates the typical erosions of the femoral head and acetabulum. Note the lack of osteophytosis and the only very minimal reactive sclerosis.

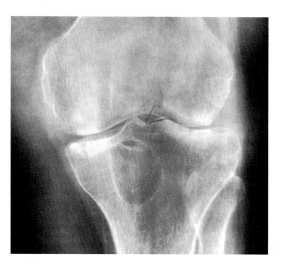

Figure 13.9 Anteroposterior radiograph of the left knee of a 35-year-old woman with rheumatoid arthritis shows a large synovial cyst in the proximal tibia.

configuration is just the opposite, with flexion in the proximal joint and extension in the distal interphalangeal joint (Fig. 13.11). The word *boutonnière* is French for "buttonhole," the term for this deformity deriving from the configuration of the finger while securing a flower to a lapel. A similar deformation of the thumb is called *hitchhiker's thumb*.

Moreover, subluxations and dislocations with malalignment of the fingers are common findings in advanced stages of rheumatoid arthritis. Particularly characteristic are ulnar deviation of the fingers in the metacarpophalangeal joints and radial deviation of the wrist in the radiocarpal articulation (Fig. 13.12). In far-advanced stages of rheumatoid arthritis, shortening of several phalanges may be encountered secondary to destructive changes in the joints associated with dislocations in the metacarpophalangeal joints. This deformity appears as a "telescoping" of the fingers, hence its name, *main en lorgnette*, from the French name for the telescoping type of opera glass (Fig. 13.13). An abnormally wide space between the lunate and scaphoid may also be encountered in advanced stages of the disease secondary to erosion and rupture of the scapholunate ligament (Fig. 13.14); this phenomenon resembles the Terry-Thomas sign seen secondary to trauma (see Figs. 6.53, 6.54). Joint deformities are also often seen in the foot; the subtalar joint is frequently affected, and subluxation in the metatarsophalangeal joints often leads to deformities such as hallux valgus and hammertoes.

Joint Ankylosis A rare finding that may be observed in advanced stages of rheumatoid arthritis, joint ankylosis is most commonly encountered in the midcarpal articulations. Ankylotic changes in the wrist are more common in patients with juvenile rheumatoid arthritis and with so-called seronegative rheumatoid arthritis.

Involvement of the Spine

The thoracic and lumbar segments are affected by rheumatoid arthritis only on rare occasions. The cervical spine, however, is involved in approximately 50% of individuals with this condition. The most characteristic radiographic features of rheumatoid arthritis in the cervical spine can be observed in the odontoid process, the atlantoaxial joints, and the apophyseal joints. Erosive changes may

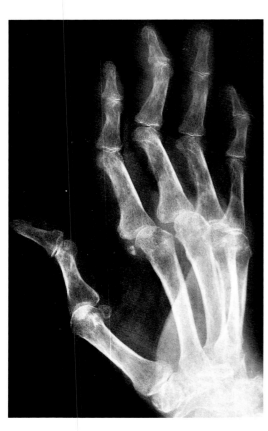

Figure 13.10 Oblique view of the hand of a 59-year-old woman shows the swan-neck deformity of the second through fifth fingers. Note the flexion in the distal interphalangeal joints and the extension in the proximal interphalangeal joints, the hallmarks of this abnormality.

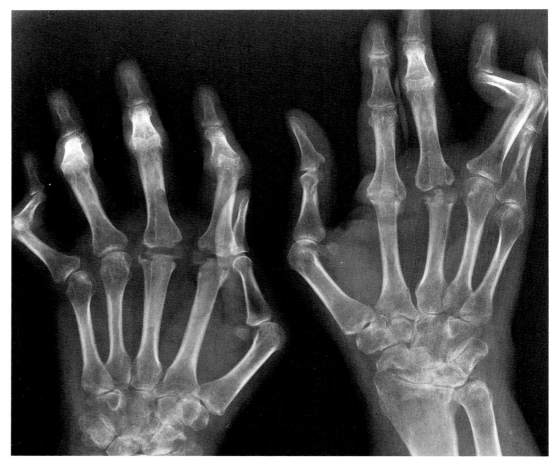

Figure 13.11 Dorsovolar view of the hands of a 48-year-old woman with rheumatoid arthritis demonstrates the boutonnière deformity in the small and ring fingers of the right hand and in the ring finger of the left hand.

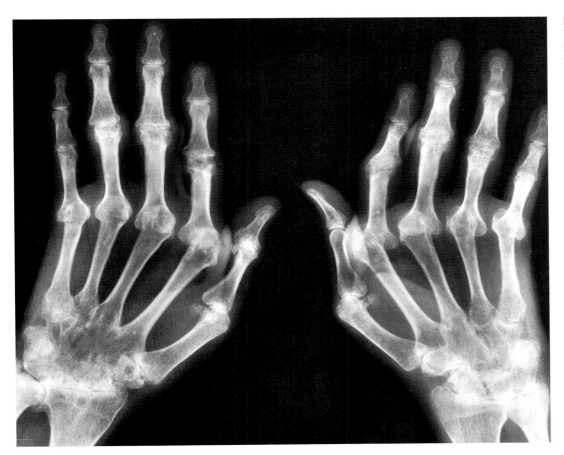

Figure 13.12 Dorsovolar projection of both hands of a 51-year-old woman shows subluxation in the metacarpophalangeal joints resulting in ulnar deviation of the fingers and radial deviation in the radiocarpal articulations.

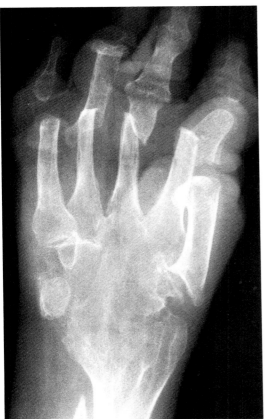

Figure 13.13
Dorsovolar view of the right hand of a 54-year-old woman with long-standing advanced rheumatoid arthritis demonstrates the *main en lorgnette* deformity. Note the telescoping of the fingers secondary to destructive joint changes and dislocations in the metacarpophalangeal joints. There is also ankylosis of the radiocarpal and intercarpal articulations and "penciling" of the distal ulna.

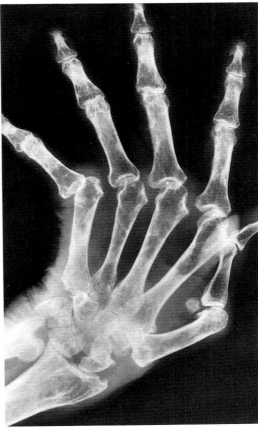

Figure 13.14
Dorsovolar view of the hand of a 60-year-old woman shows a gap between the scaphoid and lunate, indicating destruction of the scapholunate ligament. Note also the subluxation in the metacarpophalangeal joints resulting in ulnar deviation of the fingers.

be encountered in the odontoid process (see Fig. 11.32) and apophyseal joints (Fig. 13.15), while subluxation is a common finding in the atlantoaxial joint (see Fig. 11.33), frequently accompanied by superior migration of the odontoid process. The most frequent radiographic abnormality is laxity of the transverse ligament connecting the odontoid to the atlas. This laxity becomes apparent on the radiograph obtained in the lateral view of the flexed cervical spine, is expressed by subluxation in the atlantoaxial joint, and is frequently accompanied by superior migration of the odontoid process. This complication often requires surgical intervention and the most common procedure to correct this is posterior fusion.

Erosive changes may be encountered in the odontoid process and apophyseal joints. Again, it is the flexed lateral view of the cervical spine that best demonstrates the erosive changes of the apophyseal joints. Severe involvement of the joints leads to subluxations. In extremely rare cases, in a manner similar to that in juvenile rheumatoid arthritis, the apophyseal joints may ankylose.

The other structures occasionally affected by rheumatoid process are the intervertebral disks and adjacent vertebral bodies, which become involved as a result of synovitis extending from the joint of Luschka. Only a small percentage of patients with cervical disease may develop cervical myelopathy. Magnetic resonance imaging is an ideal modality to evaluate spinal cord involvement in these patients.

Complications of Rheumatoid Arthritis

The complications of rheumatoid arthritis are related not only to the inflammatory process itself but also to the sequelae of treatment (see the discussion of the complications of treatment in Chapter 11). The large doses of steroids that are commonly prescribed in therapy often lead to the development of generalized osteoporosis. Severe osteoporosis and large bony erosions may in turn precipitate pathologic fracture, a frequent complication. Tear of the rotator cuff may also occur due to erosion by inflammatory pannus in the shoulder joint (see Fig. 13.7). In the knee, a large popliteal (Baker) cyst may

complicate rheumatoid arthritic changes (Fig. 13.16); this condition may be misdiagnosed as thrombophlebitis.

Rheumatoid Nodulosis

A variant of rheumatoid arthritis, rheumatoid nodulosis occurs predominantly in men. It is a nonsystemic disorder characterized by the presence of multiple subcutaneous nodules (Fig. 13.17) and a very high rheumatoid factor titer; as a rule, there are no joint abnormalities. Occasionally, small cystic lesions may be present in various bones. Nodules are usually different in size and consistency, and distribution is over the elbows, extensor surfaces of hands and feet, and other pressure points. The most striking feature is lack of systemic manifestations of rheumatoid arthritis.

On histologic examination the nodules show typical rheumatoid changes, including central necrosis surrounded by palisading histiocytes and fibroblasts, with an outer layer of connective tissue and chronic inflammatory cells. Only occasionally will the histologic appearance be atypical. In these cases, the nodule may contain abundant cholesterol clefts and lipid-loaded macrophages, suggestive of xanthoma or even multicentric reticulohistiocytosis.

Therapy is usually limited to the occasional use of nonsteroidal anti-inflammatory drugs. Nodules that cause local pain because of nerve compression can be surgically removed. Some investigators have reported a decrease in nodule size after the use of penicillamine. These reports are controversial, however, since the regression and even disappearance of rheumatoid nodules may occur without any treatment at all.

In classic rheumatoid arthritis, small-vessel vasculitis is a primary factor in nodule development, and circulating immune complexes used by rheumatoid synovium are responsible for such extra-articular manifestations as vasculitis, polyserositis, and nodules. In rheumatoid nodulosis, however, nodules develop in the absence of active joint disease. Thus, the pathogenesis of rheumatoid nodulosis remains unclear.

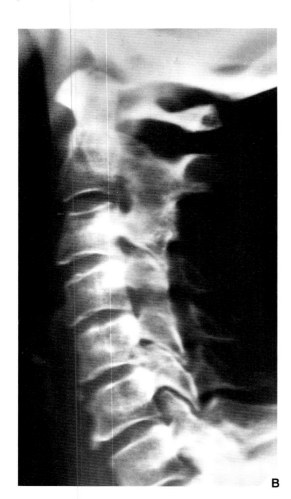

Figure 13.15 Lateral tomogram of the cervical spine in a 44-year-old woman demonstrates the erosions and narrowing of the apophyseal joints typical of rheumatoid arthritis.

B

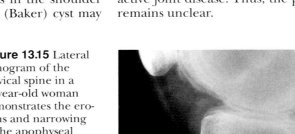

Figure 13.16
A 31-year-old woman with a two-year history of seropositive rheumatoid arthritis developed swelling of the upper calf and tenderness in the popliteal fossa. A presumptive diagnosis of thrombophlebitis was made, but a venogram failed to corroborate this. This lateral view of a knee arthrogram shows a large popliteal (Baker) cyst dissecting into the medial aspect of the calf. This condition is a well documented complication in patients with rheumatoid arthritis. (Reprinted with permission from Greenspan A, et al., 1983)

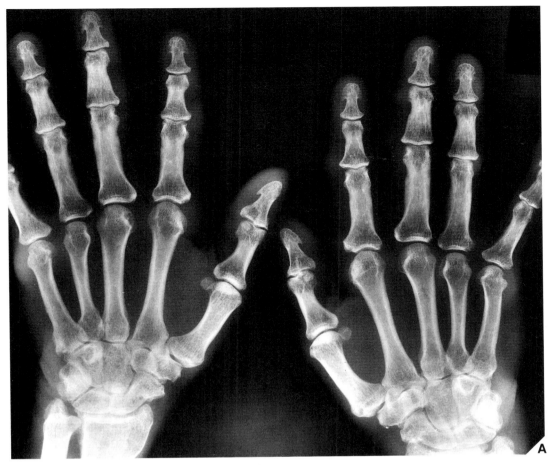

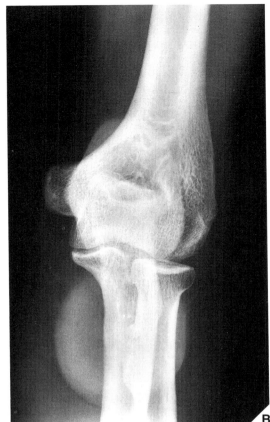

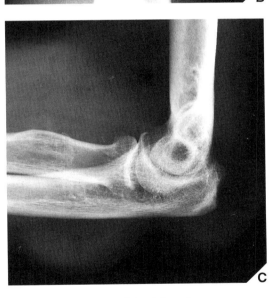

Figure 13.17 A 52-year-old man with a 15-year history of polyarthritis presented with large, fluctuant nodules on the dorsal aspect of the hands and elbows. A high titer of rheumatoid factor (1:1280) was identified in his serum. (A) Dorsovolar view of both hands shows several soft tissue nodules adjacent to joints. Note the lack of joint abnormalities. Anteroposterior (B) and lateral (C) views of the left elbow demonstrate similar soft tissue masses at the dorsal aspect of the proximal forearm. The elbow joint is intact. (Reprinted from Greenspan A, et al., 1983)

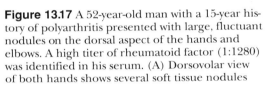

soft tissue nodules

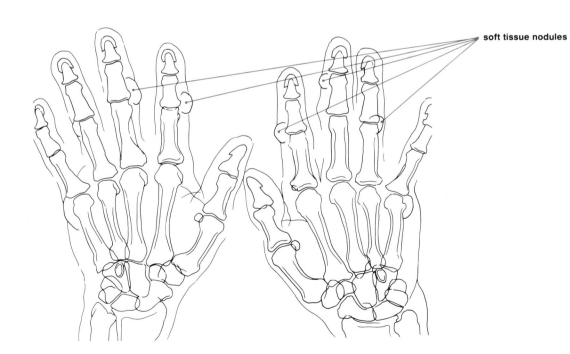

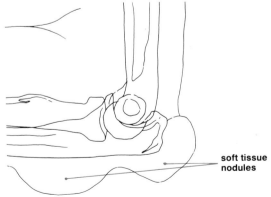

soft tissue nodules

A positive family history of rheumatoid arthritis in some patients with rheumatoid nodulosis and the occurrence of familial nodulosis suggest the involvement of hereditary factors. Investigations into tissue typing, particularly the search for DW4/DRW4 antigens, may illustrate the pathogenesis of this rheumatoid variant. The strong male preponderance suggests that androgens may modify disease expression in genetically predisposed individuals. Rheumatoid nodulosis is often misdiagnosed as gout or xanthomatosis. Moreover, it should be kept in mind when evaluating this condition that approximately 20% of patients with classic rheumatoid arthritis develop rheumatoid nodules, which are usually located at sites of pressure or stress such as the dorsal aspect of the hands and forearms (Fig. 13.18). Articular involvement in nodular rheumatoid arthritis distinguishes it from rheumatoid nodulosis, which consequently has a better prognosis.

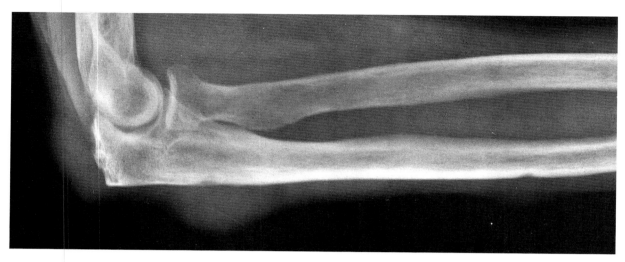

Figure 13.18 A 39-year-old man with rheumatoid arthritis was originally misdiagnosed as having gout. Lateral view of the right elbow demonstrates erosions of the olecranon process, olecranon bursitis on the left, and rheumatoid nodules on the dorsal aspect of the forearm. Note the characteristic pit-like cortical erosions at the site of the rheumatoid nodules. This presentation of rheumatoid arthritis should not be mistaken for rheumatoid nodulosis.

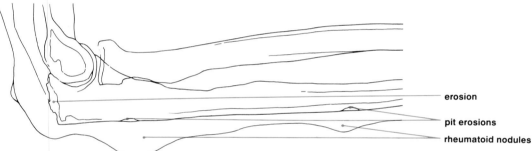

erosion

pit erosions

rheumatoid nodules

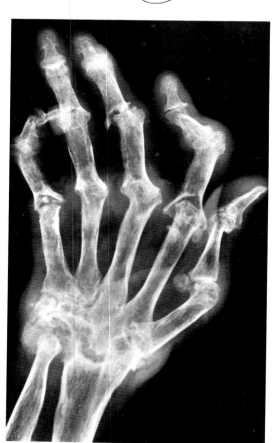

Figure 13.19
Dorsovolar view of the wrist and hand of a 26-year-old woman with a 14-year history of juvenile rheumatoid arthritis shows severe destructive changes in the wrist and in the metacarpophalangeal and proximal interphalangeal articulations. Note the ankylosis of the third and fourth metacarpophalangeal joints and periostitis involving the proximal phalanges and metacarpals.

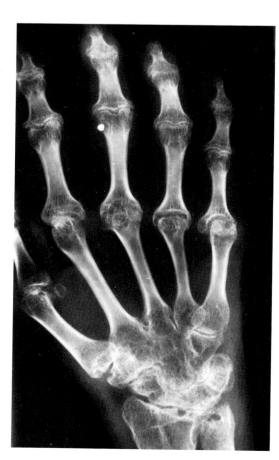

Figure 13.20
Dorsovolar projection of the left hand of a 25-year-old woman with a ten-year history of juvenile rheumatoid arthritis shows advanced destructive changes in multiple joints of the hand and wrist. Joint ankylosis is evident in several articulations.

Juvenile Rheumatoid Arthritis

Juvenile rheumatoid arthritis is a group of at least three chronic inflammatory synovial diseases that affect children; girls are more frequently affected than boys. The three defined subtypes are: Still disease, polyarticular arthritis, and pauciarticular arthritis. Each of these subgroups has distinct clinical and laboratory findings and different natural histories. There is no pathognomonic laboratory test for any of them and the diagnosis is based upon the clinical spectrum exhibited by a given patient.

Still Disease

Still disease is well known for sudden onset of spiking fever, lymphadenopathy, and an evanescent salmon-colored skin rash. Patients may exhibit hepatosplenomegaly, fatigue, anorexia, and weight loss. The majority of patients have chronic and recurrent arthralgias. A significant number of patients, depending on the series, may also subsequently develop chronic polyarthritis. Adult patients may also develop a poorly understood Still-like disease with fever and arthralgias.

Polyarticular Juvenile Rheumatoid Arthritis

Polyarticular juvenile rheumatoid arthritis consists of inflammation at four or more joints with associated findings of anorexia, weight loss, fatigue, and adenopathy. Growth retardation is common. This disorder also results in the following abnormalities: undergrowth of the mandible, early closure of the growth plates resulting in shortening of metacarpals and metatarsals, and overgrowths of the epiphyses of the knees, hips, and shoulders. A worse prognosis occurs in patients with positive rheumatoid factors.

Juvenile Rheumatoid Arthritis with Pauciarticular Onset

The third subtype of juvenile rheumatoid arthritis has pauciarticular onset, with four or fewer joints involved. About 40% of patients with juvenile rheumatoid arthritis exhibit involvement of fewer than four joints in the first six months of the disease. Some of these patients may even present with negative rheumatoid factor while others may have positive antigen HLA-B27. Pediatric rheumatologists have attempted to define other subgroups within this pauciarticular subgroup but, with the exception of HLA-B27-positive children with sacroiliitis, such definitions are broad and clinically dependent on unique systemic features such as iridocyclitis. However, involvement of the sacroiliac joints is not a feature of juvenile rheumatoid arthritis as was thought in the past; it represents rather juvenile onset of ankylosing spondylitis. Similarly, some investigators believe that patients with pauciarticular arthritis, particularly those with positive histocompatibility antigen HLA-B27, may in fact have atypical ankylosing spondylitis syndrome or spondyloarthropathy; both these conditions are different from rheumatoid arthritis.

Other Types of Juvenile Rheumatoid Arthritis

It is worthwhile to note that two new diagnostic terms currently in use in childhood arthritides—*juvenile chronic arthritis* and *juvenile arthritis*—are not equivalent to each other or to classic juvenile rheumatoid arthritis. These conditions lack any characteristic radiographic features. Much research is needed to gain a better understanding of juvenile rheumatoid arthritis before we will clearly be able to define the number of different diseases involved.

Radiographic Features

Juvenile rheumatoid arthritis exhibits many of the features of adult rheumatoid arthritis. However, some additional features that are almost pathognomonic for this condition have been identified.

PERIOSTEAL REACTION This feature is usually seen along the shafts of the proximal phalanges and metacarpals (Fig. 13.19).

JOINT ANKYLOSIS Ankylosis may occur not only in the wrist but also in the interphalangeal articulations (Fig. 13.20). Fusion in the apophyseal joints of the cervical spine is also a characteristic finding (Fig. 13.21).

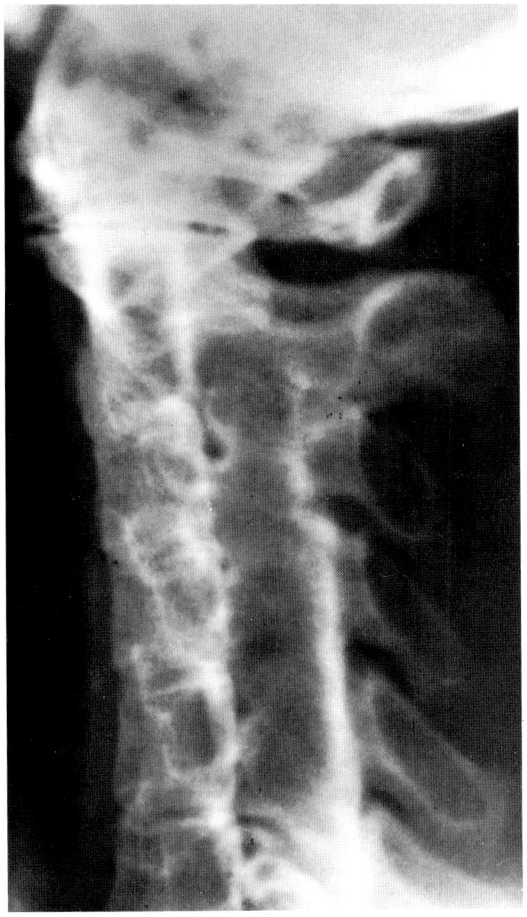

Figure 13.21 Lateral view of the cervical spine in a 25-year-old woman with a 15-year history of polyarthritis shows fusion of the apophyseal joints, a common finding in juvenile rheumatoid arthritis.

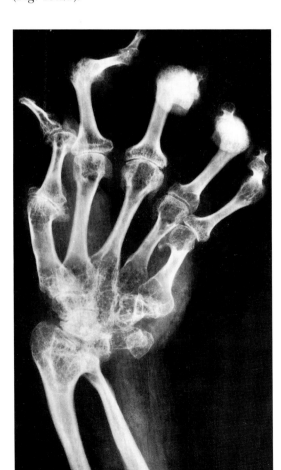

Figure 13.22 Dorsovolar view of the hand of a 24-year-old woman with advanced juvenile rheumatoid arthritis, which was diagnosed when she was seven years old, shows retarded growth of the bones due to early fusion of the growth plates. Multiple deformities of the digits include hitchhiker's thumb and a boutonnière configuration of the index finger.

GROWTH ABNORMALITIES Because the onset of juvenile rheumatoid arthritis occurs before completion of skeletal maturation, alterations in growth of the bones is a common finding. The involvement of epiphyseal sites often leads to fusion of the growth plate, with resultant retardation of bone growth (Fig. 13.22); it may also precipitate acceleration of growth due to stimulation of the growth plates by hyperemia. Enlargement of the epiphysis of the distal femur leads to characteristic overgrowth of the condyles in the knee (Fig. 13.23).

SERONEGATIVE SPONDYLOARTHROPATHIES

Ankylosing Spondylitis

Clinical Features

Ankylosing spondylitis, known in the European literature as *Bechterev disease* or *Marie-Strümpell disease*, is a chronic, progressive, inflammatory arthritis principally affecting the synovial joints of the spine and adjacent soft tissues as well as the sacroiliac joints; however, the peripheral joints such as the hips, shoulders, and knees may also be involved. It is seen seven times more frequently in men than in women, and predominantly at a young age. Patients with ankylosing spondylitis frequently exhibit extra-articular features of disease including iritis, pulmonary fibrosis, cardiac conduction defects, aortic incompetence, spinal cord compression, and amyloidosis. Patients may also have low-grade fever, anorexia, fatigue, and weight loss.

Rheumatoid factor is negative in patients with ankylosing spondylitis, which is the prototype of the seronegative spondyloarthropathies. A high percentage of patients (up to 95%), however, possess histocompatibility antigen HLA-B27. Pathologically, ankylosing spondylitis is a diffuse proliferative synovitis of the diarthrodial joints exhibiting features similar to those seen in rheumatoid arthritis.

Radiographic Features

Squaring of the anterior border of the lower thoracic and lumbar vertebrae is one of the earliest radiographic features of ankylosing spondylitis, best demonstrated on the lateral view of the spine (Fig. 13.24). As the condition progresses, syndesmophytes form, bridging the vertebral bodies (Fig. 13.25). The delicate appearance of these excrescences and their vertical rather than horizontal orientation distinguish them from the osteophytes of degenerative spine disease. Paravertebral ossifications are common in ankylosing spondylitis. When the apophyseal joints and vertebral bodies fuse late in the

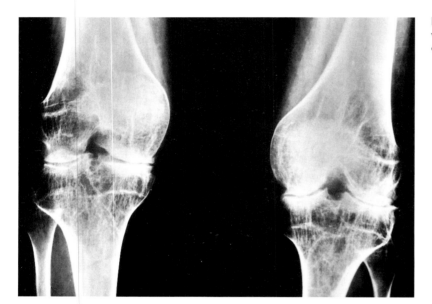

Figure 13.23 Anteroposterior view of both knees of a 20-year-old woman with juvenile rheumatoid arthritis shows overgrowth of the medial condyles, one of the characteristic features of this disorder.

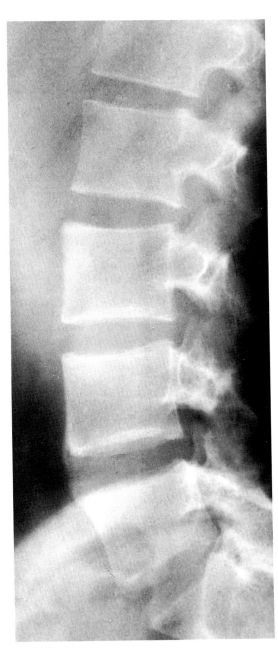

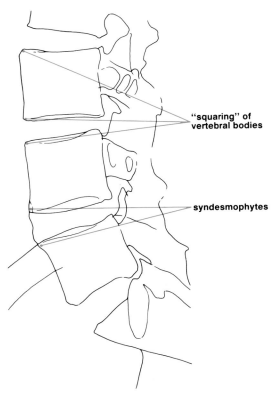

Figure 13.24 Lateral view of the lumbar spine in a 28-year-old man demonstrates squaring of the vertebral bodies secondary to small osseous erosions at the corners. This finding is an early radiographic feature of ankylosing spondylitis. Note also the formation of syndesmophytes at the L4-5 disk space.

"squaring" of vertebral bodies

syndesmophytes

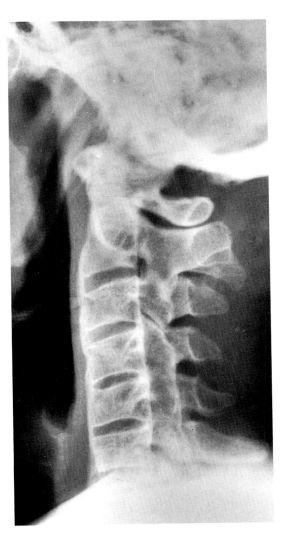

Figure 13.25 Lateral view of the cervical spine in a 31-year-old man demonstrates delicate syndesmophytes bridging the vertebral bodies, a common feature of ankylosing spondylitis. Note the fusion of several apophyseal joints.

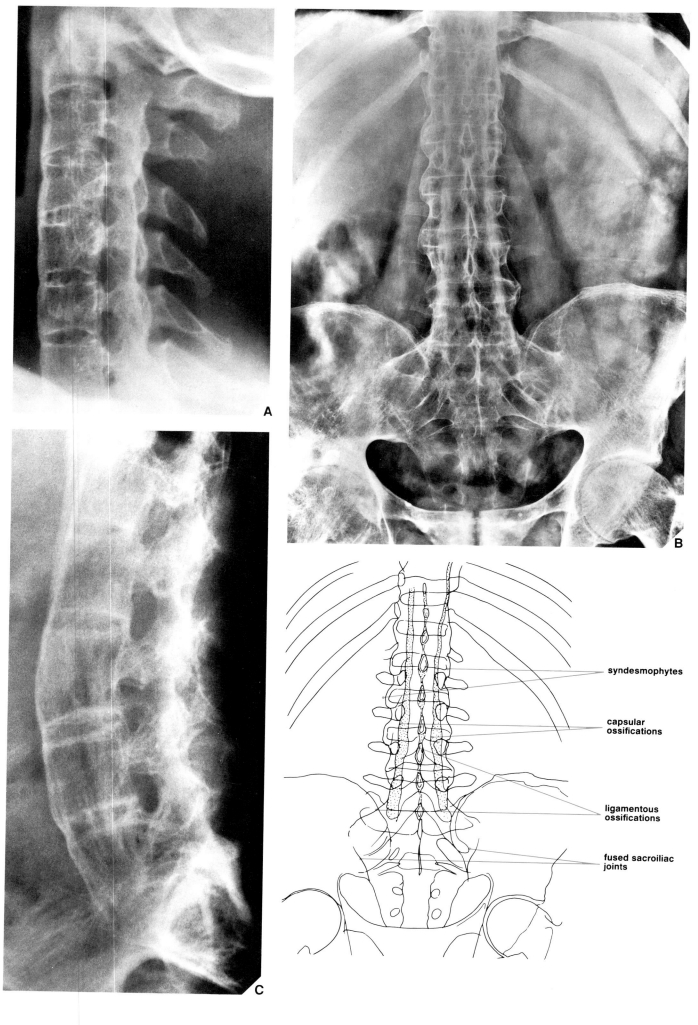

Figure 13.26 (A) Lateral view of the cervical spine in a 53-year-old man with advanced ankylosing spondylitis shows anterior syndesmophytes bridging the vertebral bodies and posterior fusion of the apophyseal joints, together with paravertebral ossifications, producing a "bamboo-spine" appearance. The same phenomenon is seen on the anteroposterior (B) and lateral (C) projections of the lumbosacral spine. Note on the anteroposterior view the fusion of the sacroiliac joints and the involvement of both hip joints, which show axial migration of the femoral heads similar to that seen in rheumatoid arthritis.

A

B

C

syndesmophytes

capsular ossifications

ligamentous ossifications

fused sacroiliac joints

course of the disease, a radiographic hallmark of this condition, the "bamboo" spine, can be observed; the sacroiliac joints are also invariably affected in this process (Fig. 13.26).

In the peripheral joints, inflammatory changes may be indistinguishable from those seen in rheumatoid arthritis (see Fig. 13.26B). In the foot, erosions characteristically occur at certain tendinous insertions, particularly in the os calcis (see Figs. 11.29, 11.30). Involvement of the ischial tuberosities and iliac crests exhibits a lace-like formation of new bone called "whiskering."

Reiter Syndrome

Clinical Features

Reiter syndrome is a clinical infectious disease that affects five times more males than females and is characterized by arthritis, conjunctivitis, and urethritis. Reiter syndrome is also well known for the presence of mucocutaneous rash, keratoderma blenorrhagica. Like ankylosing spondylitis, eye involvement is common and can include conjunctivitis, iritis, uveitis, and episcleritis. Approximately 60% to 80% of patients are HLA-B27 positive. This frequency varies according to the ethnic origin of the patient. Unlike ankylosing spondylitis, Reiter syndrome may exhibit unilateral sacroiliac diseases.

Two types of this syndrome have been identified. First, the sporadic or endemic type, which is common in the United States, is associated with nongonococcal urethritis, prostatitis, or hemorrhagic cystitis; it occurs almost exclusively in males. In Europe a second type has been identified, an epidemic form associated with bacillary (*Shigella*) dysentery; it may be seen in women as well. There has been considerable research on the putative role of *Yersina entercolitica* in inducing disease, particularly in Scandinavia, where such infections are more prevalent than in North America.

Radiographic Features

Radiographically, Reiter syndrome is marked by peripheral and usually asymmetric arthritis, with a predilection for the joints of the lower limb. The foot is the most common site of involvement, particularly the metatarsophalangeal joints and the heels (Fig. 13.27). Periosteal new bone formation is not uncommon. Involvement of the sacroiliac joints, which is frequently encountered, may be either asymmetric (unilateral or bilateral) or symmetric (bilateral) (Fig. 13.28). In the thoracic and lumbar spine, coarse syndesmophytes or paraspinal ossifications may be present, characteristically bridging adjacent vertebrae (Fig. 13.29).

Psoriatic Arthritis

Clinical Features

There are five specific subgroups of arthritic syndromes described in psoriatic arthritis.

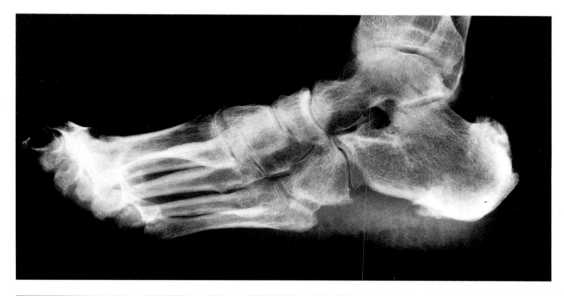

Figure 13.27 Lateral view of the foot of a 28-year-old man with Reiter syndrome demonstrates the "fluffy" periostitis of the os calcis and inflammatory changes of the metatarsophalangeal joints typical of this condition.

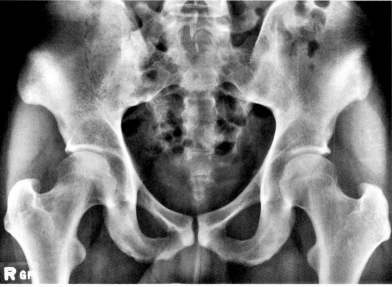

Figure 13.28 Anteroposterior view of the pelvis of the patient shown in Figure 13.27 demonstrates symmetric bilateral involvement of the sacroiliac joints.

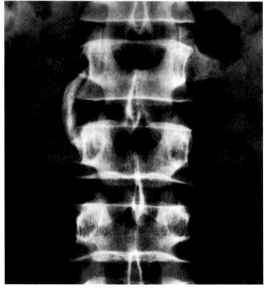

Figure 13.29 Anteroposterior view of the lumbar spine of a 23-year-old man with Reiter syndrome demonstrates a single, coarse syndesmophyte bridging the L-2 and L-3 vertebrae.

Subgroup 1, or classic psoriatic arthritis, includes nail pathology with occasional involvement of the terminal tufts and involvement of the distal and occasionally proximal interphalangeal joints of the hand (Fig. 13.30).

Subgroup 2, well known for the "opera glass" deformity of the hand, is termed *arthritis mutilans* because of the extensive destruction of the phalanges and metacarpal joints including the "pencil-in-cup" deformity (Fig.13.31); patients with arthritis mutilans often have sacroilitis.

Subgroup 3 is characterized by symmetric polyarthritis and may result in ankylosis of the proximal and distal interphalangeal joints. In this form, psoriatic arthritis is frequently indistinguishable from rheumatoid arthritis (Fig. 13.32).

Subgroup 4 is characterized by oligoarticular arthritis, and in contrast to subgroup 3 the joint involvement is asymmetric, generally including the proximal and distal interphalangeal and metacarpophalangeal articulations (Fig. 13.33). Patients with this oligoarticu-

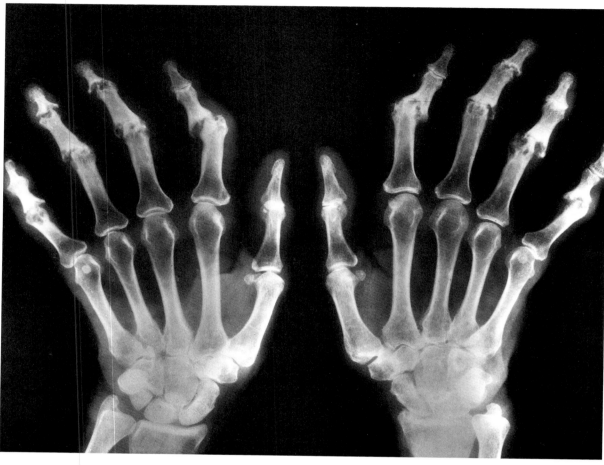

Figure 13.30 Dorsovolar view of both hands of a 55-year-old woman who presented with skin changes typical of psoriasis shows destructive changes in the proximal and distal interphalangeal joints. Note the spontaneous fusion of the distal interphalangeal joint of the small finger of the right hand and the distal interphalangeal joint of the ring finger of the left hand.

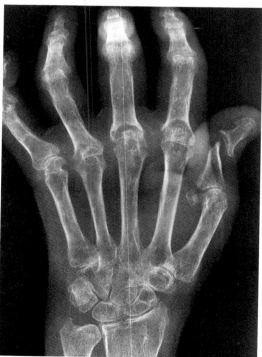

Figure 13.31
Dorsovolar view of the hand of a 57-year-old woman shows the typical presentation of psoriatic polyarthritis. The "pencil-in-cup" deformity in the interphalangeal joint of the thumb is characteristic of this form of psoriasis.

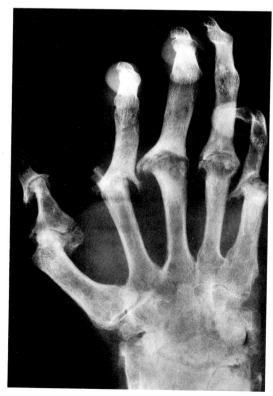

Figure 13.32
Dorsovolar view of the left hand of a 67-year-old man with the polyarthritic form of psoriatic arthritis demonstrates fusion of multiple joints. The swan-neck deformity of the small finger is similar to that seen in patients with rheumatoid arthritis.

lar arthritis are the most frequent subgroup of psoriatic arthritis and are known for the appearance of sausage-like swelling of digits.

Subgroup 5 is a spondyloarthropathy that has features similar to those of ankylosing spondylitis.

The etiology of psoriatic arthritis is unknown and its relationship to rheumatoid arthritis and spondyloarthropathies is still unsettled. It is seen in 5% to 7% of patients with psoriasis, and predominantly involves the distal interphalangeal joints of the hands and feet, although other sites of involvement—the proximal interphalangeal

joints as well as the hips, knees, ankles, shoulders, and spine—may also be encountered.

Radiographic Features

In general, there are few characteristic radiographic features of psoriatic arthritis that help to make a correct diagnosis. In the phalanges of the hand or foot, a periosteal reaction in the form of a "fluffy" new bone apposition may often be noted. If this new bone is periarticular in location and associated with erosions of

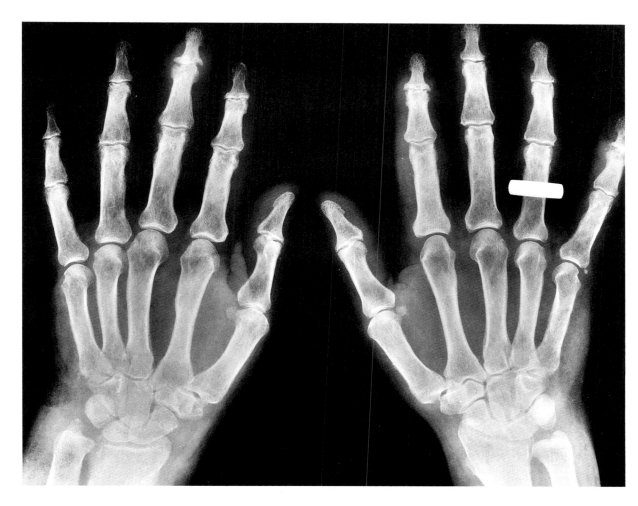

Figure 13.33 Dorsovolar view of the hands of a 33-year-old man with psoriasis and oligoarticular involvement shows destructive changes in the distal interphalangeal joints of the right middle finger and the left index and small fingers. The right middle and left index fingers presented as "sausage digits."

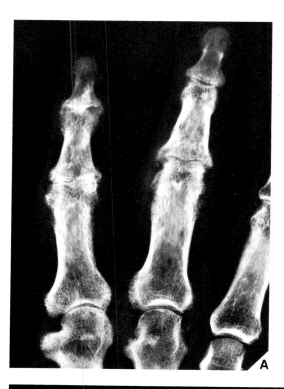

Figure 13.34 (A) Magnification study of the hand of a 48-year-old man who presented with documented psoriasis shows marginal erosions and new bone apposition in the proximal and distal interphalangeal joints, resembling mouse ears. Note the fluffy periostitis in the juxta-articular areas of the phalanges and distal metacarpals. (B) In the feet, the same process has led to a "mouse-ear" appearance of the great toes.

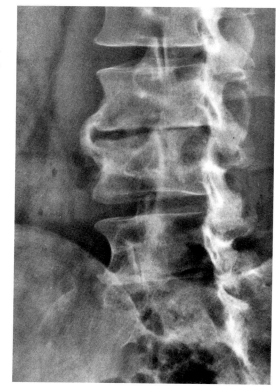

Figure 13.35 Oblique view of the lumbar spine in a 30-year-old man with psoriasis shows a characteristic single syndesmophyte bridging the bodies of L-3 and L-4. The right sacroiliac joint is also affected.

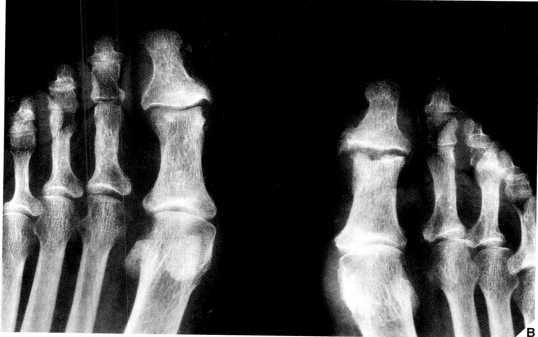

the interphalangeal joints, it exhibits a "mouse-ear" appearance (Fig. 13.34). In the advanced arthritis mutilans stage of psoriatic arthritis, severe deformities such as the "pencil-in-cup" configuration (see Fig. 13.31) and interphalangeal ankylosis may be observed (see Fig. 13.32). In the heel, late-stage changes may be seen in the formation of broad-based osteophytes and in the presence of erosions and a fluffy periostitis (see Figs. 11.29, 11.30C).

Psoriatic arthritis of the spine is associated with a particularly high incidence of sacroiliitis, which may be bilateral and symmetric, bilateral and asymmetric, or unilateral. As in Reiter syndrome, coarse asymmetric syndesmophytes and paraspinal ossifications may form (Fig. 13.35).

Enteropathic Arthropathies

This group comprises arthritides associated with inflammatory intestinal diseases such as ulcerative colitis, regional enteritis (Crohn disease), and intestinal lipodystrophy (Whipple disease), the last of which predominantly affects men in their fourth and fifth decades. The histocompatibility antigen HLA-B27 is present in most patients with enteropathic abnormalities. In all three conditions, the spine and the sacroiliac and peripheral joints may be affected. In the spine, squaring of the vertebral bodies and the formation of syndesmophytes are common features. Sacroiliitis, which is usually bilateral and symmetric, is radiographically indistinguishable from ankylosing spondylitis (Fig. 13.36). In addition, patients may also exhibit a peripheral arthritis, the activity of which generally approximates the activity of the bowel disease.

Finally, it should be noted that arthritis may follow intestinal bypass procedures. The synovitis is polyarticular and symmetric but radiographically the lesions are nonerosive.

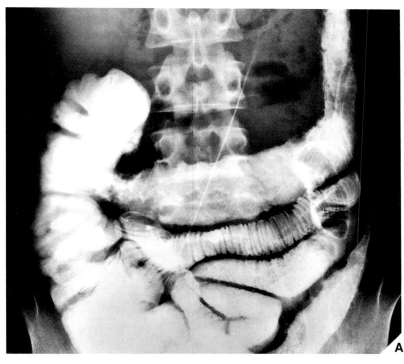
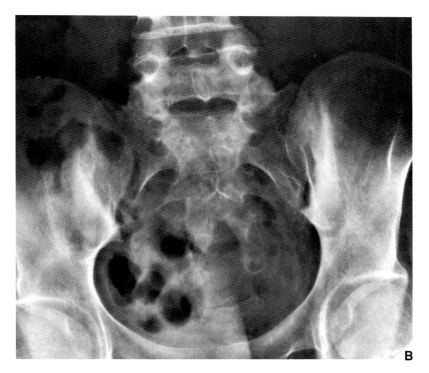

Figure 13.36 A 20-year-old woman with known ulcerative colitis developed severe low back pain localized to the sacroiliac joints. (A) Barium enema study shows extensive involvement of the transverse colon, consistent with ulcerative colitis. (B) Posteroanterior view of the pelvis shows symmetric, bilateral sacroiliitis similar to that seen in ankylosing spondylitis.

PRACTICAL POINTS TO REMEMBER

Erosive Osteoarthritis

[1] Erosive osteoarthritis, a condition seen predominantly in middle-aged women, combines the clinical manifestations of rheumatoid arthritis with the radiographic features of osteoarthritis.

[2] Erosive osteoarthritis can be recognized by:
- involvement of the proximal and distal interphalangeal joints
- a characteristic "gull-wing" configuration of articular erosions.
Spontaneous fusion (ankylosis) in the interphalangeal joints may develop.

Rheumatoid Arthritis

[1] Rheumatoid arthritis has a predilection for:
- the large joints (knees and hips)
- the small joints in the hand (metacarpophalangeal and proximal interphalangeal)
- the carpal articulations.
The distal interphalangeal and sacroiliac joints are usually spared.

[2] The radiographic hallmarks of rheumatoid arthritis include:
- diffuse, symmetric narrowing of the joint space
- periarticular osteoporosis
- fusiform soft tissue swelling
- marginal and central articular erosions
- periarticular synovial cysts
- subluxations and other joint deformities—swan-neck, boutonnière, hitchhiker's thumb.

[3] In the cervical spine, rheumatoid arthritis is characterized by:
- erosion of the odontoid process associated with subluxation in the atlantoaxial joints and, frequently, cephalad migration of C-2
- involvement of the apophyseal joints.
- erosions of vertebral bodies
- destruction of intervertebral disks.

[4] In rheumatoid arthritis,
- axial or, less frequently, medial migration of the femoral head and acetabular protrusio are characteristic in the hip joint
- rotator cuff tear is a frequent complication in the shoulder joint
- the subtalar joint is most often affected in the foot and a hallux valgus deformity is observed.

[5] Rheumatoid nodulosis, a condition occurring predominantly in men, is a variant of rheumatoid arthritis. It exhibits:
- a characteristic lack of joint abnormalities
- multiple subcutaneous nodules
- a high titer of rheumatoid factor.

[6] Juvenile rheumatoid arthritis displays several characteristic features that are not present in adult-onset disease:
- a periosteal reaction
- joint ankylosis, particularly affecting the apophyseal joints of the cervical spine
- growth abnormalities secondary to involvement of epiphyseal sites.

Other Inflammatory Arthritides

[1] Ankylosing spondylitis (Bechterev or Marie-Strümpell disease), a condition seen predominantly in young men, characteristically affects the spine and sacroiliac joints. Histocompatibility antigen HLA-B27 is invariably present in 95% of patients. The radiographic hallmarks of this condition include:
- squaring of the vertebral bodies
- the development of delicate syndesmophytes
- in a later stage of disease, complete fusion of the apophyseal joints and vertebrae, leading to "bamboo" spine.

[2] Reiter syndrome consists of inflammatory arthritis, urethritis, conjunctivitis, and mucocutaneous rash. Its radiographic features include:
- a peripheral, usually asymmetric arthritis that shows a predilection for the lower-limb joints, particularly in the foot
- coarse syndesmophytes or paraspinal ossifications bridging vertebral bodies
- sacroiliitis.

[3] Psoriatic arthritis has a predilection for the distal interphalangeal joints. Oligoarticular involvement may yield a phenomenon known as "sausage digit." Radiographically, psoriatic arthritis is marked by:
- fluffy periostitis
- "pencil-in-cup" deformity of the joints (arthritis mutilans)
- coarse syndesmophytes and paraspinal ossifications that are indistinguishable from those seen in Reiter syndrome
- involvement of the sacroiliac joints.

[4] Enteropathic arthropathies are associated with:
- ulcerative colitis
- regional enteritis
- intestinal lipodystrophy
- intestinal bypass procedures.
Characteristically, there is symmetric involvement of the sacroiliac joints.

References

Ansell BM, Wigley RAD: Arthritic manifestations in regional enteritis. *Ann Rheum Dis* 23:64, 1964.

Arnett FC, Bias WB, Stevens MB: Juvenile-onset chronic arthritis. Clinical and roentgenographic features of a unique HLA-B27 subset. *Am J Med* 69:369, 1980.

Baker H, Godling DN, Thompson M: Psoriasis and arthritis. *Ann Intern Med* 58:909, 1963.

Berens DL: Roentgen features of ankylosing spondylitis. *Clin Orthop* 74:20, 1971.

Björkengren AG, Geborek P, Rydholm U, Holtas S, Petterson H: MR imaging of the knee in acute rheumatoid arthritis: Synovial uptake of gadolinium-DOTA. *Am J Roentgenol* 155:329, 1990.

Boyle AC: The rheumatoid neck. *Proc R Soc Med* 64:1161, 1971.

Breedveld FC, Algra PR, Vielvoye CJ, Cats A: Magnetic resonance imaging in the evaluation of patients with rheumatoid arthritis and subluxations of the cervical spine. *Arthritis and Rheumatism* 30:624, 1987.

Brower AC, Allman RM: Pencil pointing: A vascular pattern of deossification. *RadioGraphics* 3:315, 1983.

Clark RL, Muhletaler CA, Margulies SI: Colitic arthritis: Clinical and radiographic manifestations. *Radiology* 101:585, 1971.

Dalinka MK, Reginato AJ, Golden DA: Calcium deposition diseases. *Semin Roentgenol* 17:39, 1982.

Eastmond CJ, Woodrow JC: The HLA system and the arthropathies associated with psoriasis. *Ann Rheum Dis* 36:112, 1977.

Ehrlich GE: Inflammatory osteoarthritis—II. The superimposition of rheumatoid arthritis. *J Chronic Dis* 25:635, 1972.

El-Khoury GY, Larson RK, Kathol MH, Berbaum KS, Furst DE: Seronegative and seropositive rheumatoid arthritis: Radiographic differences. *Radiology* 168:517, 1988.

Fam AG, Topp JR, Stein HB, Little AH: Clinical and roentgenographic aspects of pseudogout: A study of 50 cases and a review. *Can Med Assoc* 1124:545, 1981.

Genant HA: Roentgenographic aspects of calcium pyrophosphate dihydrate crystal deposition disease (pseudogout). *Arthritis Rheum* 19:307, 1976.

Green L, Meyers OL, Gordon W, Briggs B: Arthritis in psoriasis. *Ann Rheum Dis* 40:366, 1981.

Greenspan A, Baker ND, Norman A: Rheumatoid arthritis simulating other lesions. *Bull Hosp Jt Dis Orthop Inst* 43:70, 1983.

Hazes JMW, Dijkmans BAC, Hoevers JM, Janson JJM, De Vries RRP, Vandenbroucke JP, Cats A: CR4 prevalence related to the age at disease onset in female patients with rheumatoid arthritis. *Ann Rheum Dis* 48:406, 1989.

Hoffman GS: Polyarthritis: The differential diagnosis of rheumatoid arthritis. *Semin Arthritis Rheum* 8:115, 1978.

Jensen PS, Putman CE: Current concepts with respect to chondrocalcinosis and the pseudogout syndrome. *Am J Roentgenol* 123:531, 1975.

Kapasi OA, Ruby LK, Calney K: The psoriatic hand. *J Hand Surg* 7:492, 1982.

Kelly JJ III, Weisiger BB: The arthritis of Whipple's disease. *Arthritis Rheum* 6:615, 1963.

Killebrew K, Gold RH, Sholkoff SD: Psoriatic spondylitis. *Radiology* 108:9, 1973.

Ling D, Murphy WA, Kyriakos M: Tophaceous pseudogout. *Am J Roentgenol* 138:162, 1982.

Martel W, Holt JF, Cassidy JT: The roentgenologic manifestations of juvenile rheumatoid arthritis. *Am J Roentgenol* 88:400, 1962.

Martel W, Snarr JW, Horn JR: Metacarpophalangeal joints in interphalangeal osteoarthritis. *Radiology* 108:1, 1973.

Martel W, Braunstein EM, Borlaza G, Good AE, Griffin PE: Radiologic features of Reiter's disease. *Radiology* 132:1, 1979.

Martel W, Stuck KJ, Dworin AM, Hylland RG: Erosive osteoarthritis and psoriatic arthritis: A radiologic comparison in the hand, wrist and foot. *Am J Roentgenol* 134:125, 1980.

Mathews JA: Atlanto-axial subluxation in rheumatoid arthritis. A 5-year follow-up study. *Ann Rheum Dis* 33:526, 1974.

Park WM, O'Neill M, McCall IW: The radiology of rheumatoid involvement of the cervical spine. *Skeletal Radiol* 4:1, 1979.

Peterson CC Jr, Silbiger ML: Reiter's syndrome and psoriatic arthritis: Their roentgen spectra and some interesting similarities. *Am J Roentgenol* 101:860, 1967.

Pettersson H, Larsson E-M, Holtas S: MR imaging of the cervical spine in rheumatoid arthritis. *AJNR* 9:573, 1988.

Resnick D: Common disorders of synovium-lined joints: Pathogenesis, imaging abnormalities, and complications. *Am J Roentgenol* 151:1079, 1988.

Resnick D, Niwayama G, Goergen TG: Comparison of radiographic abnormalities of the sacroiliac joint in degenerative disease and ankylosing spondylitis. *Am J Roentgenol* 128:189, 1977.

Resnick D, Niwayama G: Rheumatoid arthritis and the seronegative spondyloarthropathies: Radiographic and pathologic concepts. In: Resnick D, Niwayama G (eds): *Diagnosis of Bone and Joint Disorders*, ed 2. Philadelphia, Saunders, 1988, pp 894-953.

Resnick D, Niwayama G, Goergen TG: Comparison of radiographic abnormalities of the sacroiliac joint in degenerative disease and ankylosing spondylitis. *Am J Roentgenol* 128:189, 1977.

Resnik CS, Resnick D: Radiology of disorders of the sacroiliac joints. *JAMA* 253:2863, 1985.

Resnik CS, Resnick D: Crystal deposition disease. *Semin Arthritis Rheum* 12:390, 1983.

Sanders KM, Resnik CS, Owen DS: Erosive arthritis in Cronkhite-Canada syndrome. *Radiology* 156:309, 1985.

Sartoris DJ, Resnick D: The radiographic differential diagnosis of juvenile chronic arthritis. *Aust Paediatr J* 23:273, 1987.

Schumacher HR Jr: Pathogenesis of crystal-induced synovitis. *Clin Rheum Dis* 3:105, 1977.

Seett HA, Jaffe RB, McIff EB: Popliteal cyst: Presentation as thrombophlebitis. *Radiology* 115:613, 1975.

Sharp JT: Radiologic assessment as an outcome measure in rheumatoid arthritis. *Arthritis Rheum* 32:221, 1989.

Sholkoff SD, Glickman MG, Steinbach HL: Roentgenology of Reiter's syndrome. *Radiology* 97:497, 1970.

Solomon G, Winchester R: Immunogenetic aspects of inflammatory arthritis. In: Taveras JM, Ferrucci JT (eds): *Radiology — Diagnosis, Imaging, Intervention*, vol 5, chap 45.

Steward V, Weissman BNW: Mixed connective tissue disease. In: Taveras JM, Ferrucci JT (eds): *Radiology — Diagnosis, Imaging, Intervention*, vol 5, chap 44.

Swett HA, Jaffe RB, McIff EB: Popliteal cysts: Presentation as thrombophlebitis. *Radiology* 115:613, 1975.

Weissman BN, Rappoport AS, Sosman JL, Schur PH: Radiographic findings in the hands in patients with systemic lupus erythematosus. *Radiology* 126:313, 1978.

Weissman BN, Aliabadi P, Weinfeld MS, Thomas WH, Sodman JL: Prognostic features of atlantoaxial subluxation in rheumatoid arthritis patients. *Radiology* 144:745, 1982.

Wilkinson RH, Weissman BN: Arthritis in children. *Radiol Clin North Am* 26:1247, 1988.

Wolfe BK, O'Keeffe D, Mitchell DM, Tchang SPK: Rheumatoid arthritis of the cervical spine: Early and progressive radiographic features. *Radiology* 165:145, 1987.

14

Miscellaneous Arthritides

CONNECTIVE TISSUE ARTHRITIDES

AN OVERVIEW OF THE CLINICAL and radiographic hallmarks of the forms of arthritis associated with connective tissue disorders is presented in Figure 14.1.

Systemic Lupus Erythematosus

Systemic lupus erythematosus (SLE) is a chronic, inflammatory, connective tissue disorder of unknown etiology characterized by significant immunologic abnormalities and involvement of multiple organs. Women, particularly adolescents and young adults, are affected four times as frequently as men. The clinical manifestations of SLE vary according to the distribution and extent of systemic alterations. The most common symptoms are malaise, weakness, fever, anorexia, and weight loss. Consistent and characteristic features of this disease are serologic abnormalities, including a variety of serum autoantibodies to nuclear antigens, which have been historically associated with the presence of lupus erythematosus cells and neutrophilic leukocytes filled with cytoplasmic inclusion bodies.

Antinuclear antibodies are useful in the differential diagnosis of SLE, and changes in the titer of antibodies to DNA are useful in following disease activity. Antinuclear antibodies are a heterogeneous group of antibodies directed against a number of discrete nuclear macromolecular proteins. They represent what has classically been referred to as "autoantibodies," since they are directed against components normally present in all nucleated cells. They generally lack tissue or species specificity; therefore, they will cross-react with nuclei from different sources. The primary source for study of these antibodies is patients with SLE and related systemic rheumatic diseases. Many studies have centered on defining the specificity of these antibodies and have contributed extensively to our understanding of their immunopathologic role in connective tissue disorders.

The musculoskeletal system is a frequent site of involvement in SLE, and joint abnormalities, exhibited by 90% of patients during the course of the disease, represent a significant part of the clinical and radiologic picture. Arthritic involvement is symmetric, and articular deformities without fixed contractures are a hallmark of this disorder. The hands are the predominant site of involvement. Typically, the lateral view discloses malalignments, most commonly at the metacarpophalangeal and proximal interphalangeal joints of the fingers and the interphalangeal joint of the thumb (Fig. 14.2A). These abnormalities may not be apparent on a dorsovolar radiograph (Fig. 14.2B), since the malalignments are flexible and are corrected by the pressure of the hand against the radiographic cassette. These pathognomonic deformities usually occur secondary to a loss of support from the ligamentous and capsular structures about the joint, and at least in the early stage of disease are completely reducible. Only very seldom are these abnormalities fixed and/or accompanied by articular erosions (Fig. 14.3).

Figure 14.1 Clinical and Radiographic Hallmarks of Connective Tissue Arthritides

TYPE OF ARTHRITIS	SITE	CRUCIAL ABNORMALITIES	TECHNIQUE/PROJECTION
Systemic Lupus Erythematosus (F > M; young adults; blacks > whites; skin changes: rash)	Hands Hips, ankles, shoulders	Flexible joint contractures Osteonecrosis	Lateral view Standard views of affected joints Scintigraphy Magnetic resonance imaging
Scleroderma (F > M; skin changes: edema, thickening)	Hands	Soft tissue calcifications Acro-osteolysis Tapering of distal phalanges Interphalangeal destructive changes	Dorsovolar and lateral views
	Gastrointestinal tract	Dilatation of esophagus Decreased peristalsis Dilatation of duodenum and small bowel Pseudodiverticulosis of colon	Esophagram Esophagram (cine or video study) Upper gastrointestinal and small bowel series Barium enema
Polymyositis/Dermatomyositis	Upper and lower extremities (proximal parts) Hands	Soft tissue calcifications Periarticular osteoporosis Erosions and destructive changes in distal interphalangeal articulations	Xeroradiography Dorsovolar and lateral views
Mixed Connective Tissue Disease (overlap of clinical features of SLE, scleroderma, dermatomyositis, and rheumatoid arthritis)	Hands, wrists	Erosions and destructive changes in proximal interphalangeal, metacarpophalangeal, radiocarpal and midcarpal articulations, associated with joint space narrowing Symmetric soft tissue swelling Soft tissue atrophy and calcifications	Dorsovolar and lateral views Magnetic resonance imaging
	Chest	Pleural and pericardial effusions	Posteroanterior and lateral views Sonogram

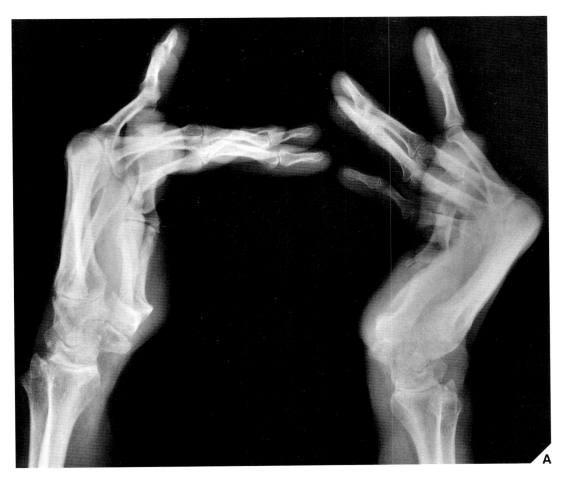

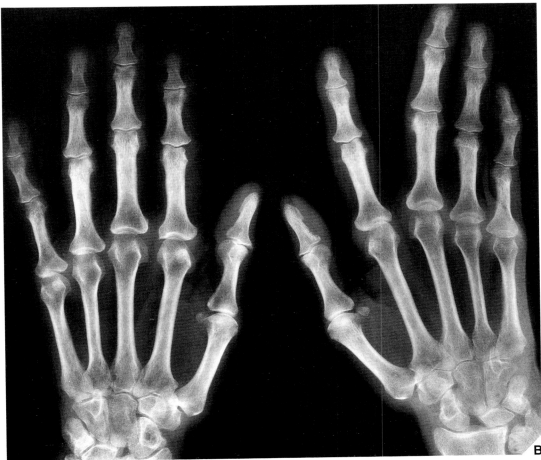

Figure 14.2 (A) Lateral view of both hands of a 42-year-old woman with documented SLE for the past four years demonstrates flexion deformities in the metacarpophalangeal joints. On the dorsovolar view (B), the flexion deformities have been corrected by the pressure of the hands against the radiographic cassette.

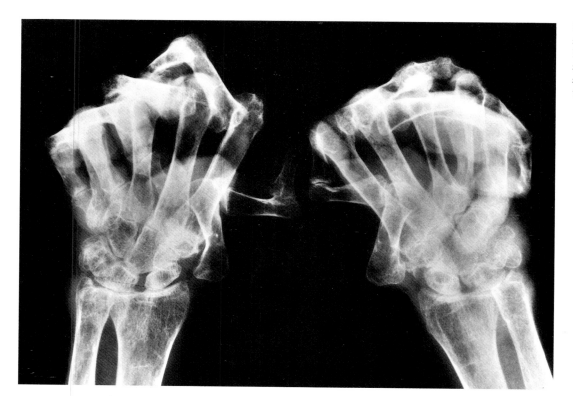

Figure 14.3 A 62-year-old woman presented with a 15-year history of SLE. Dorsovolar view of both hands shows severe deformities, subluxations, and articular erosions. Note the advanced osteoporosis secondary to disuse of the extremities and treatment with corticosteroids.

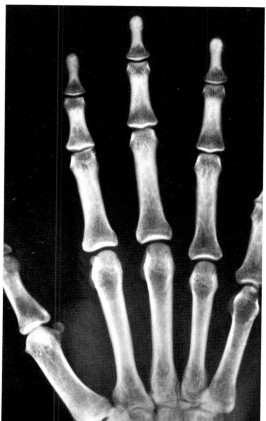

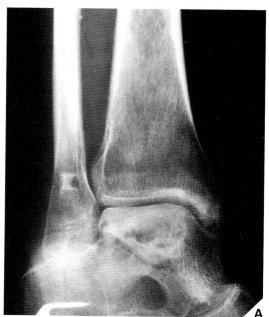

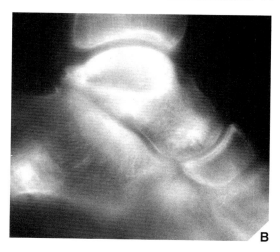

Figure 14.5 Oblique plain film (A) and lateral tomogram (B) of the ankle demonstrate osteonecrosis of the talus in a 26-year-old woman with lupus who was treated with massive doses of steroids.

Figure 14.4 Dorsovolar film of the hand of a 29-year-old woman with SLE demonstrates sclerosis of the distal phalanges (acral sclerosis). Similar sclerotic changes are also occasionally seen in rheumatoid arthritis and scleroderma.

Some patients present with sclerosis of the distal phalanges (acral sclerosis) (Fig. 14.4) or with resorption of the terminal tufts (acro-osteolysis). Osteonecrosis, which is frequently seen, has been attributed to complications of treatment with corticosteroids (Fig. 14.5). However, current investigations suggest the vital role of the inflammatory process (vasculitis) in the development of this complication.

Scleroderma

Scleroderma (progressive systemic sclerosis) is a generalized disorder of unknown etiology; it is seen predominantly in young women, usually becoming apparent in their third and fourth decades. Primarily a connective tissue disorder, it is characterized by thickening and fibrosis of the skin and subcutaneous tissues, with frequent involvement of the musculoskeletal system. The majority of patients develop the so-called CREST syndrome, which refers to the coexistence of calcinosis, Raynaud phenomenon (episodes of intermittent pallor of the fingers and toes on exposure to cold, secondary to vasoconstriction of the small blood vessels), esophageal abnormalities (dilatation and hypoperistalsis), sclerodactyly, and telangiectasia. Thirty to forty percent of patients have a positive serologic test for rheumatoid factor and a positive antinuclear antibody (ANA) test.

Radiographically, scleroderma presents with characteristic abnormalities of the bone and soft tissues. The hands usually exhibit atrophy of the soft tissues at the tips of the fingers, resorption of the distal phalanges, subcutaneous and periarticular calcifications (Fig. 14.6), and destructive changes of the small articulations, usually the interphalangeal joints (Fig. 14.7). Corroborative findings are seen in the gastrointestinal tract, where dilatation of the esophagus

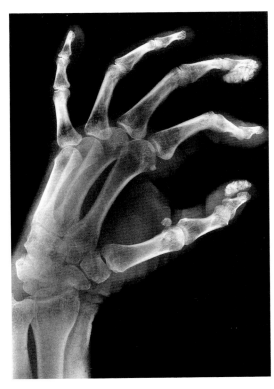

Figure 14.6 A 32-year-old woman with systemic sclerosis exhibits soft tissue calcifications in the distal phalanges of the right hand, a typical feature of this disorder.

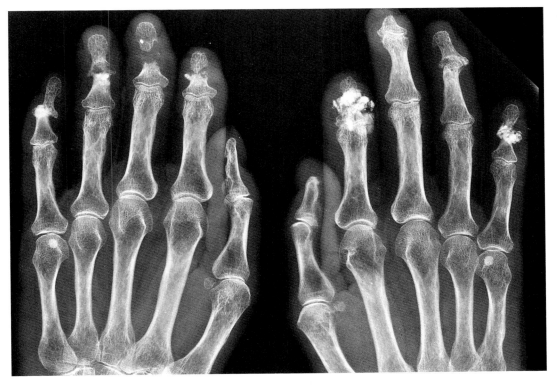

Figure 14.7 Dorsovolar view of the hands of a 50-year-old man with documented systemic sclerosis shows destructive changes in the distal interphalangeal joints, as well as soft tissue calcifications and resorption of the tip of the distal phalanx of the left middle finger.

and small bowel, together with a pseudo-obstruction pattern, is characteristic (Fig. 14.8). Pseudodiverticula in the colon are also commonly seen.

Polymyositis and Dermatomyositis

Polymyositis and dermatomyositis are disorders of striated muscle and skin and are characterized by diffuse, nonsuppurative inflammation, and degeneration. Early diagnosis and subsequent management of patients with any type of myopathy, including polymyositis and dermatomyositis, can be facilitated by the use of appropriate laboratory tests. The four tests most helpful in evaluating muscle disorders include 1) serum enzymes, 2) urinary creatine and creatinine excretion, 3) electromyogram, and 4) muscle biopsy.

Different serum enzyme determinations have been advocated, but the most valuable tests include serum creatine phosphokinase (CPK), serum aldolase (ALD), serum lactate dehydrogenase (LDH), serum glutamic oxalacetic transaminase (SGOT), and serum glutamic pyruvic transaminase (SGPT). Further, the determination of serum enzyme levels and urinary creatine excretion are helpful for the clinical management of polymyositis and determatomyositis, since the two tests provide a broader perspective than either test alone.

A positive biopsy may demonstrate not only that the disease process is myopathic, thus enabling the physician to rule out a neurogenic lower motor neuron lesion, but may also identify those patients whose muscle disease is more severe pathologically than was suspected on clinical grounds. This is important with respect to prognosis. With the aid of histochemical and electron microscopic techniques, muscle biopsy will occasionally enable the pathologist to diagnose one of the rare forms of myopathy that can clinically mimic polymyositis. Such diseases include sarcoid myopathy, central core disease, and muscle diseases associated with abnormal mitochondria.

The pathologic changes found on muscle biopsy in polymyositis have been well described. The degree of pathologic change may vary widely; one patient may show only negligible pathologic changes in muscle fibers on biopsy, whereas another patient presenting similar clinical features may show extensive necrosis and fiber replacement. This variability in histologic findings is probably responsible for the frequent normal muscle biopsies from patients with otherwise classic polymyositis. The overall rate of positive findings from muscle biopsy in several studies of polymyositis was in the range of 55% to 80%.

Radiographic abnormalities in polymyositis and dermatomyositis are divided into two types: those involving soft tissues and those involving joints. The most characteristic soft tissue abnormality in both conditions is soft tissue calcifications. The favorite sites of intermuscular calcification are the large muscles in the proximal parts of upper and lower extremities. In addition, subcutaneous calcifications similar to those of scleroderma are seen.

Articular abnormalities are rare. The most frequently reported, however, is periarticular osteoporosis. Destructive joint changes have been reported only occasionally, and primarily in the distal interphalangeal articulations of the hands.

Mixed Connective Tissue Disease (MCTD)

MCTD was first reported as a distinctive syndrome by Sharp and associates in 1972. This syndrome is characterized by clinical abnormalities that combine the features of SLE, scleroderma, dermatomyositis, and rheumatoid arthritis. The one feature that distinguishes MCTD as a separate entity is a positive serologic test for antibody to the ribonucleoprotein (RNP) component of extractable nuclear antigen

Figure 14.8 Upper gastrointestinal series and small bowel study in the patient shown in Figure 14.7 demonstrates dilatation of the second and third portions of the duodenum and jejunum, with a pseudo-obstruction pattern.

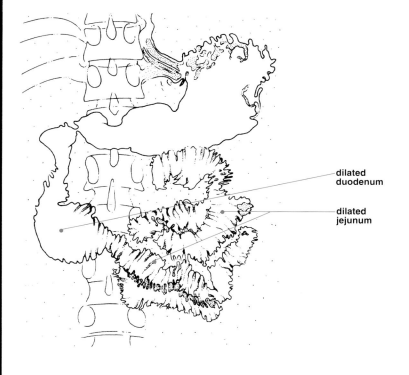

dilated duodenum

dilated jejunum

Figure 14.9 Clinical and Radiographic Hallmarks of Metabolic, Endocrine, and Miscellaneous Arthritides

TYPE OF ARTHRITIS	SITE	CRUCIAL ABNORMALITIES	TECHNIQUE/PROJECTION
Gout (M > F)	Great toe Large joints (knee, elbow) Hand	Articular erosion with preservation of part of joint Overhanging edge of erosion Lack of osteoporosis Periarticular swelling Tophi	Standard views of affected joints
CPPD Crystal Deposition Disease (M = F)	Variable joints	Chondrocalcinosis (calcification of articular cartilage and menisci) Calcifications of tendons, ligaments, and capsule	Standard views of affected joints
	Femoropatellar joint	Joint space narrowing Subchondral sclerosis Osteophytes	Lateral (knee) and axial (patella) views
	Wrists, elbows, shoulders, ankles	Degenerative changes with chondrocalcinosis	Standard views of affected joints
CHA Crystal Deposition Disease (F > M)	Variable joints, but predilection for shoulder joint (supraspinatus tendon)	Pericapsular calcifications Calcifications of tendons	Standard views of affected joints
Hemochromatosis (M > F)	Hands	Involvement of second and third metacarpophalangeal joints with beak-like osteophytes	Dorsovolar view
	Large joints	Chondrocalcinosis	Standard views of affected joints
Alkaptonuria (Ochronosis) (M = F)	Intervertebral disks, sacroiliac joints, symphysis pubis, large joints (knees, hips)	Calcification and ossification of intervertebral disks, narrowing of disks, osteoporosis, joint space narrowing, periarticular sclerosis	Anteroposterior and lateral of spine; standard views of affected joints
Hyperparathyroidism (W > M)	Hands	Destructive changes in interphalangeal joints Subperiosteal resorption	Dorsovolar view Dorsovolar and oblique views
	Multiple bones Skull Spine	Bone cysts (brown tumors) Salt-and-pepper appearance Rugger-jersey appearance	Standard views specific for locations Lateral view Lateral view
Acromegaly (M > F)	Hands	Widened joint spaces Large sesamoid Degenerative changes (beak-like osteophytes)	Dorsovolar view
	Skull Facial bones Heel Spine	Large sinuses Large mandible (prognathism) Thick heel pad (>25 mm) Thoracic kyphosis	Lateral view Lateral view Lateral view Lateral view (thoracic spine)
Amyloidosis (M > F)	Large joints (hips, knees, shoulders, elbows)	Articular and periarticular erosions, osteoporosis (periarticular), joint subluxations, pathologic fractures	Standard views of affected joints Radionuclide bone scan (scintigraphy)
Multicentric Reticulohistiocytosis (F > M)	Hands (distal and proximal interphalangeal joints) Feet	Soft-tissue swelling, articular erosions, lack of osteoporosis	Dorsovolar view Norgaard ("Allstate") view Dorsoplantar view Oblique view
Hemophilia (M = F)	Large joints (hips, knees, shoulders) Elbows, ankles	Joint effusion, osteoporosis, symmetrical and concentric joint space narrowing, articular erosions, widening of intercondylar notch, squaring of patella; very similar to changes of juvenile RA	Standard views of affected joints Magnetic resonance imaging

(ENA). The typical clinical pattern consists of Raynaud phenomenon, polyarthralgia, swelling of the hands, esophageal hypomotility, inflammatory myopathy, and pulmonary disease. Women constitute approximately 80% of affected patients. Patients with MCTD have prominent joint abnormalities, with typical involvement of the small articulations of the hand, wrist, and foot; large joints such as the knee, elbow, and shoulder may also be affected. The joint deformities mimic those seen in rheumatoid arthritis, but occasionally joint subluxation may be nonerosive, as in SLE. Soft tissue abnormalities are identical to those encountered in scleroderma.

Vasculitis

There is a diverse clinical spectrum of the vasculitides which includes systemic necrotizing vasculitis, hypersensitivity vasculitis, Wegeren granulomatosis, lymphomatoid granulomatosis, giant cell arteritis, and a variety of miscellaneous syndromes (e.g., Kawasaki disease, Behçet disease, and others). A discussion of these diverse but often overlapping diseases is far beyond the scope of this volume, but the reader is referred to several key references at the end of this chapter. The demonstration of vasculitis by angiograms can often be documented by the presence of aneurysmal dilatation in

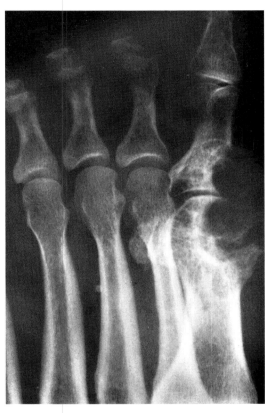

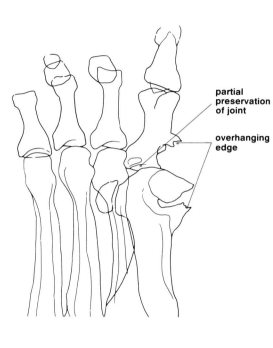

Figure 14.10 Oblique radiograph of the right foot of a 58-year-old man with a three-month history of gout shows the typical involvement of the first metatarsophalangeal joint. Note the characteristic "overhanging edge" of the erosive changes.

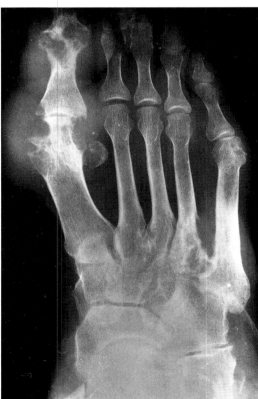

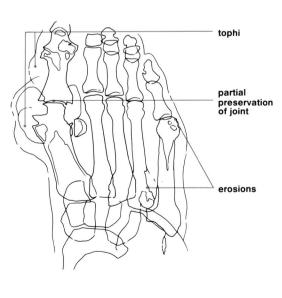

Figure 14.11 Dorsoplantar view of the left foot of a 62-year-old man with a long history of tophaceous gout shows multiple erosions involving the big and small toes and the base of the fourth and fifth metatarsals. The first metatarsophalangeal joint is partially preserved, a characteristic feature of gouty arthritis. A large soft tissue swelling of the great toe represents a tophus.

affected vessels. Generally, an angiogram is performed when the diagnosis cannot be established by tissue biopsy.

METABOLIC AND ENDOCRINE ARTHRITIDES

An overview of the clinical and radiographic hallmarks of the arthritides associated with metabolic and endocrine abnormalities is shown in Figure 14.9.

Gout

Gout is a metabolic disorder characterized by recurrent episodes of arthritis associated with the presence of monosodium urate monohydrate crystals in the synovial fluid leukocytes and, in many cases, gross deposits of sodium urate (tophi) in periarticular soft tissues. Serum uric acid concentrations are elevated.

The great toe is the most common site of involvement in gouty arthritis; the condition known as *podagra*, which involves the first metatarsophalangeal joint, occurs in about 75% of patients. Other frequently affected sites include the ankle, knee, elbow, and wrist. The majority of patients are males, but gouty arthritis is seen in postmenopausal women as well.

Hyperuricemia

An increased miscible pool of uric acid with resulting hyperuricemia can occur in two principal ways. First, urate is produced in such large quantities that, even though excretion routes are of normal capacity, they are inadequate to handle the excessive load. Second, the capacity for uric acid excretion is critically reduced, so that even a normal quantity of uric acid cannot be eliminated.

In 25% to 30% of gouty patients, a primary defect in the rate of purine synthesis causes excessive uric acid formation, as reflected in excessive urinary uric acid excretion (over 600 mg/day) measured while the patient is maintained on a standard purine-free diet. Increased production can also be seen in gout secondary to myeloproliferative disorders associated with increased destruction of cells and result in increased breakdown of nucleic acids. Decreased excretion occurs in primary gout in patients with a dysfunction in the renal tubular capacity to secrete urate and in patients with chronic renal disease. In most patients, however, there is evidence of both uric acid overproduction and diminished renal excretion of uric acid.

The chance of development of gouty arthritis in hyperuricemic individuals should increase in proportion to the duration and, even more, to the degree of hyperuricemia. Monosodium urate, however, has a marked tendency to form relatively stable supersaturated solutions; therefore, the proportion of hyperuricemic patients who actually develop gouty arthritis is relatively low. The clinical development of gouty arthritis in the hyperuricemic subject is also substantially influenced by other factors, such as binding of urate to plasma proteins or the presence of promoters or inhibitors of crystallization.

Examination of Synovial Fluid

A wet preparation of fresh synovial fluid is best for examination of crystals. Although crystals may often be seen by ordinary light microscopy, reliable identification requires polarization equipment. To differentiate between urate and pyrophosphate crystals—characteristics of gout and pseudogout, respectively—a compensated, polarized light microscope is advisable. Since both types of crystals are birefringent, they refract the polarized light that passes through them. The birefringence phenomenon is due to the refractive index for light, which vibrates either parallel or perpendicular to the axis of the crystal being viewed. Color is the key to negative or positive birefringence. Urates are strongly birefringent; therefore, they are brightly colored in polarized light, with a red compensator. They are usually seen as needles. During an acute gouty attack, many intraleukocytic crystals are seen. Monosodium urate crystals are negatively birefringent, i.e., they appear yellow when the longitudinal axis of the crystal is parallel to the axis of slow vibrations of the red compensator on the polarizing system, and they appear blue when perpendicular.

Monosodium urate crystals, the pathogens of gouty arthritis, range in length from 2 μ to 10 μ and are found within synovial leukocytes or extracellularly in virtually every case of acute gout, although the likelihood of finding such crystals varies inversely with the amount of time elapsed from onset of symptoms to the time of examination. Crystals from tophi may be larger.

Radiographic Features

Gouty arthritis has several characteristic radiographic features. Erosions, which are usually sharply marginated, are initially periarticular in location and are later seen to extend into the joint; an "overhanging edge" of erosion is a frequent identifying feature (Fig. 14.10). Usually, there is a striking lack of osteoporosis, which helps differentiate this condition from rheumatoid arthritis. The reason for the absence of osteoporosis is that the duration of an acute gouty attack is too short to allow the development of the disuse osteoporosis so often seen in patients with rheumatoid arthritis. If erosion involves the articular end of the bone and extends into the joint, part of the joint is usually preserved (Fig. 14.11). In chronic tophaceous gout, sodium urate deposits in and around the joint are seen, creating a dense mass in the soft tissues called a tophus, which frequently exhibits calcifications (Fig. 14.12). Characteristically, tophi are randomly distributed and are usually asymmetric; if they occur in the hands or feet, they are more often seen on the dorsal aspect.

Figure 14.12 Lateral view of the elbow of a 73-year-old man with a 30-year history of gout shows a tophus with dense calcifications adjacent to the olecranon process, which exhibits a small erosion.

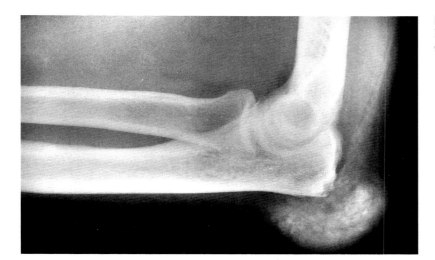

Unlike rheumatoid arthritis, periarticular and articular erosions are asymmetric in distribution (Fig. 14.13).

CPPD Crystal Deposition Disease

Clinical Features

Resulting from the intra-articular presence of calcium pyrophosphate dihydrate (CPPD) crystals, CPPD crystal deposition disease affects men and women equally; most commonly, patients are middle-aged and older. The condition may be asymptomatic, in which case it is commonly referred to as *chondrocalcinosis*; when symptomatic, it is called *pseudogout*. There is, however, a great deal of con-

Radiographic Features

Radiographically, the arthritic changes encountered in this condition are similar to those seen in osteoarthritis, but the wrist, elbow, shoulder, ankle, and the femoropatellar joint compartment are also characteristically involved. As mentioned above, CPPD crystal deposition disease is characterized by calcification of the articular cartilage and menisci; the tendons, ligaments, and joint capsule may exhibit calcifications as well (Fig. 14.14).

Rarely, calcium pyrophosphate dihydrate deposits can assume the form of bulky tumor-like masses located in the joint and paraarticular soft tissues. In these instances, it may mimic a malignant tumor; hence, this form of CPPD deposition was termed by Sissons and associates "tumoral calcium pyrophosphate deposition disease,"

PRACTICAL POINTS TO REMEMBER

Connective Tissue Arthritides

[1] Systemic lupus erythematosus (SLE) is characterized by flexible joint contractures and malalignments of the metacarpophalangeal and proximal interphalangeal joints. These abnormalities are better demonstrated on the lateral projection, since they can easily be reduced during positioning of the hand for the dorsovolar view.

[2] Osteonecrosis is a frequent complication of SLE.

[3] Radiographically, the musculoskeletal abnormalities associated with scleroderma are recognized by:
  • atrophy of the soft tissues, particularly the tips of fingers
  • resorption of the distal phalanges
  • subcutaneous and periarticular calcifications
  • destructive changes in the interphalangeal joints.

[4] In scleroderma, corroborative findings are seen in the gastrointestinal tract, where characteristically there is:
  • dilatation and hypomotility of the esophagus
  • dilatation of the duodenum and small bowel, with a pseudo-obstruction pattern
  • pseudodiverticula of the colon.

[5] Mixed connective tissue disease is characterized by the clinical and radiologic features that combine the findings of systemic lupus erythematosus, scleroderma, dermatomyositis, and rheumatoid arthritis.

Metabolic and Endocrine Arthritides

[1] Gout is a metabolic disorder characterized by recurrent episodes of arthritis associated with the presence of monosodium urate monohydrate crystals in the synovial fluid.

[2] Hyperuricemia may result from either increased uric acid production or decreased renal excretion.

[3] Gouty arthritis can be recognized radiographically by:
  • sharply marginated periarticular and articular erosions, with an "overhanging edge" phenomenon
  • partial preservation of the joint space
  • asymmetric joint involvement
  • asymmetric distribution of tophi
  • the absence of osteoporosis.

[4] CPPD crystal deposition disease consists of three distinct entities:
  • chondrocalcinosis
  • calcium pyrophosphate arthropathy
  • the pseudogout syndrome.

[5] The presence of intra-articular crystals and calcifications of hyaline and fibrocartilage, occasionally associated with painful attacks similar to gout, are characteristic features of CPPD crystal deposition disease.

[6] Chondrocalcinosis may also be seen in other conditions, such as hyperparathyroidism, hemochromatosis, Wilson disease, and degenerative joint disease.

[7] Calcium hydroxyapatite (CHA) crystal deposition disease results from abnormal deposition of mineral crystals in and around the joints. The most common location is around the shoulder joint, at the site of supraspinatus tendon.

[8] Hemochromatosis is a disorder resulting from an error of metabolism of iron or due to iron overload. The arthropathy starts in the small joints of the hand with characteristic involvement of the heads of second and third metacarpals.

[9] Alkaptonuria (ochronosis) is characterized by narrowing of the intervertebral disk spaces, disk calcification and ossification, involvement of sacroiliac joints and symphysis pubis, and joint space narrowing with periarticular osteosclerosis. The radiographic appearance may occasionally mimic degenerative joint disease or CPPD.

[10] Hyperparathyroidism arthropathy results from subperiosteal and subchondral resorption at the site of small joints of the hand. This accounts for articular manifestation of this disorder.

[11] Acromegaly arthropathy is the result of overgrowth of the articular cartilage and secondary degenerative changes (secondary osteoarthritis).

Miscellaneous Arthropathies

[1] Amyloid arthropathy is a noninflammatory symmetric polyarthritis. The articular ends of the bone can be destroyed and subluxations and pathologic fractures occur. Focal osteolytic lesions, particularly of the bones of the upper extremities and in the proximal ends of the femora, can be seen.

[2] Multicentric reticulohistiocytosis is characterized by proliferation of histiocytes in the skin, mucosa, subcutaneous tissue, and synovium. This may lead to severe articular destruction, but there is neither periarticular osteoporosis nor periosteal bone formation.

[3] The articular changes in hemophilia are due to repetitive bleeding into the joints and bone. The radiographic presentation is similar to that of juvenile rheumatoid arthritis.

[4] Jaccoud arthritis is a poorly defined entity resulting in periarticular stiffness in patients with repeated attacks of rheumatic fever. The articular changes are not erosive.

[5] There is an increased prevalence of rheumatologic disorders in patients with acquired immune deficiency syndrome (AIDS), particularly Reiter syndrome, psoriatic arthritis, and vasculitis.

[6] Infectious arthritis is characterized by the complete destruction of both articular ends of the bones forming the joint. All communicating joint compartments are invariably involved, with diffuse osteoporosis, joint effusion, and periarticular soft tissue swelling.

References

Adams PC, Searle J: Neonatal hemochromatosis: A case and review of the literature. *Am J Gastroenterol*, 83:422, 1988.

Adamson TC III, Resnik CS, Guerra J Jr, Vint VC, Weisman MH, Resnick D: Hand and wrist arthropathies of hemochromatosis and calcium pyrophosphate deposition disease: Distinct radiographic features. *Radiology* 147:377, 1983.

Amor B, Cherot A, Delbarre F, Roldan AN, Hors J: Hydroxyapatite rheumatism and HLA markers. *J Rheumatol* 4 (Suppl 3):101, 1977.

Anderson HC: Mechanisms of pathologic calcification. *Rheum Dis Clin North Am* 14:303, 1988.

Baker ND: Hemochromatosis. In: Taveras JM, Ferrucci JT (eds): *Radiology—Diagnosis, Imaging, Intervention*. Philadelphia, Lippincott, 1986.

Barrow MV, Holubar K: Multicentric reticulohistiocytosis. A review of 33 patients. *Medicine* 48:287, 1969.

Barthelemy CR, Nakayama DA, Carrera GF, Lightfoot RW Jr, Wortmann RL: Gouty arthritis: A prospective radiographic evaluation of sixty patients. *Skeletal Radiol* 11:1, 1984.

Berman A, Espinoza LR, Diaz JD, et al: Rheumatic manifestations of human immunodeficiency virus infections. *Am J Med* 85:59, 1988.

Bonavita JA, Dalinka MK, Schumacher HR Jr: Hydroxyapatite deposition disease. *Radiology* 134:781, 1980.

Boskey AL, Vigorita VJ, Spencer O, Stuchin SA, Lane JM: Chemical, microscopic, and ultrastructural characterization of the mineral deposits in tumoral calcinosis. *Clin Orthop* 178:258, 1983.

Bywaters EGL: The relation between heart and joint disease including "rheumatoid heart disease" and chronic post-rheumatic arthritis (type Jaccoud). *Br Heart J* 12:101, 1950.

Bywaters EGL, Dixon ASJ, Scott JT: Joint lesions of hyperparathyroidism. *Ann Rheum Dis* 22:171, 1963.

Campbell SM: Gout: How presentation, diagnosis, and treatment differ in the elderly. *Geriatrics* 43:71, 1988.

Dalinka MK, Reginato AJ, Golden DA: Calcium deposition diseases. *Semin Roentgenol* 17:39, 1982.

Fam AG, Topp JR, Stein HB, Little AH: Clinical and roentgenographic aspects of pseudogout: A study of 50 cases and a review. *Can Med Assoc J* 124:545, 1981.

Genant HK: Roentgenographic aspects of calcium pyrophosphate dihydrate crystal deposition disease (pseudogout). *Arthritis Rheum* 19:307, 1976.

Goldman AB, Pavlov H, Bullough P: Primary amyloidosis involving the skeletal system. *Skeletal Radiol* 6:69, 1979.

Grossman RE, Hensley GT: Bone lesions in primary amyloidosis. *Am J Roentgenol* 101:872, 1967.

Helms CA, Vogler JB III, Simms DA, Genant HK: CPPD crystal deposition disease or pseudogout. *RadioGraphics* 2:40, 1982.

Hirsch JH, Killien FC, Troupin RH: The arthropathy of hemochromatosis. *Radiology* 118:591, 1976.

Huaux JP, Vandenbroucke JM, Noel H: Amyloidosis 1970-1985 with special reference to amyloid arthropathy. A discussion about 106 cases. *Acta Clin Belg* 42:365,1987.

Jensen PS: Chondrocalcinosis and other calcifications. *Radiol Clin North Am* 26:1315,1988.

Jensen PS, Putman CE: Current concepts with respect to chondrocalcinosis and the pseudogout syndrome. *Am J Roentgenol* 123:531, 1975.

Justesen P, Andersen PE Jr: Radiologic manifestations in alkaptonura. *Skeletal Radiol* 11:204, 1984.

Laborde MJ, Green DL, Ascari AD, Muir A: Arthritis in hemochromatosis. *J Bone Joint Surg* 59-A:8, 1977.

Lawson JP, Steere AC: Lyme arthritis: Radiologic findings. *Radiology* 154:37, 1985.

Ling D, Murphy WA, Kyriakos M: Tophaceous pseudogout *Am J Roentgenol* 138:162,1982.

Madhok R, Bennett D, Sturrock RD, Forbes CD: Mechanisms of joint damage in an experimental model of hemophilic arthritis. *Arthritis Rheum* 31:1148, 1988.

Martel W: The overhanging margin of bone: A roentgenologic manifestation of gout. *Radiology* 91:755, 1968.

Melton JW III, Irby R: Multicentric reticulohistiocytosis. *Arthritis Rheum* 15:221, 1972.

Resnik CS, Resnick D: Crystal deposition disease. *Semin Arthritis Rheum* 12:390, 1983.

Resnick D: Bleeding disorders. In: Resnick D, Niwayama G (eds): *Diagnosis of Bone and Joint Disorders, vol. 2*. Philadelphia, Saunders, 1981.

Resnick D, Niwayama G: Calcium pyrophosphate dihydrate (CPPD) crystal deposition disease. In: Resnick D, Niwayama G (eds): *Diagnosis of Bone and Joint Disorders, vol 2*. Philadelphia, Saunders, 1981.

Rosenberg ZS, Norman A, Solomon G: Arthritis associated with HIV infection: Radiographic manifestations. *Radiology* 173:171, 1989.

Rubenstein J, Pritzker KPH: Crystal-associated arthropathies. *Am J Roentgenol* 152:685, 1989.

Shumacher HR: Articular cartilage in the degenerative arthropathy of hemochromatosis. *Arthritis Rheum* 25:1460, 1982.

Schumacher HR, Straka PC, Krikker MA, Dudley AT: The arthropathy of hemochromatosis. Recent studies. *Ann NY Acad Sci* 526:224, 1988.

Schumacher HR Jr: Crystals, inflammation, and osteoarthritis. *Am J Med* 83:11–6, 1987.

Sharp GC, Irvin WS, Tan EM, Gould RG, Holman HR: Mixed connective tissue disease—an apparently distinct rheumatic disease syndrome associated with a specific antibody to an extractable nuclear antigen (ENA). *Am J Med* 52:148, 1972.

Sissons HA, Steiner GC, Bonar F, May F, Rosenberg ZS, Samuels H, Present D: Tumoral calcium pyrophosphate deposition disease. *Skeletal Radiol* 18:79, 1989.

Stoker DJ, Murray RO: Skeletal changes in hemophilia and other bleeding disorders. *Semin Roentgenol* 9:185, 1974.

Talbott JH, Altman RD, Yu TF: Gouty arthritis masquerading as rheumatoid arthritis or vice versa. *Semin Arthritis Rheum* 8:77, 1978.

Udoff EJ, Genant HK, Kozin F, Ginsberg M: Mixed connective tissue disease: the spectrum of radiographic manifestations. *Radiology* 124:613, 1977.

Yulish BS, Lieberman JM, Strandjord SE, Bryan PJ, Mulopulos GP, Modic MT: Hemophilic arthropathy: Assessment with MR imaging. *Radiology* 164:759, 1987.

PART IV

Tumors and Tumor-Like Lesions

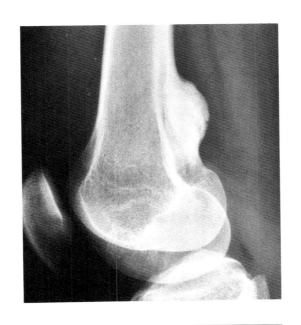

15

Radiologic Evaluation of Tumors and Tumor-Like Lesions

CLASSIFICATION OF TUMORS AND TUMOR-LIKE LESIONS

TUMORS, INCLUDING TUMOR-LIKE lesions, can generally be divided into two groups: benign and malignant. The latter group can be further subclassified into primary malignant tumors, secondary malignant tumors (from the transformation of benign conditions), and metastatic tumors (Fig. 15.1). All of these lesions can be still further classified according to their tissue of origin (Fig. 15.2). Figure 15.3 lists benign conditions that have the potential for malignant transformation.

In order to understand the terminology applied to tumors and tumor-like lesions of the bone, it is important to redefine certain terms pertinent to lesions and their location in the bone. The term *tumor* generally means *mass*; in common radiologic and orthopedic parlance, however, it is the equivalent of the term *neoplasm*. By definition, a neoplasm demonstrates autonomous growth; if in addition it produces local or remote metastases, it is defined as a *malignant neoplasm* or *malignant tumor*. Beyond this (and not dealt with in this chapter) are specific histopathologic criteria for defining a tumor as benign or malignant. It is nevertheless worth mentioning that cer-

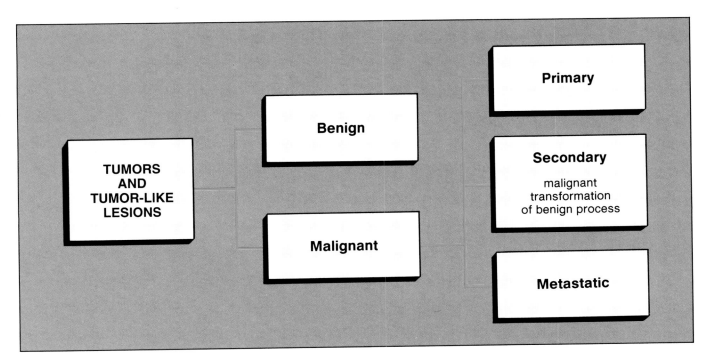

Figure 15.1
Classification of tumors and tumor-like lesions.

tain giant cell tumors, despite a "benign" histopathology, may produce distant metastases, and that certain cartilage tumors, despite adhering to a "benign" histopathologic pattern, can behave locally like malignant neoplasms, even though this is detectable only radiographically. Moreover, certain lesions discussed here and termed *tumor-like lesions* are not true neoplasms, but rather have a developmental or inflammatory origin. They are included in this chapter because they display a radiographic pattern that is almost indistinguishable from that of true neoplasms. Their etiology is in some cases still being debated.

Equally important is the redefinition of certain terms pertinent to the location of a lesion in the bone. In the growing skeleton, one can clearly distinguish the epiphysis, growth plate, metaphysis, and diaphysis (Fig. 15.4A), and when lesions are located at these sites they are named accordingly. The greatest confusion is in the use of the term *metaphysis*. The metaphysis is a histologically very thin zone of active bone growth, adjacent to the physis (growth plate). Consequently, for a lesion to be called metaphyseal in location, it must extend into and abut the growth plate. Yet it is customary—however incorrect—to use the same term for locating a lesion after skeletal maturity has occurred. By the time of maturity, the growth plate is scarred and neither the epiphysis nor metaphysis remains. More proper and less confusing would be a terminology (Fig. 15.4B) such as *articular end of the bone* and *shaft* for locating lesions in the bone whose growth plate has been obliterated and whose metaphysis has ceased to exist. Some other terms used to describe the location of bone lesions are illustrated in Figure 15.5.

RADIOLOGIC IMAGING MODALITIES

The radiologic modalities most often used in analyzing tumors and tumor-like lesions include: 1) conventional radiography, 2) magnification radiography, 3) tomography, 4) angiography (usually arteriography), 5) computed tomography (CT), 6) magnetic resonance imaging (MRI), 7) scintigraphy (radionuclide bone scan), and 8) fluoroscopy- or CT-guided percutaneous soft tissue and bone biopsy.

Figure 15.2 Classification of Tumors and Tumor-Like Lesions by Tissue of Origin

TISSUE OF ORIGIN	BENIGN LESION	MALIGNANT LESION
Bone-forming (osteogenic)	Osteoma Osteoid osteoma Osteoblastoma	Osteosarcoma (and variants) Juxtacortical osteosarcoma (and variants)

Cartilage-forming (chondrogenic)	Enchondroma (chondroma)
	Periosteal (juxtacortical) chondroma
	Enchondromatosis (Ollier disease)
	Osteochondroma (osteocartilaginous exostosis, single or multiple)
	Chondroblastoma
	Chondromyxoid fibroma
		Chondrosarcoma (central)
		   Conventional
		   Mesenchymal
		   Clear cell
		   Dedifferentiated
		Chondrosarcoma (peripheral)
		   Periosteal (juxtacortical)

Fibrous, osteofibrous, and fibrohistiocytic (fibrogenic)	Fibrous cortical defect (metaphyseal fibrous defect) Nonossifying fibroma Benign fibrous histiocytoma Fibrous dysplasia (mono- and polyostotic) Periosteal desmoid Desmoplastic fibroma Osteofibrous dysplasia (Kempson-Campanacci lesion) Ossifying fibroma (Sissons lesion)	Fibrosarcoma Malignant fibrous histiocytoma
Vascular	Hemangioma Glomus tumor Cystic angiomatosis	Angiosarcoma Hemangioendothelioma Hemangiopericytoma
Hematopoietic, reticuloendothelial, and lymphatic	Giant cell tumor (osteoclastoma) Eosinophilic granuloma Lymphangioma	Malignant giant cell tumor Histiocytic lymphoma Hodgkin lymphoma Leukemia Myeloma (plasmacytoma) Ewing sarcoma
Neural (neurogenic)	Neurofibroma Neurilemoma	Malignant schwannoma Neuroblastoma Primitive neuroectodermal tumor (PNET)
Notochordal		Chordoma
Fat (lipogenic)	Lipoma	Liposarcoma
Unknown	Simple bone cyst Aneurysmal bone cyst Intraosseous ganglion	Adamantinoma

Figure 15.3 Benign Conditions With Potential for Malignant Transformation

BENIGN LESION	MALIGNANCY
Enchondroma (in the long or flat bones*; in the short, tubular bones only as a part of Ollier disease or Maffucci syndrome)	Chondrosarcoma
Osteochondroma	Peripheral chondrosarcoma
Synovial chondromatosis	Chondrosarcoma
Fibrous dysplasia (usually polyostotic, or treated with radiation)	Fibrosarcoma Malignant fibrous histiocytoma Osteosarcoma
Osteofibrous dysplasia** (Kempson-Campanacci lesion)	Adamantinoma
Neurofibroma (in plexiform neurofibromatosis)**	Malignant schwannoma Liposarcoma Malignant mesenchymoma
Bone infarct	Fibrosarcoma Malignant fibrous histiocytoma
Osteomyelitis with chronic draining sinus tract (usually more than 15-20 years duration)	Squamous cell carcinoma Fibrosarcoma
Paget disease	Osteosarcoma Chondrosarcoma Fibrosarcoma Malignant fibrous histiocytoma

*Some authorities believe that, at least in some "malignant transformations" of enchondroma to chondrosarcoma, there was in fact from the very beginning a malignant lesion masquerading as benign and not recognized as such.

**Some authorities believe that this is not a true malignant transformation, but independent development of malignancy in the benign condition.

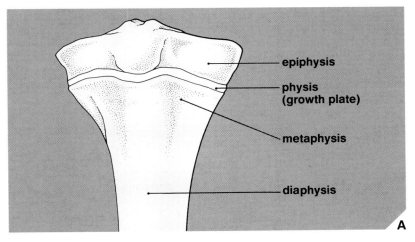

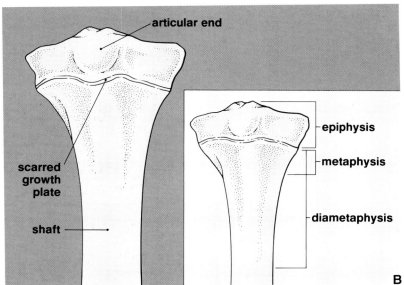

Figure 15.4 (A) In the maturing skeleton, the epiphysis, growth plate, metaphysis, and diaphysis are clearly recognizable areas. (B) With skeletal maturity, distinct epiphyseal and metaphyseal zones have ceased to exist. The terminology for describing the location of lesions should alter accordingly. The inset illustrates an alternate terminology.

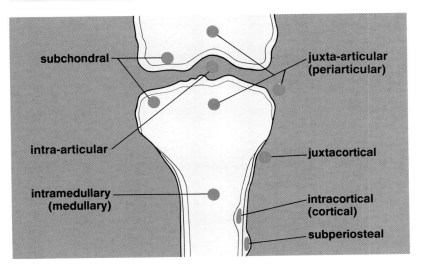

Figure 15.5 Terminology used to describe the location of lesions in the bone.

In most instances, the standard radiographic views specific for the anatomic site under investigation, in conjunction with conventional tomography, suffice to make a correct diagnosis (Fig. 15.6), which can subsequently be confirmed by biopsy and histopathologic examination. Chest radiography may also be required in cases of suspected metastasis, the most frequent complication of malignant lesions. This should be done before any treatment of a malignant primary bone tumor, since most bone malignancies metastasize to the lung. Magnification radiography may reveal small details not sufficiently outlined on routine films. Although CT by itself is rarely helpful in making a specific diagnosis, it can provide a precise evaluation of the extent of a bone lesion and may demonstrate breakthrough of the cortex and involvement of surrounding soft tissues (Fig. 15.7). CT is moreover very helpful in delineating a bone tumor having a complex anatomic structure. The scapula (Fig. 15.8), pelvis (Fig. 15.9), and sacrum, for example, may be difficult to image fully with conventional radiographic techniques. CT examination is crucial in determining the extent and spread of a tumor in the bone if limb salvage is contemplated, so that a safe margin of resection can be planned (Fig. 15.10). It can effectively demonstrate the intraosseous

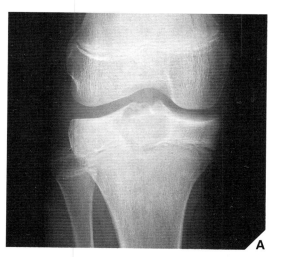

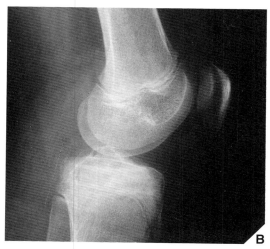

Figure 15.6
Anteroposterior (A) and lateral (B) views of the right knee of a 13-year-old girl reveal a radiolucent lesion located eccentrically in the proximal epiphysis of the tibia, with sharply defined borders and a thin, sclerotic margin. Here the standard projections led to the radiographic diagnosis of chondroblastoma.

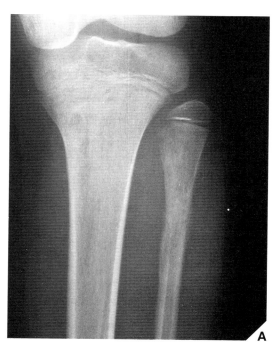

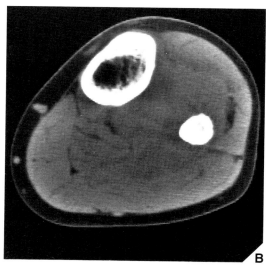

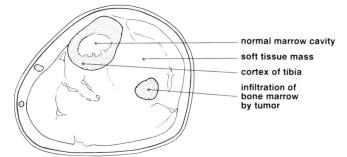

Figure 15.7
(A) Anteroposterior film demonstrates a malignant lesion that proved to be Ewing sarcoma in the proximal diaphysis of the left fibula of a 12-year-old boy.
(B) On CT examination, there is involvement of the bone marrow and extension of the tumor into the soft tissues.

normal marrow cavity
soft tissue mass
cortex of tibia
infiltration of bone marrow by tumor

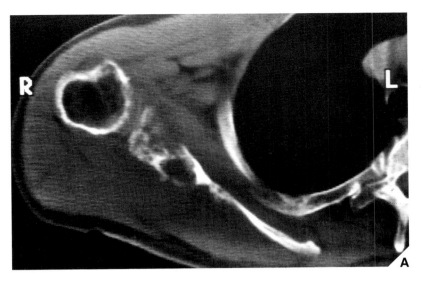

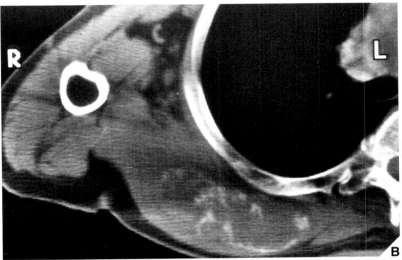

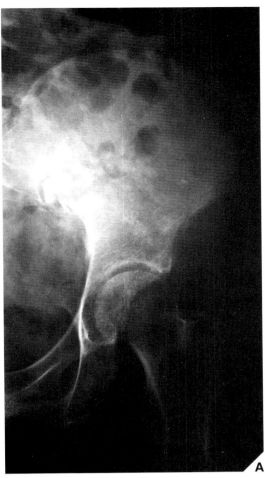

Figure 15.9
(A) Standard plain film of the pelvis was not sufficient to delineate the full extent of the destructive lesion of the iliac bone in this 66-year-old woman. (B) A CT section, however, showed a pathologic fracture of the ilium and the full extent of soft tissue involvement. The high Hounsfield values of the multiple soft tissue densities suggested bone formation. Enhancement of the CT images with contrast medium showed an increased vascularity of the lesion. Collectively, the CT findings suggested a diagnosis of osteosarcoma that, although unusual for a person of this age, was confirmed by open biopsy.

Figure 15.8 Standard radiographs were ambiguous in this 70-year-old man with a palpable mass over the right scapula. However, two CT sections demonstrate a destructive lesion of the glenoid portion and body of the scapula (A), with a large soft tissue mass extending to the rib cage and containing calcifications (B). The lesion proved on biopsy to be a chondrosarcoma.

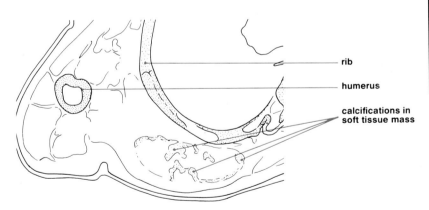

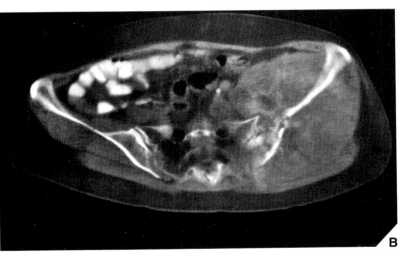

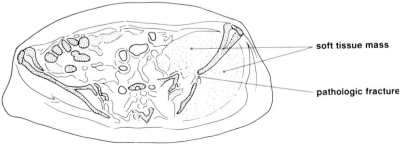

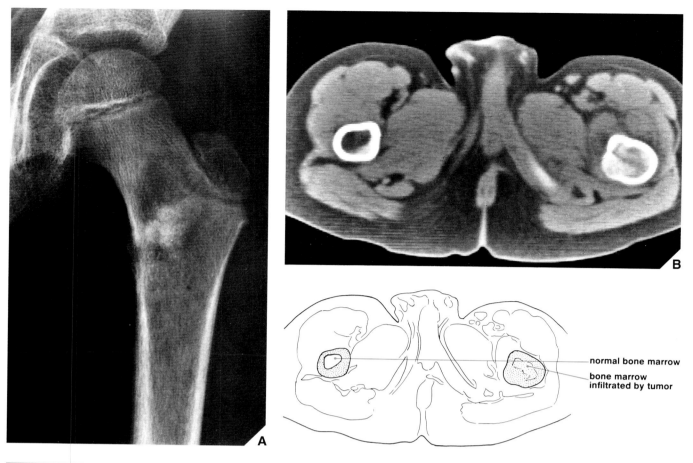

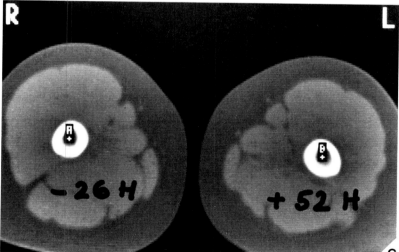

Figure 15.10 (A) Anteroposterior view of the left proximal femur of a 12-year-old boy demonstrates an osteolytic lesion in the intertrochanteric region, with a poorly defined margin and amorphous densities in the center associated with a periosteal reaction medially—features suggesting osteosarcoma, which was confirmed on biopsy. Because a limb-salvage procedure was contemplated, a CT scan was done to determine the extent of marrow infiltration and the required level of bone resection. The most proximal section (B) shows obvious gross tumor involvement of the marrow cavity of the left femur. A more distal section (C) shows no gross marrow abnormality, but a positive Hounsfield value of 52 units indicates tumor involvement of the marrow, which was not shown on the standard radiographs. By comparison, the section of the right femur shows a normal Hounsfield value of –26 for bone marrow.

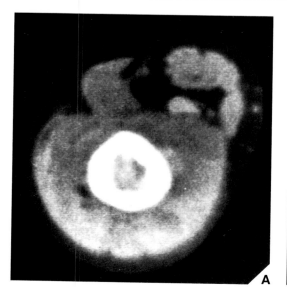

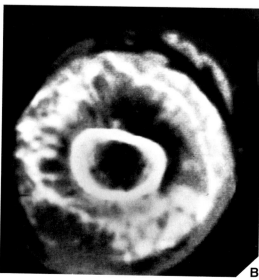

Figure 15.11 Prior to surgery, this 14-year-old girl with an osteosarcoma of the left femur underwent a full course of chemotherapy. (A) CT section before the therapy was begun shows involvement of the bone and marrow cavity. Note the soft tissue extension of the tumor, with nonhomogeneous, amorphous tumor bone formation. After combined treatment with doxorubicin hydrochloride, vincristine, methotrexate, and cisplatin, a repeat CT scan (B) shows calcifications and ossifications in the periphery of the lesion, which represents reactive rather than tumor bone and demonstrates the success of chemotherapy. Radical excision of the femur and a subsequent histopathologic examination showed almost complete eradication of malignant cells, confirming the CT findings.

extension of a tumor and its extraosseous involvement of soft tissues such as muscles and neurovascular bundles. CT is also useful for monitoring the results of treatment, evaluating for recurrence of a resected tumor, and demonstrating the effect of nonsurgical treatment such as radiation therapy or chemotherapy (Fig. 15.11). It is also indispensable in evaluating soft tissue tumors (Fig. 15.12), which on standard radiographs are indistinguishable from one another (with the exception of lipomas, which usually demonstrate low-density features), blending imperceptibly into the surrounding normal tissue.

Contrast enhancement of CT images aids in the identification of major neurovascular structures and well vascularized lesions.

Evaluating the relationship between the tumor and the surrounding soft tissues and neurovascular structures is particularly important for planning limb-salvage surgery.

Arteriography is used mainly to map out bone lesions and to assess the extent of disease. It is also used to demonstrate the vascular supply of a tumor and to locate vessels suitable for preoperative intra-arterial chemotherapy, as well as to demonstrate the area suitable for open biopsy, since the most vascular area of a tumor contains the most aggressive component. Occasionally, arteriography can be used to demonstrate abnormal tumor vessels, corroborating findings with plain-film radiography and tomography (Fig. 15.13). Arteriography is often useful in planning for limb-salvage procedures because it

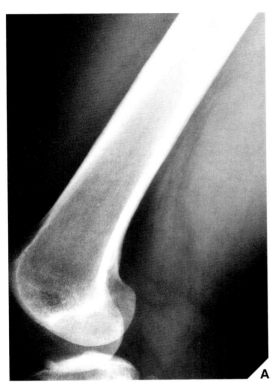

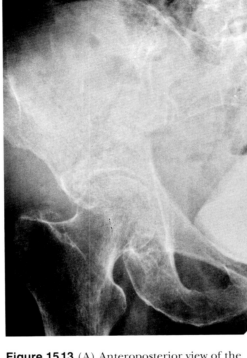

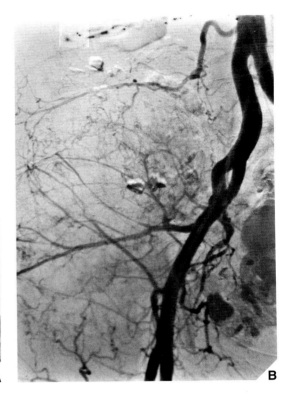

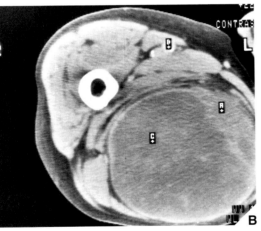

Figure 15.13 (A) Anteroposterior view of the pelvis in a 79-year-old woman with an eight-month history of pain in the right buttock and weight loss demonstrates a poorly defined destructive lesion of the right iliac bone, with multiple small calcifications and a soft tissue mass extending into the pelvis. Note the effect of the mass on the urinary bladder. A chondrosarcoma was suspected, and a femoral arteriogram was performed as part of the diagnostic workup.

(B) Subtraction study of an arteriogram demonstrates hypervascularity of the tumor. Note the abnormal tumor vessels, encasement and stretching of some vessels, and "pulling" of contrast medium into small "lakes"—all characteristic signs of a malignant lesion. Biopsy revealed a highly malignant, dedifferentiated chondrosarcoma. In this case the vascular study corroborated the plain-film findings of a malignant bone tumor.

Figure 15.12 A 56-year-old woman presented with a soft tissue mass on the posteromedial aspect of the right thigh. (A) Lateral plain film of the femur demonstrates only a soft tissue prominence posteriorly. (B) CT section shows an axial image of the mass, which is contained by a fibrotic capsule. The overlying skin is not infiltrated. Despite the benign appearance, the mass proved on biopsy to be a malignant fibrous histiocytoma.

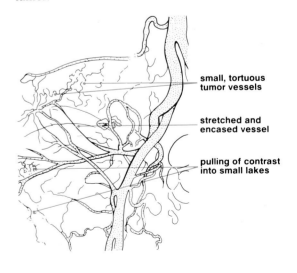

displacement of major neurovascular bundles, and the extent of joint involvement. Spin-echo T1-weighted images enhance tumor contrast with bone, bone marrow, and fatty tissue, while spin-echo T2-weighted images enhance tumor contrast with muscle and accentuate peritumoral edema. Axial and coronal images have been employed in determining the extent of soft tissue invasion in relation to important vascular structures. On the other hand, in comparison with CT, MR images do not clearly demonstrate calcification in the tumor matrix; in fact, large amounts of calcification or ossification may be almost undetectable. Moreover, MRI has shown itself less satisfactory than CT, or even than plain films and tomography, in the demonstration of cortical destruction. It is important to realize that both MRI and CT have advantages and disadvantages, and circumstances exist in which either can be the preferential or complementary study. But it is even more important that the surgeon communicate the information he needs to the radiologist who is performing and interpreting the study.

Recently, several investigators have stressed the superior contrast enhancement of MR images using intravenous injection of gadopentate dimeglumine (gadolinium diethylenetriamine-penta-acetic acid, or Gd-DTPA). Enhancement was found to give better delineation of the tumor's richly vascularized parts and of the compressed tissue immediately surrounding the tumor. It was also found to assist in differentiation of intra-articular tumor extension from joint effusion, and, as Erlemann pointed out, improved the differentiation of necrotic tissue from viable areas in various malignant tumors.

According to the recent investigations, MRI may have an additional application in evaluating both the tumor's response to radiation and chemotherapy and any local recurrence. On gadolinium-enhanced T1-weighted images, signal intensity remains low in avascular, necrotic areas of tumor, while it increases in viable tissue. Although static MRI was of little value for assessment of response to the treatment, dynamic MRI using Gd-DTPA as a contrast enhancement, according to Erlemann, had the highest degree of accuracy (85.7%) and was superior to scintigraphy, particularly in patients who were receiving intra-arterial chemotherapy. In general, drug-sensitive tumors display slower uptake of Gd-DTPA after preoperative chemotherapy than do nonresponsive lesions. As Vaupel contended, the rapid uptake of Gd-DTPA by malignant tissues may be due to increased vascularity and more rapid perfusion of the contrast material through an expanded interstitial space. The latest observation by Dewhirst and Kautcher suggests that MR spectroscopy may also be useful in the evaluation of patients undergoing chemotherapy.

It must be stressed, however, that most of the time MRI is not suitable for establishing the precise nature of a bone tumor. In particular, too much faith has been placed in MRI as a method of distinguishing benign lesions from malignant ones. Trials using combined hydrogen-1 MRI and P-31 MR spectroscopy also failed to distinguish most benign lesions from malignant tumors (Negendank, 1989). Despite the use of various criteria, the application of MRI to tissue diagnosis has rarely brought satisfactory results. This is because, in general, the small number of protons in calcified structures renders MRI less effective in diagnosing bone lesions, and

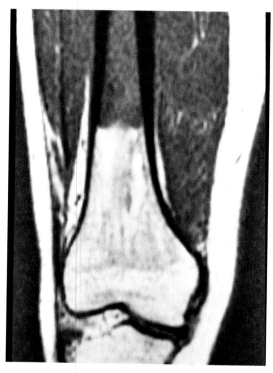

Figure 15.19 Coronal T1-weighted MRI (SE, TR 500/TE 20) demonstrates involvement of the medullary cavity of the right femur in this 16-year-old female with malignant fibrous histiocytoma. Note the excellent demonstration of the interface between normal bone displaying high signal intensity and a tumor displaying intermediate signal intensity.

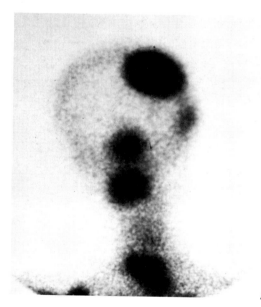

A

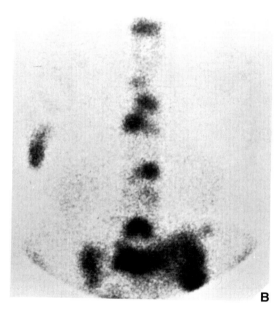

B

Figure 15.20 A radionuclide bone scan was performed on a 68-year-old woman with metastatic breast carcinoma to determine the distribution of metastases. After an intravenous injection of 15 mCi (555 MBq) of technetium-99m diphos-phonate, an increased uptake of the radiopharmaceutical is seen in the skull and cervical spine (A) and lumbar spine and pelvis (B), localizing the multiple metastases.

hence valuable evidence concerning the production of the tumor matrix can be missed. Moreover, as several investigations have shown, MRI is an imaging modality of low specificity. T1 and T2 measurements are generally of limited value for histologic characterization of musculoskeletal tumors. Quantitative determination of relaxation times has not proved to be clinically valuable in identifying various tumor types, although, as noted by Sundaram, it has proved to be an important technique in the staging of osteosarcoma and chondrosarcoma. T2-weighted images in particular are a crucial factor in delineating extraosseous tumor extension and peritumoral edema, as well as in assessing the involvement of major neurovascular bundles. Necrotic areas change from a low-intensity signal in the T1-weighted image to a very bright, intense signal in the T2-weighted image and can be differentiated from viable, solid tumor tissue. Although MRI cannot predict the histology of bone tumors, as Sundaram pointed out, it is a useful tool for distinguishing round cell tumors and metastases from stress fractures or medullary infarcts in symptomatic patients with normal radiographs, and, according to Baker, it can occasionally differentiate benign from pathologic fracture.

The radionuclide bone scan is an indicator of mineral turnover, and because there is usually enhanced deposition of bone-seeking radiopharmaceuticals in areas of bone undergoing change and repair, a bone scan is useful in localizing tumors and tumor-like lesions in the skeleton, particularly in such conditions as fibrous dysplasia, eosinophilic granuloma, or metastatic cancer where more than one lesion is encountered (Fig. 15.20). It also plays an important role in localizing small lesions such as osteoid osteomas, which

may not always be seen on plain-film studies (see Fig. 16.10). Although in most instances a radionuclide bone scan cannot distinguish benign lesions from malignant tumors, since increased blood flow with increased isotope deposition and increased osteoblastic activity takes place in both benign and malignant conditions, it is still occasionally capable of making such differentiation in benign lesions that do not absorb the radioactive isotope (Fig. 15.21). The radionuclide bone scan is sometimes also useful for differentiating multiple myeloma, which usually shows no significant uptake of the tracer, from metastatic cancer, which usually does.

Aside from routine radionucleide scans performed using technetium-99m-labeled phosphate compounds, occasionally gallium-67 is used for detection and staging of bone and soft tissue neoplasms. Gallium is handled by the body much like iron in that the protein transferrin carries it in the plasma, and it also competes for extravascular iron-binding proteins such as lactoferrin. The administrated dose for adults ranges from 3mCi (111 MBq) to 10mCi (370 MBq) per study. The exact mechanism of tumor uptake of gallium remains unsettled and its uptake varies with tumor type. In particular, Hodgkin lymphomas and histiocytic lymphomas are prone to significant gallium uptake.

Percutaneous bone and soft tissue biopsy done in the radiology department has in recent years gained its place in the diagnostic workup for various neoplastic diseases, including bone tumors. In patients with primary bone neoplasms, it is a helpful diagnostic and evaluative tool, allowing rapid histologic diagnosis, which is now considered essential, particularly in the planning of a limb-salvage procedure. It also helps assess the effect of chemotherapy and radia-

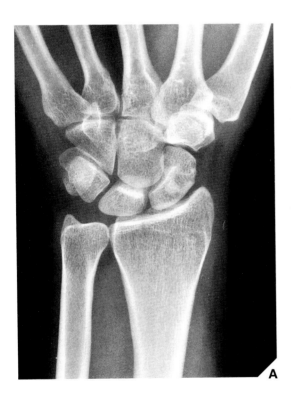
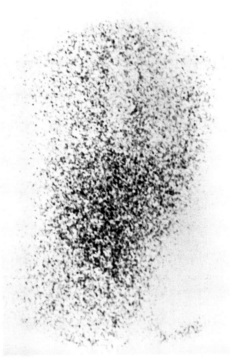

A   **B**

Figure 15.21 A 32-year-old woman presented with pain localized in the wrist area. (A) Dorsovolar plain film of the wrist demonstrates a dense, round lesion in the scaphoid, and a diagnosis of osteoid osteoma was considered. (B) Bone scan reveals normal isotope uptake, ruling out osteoid osteoma, which is invariably associated with an increased uptake of radiopharmaceutical. The lesion instead proved to be a bone island (enostosis), an asymptomatic developmental error of endochondral ossification without any consequence to the patient. The pain was unrelated to the island, coming instead from tenosynovitis; it disappeared after the patient was treated for the latter condition.

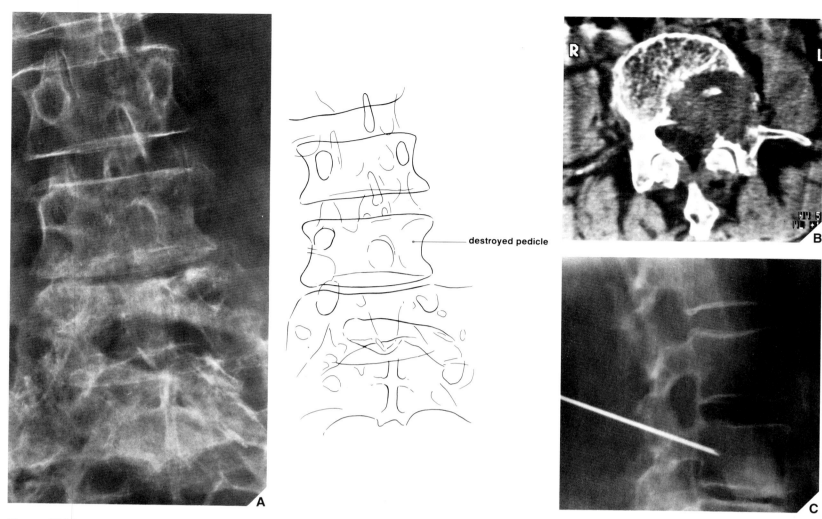

destroyed pedicle

Figure 15.22 (A) Anteroposterior plain film of the lumbar spine in a 67-year-old woman with lower-back pain for four months demonstrates destruction of the left pedicle of the L-4 vertebra. (B) CT section shows, in addition, involvement of the vertebral body by the tumor. (C) Percutaneous biopsy of the lesion, performed in the radiology suite for the purpose of rapid histopathologic diagnosis, revealed a metastatic adenocarcinoma from the colon.

tion therapy and helps locate the site of the primary tumor in cases of metastatic disease (Fig. 15.22). In addition, percutaneous bone and soft tissue biopsy performed in the radiology suite is simpler and costs less than a biopsy done in the operating room.

Finally, it is important to compare recent radiographic studies with earlier films; this point cannot be emphasized enough. The comparison can reveal not only the nature of a bone lesion (Fig. 15.23), but also its aggressiveness, a critical factor in a diagnostic workup.

TUMORS AND TUMOR-LIKE LESIONS OF THE BONE

Diagnosis

Clinical Information

The age of the patient is probably the single most important item of clinical data in radiographically establishing the diagnosis of a tumor (Fig. 15.24). Certain tumors have a predilection for specific age groups; aneurysmal bone cysts, for example, rarely occur beyond

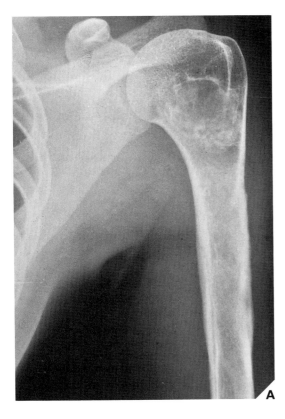 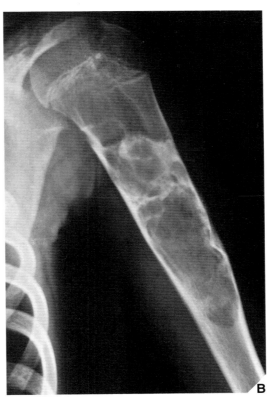

Figure 15.23 (A) Anteroposterior plain film of the humerus in a 26-year-old woman with vague pain in the left upper humerus for two months shows an ill defined lesion in the medullary region, with a periosteal reaction medially and laterally. There appear to be scattered calcifications in the proximal portion of the lesion. The possibility of a cartilage tumor such as chondrosarcoma was considered, but a film made seventeen years earlier (B) shows an unquestionably benign lesion (a simple bone cyst) that had been treated by curettage and the application of bone chips. In view of this, the later findings were interpreted as representing a healed bone cyst. The patient's pain was found to be related to muscular strain.

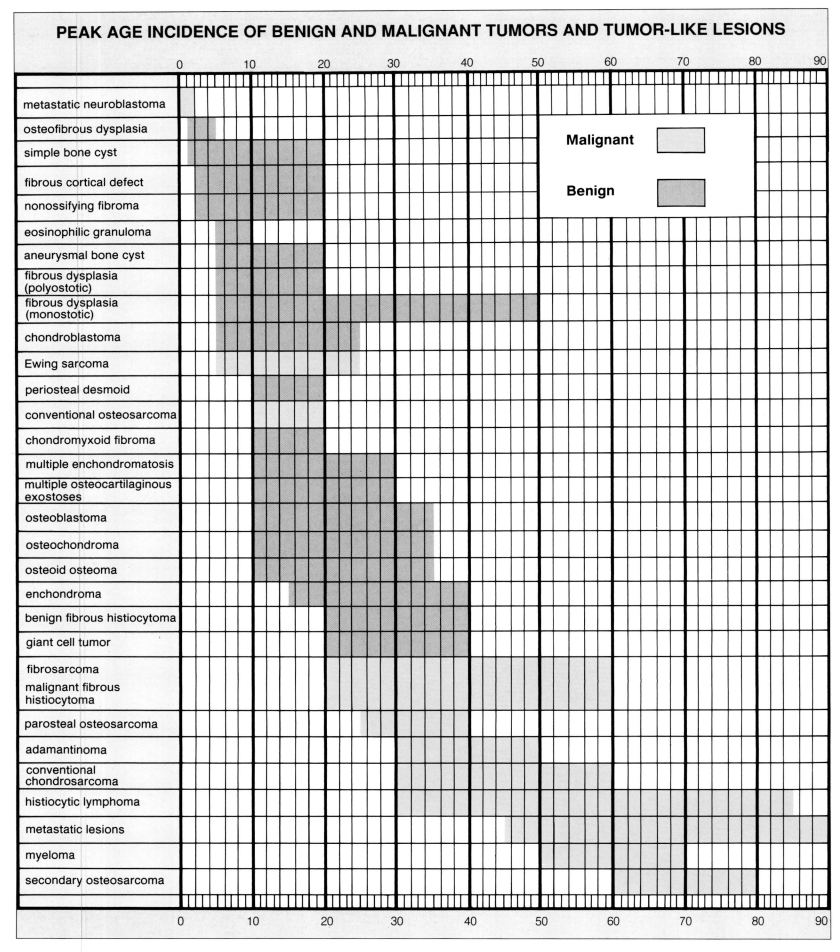

Figure 15.24 Peak age incidence of benign and malignant tumors and tumor-like lesions. (Sources: Dahlin DC, 1986; Huvos AG, 1979; Jaffe HL, 1968; Mirra JM, 1989; Moser RP, 1990; Schajowicz F, 1981; Wilner D, 1982)

age 20, and giant cell tumors as a rule are found only after the growth plate is closed. Other lesions may have different radiographic presentations or occur in different locations in patients of different ages. Simple bone cysts, which before skeletal maturity present almost exclusively in the long bones such as the proximal humerus and proximal femur, may appear in other locations (pelvis, scapula, os calcis) and have unconventional radiographic presentations with progressing age (Fig. 15.25).

Also important for clinically differentiating lesions of similar radiographic presentation—such as eosinophilic granuloma, osteomyelitis, and Ewing sarcoma—is the duration of the patient's symptoms. In eosinophilic granuloma, for example, the amount of bone destruction seen radiographically after one week of symptoms is usually the same as that seen after four to six weeks of symptoms in osteomyelitis and three to four months in Ewing sarcoma.

Occasionally, race may also be an important differential diagnostic factor, since certain lesions, such as tumoral calcinosis or bone infarctions, are seen more commonly in blacks than in whites, while others, such as Ewing sarcoma, are almost never seen in blacks.

The growth rate of the tumor may be an additional factor in differentiating malignant tumors (usually rapid-growing) from benign tumors (usually slow-growing).

Laboratory data, such as an increased erythrocyte sedimentation rate, an elevated alkaline or acid phosphatose level in the serum, occasionally can be a corraborative factor in diagnosis.

Imaging Modalities

With so many imaging techniques available to diagnose and further characterize the bone tumor, radiologists and clinicians are frequently at a loss as to how to proceed in a given case, what modality to use for this particular problem, in what order of preference to use the modalities, and when to stop. It is important to keep in mind that the choice of techniques for imaging the bone or soft tissue tumor should be dictated not only by the clinical presentation and the technique's expected effectiveness, but also by equipment availability, expertise, cost, and restrictions applicable to individual patients (for example, allergy to ionic or nonionic iodinated contrast agents, may preclude the use of arthrography; presence of a pacemaker, may preclude the use of MRI; or physiologic states such as pregnancy, warrant the use of sonography over the use of ionized radiation). Some of these problems were discussed in general in Chapters 1 and 2. Here I would attempt to give a general guideline related to the most effective modality for diagnosing and evaluating bone and soft tissue tumors. In the evaluation of bone tumors, plain-film radiography and tomography are still the standard diagnostic procedures. No matter what ancillary technique is used, the plain film should always be available for comparison. Most of the time, the choice of imaging technique is dictated by the type of suspected tumor. For instance, if osteoid osteoma is suspected based on the clinical history (see Fig. 1.5), plain-film radiography followed by scintigraphy should be performed first, and after the lesion is localized to the particular bone, CT should be employed for more specific localization and for obtaining quantitative information (measurements). On the other hand, if a soft tissue tumor is suspected, MRI is the only technique able to localize and characterize the lesion accurately. Likewise, if plain films are suggestive of a malignant bone tumor, MRI or CT should be employed next to evaluate both the intraosseous extent of the tumor and the extraosseous involvement of the soft tissues.

The use of CT versus MRI is based on the plain radiographs: If there is no definite evidence of soft tissue extension, CT is superior to MRI for detecting subtle cortical erosions and periosteal reaction, while providing at the same time an accurate means of determining the intraosseous extension of the tumor; if, however, the plain radiographs suggest cortical destruction and soft tissue mass, MRI would be the preferred modality since it provides an excellent soft tissue contrast and can determine the extraosseous extension of the tumor much better than CT.

In evaluating the results of malignant tumors treated by radiotherapy and chemotherapy, dynamic MRI using Gd-DTPA as a contrast enhancement is much superior to scintigraphy, CT, or even plain MRI.

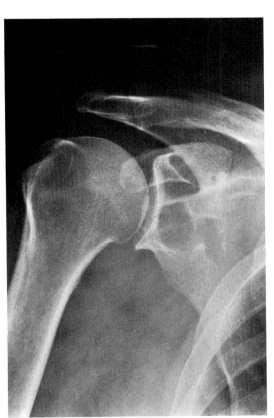

Figure 15.25 Anteroposterior view of the right shoulder of a 69-year-old man with shoulder pain for eight months demonstrates a well defined radiolucent lesion with a sclerotic border in the glenoid portion of the scapula. Because the patient had a history of gout, the lesion was thought to represent an intraosseous tophus. In the differential diagnosis, an intraosseous ganglion and even a cartilage tumor were also considered. An excision biopsy, however, revealed a simple bone cyst, which is very unusual in the glenoid part of the scapula.

Figure 15.26 depicts an algorithm for evaluating a bone lesion discovered on the standard plain radiographs. Note that the proper order of the various imaging modalities depends upon two main factors: 1) whether the plain-film findings are or are not diagnostic for any particular tumor, and 2) the lesion's uptake of a tracer on the radionuclide bone scan. Scintigraphy plays a crucial role here, dictating further steps in using the different techniques.

Radiographic Features of Bone Lesions
The radiographic features that help the radiologist diagnose a tumor or tumor-like bone lesion include: 1) the site of the lesion (location in the skeleton and in the individual bone), 2) the borders of the lesion (the so-called zone of transition), 3) the type of matrix of the lesion (composition of the tumor tissue), 4) the type of bone destruction, 5) the type of periosteal response to the lesion (periosteal reaction), 6) the nature and extent of soft tissue involvement, and 7) the single or multiple nature of the lesion (Fig. 15.27).

SITE OF THE LESION The site of a bone lesion is an important feature, since some tumors have a predilection for specific bones or specific sites in the bone (Figs. 15.28, 15.29). The sites of some lesions are so characteristic that a diagnosis can be suggested on this basis alone, as in the case of parosteal osteosarcoma (Fig. 15.30) or chondroblastoma (see Fig. 15.6). Moreover, certain entities can be readily excluded from the differential diagnosis on the basis of the lesion's location. Thus, for example, the diagnosis of a giant cell tumor should not be made for a lesion that does not reach the articular end of the bone, since very few of these tumors develop in sites remote from the joint.

Figure 15.26 Algorithm to evaluate and manage a bone lesion discovered on standard radiograph.

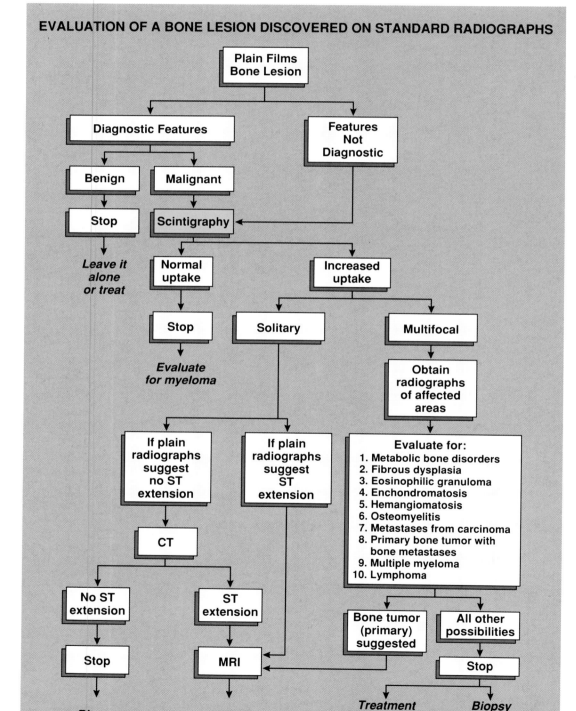

EVALUATION OF A BONE LESION DISCOVERED ON STANDARD RADIOGRAPHS

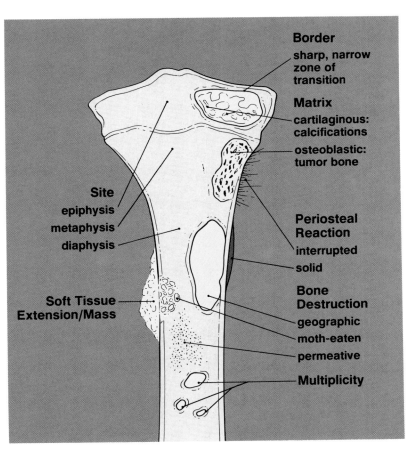

Border
sharp, narrow zone of transition

Matrix
cartilaginous: calcifications
osteoblastic: tumor bone

Site
epiphysis
metaphysis
diaphysis

Soft Tissue Extension/Mass

Periosteal Reaction
interrupted
solid

Bone Destruction
geographic
moth-eaten
permeative

Multiplicity

Figure 15.28 Examples of Tumors and Tumor-Like Lesions With a Predilection for Specific Bones, Sites in Bones, and Location*

LESION	BONE	ANATOMIC SITE	LOCATION
Simple bone cyst	Humerus Femur	Metaphysis Proximal diaphysis (see Figs. 17.26, 17.27)	Central
Osteoid osteoma	Femur Tibia	Neck of femur (see Figs. 16.4, 16.16)	
Chondroblastoma		Epiphysis (see Figs. 15.6, 16.52, 16.53)	Eccentric
Parosteal osteosarcoma	Femur	Posterior aspect, distal end (see Figs. 15.18, 18.14)	
Chordoma	Clivus C-2 Sacrum		Central
Osteofibrous dysplasia Adamantinoma	Tibia	Anterior aspect (see Fig. 17.20)	
Giant cell tumor	Femur Tibia Radius	Articular end (see Figs. 17.36, 17.39, 17.41, 17.42, 17.43)	Eccentric
Aneurysmal bone cyst	Tibia Humerus	Metaphysis (see Fig. 17.32)	Eccentric
Chondromyxoid fibroma	Tibia	Metaphysis (see Figs. 16.55, 16.56)	Eccentric
Multiple myeloma	Pelvis Spine Skull	Vertebral body Calvaria (see Figs. 18.43, 18.45)	

*See also Figs. 16.3, 16.20, 16.28, 16.36, 16.39, 16.48, 16.51, 16.54, 17.1, 17.12, 17.24, 17.30, 17.35, 17.45, 18.2, 18.13, 18.20, 18.27, 18.31, 18.37, 18.41, 18.48, 18.56

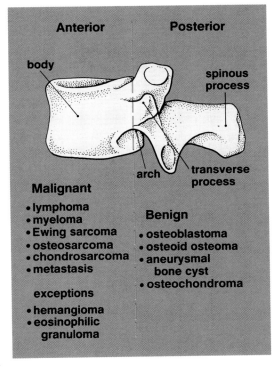

Anterior   **Posterior**

body
spinous process
arch   transverse process

Malignant
• lymphoma
• myeloma
• Ewing sarcoma
• osteosarcoma
• chondrosarcoma
• metastasis

exceptions
• hemangioma
• eosinophilic granuloma

Benign
• osteoblastoma
• osteoid osteoma
• aneurysmal bone cyst
• osteochondroma

Figure 15.29 Distribution of various tumors and tumor-like lesions in a vertebra. Malignant lesions are seen predominantly in its anterior part (body), while benign lesions predominate in its posterior elements (neural arch).

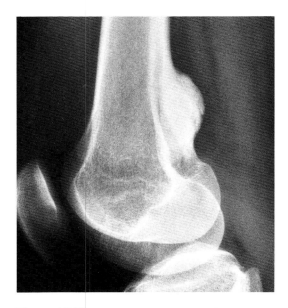

Figure 15.30 Parosteal osteosarcoma has a predilection for the posterior aspect of the distal femur.

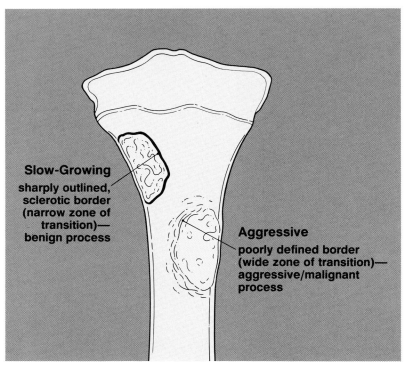

Figure 15.31 The radiographic features of the borders of a lesion characterize it as either slow-growing (and most likely benign) or aggressive (and most likely malignant).

Slow-Growing
sharply outlined, sclerotic border (narrow zone of transition)—benign process

Aggressive
poorly defined border (wide zone of transition)—aggressive/malignant process

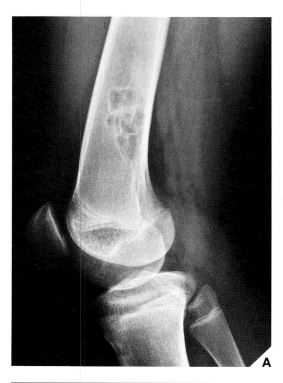

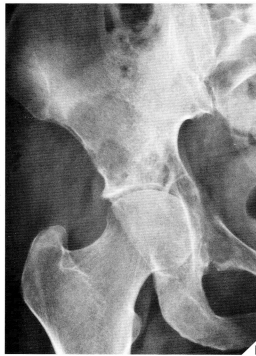

A

B

Figure 15.32 (A) A sclerotic border or narrow zone of transition from normal to abnormal bone typifies a benign lesion, as in this example of nonossifying fibroma. (B) A wide zone of transition typifies an aggressive/malignant lesion, in this case a solitary plasmacytoma involving the pubic bone and the supra-acetabular portion of the right ilium.

Figure 15.33 Bone Lesions Usually Lacking a Sclerotic Border

BENIGN	MALIGNANT
Giant cell tumor	Myeloma (plasmacytoma)
Brown tumor of	Fibrosarcoma
hyperparathyroidism	Malignant fibrous histiocytoma
	Lymphoma
	Metastatic tumor from primary in lung, gastrointestinal tract, kidney, breast, or thyroid

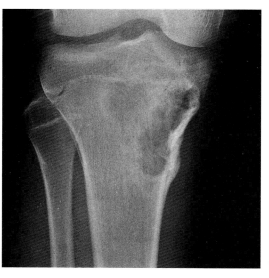

Figure 15.34 After three months of combined therapy with methotrexate, doxorubicin hydrochloride, and vincristine, the anteroposterior view of the knee of this 16-year-old boy with a conventional osteosarcoma of the right tibia reveals reactive sclerosis at the borders of the tumor and a narrow zone of transition, features more often seen in benign lesions. The patient underwent a limb-salvage procedure.

BORDERS OF THE LESION Evaluation of the borders or margins of a lesion is crucial in determining whether it is slow-growing or fast-growing (aggressive) (Fig. 15.31). Slow-growing lesions, which are usually benign, have sharply outlined sclerotic borders (a narrow zone of transition) (Fig. 15.32A), whereas malignant or aggressive lesions typically have indistinct borders (a wide zone of transition) with either minimal or no reactive sclerosis (Fig. 15.32B). Some lesions ordinarily lack a sclerotic border (Fig. 15.33). It must be emphasized that treatment can alter the appearance of malignant bone tumors; following radiation or chemotherapy they may exhibit significant sclerosis as well as a narrow zone of transition (Fig. 15.34).

TYPE OF MATRIX All bone tumors are composed of characteristic tissue components, the so-called tumor matrix. Only two of these—osteoblastic and cartilaginous tissue—can usually be clearly demonstrated radiographically. If one can identify bone or cartilage within a tumor, one can assume that it is osteoblastic or cartilaginous (Fig. 15.35). The identification of tumor bone within or adjacent to the area of destruction should alert the radiologist to the possibility of osteosarcoma. However, the deposition of new bone may also be the result of a reparative process secondary to bone destruction—so-called reactive sclerosis—rather than production of osteoid or bone by malignant cells. This new tumor bone is often radiographically indistinguishable from reactive bone; however, fluffy, cotton-like or cloud-like densities within the medullary cavity and in the adjacent soft tissue should suggest the presence of tumorous bone and hence the diagnosis of osteosarcoma (Fig. 15.36A).

Cartilage is identified by the presence of typically popcorn-like, punctate, annular, or comma-shaped calcifications (Fig. 15.36B). Since cartilage usually grows in lobules, a tumor of cartilaginous ori-

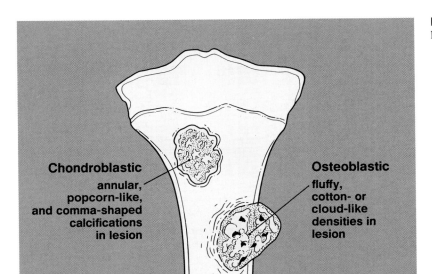

Figure 15.35 Radiographic features of the matrix of tumors and tumor-like lesions that characterize a lesion as cartilage-forming or bone-forming.

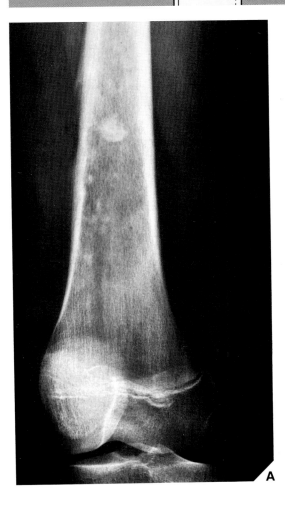
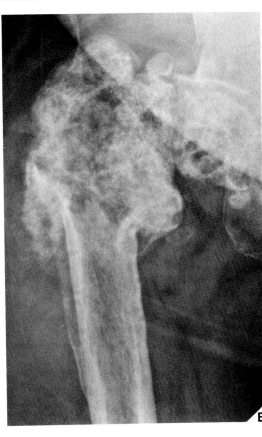

Figure 15.36 (A) The matrix of a typical osteoblastic lesion, in this case an osteosarcoma, is characterized by the presence of fluffy, cotton-like densities within the medullary cavity of the distal femur. (B) The matrix of the typical cartilage tumor, in this case chondrosarcoma, is characterized by punctate, annular, and popcorn-like calcifications within the osteolytic lesion in the proximal femur. Note also the endosteal scalloping and lobular appearance of the tumor. Periosteal reaction and pathologic fracture of the femoral neck are evident.

gin can often be suggested by lobulated growth. A completely radiolucent lesion may be either fibrous or cartilaginous in origin, although hollow structures produced by tumor-like lesions, such as simple bone cysts or intraosseous ganglia, can also present as radiolucent areas (Fig. 15.37).

TYPE OF BONE DESTRUCTION The type of bone destruction caused by a tumor is primarily related to the tumor growth rate. While not pathognomonic for any specific neoplasm, the type of destruction, which can be described as geographic, moth-eaten, or permeative (Fig. 15.38), may suggest not only a benign or malignant neoplastic process (Fig. 15.39A,B) but sometimes even the histologic type of a tumor, as in the permeative type of bone destruction characteristically produced by the so-called round cell tumors—Ewing sarcoma (Fig. 15.39C) and lymphoma.

PERIOSTEAL RESPONSE The periosteal reaction to a neoplastic process in the bone is usually categorized as uninterrupted or inter-

---

Figure 15.37 Tumors and Pseudotumors That May Present as Radiolucent Lesions

A. SOLID

Osteoblastic (osteoid osteoma, osteoblastoma, telangiectatic osteosarcoma)

Cartilaginous (enchondroma, chondroblastoma, chondromyxoid fibroma, chondrosarcoma)

Fibrous and histiocytic (nonossifying fibroma, fibrous dysplasia, osteofibrous dysplasia, desmoplastic fibroma, fibrosarcoma, malignant fibrous histiocytoma)

Lymphoma

Myeloma (plasmacytoma)

Ewing sarcoma

Metastatic (from lung, breast, gastrointestinal tract, kidney, thyroid)

Giant cell tumor

Eosinophilic granuloma

Paget disease (osteolytic phase—osteoporosis circumscripta)

B. CYSTIC

Simple bone cyst

Aneurysmal bone cyst

Various bone cysts (synovial, degenerative)

Intraosseous lipoma

Brown tumor of hyperparathyroidism

Vascular lesions

Hydatid cyst

Hemophilic pseudotumor

Intraosseous ganglion

Bone abscess

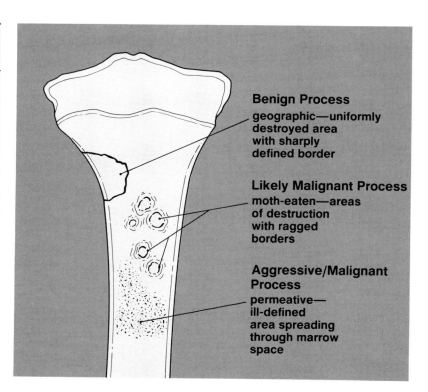

Benign Process
geographic—uniformly destroyed area with sharply defined border

Likely Malignant Process
moth-eaten—areas of destruction with ragged borders

Aggressive/Malignant Process
permeative—ill-defined area spreading through marrow space

Figure 15.38 The radiographic features of the type of bone destruction may suggest a benign or malignant neoplastic process.

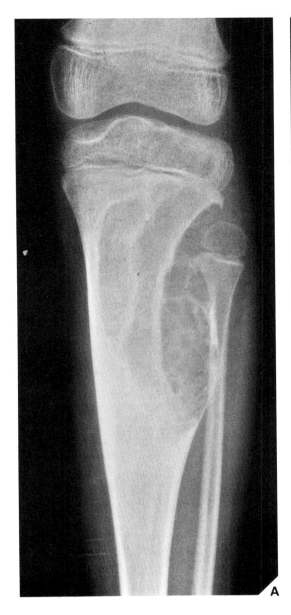

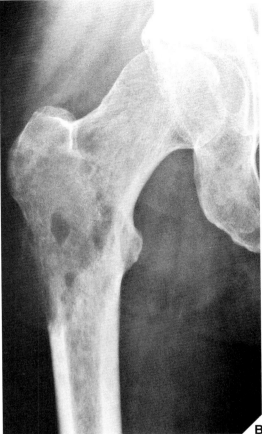

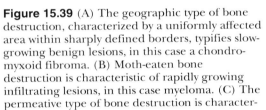

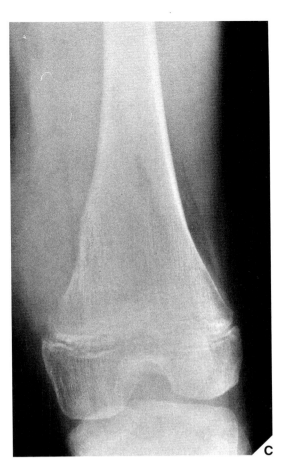

Figure 15.39 (A) The geographic type of bone destruction, characterized by a uniformly affected area within sharply defined borders, typifies slow-growing benign lesions, in this case a chondro-myxoid fibroma. (B) Moth-eaten bone destruction is characteristic of rapidly growing infiltrating lesions, in this case myeloma. (C) The permeative type of bone destruction is character-istic of round cell tumors, in this case Ewing sarcoma. Note the almost imperceptible destruction of the metaphysis of the femur by a tumor that has infiltrated the medullary cavity and cortex and extended into the surrounding soft tissues, forming a large mass. (A: Reproduced with permission from Lewis MM, et al., 1987)

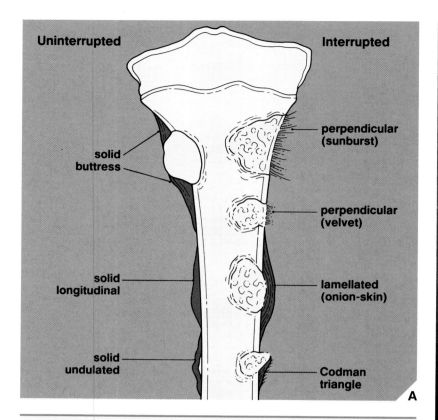

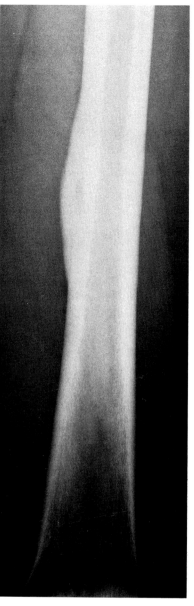

Figure 15.41 An uninterrupted solid periosteal reaction is characteristic of benign lesions, in this case a cortical osteoid osteoma.

Figure 15.40B Examples of Non-Neoplastic and Neoplastic Processes Categorized by Type of Periosteal Reaction

UNINTERRUPTED PERIOSTEAL REACTION

Benign Tumors and Tumor-Like Lesions	*Non-Neoplastic Conditions*
Osteoid osteoma	Osteomyelitis
Osteoblastoma	Eosinophilic granuloma
Aneurysmal bone cyst	Healing fracture
Chondromyxoid fibroma	Juxtacortical myositis ossificans
Periosteal chondroma	Hypertrophic pulmonary
Chondroblastoma	osteoarthropathy
	Hemophilia (subperiosteal bleeding)
	Varicose veins and peripheral vascular insufficiency
Malignant Tumors	Caffey disease
Chondrosarcoma (rare)	Thyroid acropachy
	Treated scurvy
	Pachydermoperiostosis
	Gaucher disease

INTERRUPTED PERIOSTEAL REACTION

Malignant Tumors	*Non-Neoplastic Conditions*
Osteosarcoma	Osteomyelitis (occasionally)
Ewing sarcoma	Eosinophilic granuloma (occasionally)
Chondrosarcoma	Subperiosteal hemorrhage (occasionally)
Lymphoma (rare)	
Fibrosarcoma (rare)	
MFH (rare)	
Metastatic carcinoma	

B

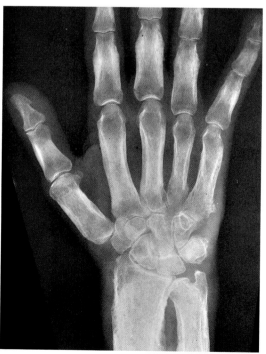

Figure 15.42 An uninterrupted periosteal reaction typifies changes of hypertrophic pulmonary osteoarthropathy as seen here in the distal forearm and hand in a patient with carcinoma of the lung.

Figure 15.40 (A) Radiographic characteristics of uninterrupted and interrupted types of periosteal reaction. Uninterrupted periosteal reaction indicates a benign process, while interrupted reaction indicates a malignant or aggressive nonmalignant process. (B) Some examples of non-neoplastic and neoplastic conditions in which these types of periosteal reaction may be seen.

rupted (Fig. 15.40). The first type of reaction is marked by solid layers of periosteal density, indicating a longstanding benign process, such as that seen in osteoid osteoma (Fig. 15.41) or osteoblastoma. Uninterrupted reaction is also seen in non-neoplastic processes such as eosinophilic granuloma, osteomyelitis, pachydermoperiostosis, in fractures in the healing stage, or in hypertrophic pulmonary osteoarthropathy (Fig. 15.42). The interrupted type of periosteal reaction suggests malignancy or a highly aggressive nonmalignant process. It may present as a sunburst pattern, a lamellated (onion-skin) pattern, velvet pattern, or Codman triangle, and is commonly seen in malignant primary tumors such as osteosarcoma or Ewing sarcoma (Fig. 15.43).

SOFT TISSUE EXTENSION   With few exceptions—such as giant cell tumors, aneurysmal bone cysts, osteoblastomas, or desmoplastic fibromas—benign tumors and tumor-like bone lesions usually do not exhibit soft tissue extension; thus almost invariably, a soft tissue mass indicates an aggressive lesion and one that is in many instances

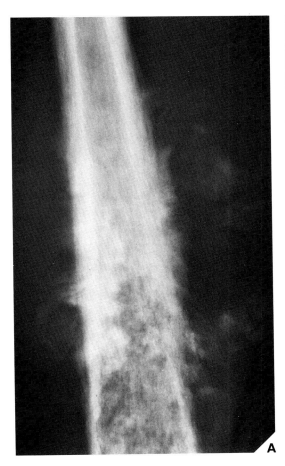

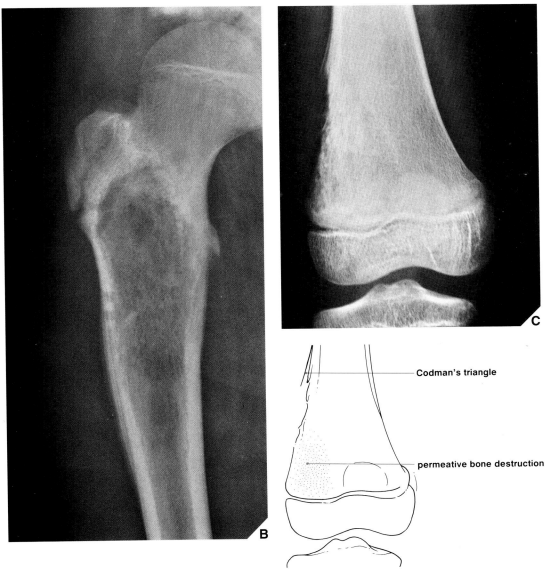

Figure 15.43 Highly aggressive and malignant lesions may present radiographically with a sunburst pattern of periosteal reaction, as seen in this case of osteosarcoma (A). Other patterns of interrupted periosteal reaction may also be encountered, such as the lamellated or onion-skin type (B), seen here in Ewing sarcoma involving the proximal femur, or Codman triangle (C), seen here in the distal femoral diaphysis (also in Ewing sarcoma).

malignant (Fig. 15.44). It should be kept in mind, however, that non-neoplastic conditions such as osteomyelitis also exhibit a soft tissue component, but the involvement of the soft tissues is usually poorly defined, with obliteration of fatty tissue layers. In malignant processes, on the other hand, the tumor mass is sharply defined, extending through the destroyed cortex with preservation of the tissue planes (Fig. 15.45).

In the case of a bone lesion associated with a soft tissue mass, it is always helpful to determine which condition arose first: Is the soft tissue lesion, in other words, an extension of a primary bone tumor or itself a primary lesion that has invaded the bone? Although not always applicable, certain radiographic criteria may help in deciding this issue (Fig. 15.46). In most instances, for example, a large soft tissue mass and a smaller bone lesion indicate secondary skeletal involvement. Ewing sarcoma breaks this rule, however; its destruc-

tive primary bone lesion may be small and often accompanied by a large soft tissue mass. A destructive lesion of bone lacking a periosteal reaction and adjacent to a soft tissue mass may indicate secondary invasion by a primary soft tissue tumor, which usually destroys the neighboring periosteum. This contrasts with primary bone lesions, which usually prompt a periosteal reaction when they break through the cortex and extend into adjacent soft tissues. Since these observations are not universally applicable, however, they should be taken only as indicators and not as pathognomonic features.

MULTIPLICITY OF LESIONS A multiplicity of malignant lesions usually indicates metastatic disease, multiple myeloma, or lymphoma (Fig. 15.47). Very rarely do primary malignant lesions, such as an osteosarcoma or Ewing sarcoma, present as multifocal disease. Benign

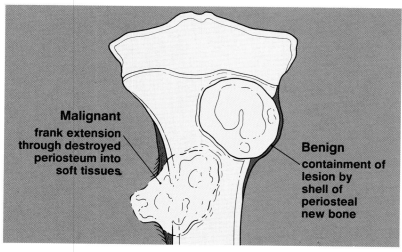

Figure 15.44 Radiographic features of soft tissue extension characterizing malignant/aggressive bone lesions and benign neoplastic processes.

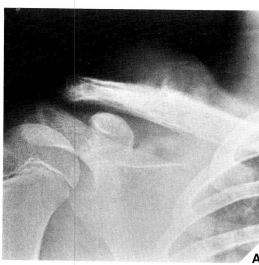

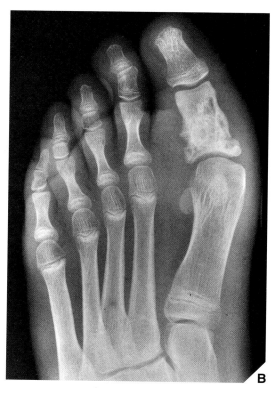

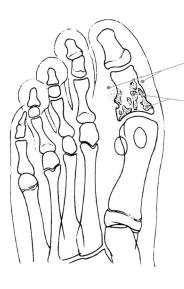

Figure 15.45 (A) A malignant tumor of the clavicle, in this case Ewing sarcoma, exhibits a distinct, sharply outlined soft tissue mass. (B) In osteomyelitis, on the other hand, the tissue planes are obliterated and the soft tissue mass has an indistinct border.

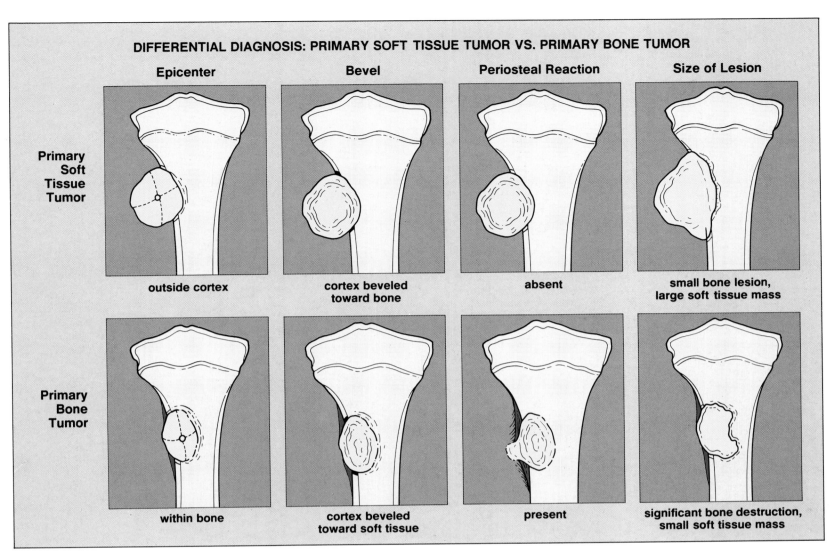

DIFFERENTIAL DIAGNOSIS: PRIMARY SOFT TISSUE TUMOR VS. PRIMARY BONE TUMOR

	Epicenter	Bevel	Periosteal Reaction	Size of Lesion
Primary Soft Tissue Tumor	outside cortex	cortex beveled toward bone	absent	small bone lesion, large soft tissue mass
Primary Bone Tumor	within bone	cortex beveled toward soft tissue	present	significant bone destruction, small soft tissue mass

Figure 15.46 Certain radiographic features of bone and soft tissue lesions may help differentiate a primary soft tissue tumor invading the bone from a primary bone tumor invading soft tissues.

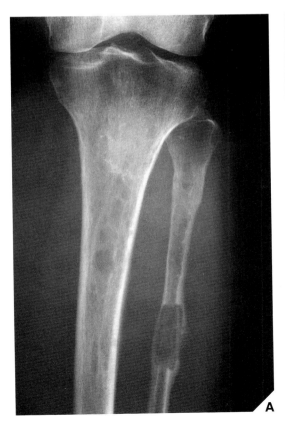

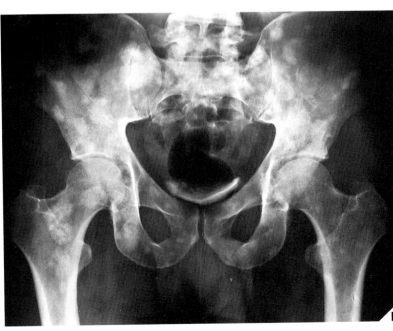

Figure 15.47
(A) Multiple myeloma is characterized by numerous osteolytic lesions.
(B) Metastatic disease may also present with multiple foci, as seen in this 66-year-old man with carcinoma of the prostate. Note several osteoblastic lesions scattered throughout the pelvis and both femora.

lesions, on the other hand, tend to involve multiple sites, as in polyostotic fibrous dysplasia (Fig. 15.48), multiple osteochondromas, enchondromatosis, eosinophilic granulomas, hemangiomatosis, and fibromatosis.

BENIGN VERSUS MALIGNANT Although it is sometimes very difficult to distinguish benign from malignant bone lesions on the basis of radiography alone, certain characteristic features favor one designation over the other (Fig. 15.49). Benign tumors usually present with well defined, sclerotic borders, a geographic type of bone destruction, an uninterrupted, solid periosteal reaction, and no soft tissue mass (see Figs. 15.25, 15.32A, 15.39A, 15.41). Malignant lesions, on the other hand, tend to demonstrate poorly defined borders with a wide zone of transition, a moth-eaten or permeative pattern of bone destruction, an interrupted periosteal reaction of the sunburst or onion-skin type, and an adjacent soft tissue mass (see Figs. 15.32B, 15.36, 15.39B,C, 15.43, 15.45A). It should be kept in mind, however, that some benign lesions may also exhibit aggressive features (Fig. 15.50).

Management

When all of the clinical and radiographic information concerning a patient with a bone lesion has been analyzed, the most important diagnostic decision is whether the lesion is definitely benign and not to be biopsied, but rather merely monitored or completely ignored—a "don't touch" lesion (Figs. 15.51, 15.52)—or whether it has an aggressive or ambiguous appearance and should be further

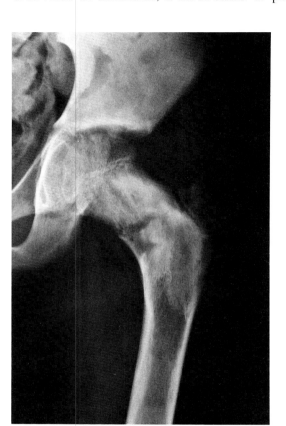

Figure 15.48
Anteroposterior view of the hip in a 10-year-old boy with polyostotic fibrous dysplasia shows numerous sites of involvement in the left femur and ilium. Scintigraphy demonstrated involvement of additional sites.

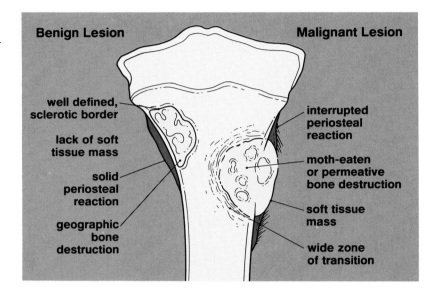

Figure 15.49 Radiographic features that may help differentiate benign from malignant lesions.

Figure 15.50 Benign Lesions With Aggressive Features

LESION	RADIOGRAPHIC PRESENTATION	LESION	RADIOGRAPHIC PRESENTATION
Osteoblastoma (aggressive)	Bone destruction and soft tissue extension similar to osteosarcoma	Osteomyelitis	Bone destruction, aggressive periosteal reaction Occasionally, features resembling osteosarcoma, Ewing sarcoma, or lymphoma
Desmoplastic fibroma	Expansile, destructive lesion, frequently trabeculated	Eosinophilic granuloma	Bone destruction, aggressive periosteal reaction Occasionally, features resembling Ewing sarcoma
Periosteal desmoid	Irregular cortical outline, mimics osteosarcoma or Ewing sarcoma	Pseudotumor of hemophilia	Bone destruction, periosteal reaction occasionally mimics malignant tumor
Giant cell tumor	Occasionally, aggressive features such as osteolytic bone destruction, cortical penetration, and soft tissue extension	Myositis ossificans	Features of parosteal or periosteal osteosarcoma, soft tissue osteosarcoma, or liposarcoma
Aneurysmal bone cyst	Soft tissue extension, occasionally mimicking malignant tumor	Brown tumor of hyperparathyroidism	Lytic bone lesion, resembling malignant tumor

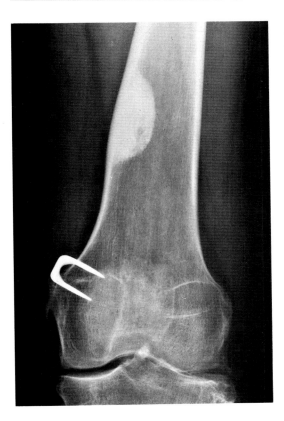

Figure 15.51 A typical benign "don't touch" lesion, in this case a nonossifying fibroma in healing-phase, should not be mistaken for a malignant tumor of bone.

Figure 15.52 "Don't Touch" Lesions That Should Not Be Biopsied

TUMORS AND TUMOR-LIKE LESIONS	NON-NEOPLASTIC PROCESSES
Fibrous cortical defect	Stress fracture
Nonossifying fibroma (healing phase)	Avulsion fracture (healing stage)
Periosteal desmoid	Bone infarct
Small, solitary focus of fibrous dysplasia	Bone island (enostosis)
	Myositis ossificans
Intraosseous ganglion	Degenerative and post-traumatic cysts
Enchondroma in a short, tubular bone	Brown tumor of hyperparathyroidism

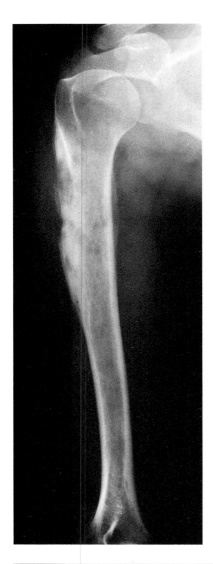

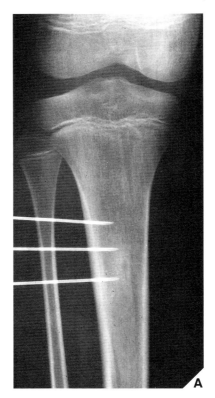

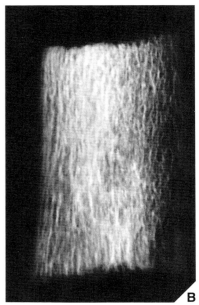

Figure 15.53 A typical "ambiguous" lesion exhibiting aggressive characteristics requires biopsy. The radiographic differential diagnosis in this case included osteosarcoma, Ewing sarcoma, lymphoma, and bone infection. Biopsy revealed chronic osteomyelitis.

Figure 15.54 (A) During surgery for resection of a nidus of osteoid osteoma in the proximal diaphysis of the tibia of a 10-year-old boy, needles are taped into the skin to localize the nidus. (B) Radiograph of the resected specimen demonstrates complete excision of the lesion.

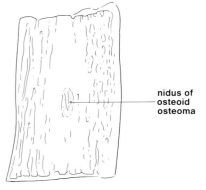

nidus of osteoid osteoma

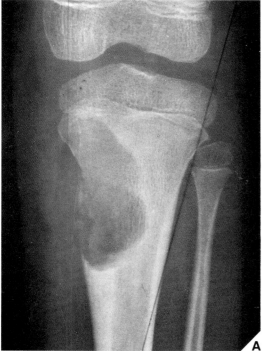

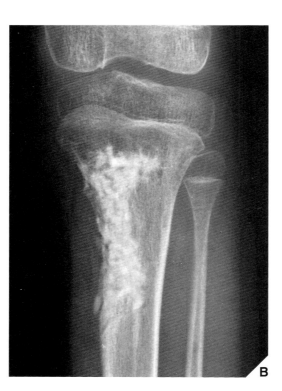

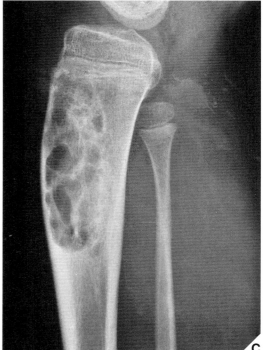

Figure 15.55 A 9-year-old boy was treated for a chondromyxoid fibroma, a benign cartilaginous lesion, in the proximal left tibia. (A) Preoperative film shows a lesion exhibiting a thin sclerotic border with endosteal scalloping, a geographic-type bone destruction, and a solid buttress of periosteal new bone formation at its distal part. (B) Postoperative film shows the lesion's cavity packed with bone chips following curettage. (C) Two years later the tumor recurred.

investigated via percutaneous or open biopsy (Fig. 15.53). The results of the histopathologic examination of a specimen determine whether the further management in a given case should be surgical, chemotherapeutic, radiotherapeutic, or a combination of these.

Monitoring Treatment Results
Five modalities—plain-film radiography, CT, MRI, scintigraphy, and arteriography—are commonly used to monitor the results of treatment for bone tumors. Of these five, plain-film radiography is used mainly to document the results of surgical resection of benign

lesions such as osteochondroma or osteoid osteoma (Fig. 15.54), or to follow-up after curettage of benign tumors or tumor-like lesions and application of bone graft (Fig. 15.55). In the case of malignant tumors, plain films permit one to demonstrate the position of endoprostheses (Fig. 15.56) or bone grafts (Fig. 15.57) in limb-salvage procedures. The effectiveness of chemotherapy is best monitored by a combination of plain-film radiography, arteriography (Fig. 15.58), CT (see Fig. 15.11), and MRI. Recurrence or metastatic spread of a tumor can be effectively shown at an early stage on scintigraphy, CT, or MRI.

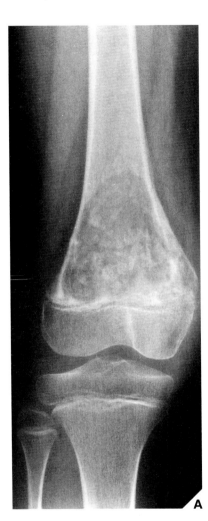

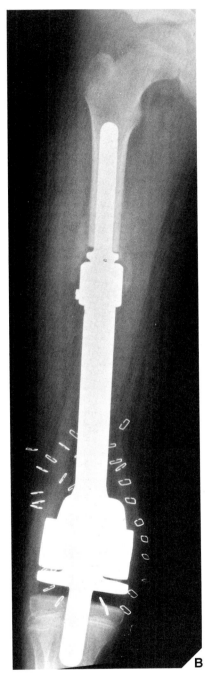

Figure 15.56 After a course of chemotherapy, an 8-year-old girl with an osteosarcoma of the right femur (A) underwent radical resection of the distal three-quarters of the femur, with insertion of an expandable (LEAP) prosthesis (B), which can be lengthened as the child grows. (Courtesy of Dr. MM Lewis, New York, NY)

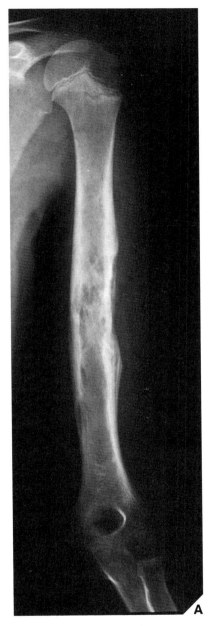

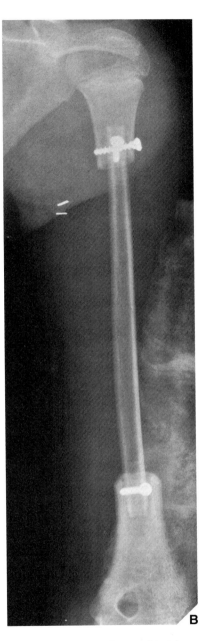

Figure 15.57 After a course of radio- and chemotherapy, a 9-year-old girl with a Ewing sarcoma in the diaphysis of the left humerus (A) underwent radical resection of the middle segment of the humerus. (B) Reconstruction was accomplished with the application of a fibular autograft.

Complications

While the most frequent direct complication of malignant bone tumors is metastasis, particularly to the lung, the most serious complication of some benign lesions is their potential for malignant transformation (Fig. 15.59; see also Fig. 15.3). Moreover, some benign lesions, such as those seen in multiple cartilaginous exostoses (Fig. 15.60) or enchondromatosis, may result in severe growth disturbance. The most common complication of tumors and tumor-like lesions in general, however, is pathologic fracture. Although not a diagnostic feature, this may complicate both benign and malignant lesions. Among lesions with a high potential for fracture are simple bone cysts, giant nonossifying fibromas (Fig. 15.61), fibrous dysplasia, and enchondromas. Occasionally, pathologic fracture is the first sign of a neoplastic process. Other complications, such as pressure erosion of adjacent bone (Fig. 15.62) or compression of adjacent blood vessels or nerves (see Fig. 16.42), may occur with growth of a lesion beyond the cortical outline.

SOFT TISSUE TUMORS AND TUMOR-LIKE LESIONS OF THE JOINT
Soft Tissue Tumors

Unlike tumors and tumor-like lesions of bone, most soft tissue tumors (Fig. 15.63) lack specific radiographic characteristics that might be helpful in their diagnosis. Some findings, however, may point to a particular kind of lesion. For instance, calcified phleboliths in a soft tissue mass suggest a hemangioma or hemangiomatosis (Fig. 15.64); radiolucency within a mass suggests a lipoma

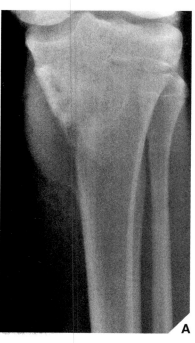 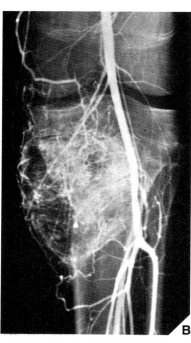 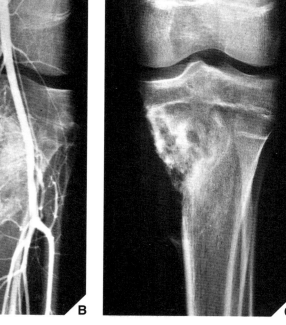 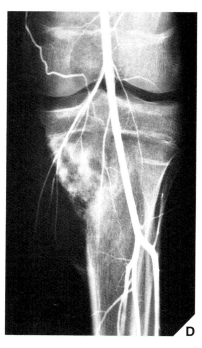

Figure 15.58 (A) Anteroposterior view of the proximal left tibia of a 15-year-old boy demonstrates an osteosarcoma in the metaphysis associated with a large soft tissue mass. (B) An arteriogram done prior to treatment shows the soft tissue mass to be hypervascular. After combination chemotherapy with methotrexate, vincristine, doxorubicin hydrochloride, and cisplatin, a repeated plain film (C) and arteriogram (D) show marked reduction of the tumor mass. Subsequently, a wide resection of the proximal tibia was done, and a metallic spacer similar to the one shown in Figure 15.56B was implanted.

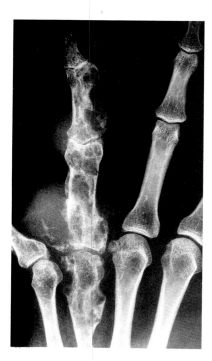

Figure 15.59 An enchondroma at the base of the ring finger of this 32-year-old man with multiple enchondromatosis underwent sarcomatous transformation to a chondrosarcoma.

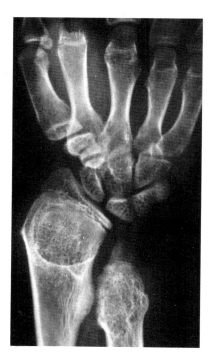

Figure 15.60 Anteroposterior view of the forearm of a 14-year-old boy with multiple cartilaginous exostoses (osteochondromas) shows marked growth disturbance of the distal ends of the radius and ulna.

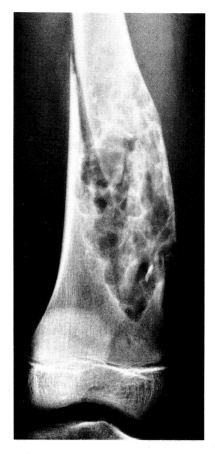

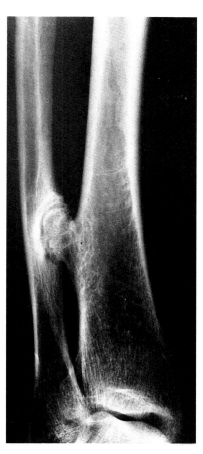

Fig.15.61 A 9-year-old boy with a giant nonossifying fibroma of the distal diaphysis of the right femur developed a pathologic fracture, a common complication of this lesion.

Figure 15.62 Extension of a lesion arising from the posterolateral aspect of the distal tibia in a 24-year-old man with an osteochondroma erodes the adjacent fibula.

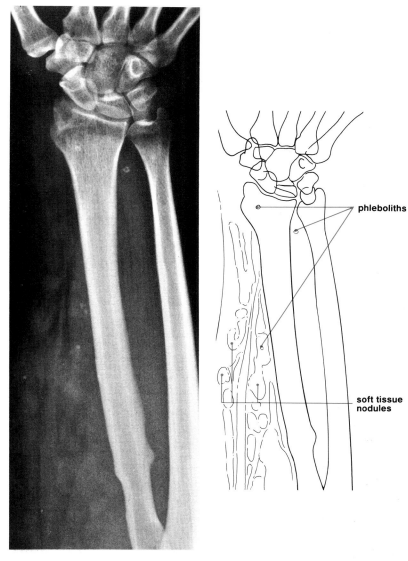

phleboliths

soft tissue nodules

Figure 15.64 Plain film in a 39-year-old woman with a nodular swelling of the left forearm demonstrates multiple small calcified phleboliths, suggesting the diagnosis of hemangiomatosis.

Figure 15.63 Most Common Benign and Malignant Soft Tissue Tumors

BENIGN	MALIGNANT
Ganglion	Rhabdomyosarcoma
Lipoma	Leiomyosarcoma
Myoma, leiomyoma	Malignant fibrous
Fibroma	histiocytoma
Myxoma	Fibrosarcoma
Hemangioma,	Liposarcoma
hemangiomatosis	Synovial sarcoma
Chondroma	Extraskeletal osteosarcoma
Neurofibroma	

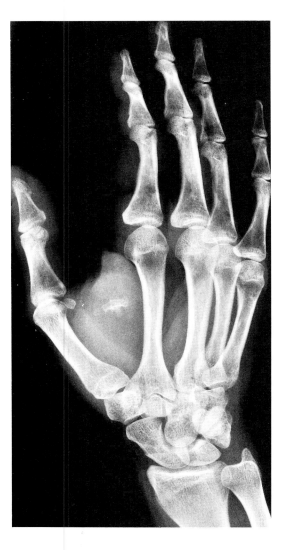

Figure 15.65 Oblique view of the hand of a 27-year-old woman with a soft tissue mass in the dorsal aspect shows a radiolucent lesion in the soft tissues adjacent to the radial aspect of the second metacarpal bone. Within the radiolucent area there is evidence of bone formation. The lesion proved to be a lipoma.

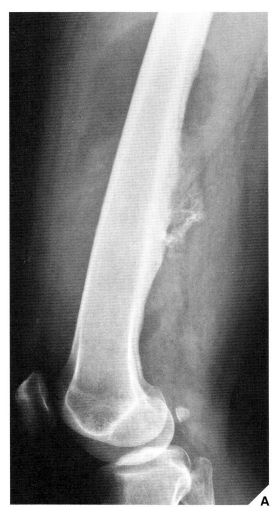

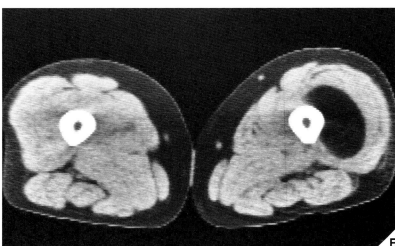

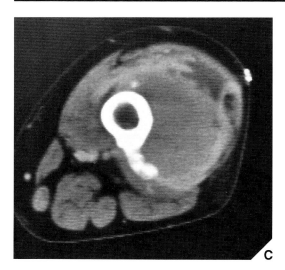

Figure 15.66 (A) Lateral plain film in a 54-year-old man with a slowly enlarging mass on the posterior aspect of the thigh demonstrates a poorly defined soft tissue mass with radiolucent areas and bone formation at the site of the posterior cortex of the femur. (B) CT section at the level of the radiolucency confirms the presence of fatty tissue. (C) A section through the bone formation discloses a more dense mass infiltrating surrounding muscular structures. A liposarcoma was suggested as a possible diagnosis and was later confirmed on excision biopsy.

(Fig. 15.65); mottled lucencies within a dense mass, in association with bone formation, suggest liposarcoma (Fig. 15.66); popcorn-like calcifications suggest soft tissue chondroma or chondrosarcoma; similar calcifications in the vicinity of a joint, particularly when associated with bone destruction, suggest synovial sarcoma; and ill defined, nonhomogeneous, smudgy bone in a soft tissue mass may indicate a soft tissue osteosarcoma (Fig. 15.67). Several investigators implied the efficacy of MRI in the characterization and evaluation of soft tissue masses; its superiority over CT stems from lack of ionizing radiation, its capability of multidirectional and multiplanar imaging, and its excellent contrast resolution and accurate anatomic definition of soft tissue tumors. On T1-weighted pulsing sequences, the majority of soft tissue masses display low-to-intermediate signal intensity, while on T2-weighted images they display high signal intensity. There are, however, masses that show high signal intensity on T1-weighting due to blood or fat content, such as lipomas, hemangiomas, and chronic hematomas. One of the fatty tumors that does not show a high signal on T1-weighting is myxoid liposarcoma. At present, however, as Sundaram contended based on MRI results, neither visual characteristics nor signal intensity values permit one to distinguish or predict the histology of soft tissue masses.

The main role of the radiologist is not to make a specific diagnosis, but rather to demonstrate the extent of the lesion and decide whether the lesion is a primary soft tissue tumor invading the bone or an extracortical extension of a primary bone tumor (see Fig. 15.46). Most often, this is achieved by using arteriography (Fig. 15.68), CT scan (Fig. 15.69), and MRI (Fig. 15.70). After this, the radiologist's role may become more active, involving fluoroscopy- or

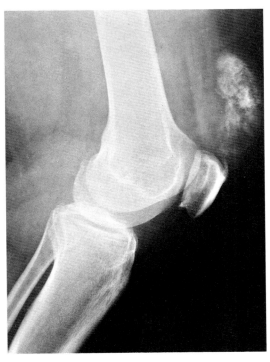

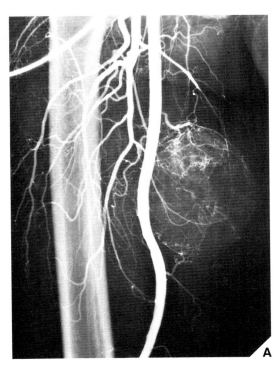

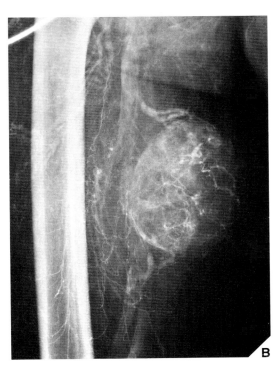

Figure 15.67 A 51-year-old woman presented with a large suprapatellar soft tissue mass. Lateral radiograph of the knee demonstrates a mass with ill defined nonhomogeneous bone formation in the central part of the lesion. Biopsy revealed a soft tissue osteosarcoma. (Reproduced with permission from Greenspan A, et al., 1987)

Figure 15.68 Femoral arteriography was performed on a 56-year-old man with a tumor on the medial aspect of the right thigh, which proved to be a malignant fibrous histiocytoma of the soft tissues. (A) The arterial phase demonstrates the displacement of the superficial femoral artery by the tumor, the extent of the tumor and area of neovascularity, and the accumulation of contrast medium within the tumor. (B) The venous phase shows the accumulation of contrast in abnormal vessels and a tumor "stain," as well as the topography of venous structures.

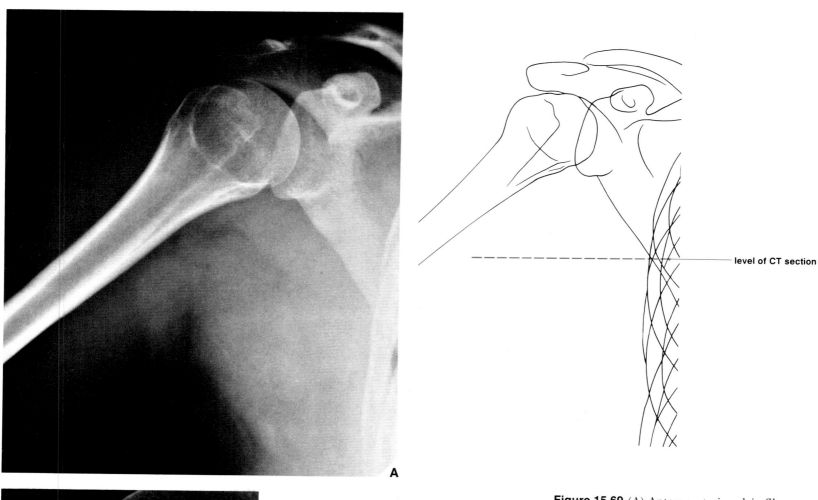

A

level of CT section

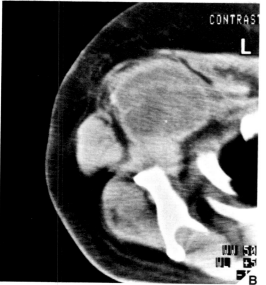

B

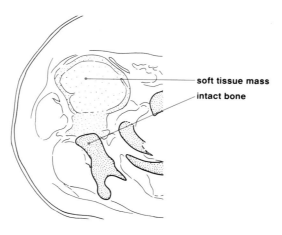

soft tissue mass

intact bone

Figure 15.69 (A) Anteroposterior plain film of the shoulder of a 40-year-old woman with a history of an enlarging mass in the right axilla shows an ill defined mass adjacent to the lateral border of the scapula. (B) CT section with contrast enhancement shows the extent of the mass and the lack of bone involvement. The tumor proved to be a fibrosarcoma.

CT-guided percutaneous biopsy of the lesion. In this respect, prior arteriography helps select the proper area for biopsy, with the specimen usually taken from the most vascular part of the lesion (Fig. 15.71).

Tumor-Like Lesions of the Joint

Within the category of tumor-like conditions of the joint, two types are often seen: synovial chondromatosis and pigmented villonodular synovitis. Although the plain-film characteristics of these two condi-

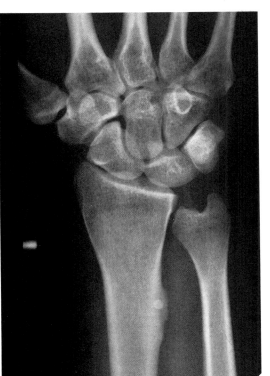

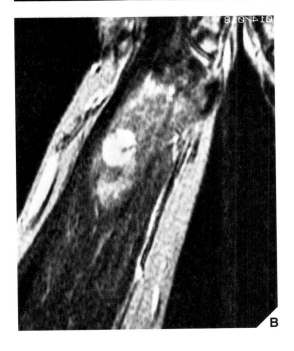

Figure 15.70
A 34-year-old woman presented with pain in the distal left forearm. The plain radiograph (A) demonstrates periosteal reaction at the ulnar border of the distal radius, associated with a phlebolith. (B) Coronal T2-weighted MRI (SE, TR 2000/TE 80) shows a large mass situated in the pronator quadratus muscle of the distal forearm, displaying inhomogenous signal ranging from intermediate to high intensity. The lesion proved to be an intramuscular hemangioma. (Reprinted with permission from Greenspan A, et al., 1992)

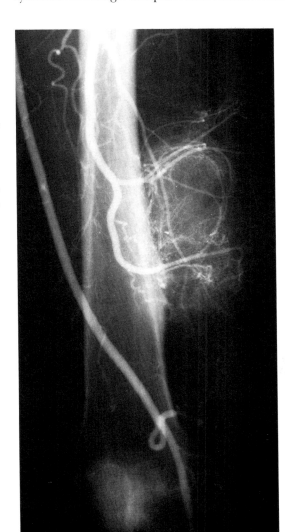

Figure 15.71 Vascular study of the patient shown in Figure 15.66 shows that the lesion consists of two parts: The proximal part is more radiolucent and hypovascular, while the distal is more dense and hypervascular. The biopsy specimen on which the diagnosis of liposarcoma was made was obtained from the more vascular segment of the tumor. After radical resection and examination of the entire specimen, the more radiolucent hypovascular area revealed almost no malignant component. Had the biopsy been obtained only from that part of the tumor, the result probably would not have been consistent with the final diagnosis.

tions are usually sufficient to indicate their nature, contrast arthrography and MRI are the most reliable means of establishing the diagnosis. Synovial chondromatosis, a condition marked by cartilage formation by the synovial membrane or joint capsule, is characterized by multiple foci of cartilaginous metaplasia within the synovium and multiple osteochondral bodies of relatively uniform size and shape within the joint capsule (Fig. 15.72). Occasionally, the lesion may also arise from the tendon sheaths. The knee is the most commonly affected joint, but hip, shoulder, elbow, and ankle involvement have been reported. Radiographically, synovial chondromatosis presents as multiple calcified bodies that are regular in outline and usually uniform in size, ranging from a few millimeters to several centimeters. This condition is seen in adults, and males are twice as often affected as females. Associated bony ero-

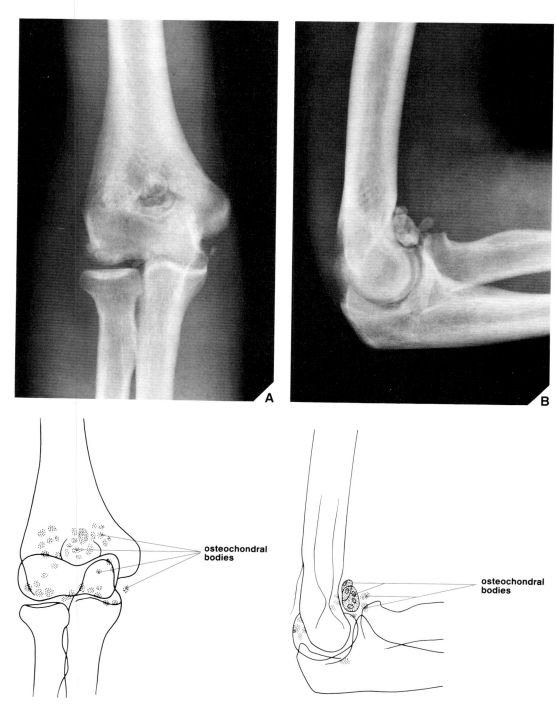

Figure 15.73 Lateral view of the knee of a 58-year-old man shows a large suprapatellar joint effusion and a dense, lumpy soft tissue mass eroding the posterior aspect of the lateral femoral condyle, features suggesting pigmented villonodular synovitis.

Figure 15.72 A 23-year-old man complained of pain and occasional locking in the elbow joint; he had no history of trauma. Anteroposterior (A) and lateral (B) views demonstrate multiple osteochondral bodies in the elbow joint, which are regularly shaped and uniform in size. This finding is characteristic of synovial chondromatosis.

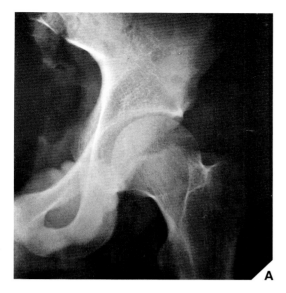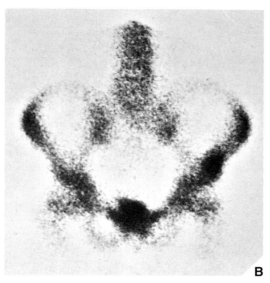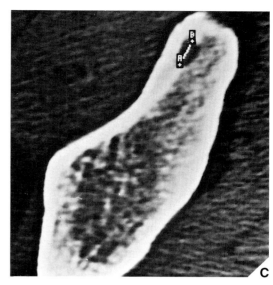

Figure 16.10 (A) Anteroposterior view of the left hip of a 16-year-old boy with a typical history of osteoid osteoma is equivocal, although there is the suggestion of a radiolucency in the supra-acetabular portion of the ilium.

(B) Radionuclide bone scan shows an increased uptake of isotope in the supra-acetabular portion of the left ilium. (C) Subsequent CT scan not only demonstrates the lesion but also allows its measurement (6.8 mm).

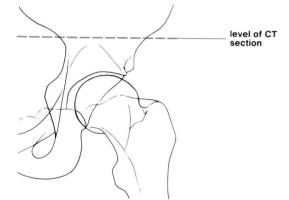

level of CT section

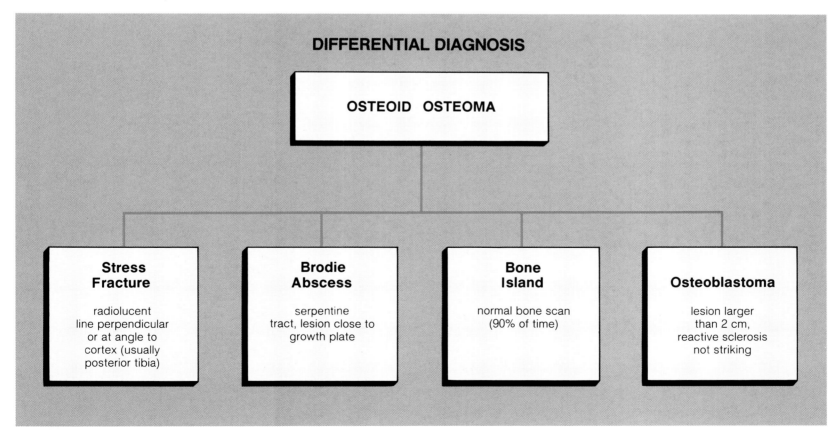

DIFFERENTIAL DIAGNOSIS

OSTEOID OSTEOMA

Stress Fracture	**Brodie Abscess**	**Bone Island**	**Osteoblastoma**
radiolucent line perpendicular or at angle to cortex (usually posterior tibia)	serpentine tract, lesion close to growth plate	normal bone scan (90% of time)	lesion larger than 2 cm, reactive sclerosis not striking

Figure 16.11 Differential diagnosis of osteoid osteoma.

rather than parallel to it (Fig. 16.12). A bone abscess may have a similar radiographic appearance, but one can usually detect a linear, serpentine tract extending from the abscess cavity toward the closest growth plate (Fig. 16.13). A bone island usually shows no increase in isotope uptake on radionuclide bone scan (see Fig. 15.21).

COMPLICATIONS Osteoid osteoma may be accompanied by a few complications. Accelerated bone growth may occur if the nidus is located near the growth plate, particularly in young children (Fig. 16.14). A vertebral lesion, particularly in the neural arch, may lead to painful scoliosis, with concavity of the curvature directed toward the side of the lesion (Fig. 16.15).

Moreover, an intracapsular lesion may result in arthritis of precocious onset (Fig. 16.16). As observed by Norman and associates, this latter complication may serve as an important diagnostic clue to an osteoid osteoma when a typical history of the condition is elicited from the patient but the nidus is not recognizable radiographically (Fig. 16.17).

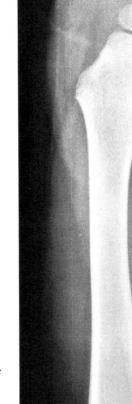

Figure 16.12 Lateral magnification view demonstrates a stress fracture of the tibia. Note the perpendicular direction of the radiolucency to the long axis of the tibial cortex. In osteoid osteoma, the radiolucent nidus is oriented parallel to the cortex.

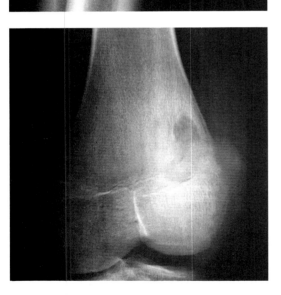

Figure 16.13 In a bone abscess, seen here in the distal femoral diaphysis, a serpentine tract extends from an abscess cavity toward the growth plate. This feature distinguishes the lesion from osteoid osteoma.

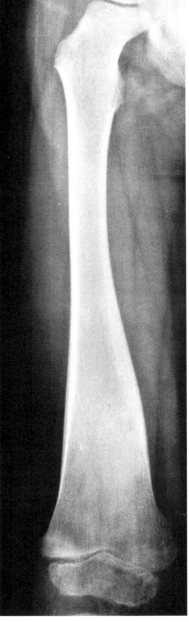

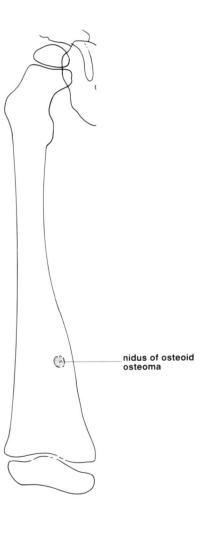

Figure 16.14 A 2-year-old boy had an osteoid osteoma of the distal femoral diaphysis. The proximity of the nidus to the growth plate caused accelerated growth of the bone, with marked widening of the distal end of the femur.

nidus of osteoid osteoma

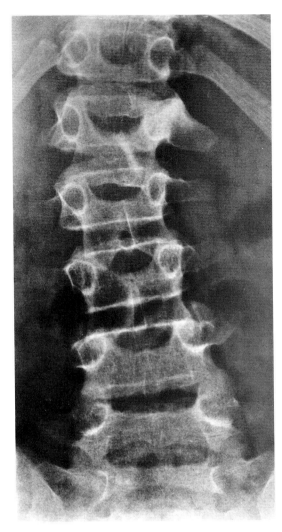

Figure 16.15 Anteroposterior plain film of the spine shows an osteoid osteoma in the left pedicle of L-l in a 12-year-old boy. Note the shallow-curve scoliosis, with concavity directed toward the lesion.

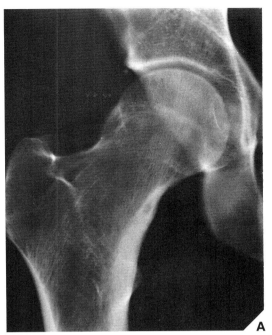

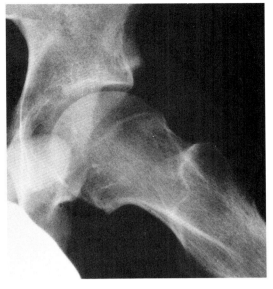

Figure 16.17 A 14-year-old boy presented with pain in the left hip for eight months; it was more severe at night and was relieved by aspirin within 15 to 20 minutes. Several previous radiographic examinations, including conventional and computed tomographic scans, had failed to demonstrate the nidus. A frog-lateral view shows evidence of periarticular osteoporosis and early degenerative changes, both presumptive features of osteoid osteoma.

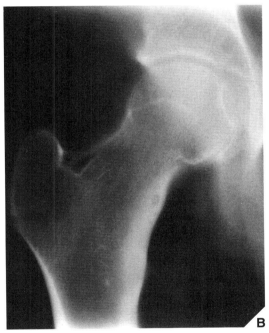

Figure 16.16 (A) Anteroposterior view of the right hip demonstrates an intracapsular osteoid osteoma located in the medial aspect of the neck of the right femur in a 28-year-old man. (B) Tomographic cut shows the early changes of osteoarthritis. Note a collar osteophyte and slight narrowing of the weight-bearing segment of the hip joint. A radionuclide bone scan showed increased uptake not only at the site of the lesion but also at the site of the reactive bone formation resulting from the osteoarthritis.

TREATMENT The treatment of osteoid osteoma consists of complete en bloc resection of the nidus. The resected specimen and the involved bone should be radiographed promptly (Fig. 16.18) so as to exclude the possibility of incomplete resection, which can lead to recurrence (Fig. 16.19).

Osteoblastoma

Osteoblastoma, which accounts for approximately 1% of all primary bone tumors and 3% of all benign bone tumors, is a lesion histologically similar to osteoid osteoma but characterized by a larger size (more than 1.5 cm in diameter and usually above 2 cm). The age range of its occurrence is also similar to that of osteoid osteoma: 75% of osteoblastomas are found in patients in their first, second, or third decade. Although the long bones are frequently involved, the lesion has a predilection for the vertebral column (Fig. 16.20). Its clinical presentation, however, is different from that of osteoid osteoma: not only are some patients asymptomatic, but pain is not as readily relieved by salicylates.

Plain-film radiography and conventional tomography are usually sufficient to demonstrate the lesion and suggest the diagnosis. On those rare occasions when the tumor penetrates the cortex and extends into the soft tissues, MRI may demonstrate these features (Fig. 16.21).

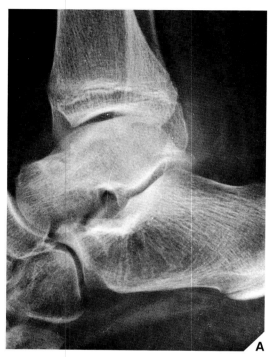
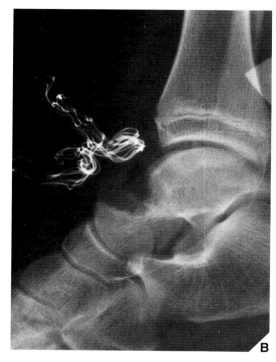
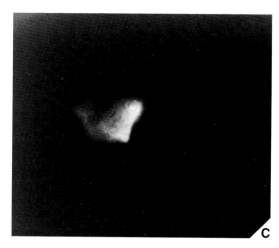

Figure 16.18 (A) Preoperative lateral film of the ankle of a 13-year-old boy demonstrates the nidus of osteoid osteoma in the talar bone. Intraoperative films demonstrate the area of resection (B) and the resected specimen (C), confirming that the lesion was totally excised.

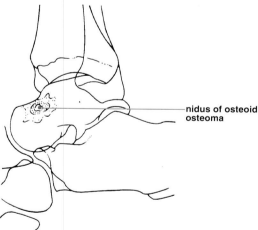

nidus of osteoid osteoma

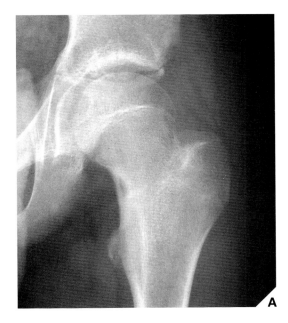

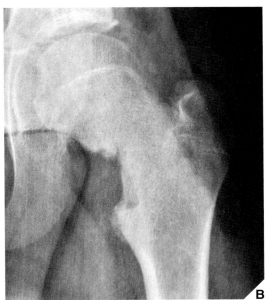

Figure 16.19 (A) Plain radiograph of the left hip in a 17-year-old boy with pain in the left groin relieved promptly by salicylates demonstrates a nidus of osteoid osteoma in the medial cortex of the femoral neck. (B) The lesion was incompletely resected; note its remnants. Two years later the symptoms recurred. (C) Plain film of the left hip demonstrates a radiolucent area in the medial femoral cortex at the junction of the head and neck, and a CT section (D) demonstrates the nidus.

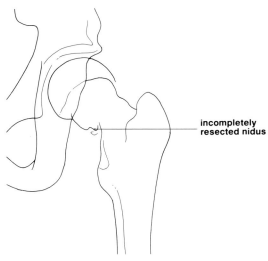

incompletely resected nidus

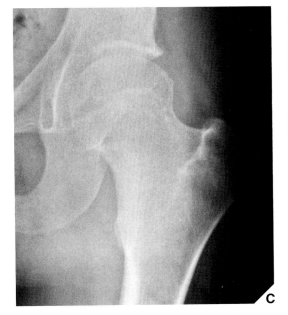

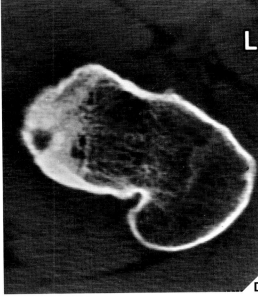

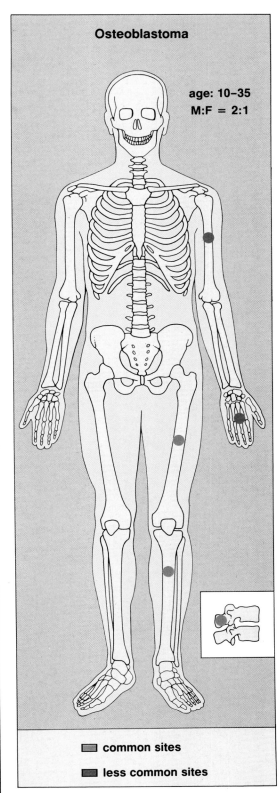

Osteoblastoma

age: 10–35
M:F = 2:1

common sites

less common sites

Figure 16.20 Skeletal sites of predilection, peak age range, and male-to-female ratio in osteoblastoma.

Osteoblastoma has three distinctive radiographic presentations:

1. A giant osteoid osteoma. The lesion is usually more than 2 cm in diameter and exhibits less reactive sclerosis and a possibly more prominent periosteal response than does osteoid osteoma (Fig. 16.22).
2. A blow-out expansion similar to an aneurysmal bone cyst with small radiopacities in the center. This pattern is particularly common in lesions involving the spine (Fig. 16.23).
3. An aggressive lesion simulating a malignant tumor (Fig. 16.24). Histologic differentiation between osteoid osteoma and osteoblas-

toma can be very difficult, and in a considerable number of patients it can be impossible. Both are osteoid-producing lesions, but in the typical osteoblastoma the bone trabeculae are broader and longer and seem less densely packed and less coherent than those in osteoid osteoma.

DIFFERENTIAL DIAGNOSIS The differential diagnosis of osteoblastoma should include a bone abscess. The latter lesion is usually marked by a serpentine tract (see Fig. 16.13) or it is seen to cross the growth plate (Fig. 16.25), phenomena almost never seen in osteoblastoma.

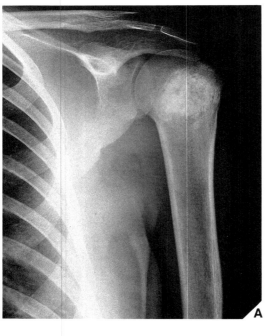
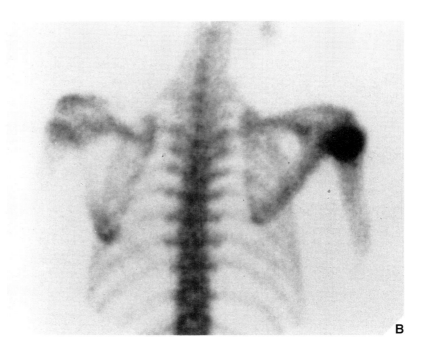
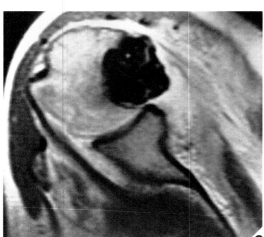
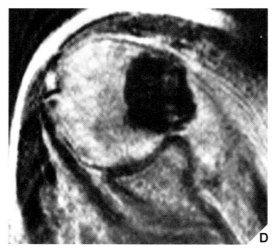

Figure 16.21 A 15-year-old girl presented with pain in her left shoulder. (A) Plain film demonstrates a sharply demarcated sclerotic lesion in the proximal metaphysis of the left humerus abutting the growth plate. (B) Radionuclide bone scan obtained after injection of 15 mCi (555 MBq) of technetium-99m-labeled MDP shows an increased uptake of tracer localized to the site of the lesion. (C) Axial spin-echo T1-weighted MR image (TR 700/TE 20) demonstrates that the lesion is located posteriorly. The cortex is destroyed and the tumor extends into the soft tissues. (D) Axial spin-echo T2-weighted MR image (TR 2200/TE 60) shows that the lesion remains of low signal intensity, indicating bony matrix. The rim of high signal intensity adjacent to the posterolateral margin of the tumor reflects peritumoral edema. Biopsy confirmed the diagnosis of osteoblastoma.

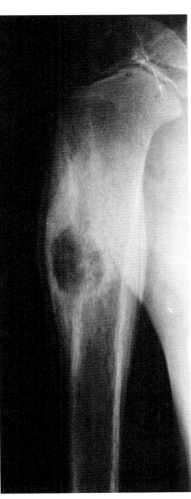

Figure 16.22 The osteoblastoma in the upper humerus of this 8-year-old boy is similar to the lesion of osteoid osteoma. This lesion, however, is larger (2.5 cm in its largest dimension), and there is a more pronounced periosteal response in the medial and lateral humeral cortices. On the other hand, the extent of reactive bone surrounding the radiolucent nidus is less than that usually seen in osteoid osteoma. This type of osteoblastoma is frequently called a giant osteoid osteoma.

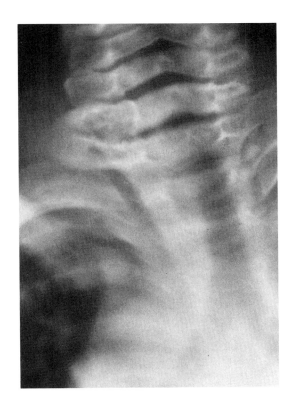

Figure 16.23 Tomographic section of the cervical spine shows an expanding, blow-out lesion of osteoblastoma, with several small central opacities, in the lamina of C-6.

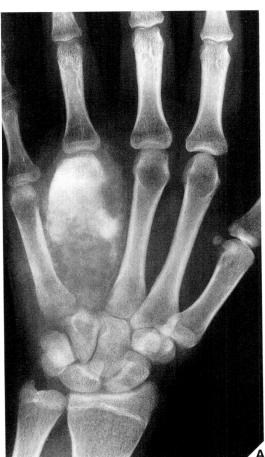

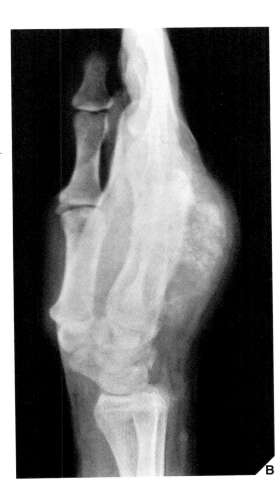

Figure 16.24 Posteroanterior (A) and lateral (B) views of the hand demonstrate an aggressive osteoblastoma. Note the destruction of the entire fourth metacarpal with massive bone formation, particularly in the distal portion. Although very similar in appearance to osteosarcoma, the lesion still appears to be contained by periosteal new bone formation.

Aggressive osteoblastoma should be differentiated from osteosarcoma, for which tomography may be helpful (Fig. 16.26). CT may also help in the differential diagnosis of lesions located in complex anatomic regions such as the vertebrae. If there is tumor extension into the thecal sac, myelography or MRI may be needed.

TREATMENT The treatment for osteoblastoma is similar to that for osteoid osteoma; en bloc resection should be performed. Larger lesions may require additional bone grafting and internal fixation.

BENIGN CHONDROBLASTIC LESIONS
Enchondroma (Chondroma)

This benign lesion is characterized by the formation of mature hyaline cartilage. When it is located centrally in the bone, it is termed an *enchondroma* (Fig. 16.27); if it is extracortical (periosteal) in location, it is called a *chondroma* (periosteal or juxtacortical) (see Fig. 16.33). Although occurring throughout life, enchondromas are usually seen in patients in their second through fourth decades. There is no sex

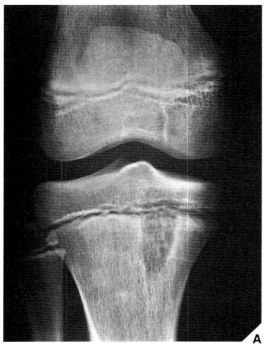

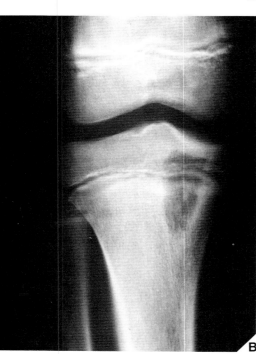

Figure 16.25 (A) Anteroposterior view of the knee of a 10-year-old boy demonstrates an oval radiolucent lesion abutting and crossing the growth plate of the proximal tibia. Confirmation of extension of the lesion into the epiphysis is shown on an anteroposterior tomographic section (B). The lesion proved to be a bone abscess.

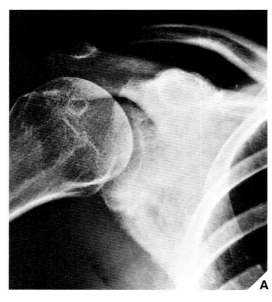

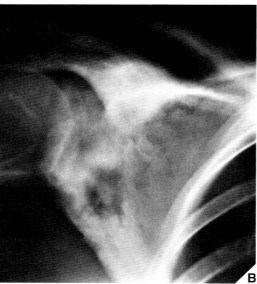

Figure 16.26 (A) Anteroposterior plain radiograph of the right shoulder of a 28-year-old woman with progressive pain in the right scapula demonstrates a sclerotic area in the scapula with a periosteal reaction—signs highly suggestive of a malignant tumor, such as osteosarcoma. (B) Conventional tomogram clearly demonstrates a radiolucent nidus with a sclerotic center resembling an osteoid osteoma. The size of this lesion (3 cm x 3 cm), however, marks it as an osteoblastoma.

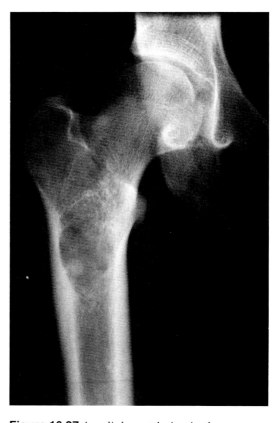

Figure 16.27 A radiolucent lesion in the medullary portion of the proximal femur of a 22-year-old man is seen eroding the inner aspect of the lateral cortex. It proved on biopsy to be an enchondroma.

predilection. The short tubular bones of the hand (phalanges and metacarpals) are the most frequent sites of occurrence, although the lesions may also be encountered in the long tubular bones (Fig. 16.28). Enchondromas are often asymptomatic; a pathologic fracture through the tumor (Fig. 16.29) often calls attention to the lesion.

Enchondroma protuberans is a rare variant, a lesion that arises in the intramedullary cavity of a long bone and forms a prominent exo-phytic mass on the cortical surface. This lesion must be distinguished from an osteochondroma or central chondrosarcoma that penetrates the cortex and forms a juxtacortical mass.

In most instances, plain-film radiography and conventional tomography suffice to demonstrate the lesion. In the short bones, the lesion is often entirely radiolucent (Fig. 16.30), while in the long bones it may display visible calcifications. If the calcifications are

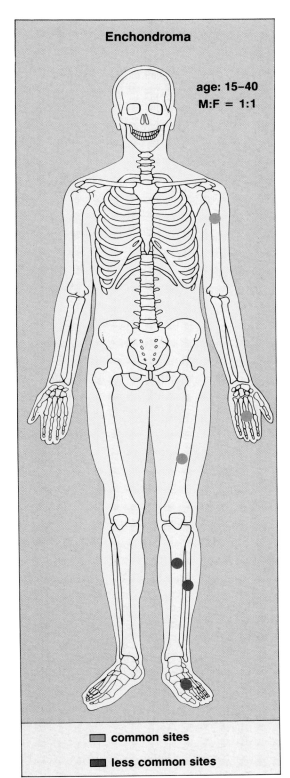

Figure 16.28 Skeletal sites of predilection, peak age range, and male-to-female ratio in enchondroma.

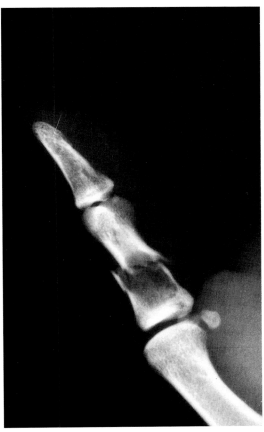

Figure 16.29 Plain film in a 31-year-old man who had injured his left thumb reveals a pathologic fracture through an otherwise asymptomatic enchondroma.

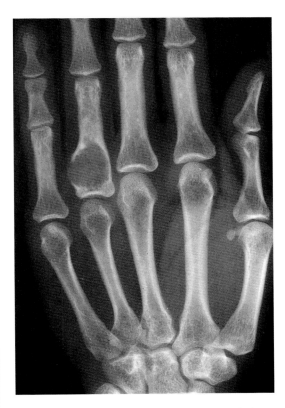

Figure 16.30 A typical, purely radiolucent lesion at the base of the proximal phalanx of the ring finger of a 37-year-old woman represents an enchondroma. Note the marked attenuation of the ulnar side of the cortex.

extensive, enchondromas are called "calcifying" (Fig. 16.31). The lesions can also be recognized by scalloping of the inner cortical margins, since the cartilage in general grows in a lobular pattern (see Figs. 16.27, 16.31).

CT and MRI may further delineate the tumor and more precisely localize it in the bone. On spin-echo T1-weighted MR images enchondromas demonstrate intermediate-to-low signal intensity, while on T2-weighted images they demonstrate high signal intensity. The calcifications within the tumor will image as low signal intensity structures (Fig. 16.32). It must be stressed, however, that most of the time neither CT nor MRI is suitable for establishing the precise nature of a cartilaginous lesion, nor can CT or MRI distinguish

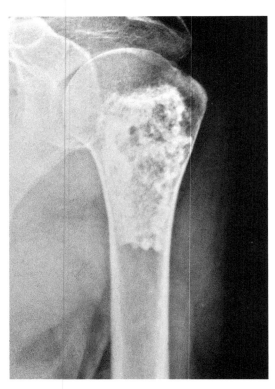

Figure 16.31 In this heavily calcified enchondroma of the proximal humerus of a 58-year-old woman, note the lobular appearance of the lesion and the scalloping of the endocortex.

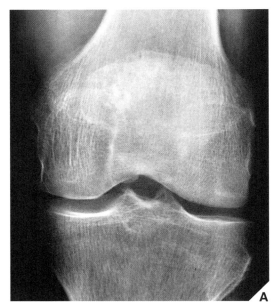

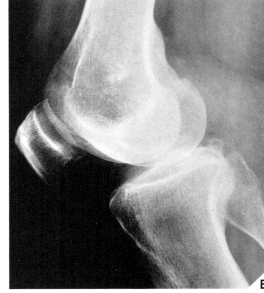

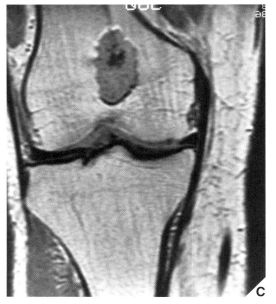

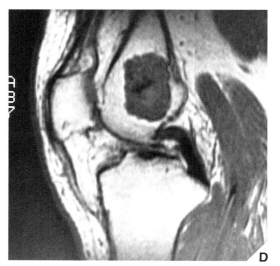

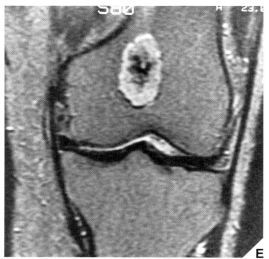

Figure 16.32 A 61-year-old man sustained a trauma to the left knee. Anteroposterior (A) and lateral (B) films demonstrate only a few calcifications in the distal femur. The extent of the lesion cannot be determined. Coronal (C) and sagittal (D) T1-weighted MR images demonstrate a well circumscribed, lobulated lesion displaying an intermediate signal intensity. The darker area in the center represents calcifications. Coronal T2-weighted image (E) shows the lesion displaying a mixed-intensity signal: the brighter areas represent cartilaginous tumor, the darker areas calcifications. The biopsy of the lesion revealed enchondroma.

benign from malignant lesions. Despite the use of various criteria, the application of MRI to the tissue diagnosis of cartilaginous lesions has not brought satisfactory results.

Periosteal chondroma is a slow-growing, benign cartilaginous lesion that arises on the surface of a bone. It occurs in children as well as adults, with no sex predilection. There is usually a history of pain and tenderness, often accompanied by swelling at the site of the lesion, which is most commonly located in the proximal humerus. As the tumor enlarges, it is seen radiographically eroding the cortex in a saucer-like fashion, producing a solid buttress of periosteal new bone. The lesion has a sharp sclerotic inner margin demarcating it from the buttress of periosteal new bone (Fig. 16.33). Scattered calcifications are often seen within the lesion.

Histologically, enchondroma consists of lobules of hyaline cartilage of varying cellularity and is recognized by the features of its intercellular matrix, which has a uniformly translucent appearance and contains relatively little collagen. The tissue is sparsely cellular and the cells contain small and darkly staining nuclei. The tumor cells are located in rounded spaces known as lacunae.

DIFFERENTIAL DIAGNOSIS The main differential diagnosis of enchondroma, particularly in lesions of the long bones, is a medullary bone infarct (Fig. 16.34). At times, the two lesions may be difficult to distinguish from one another, particularly if the enchondroma is small, since both lesions present with similar calcifications. The radiographic features helpful in the differential diagnosis are the lobulation of the inner cortical margins in enchondroma, the annular, punctate, and comma-shaped calcifications in the matrix, and the lack of sclerotic rim that is usually seen in bone infarcts.

COMPLICATIONS The single most important complication of enchondroma, aside from pathologic fracture (see Fig. 16.29), is its malignant transformation to chondrosarcoma. With solitary enchondromas, this occurs almost exclusively in a long or flat bone

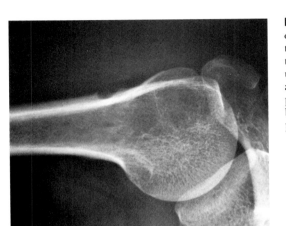

Figure 16.33 A radiolucent lesion eroding the external surface of the cortex of the upper humerus of a 24-year-old man proved on excision biopsy to be a periosteal chondroma.

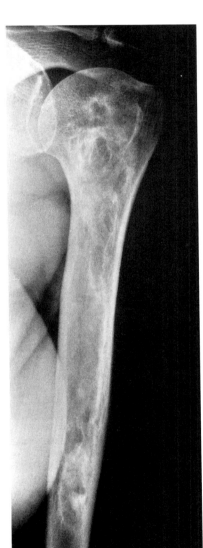

Figure 16.34 In a medullary bone infarct, seen here in the proximal humerus of a 36-year-old man with sickle-cell disease, there is no endosteal scalloping of the cortex, and the calcified area is surrounded by a thin, dense sclerotic rim, the hallmark of a bone infarct.

strong predilection for one side of the body. Maffucci syndrome is recognized radiographically by multiple calcified phleboliths.

Osteochondroma

Also known as osteocartilaginous exostosis, this lesion is characterized by a cartilage-capped bony projection on the external surface of a bone. It is the most common benign bone lesion and is usually diagnosed in patients before their third decade. Osteochondroma, which has its own growth plate, usually stops growing at skeletal maturity. The most common sites of involvement are the metaphysis of the long bones, particularly in the region around the knee and the proximal humerus (Fig. 16.39).

The radiographic presentation of osteochondroma is characteristic according to whether the lesion is pedunculated, with a slender pedicle usually directed away from the neighboring growth plate (Fig. 16.40A), or sessile, with a broad base attached to the cortex (Fig. 16.40B). The most important characteristic feature of either type of lesion is uninterrupted merging of the cortex of the host bone with the cortex of the osteochondroma; additionally, the medullary portion

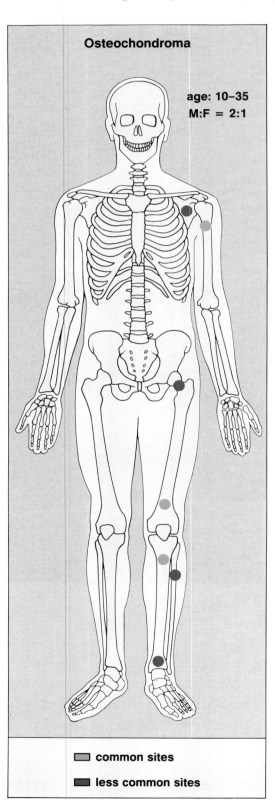

Osteochondroma

age: 10–35
M:F = 2:1

◻ common sites
◼ less common sites

Figure 16.39 Skeletal sites of predilection, peak age range, and male-to-female ratio in osteochondroma (osteocartilaginous exostosis).

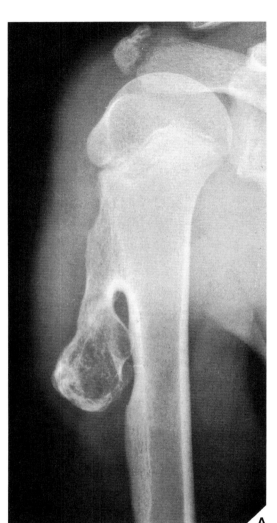

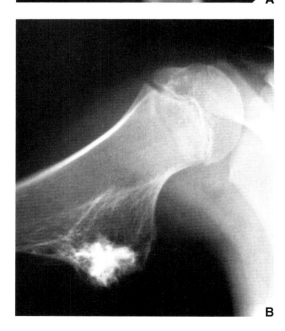

Figure 16.40 (A) The typical pedunculated type of osteochondroma is seen arising near the proximal growth plate of the right humerus in a 13-year-old boy. (B) In the typical sessile or broad-based variant, seen here arising from the medial cortex of the proximal diaphysis of the right humerus in a 14-year-old boy, the cortex of the host bone merges without interruption with the cortex of the lesion. The cartilaginous cap is not visible on the plain films, but dense calcifications in the stalk can be seen.

of the lesion and the medullary cavity of the adjacent bone communicate. These are important features that distinguish this lesion from the occasionally similar looking bone masses of osteoma, periosteal chondroma, juxtacortical osteosarcoma, soft tissue osteosarcoma, and juxtacortical myositis ossicans (Fig. 16.41). The other characteristic feature of osteochondroma involves calcifications in the chondro-osseous portion of the stalk of the lesion (see Fig. 16.40).

Histologically, the osteochondroma cap is composed of hyaline cartilage arranged similarly to that of a growth plate. A zone of calci-fication in the chondro-osseous portion of the stalk corresponds to the zone of provisional calcification in the physis. Beneath this zone, there is vascular invasion and replacement of the calcified cartilage by new bone formation, which undergoes maturation and merges with the cancellous bone of the host bone's medullary cavity.

COMPLICATIONS Osteochondroma may be complicated by a number of secondary abnormalities, including pressure on nerves or blood vessels (Fig. 16.42), pressure on the adjacent bone, with occasional

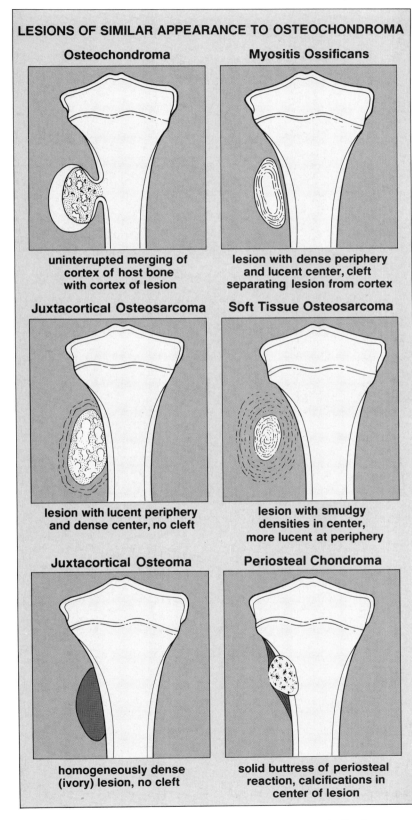

Figure 16.41 Radiographic features characterizing lesions similar in appearance to osteochondroma.

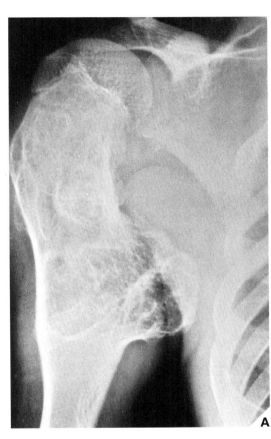

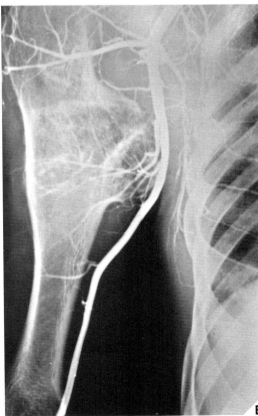

Figure 16.42
A 14-year-old boy with a known osteochondroma of the right humerus complained of pain and numbness of the hand and fingers. (A) Plain film of the shoulder demonstrates a sessile-type osteochondroma arising from the medial aspect of the proximal diaphysis of the humerus. (B) Arteriography reveals compression and displacement of the brachial artery.

fracture (Fig. 16.43), fracture through the lesion itself, and inflammatory changes of the bursa exostotica covering the cartilaginous cap (Fig. 16.44).

The least common complication of osteochondroma, seen in solitary lesions in less than 1% of cases, is malignant transformation to chondrosarcoma. Nevertheless, it is important to recognize this complication at an early stage. The chief clinical features suggesting malignant transformation are pain (in the absence of a fracture, bursitis, or pressure on nearby nerves) and a growth spurt or continued growth of the lesion beyond the age of skeletal maturity. Certain radiographic features have also been identified that may help in the determination of malignancy (Fig. 16.45).

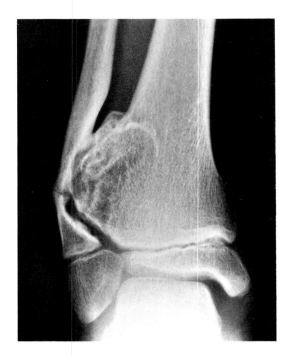

Figure 16.43 A 9-year-old boy had a sessile osteochondroma of the distal tibia. The lesion produced pressure erosion, and later bowing and attenuation of the fibula, with subsequent fracture of the bone. (Reproduced with permission from Norman A, Greenspan A, 1982)

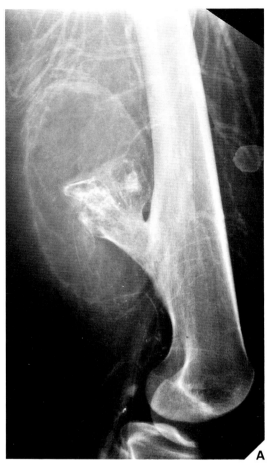

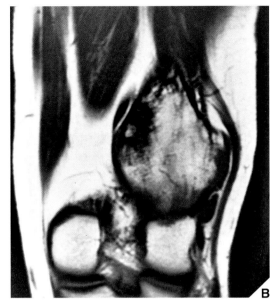

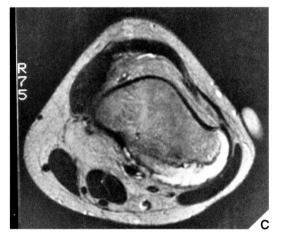

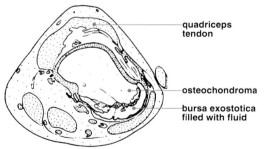

quadriceps tendon

osteochondroma

bursa exostotica filled with fluid

Figure 16.44 (A) A 25-year-old man with a known solitary osteochondroma of the distal right femur complained of gradually increasing pain. The capillary phase of an arteriogram reveals a huge bursa exostotica. Inflammation of the bursa, with the accumulation of a large amount of fluid (bursitis), was the cause of the patient's symptoms. (B) Another patient, a 12-year-old girl, presented with pain in the popliteal fossa. Coronal T1-weighted MR image (SE, TR 650/TE 25) demonstrates a large osteochondroma arising from the posterolateral aspect of distal femur. (C) Axial T2-weighted image (SE, TR 2200/TE 70) demonstrates a bursa exostotica distended with fluid.

The most reliable imaging modalities for evaluating the possible malignant transformation of an osteochondroma are plain radiography, conventional tomography, CT, and MRI; the results of a radionuclide bone scan, which may show increased uptake of radiopharmaceutical at the site of the lesion, may not be reliable. The plain film usually demonstrates whether or not the calcifications in an osteochondroma are contained within the stalk of the lesion—a clear indication of benignity (see Fig. 16.40)—but conventional tomography can occasionally also be helpful in this respect (Fig. 16.46). Similarly, CT can demonstrate both dispersed calcifications in

Fig. 16.45 Clinical and Radiologic Features Suggesting Malignant Transformation of Osteochondroma

CLINICAL FEATURES	RADIOLOGIC FINDINGS	IMAGING MODALITY
Pain (in the absence of fracture, bursitis, or pressure on nearby nerves)	Enlargement of the lesion	Plain films (comparison with earlier radiographs)
	Development of a bulky carilaginous cap, usually 2-3 cm thick	CT, MRI
Growth spurt (after skeletal maturity)	Dispersed calcifications in the cartilaginous cap	Conventional tomography
	Development of a soft tissue mass with or without calcifications	Plain films, CT, MRI
	Increased uptake of isotope after closure of growth plate (not always reliable)	Scintigraphy

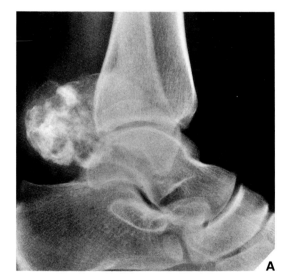 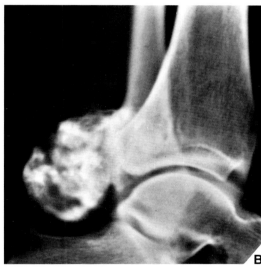

A   B

Figure 16.46 (A) Lateral view of the left ankle of a 26-year-old woman with a painful osteochondroma around the ankle shows a sessile lesion arising from the posterior aspect of the distal tibia. In the interpretation of this radiograph, uncertainties were raised that some of the calcifications might not be contained within the stalk, and tomographic examination was suggested. (B) Tomographic section demonstrates lack of separation of calcifications from the main mass, suggesting a benign lesion. The osteochondroma was resected, and a histopathologic examination confirmed the lack of malignant transformation. The symptoms were apparently caused by pressure on a nerve.

the cartilaginous cap and increased thickness of the cap, cardinal signs of malignant transformation of the lesion, as Norman and Sissons (1984) have pointed out (Fig. 16.47).

The unreliability of radionuclide imaging is related to the fact that even benign exostoses exhibit increased uptake of radiopharmaceutical due to endochondral ossification. Exostotic chondrosarcoma is also marked by isotope uptake, which is related to active ossification, osteoblastic activity, and hyperemia within the cartilage and bony stalk of the tumor. Thus, although the uptake is more intense in exostotic chondrosarcomas than in benign exostoses, various investigations show that this is not always a reliable feature distinguishing these lesions.

TREATMENT   Solitary lesions of osteochondroma usually can simply be monitored if they do not cause clinical problems. Surgical resec-tion is indicated if the lesion becomes painful, if there is suspected encroachment on adjacent nerves or blood vessels, if pathologic fracture occurs, or if there is concern about the diagnosis.

Multiple Osteocartilaginous Exostoses

This condition is classified by some authorities in the category of bone dysplasias; it is a hereditary, autosomal-dominant disorder. The knees, ankles, and shoulders are the sites most frequently affected by the development of multiple osteochondromas (Fig. 16.48). The radiographic features are similar to those of single osteochondromas (see Fig. 16.40), but the lesions are more frequently of the sessile type (Fig. 16.49). The histopathologic features of multiple osteochondromas are the same as those of solitary lesions.

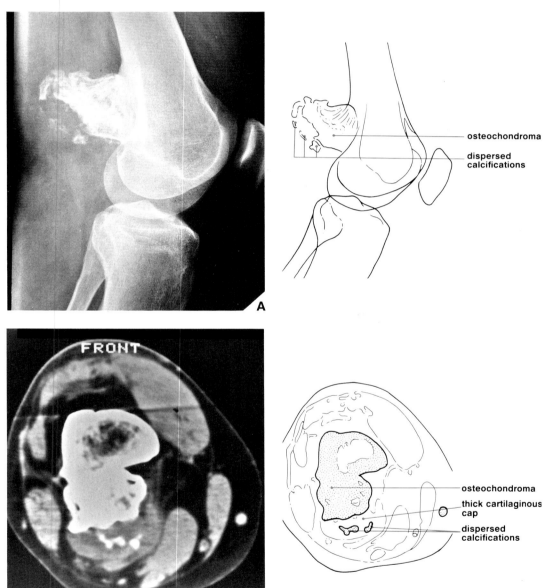

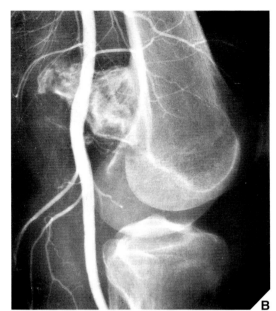

Figure 16.47 A 28-year-old man developed pain in the popliteal region and also noticed an increase in a mass he had been aware of for 15 years—important clinical information that warranted further investigation to rule out the malignant transformation of an osteochondroma. (A) Lateral view of the knee demonstrates a sessile-type osteochondroma arising from the posterior cortex of the distal femur. Note that calcifications are present not only in the stalk of the lesion but also are dispersed in the cartilaginous cap. (B) An arteriogram demonstrates displacement of the small vessels, which are draped over the invisible cartilaginous cap. (C) CT section confirms the increased thickness of the cartilaginous cap (2.5 cm) and dispersed calcifications within the cap. These radiographic features are consistent with a diagnosis of malignant transformation to chondrosarcoma, which was confirmed by histopathologic examination.

COMPLICATIONS There is a greater incidence of growth disturbance in multiple osteocartilaginous exostoses than in single osteochondromas. Growth abnormalities are primarily seen in the forearms (Fig. 16.50) and legs. Malignant transformation to chondrosarcoma is also more common, seen in 5% to 15% of cases, with lesions at the shoulder girdle and around the pelvis at greater risk of undergoing transformation. The clinical and radiographic signs of this complication are identical to those in malignant transformation of a solitary osteochondroma (see Figs. 16.45-16.47).

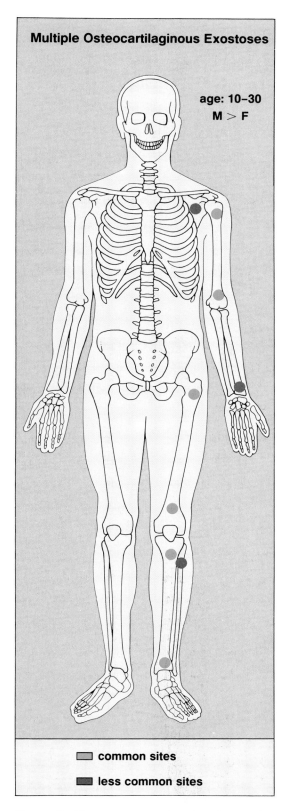

Multiple Osteocartilaginous Exostoses

age: 10–30
M > F

☐ common sites
■ less common sites

Figure 16.48 Skeletal sites of predilection, peak age range, and male-to-female ratio in multiple osteocartilaginous exostoses (multiple osteochondromatosis, diaphyseal aclasis).

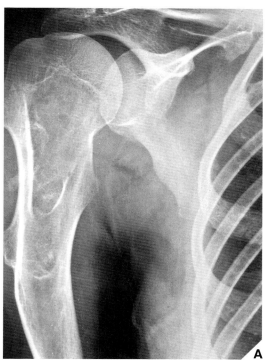

A

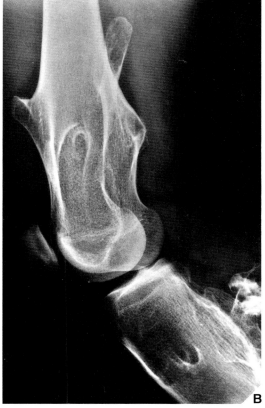

B

Figure 16.49 (A) Anteroposterior view of the shoulder of a 22-year-old man with familial multiple osteochondromatosis demonstrates multiple sessile lesions involving the proximal humerus, scapula, and ribs. (B) Involvement of the distal femur and proximal tibia is characteristic of this disorder.

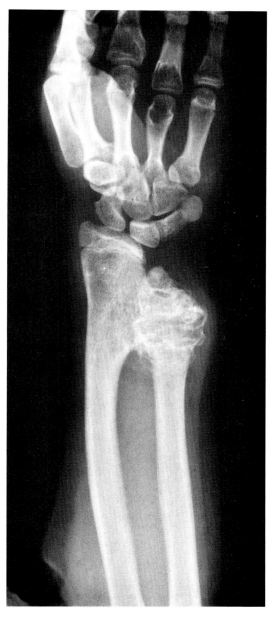

Figure 16.50 Posteroanterior view of the forearm of an 8-year-old boy with multiple osteochondromas shows a growth disturbance in the distal radius and ulna, which is frequently seen as a complication in this disorder.

TREATMENT Multiple osteochondromas are treated individually. Like solitary lesions, they are likely to recur in younger children, and surgery may be deferred to a later date.

Chondroblastoma

Also known as a Codman tumor, chondroblastoma is a benign lesion occurring before skeletal maturity, characteristically presenting in the epiphyses of long bones such as the humerus, tibia, and femur (Fig. 16.51). It represents fewer than 1% of all primary bone tumors. It is usually located eccentrically, shows a sclerotic border, and often demonstrates scattered calcifications of the matrix (25% of cases). Brower and colleagues noticed a distinctively thick, solid periosteal reaction distal to the lesion in 57% of chondroblastomas in long bones. This most likely represents an inflammatory reaction to the tumor. In most cases plain films and conventional tomography suffice to demonstrate the lesion (Fig. 16.52), but CT scan can help demonstrate the calcifications if they are not visible on the standard radiographs (Fig. 16.53).

Histologically, chondroblastoma is composed of uniformly large round cells with ovoid nuclei and clear cytoplasm. Multinucleated osteoclast-like giant cells are a frequent finding. The matrix shows characteristic fine calcifications surrounding apposing chondroblasts, having a spatial arrangement resembling the hexagonal configuration of chicken wire.

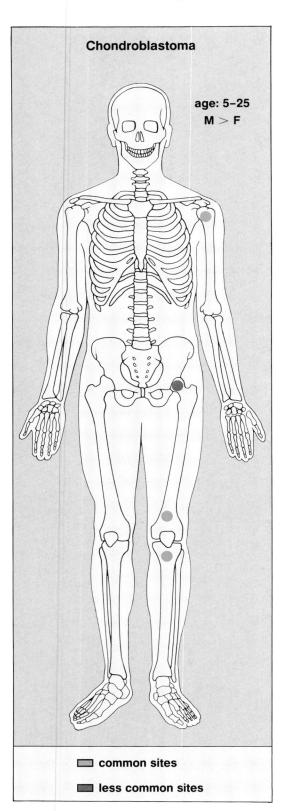

Chondroblastoma

age: 5–25
M > F

common sites

less common sites

Figure 16.51 Skeletal sites of predilection, peak age incidence, and male-to-female ratio in chondroblastoma.

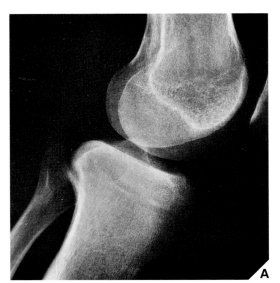

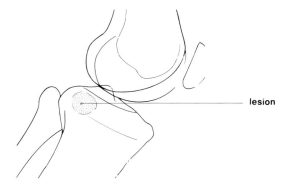

lesion

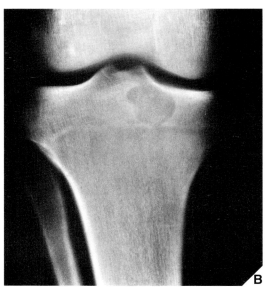

Figure 16.52 Lateral plain film (A) and anteroposterior tomogram (B) of the knee show the typical appearance of a chondroblastoma in the proximal epiphysis of the tibia. Note the radiolucent, eccentrically located lesion with a thin, sclerotic margin. There are small, scattered calcifications in the center of the lesion, which are better seen on the tomogram.

TREATMENT AND COMPLICATIONS Chondroblastomas are usually treated by curettage and bone grafting. They rarely recur.

In rare cases, pulmonary metastases develop in the absence of any histologic evidence of malignancy in either the primary bone tumor or the pulmonary lesions.

Chondromyxoid Fibroma

Chondromyxoid fibroma is a rare tumor of cartilaginous derivation, characterized by the production of chondroid, fibrous, and myxoid tissues in variable proportions, and accounting for 0.5% of all primary bone tumors and 2% of all benign bone tumors. It occurs predominantly in adolescents and young adults (males more than females), most commonly in the patient's second or third decade. It has a predilection for the bones of the lower extremities, with preferred sites in the proximal tibia (32%) and distal femur (17%) (Fig. 16.54). Its clinical symptoms include local swelling and pain, which is occasionally due to pressure on adjacent neurovascular structures by a peripherally located mass.

Its characteristic radiographic picture is that of an eccentrically located radiolucent lesion in the bone, with a sclerotic scalloped margin often eroding or ballooning out the cortex (Fig. 16.55). The lesion

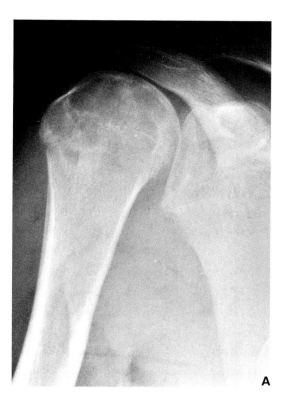

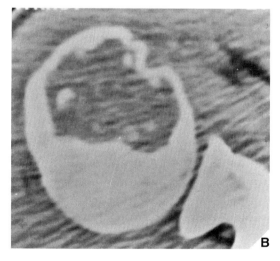

Figure 16.53 (A) Anteroposterior film of the right shoulder of a 16-year-old boy shows a lesion in the proximal humeral epiphysis, but calcifications are not well demonstrated. Note the well organized layer of periosteal reaction at the lateral cortex. (B) CT section shows the calcifications clearly. The tumor was removed by curettage, and a histopathologic examination confirmed the radiographic diagnosis of chondroblastoma.

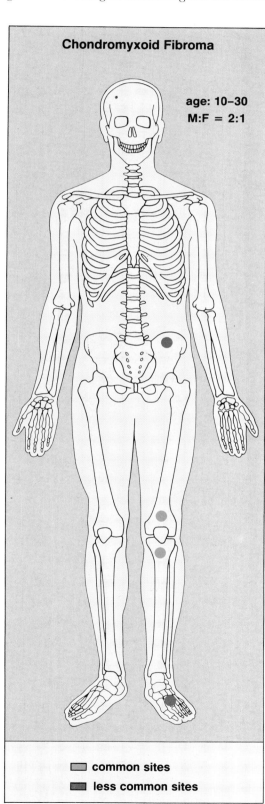

Figure 16.54 Skeletal sites of predilection, peak age range, and male-to-female ratio in chondromyxoid fibroma.

may range from 1 cm to 10 cm in size, with an average of 3 cm to 4 cm. Calcifications are not apparent radiographically, but focal microscopic calcifications have been reported in as many as 27% of cases. Frequently, a buttress of periosteal new bone can be observed.

Pathologically, the most important feature of the lesion is its lobular or pseudolobular arrangement into zones of varying cellularity. The center of the lobule is hypocellular. Within the matrix, loosely arranged spindle-shaped and stellate cells with elongated processes are present. The periphery of the lobule is densely cellular, containing a mixture of mononuclear spindle-shaped and polyhedral stromal cells with a variable number of multinucleated giant cells.

DIFFERENTIAL DIAGNOSIS Frequently, one can observe a characteristic buttress of periosteal new bone formation (Fig. 16.56), in which case a chondromyxoid fibroma may be radiographically indistinguishable from an aneurysmal bone cyst. In unusual locations such as in short tubular or flat bones it may mimic a giant cell tumor or desmoplastic fibroma.

TREATMENT The treatment of this lesion usually consists of curettage and a bone graft. Recurrences are frequent, with the reported rate between 20% and 80% (see Fig. 15.55).

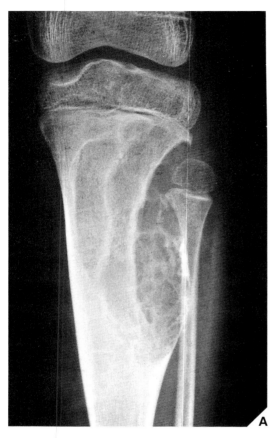
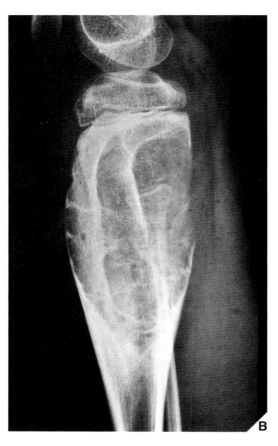

Figure 16.55 Anteroposterior (A) and lateral (B) views of the left leg of an 8-year-old girl with a chondromyxoid fibroma demonstrate a radiolucent lesion extending from the metaphysis into the diaphysis of the tibia, with a geographic type of bone destruction and a sclerotic scalloped border.

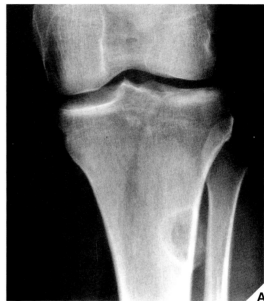
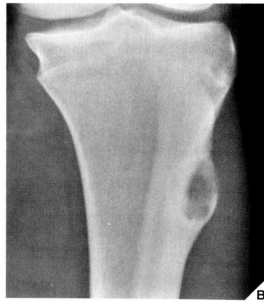

Figure 16.56 (A) Anteroposterior plain film of the knee of an 18-year-old woman shows a chondromyxoid fibroma in the lateral aspect of the proximal tibia. The lesion balloons out from the cortex and is supported by a solid periosteal buttress resembling that seen in an aneurysmal bone cyst. The periosteal buttress is better appreciated on a tomographic cut (B).

PRACTICAL POINTS TO REMEMBER

Benign Osteoblastic Lesions

[1] The most characteristic clinical symptom of osteoid osteoma is pain that is most severe at night and is promptly relieved by salicylates (aspirin).

[2] In the radiographic evaluation of osteoid osteoma:
- the lesion (nidus) consists of a small radiolucent area, sometimes with a sclerotic center. The dense zone surrounding the nidus represents reactive sclerosis, not a tumor
- the radiographic characteristics depend on the location of the lesion: intracortical, intramedullary, subperiosteal, or periarticular (intracapsular)
- the differential diagnoses of osteoid osteoma should include osteoblastoma, stress fracture, bone abscess (Brodie abscess), and a bone island.

[3] The complications of osteoid osteoma include:
- recurrence of the lesion (if not completely resected)
- accelerated growth (if the lesion is close to the growth plate)
- scoliosis
- arthritis of precocious onset (if nidus is intracapsular).

[4] A well prepared surgical approach to the treatment of osteoid osteoma requires:
- radiologic localization of the lesion (by scintigraphy, plain-film radiography, conventional tomography, CT)
- verification of total excision of the lesion in vivo (by examination of the host bone) and in vitro (by examination of the resected specimen).

[5] Osteoblastoma, histologically almost identical with osteoid osteoma, is nevertheless a distinct clinical entity. Its radiographic appearance is characterized by:
- features similar to a giant osteoid osteoma
- a "blow-out" type of expansile lesion with small radiopacities in the center, resembling aneurysmal bone cyst
- a lesion exhibiting aggressive features resembling a malignant tumor (osteosarcoma).

Benign Chondroblastic Lesions

[1] Enchondroma is characterized by the formation of mature hyaline cartilage and is seen:
- most commonly in the short tubular bones of the hand, where the lesion is usually radiolucent
- in the long bones, where scattered calcifications may be seen, resembling a medullary bone infarct.

[2] The characteristic radiographic features of enchondroma include:
- popcorn-like or annular calcifications
- a lobulated growth pattern with frequent scalloping of the endosteal cortex.

[3] Important clinical and radiographic features of the malignant transformation of an enchondroma include:
- the development of pain, in the absence of a fracture, in a previously asymptomatic lesion
- thickening or destruction of the cortex
- development of a soft tissue mass.

[4] Ollier disease and Maffucci syndrome (an association of Ollier disease with soft tissue hemangiomatosis) both carry an increased risk for malignant transformation to chondrosarcoma.

[5] In the radiographic evaluation of osteochondroma, the most common benign bone lesion, note that:
- it can be seen as pedunculated or sessile (broad-based) variants
- its two important radiographic features are uninterrupted merging of the lesion's cortex with the host bone cortex and continuity of the cancellous portion of the lesion with the medullary cavity of the host bone.

[6] The most important differential diagnoses in suspected osteochondroma include:
- juxtacortical osteoma
- juxtacortical osteosarcoma
- soft tissue osteosarcoma
- juxtacortical myositis ossificans.

[7] Osteochondroma may be complicated by:
- pressure on adjacent nerves or blood vessels
- pressure on the adjacent bone, frequently leading to fracture
- bursitis exostotica
- malignant transformation to chondrosarcoma

[8] In the malignant transformation of osteochondroma, radiologic signs include:
- enlargement of the lesion
- marked thickening of the cartilaginous cap of the lesion
- dispersion of calcifications into the cartilaginous cap
- development of a soft tissue mass
- increased isotope uptake by the lesion after skeletal maturity.

[9] Multiple osteocartilaginous exostoses, a familial hereditary condition, carries the increased risk of malignant transformation of an osteochondroma to a chondrosarcoma, particularly in the shoulder girdle and pelvis.

[10] Chondroblastoma is characterized radiographically by:
- its eccentric epiphyseal location
- sclerotic margin
- scattered calcifications
- periosteal reaction (>50% cases).

[11] Chondromyxoid fibroma is characterized radiographically by:
- its location close to the growth plate
- its scalloped, sclerotic border
- a buttress of periosteal new bone
- lack of visible calcifications.

It may mimic an aneurysmal bone cyst.

References

Bloem JL, Mulder JD: Chondroblastoma: A clinical and radiological study of 104 cases. *Skeletal Radiol* 14:1, 1985.

Brower AC, Moser RP, Kransdorf MG: The frequency and diagnostic significance of periostitis in chondroblastoma. *Am J Roentgenol* 154:309, 1990.

Caballes R: Enchondroma protuberans masquerading as osteochondroma. *Hum Pathol* 13:734, 1982.

Crim JR, Mirra JM: Enchondroma protuberans. Report of a case and its distinction from chondrosarcoma and osteochondroma adjacent to an enchondroma. *Skeletal Radiol* 19:431, 1990.

Dahlin DC: *Bone Tumors. General Aspects and Data on 6221 Cases,* ed 3. Springfield,Ill, Charles C. Thomas, 1981.

Feldman F, Hecht HI, Johnston AD: Chondromyxoid fibroma of bone. *Radiology* 94:249, 1970.

Freiberger RH, Loitman BS, Halpern M, Thompson TC: Osteoid osteoma: Report of 80 cases. *Am J Roentgenol* 82:194, 1959.

Gardner EJ, Richards RE: Multiple cutaneous and subcutaneous lesions occurring simultaneously with hereditary polyposis and osteomatosis. *Am J Hum Genet* 5:139, 1953.

Gohel VK, Dalinka MK, Edeiken J: The serpiginous tract: A sign of subacute osteomyelitis. *J Can Assoc Radiol* 24:337, 1973.

Greenspan A, Elguezabel A, Bryk D: Multifocal osteoid osteoma. A case report and review of the literature. *Am J Roentgenol* 121:103, 1974.

Helms CA: Osteoid osteoma. The double density sign. *Clin Orthop* 222:167, 1987.

Hudson TM, Chew FS, Manaster BJ: Scintigraphy of benign exostoses and exostotic chondrosarcomas. *Am J Roentgenol* 140:581, 1983.

Hudson TM, Hawkins IF Jr: Radiological evaluation of chondroblastoma. *Radiology* 139:1, 1981.

Hudson TM, Spriengfield DS, Spanier SS, Enneking WF, Derek HJ: Benign exostoses and exostotic chondrosarcomas: Evaluation of cartilage thickness by CT. *Radiology* 152:595, 1984.

Huvos AG, Marcove RC: Chondroblastoma of bone. A critical review. *Clin Orthop Rel Review* 95:300, 1973.

Jackson RP: Recurrent osteoblastoma: A review. *Clin Orthop* 131:229, 1987.

Jaffe HL: Osteoid osteoma. *Arch Surg* 31:709, 1935.

Jaffe HL: Benign osteoblastoma. *Bull Hosp Jt Dis Orthop Inst* 17:141, 1956.

Kransdorf MJ, Stull MA, Gilkey FW, Moser RP: Osteoid osteoma. *RadioGraphics* 11:671, 1991.

Kroon HM, Schurmans J: Osteoblastoma: Clinical and radiologic findings in 98 new cases. *Radiology* 175:783, 1990.

Lewis MM, Sissons H, Norman A, Greenspan A: Benign and malignant cartilage tumors. In: Griffin PP (ed): *Instructional Course Lectures, AAOS, vol 36.* Chicago, American Academy of Orthopaedic Surgeons, 1987, p 87.

Marsh BW, Bonfiglio M, Brady LP, Enneking WF: Benign osteoblastoma: Range of manifestations. *J Bone Joint Dis* A57:1, 1957.

McLeod RA, Beabout JW: The roentgenographic features of chondroblastoma. *Am J Roentgenol* 118:464, 1973.

McLeod RA, Dahlin DC, Beabout JW: The spectrum of osteoblastoma. *Am J Roentgenol* 126:321, 1976.

Milgram JW: The origins of osteochondromas and enchondromas: A histopathologic study. *Clin Orthop* 174:264, 1983.

Mirra J, Gold RH, Downs J, Eckardt JJ: A new histologic approach to the differentiation of enchondroma and chondrosarcoma of the bones. *Clin Orthop* 201:214, 1985.

Norman A: Persistence or recurrence of pain: A sign of surgical failure in osteoid osteoma. *Clin Orthop* 130:263, 1978.

Norman A, Dorfman HD: Osteoid osteoma inducing pronounced overgrowth and deformity of bone. *Clin Orthop* 110:233, 1975.

Norman A, Greenspan A: Bone dysplasias. In: Jahss MH (ed): *Disorders of the Foot, vol 1.* Philadelphia, Saunders, 1982.

Norman A, Sissons HA: Radiographic hallmarks of peripheral chondrosarcoma. *Radiology* 151:589, 1984.

Norman A, Abdelwahab IF, Buyon J, Matzkin E: Osteoid osteoma of the hip stimulating an early onset osteoarthritis. *Radiology* 158:417, 1986.

Pettine KA, Klasen RA: Osteoid osteoma and osteoblastoma of the spine. *J Bone Joint Surg* 68A:354, 1986.

Schajowicz F: *Tumors and Tumorlike Lesions of Bone and Joints.* New York, Springer-Verlag, 1981.

Schajowicz F, Lemos C: Osteoid osteoma and osteoblastoma: Closely related entities of osteoblastic derivation. *Acta Orthop Scand* 41:272, 1970.

Turcotte B, Pugh DG, Dahlin DC: The roentgenologic aspect of chondromyxoid fibroma of bone. *Am J Roentgenol* 87:1085, 1962.

Unni KK, Dahlin DC: Premalignant tumors and conditions of bone. *Am J Surg Pathol* 3:47, 1979.

Benign Tumors and Tumor-Like Lesions II: Fibrous and Fibro-Osseous Lesions and Other Benign Conditions

BENIGN FIBROUS AND FIBRO-OSSEOUS LESIONS
Fibrous Cortical Defect and Nonossifying Fibroma

FIBROUS CORTICAL DEFECTS and nonossifying (nonosteogenic) fibromas are the most common fibrous lesions of bone and are predominantly seen in children and adolescents. More common in boys than in girls, they have a predilection for the long bones, particularly the femur and tibia (Fig. 17.1).

Fibrous cortical defect (metaphyseal fibrous defect) is a small asymptomatic lesion found in 30% of normal individuals in the first and second decades of life. The radiolucent lesion is elliptical and confined to the cortex of a long bone near the growth plate; it is demarcated by a thin margin of sclerosis (Fig. 17.2). Most of these lesions disappear spontaneously, but a few may continue to enlarge; when they encroach on the medullary region of a bone, they are designated nonossifying fibroma (Fig. 17.3). With continued

Monostotic Fibrous Dysplasia

Monostotic fibrous dysplasia most commonly affects the femur—particularly the femoral neck—as well as the tibia and ribs (Fig. 17.9). The lesion arises centrally in the bone, usually sparing the epiphysis in children, and it is very rarely seen in the articular end of the bone in adults (Fig. 17.10). As the lesion enlarges, it expands the medullary cavity. The radiographic appearance of monostotic fibrous dysplasia varies, depending on the proportion of osseous-to-fibrous content. Lesions with greater osseous content are more dense and sclerotic, while those with greater fibrous content are more radiolucent, with a characteristic "ground-glass" appearance (Fig. 17.11). Pathologic fracture of the structurally

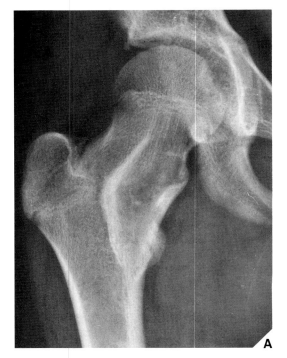 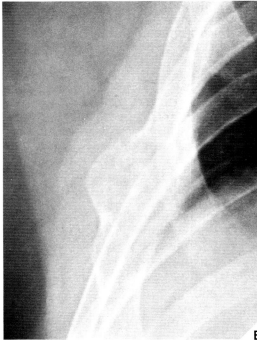

Figure 17.9 (A) Typically, the focus of fibrous dysplasia is located in the femoral neck, as seen here in a 13-year-old girl. Note a characteristic sclerotic "rind" encapsulating the lesion. (B) The rib is a frequent site of fibrous dysplasia.

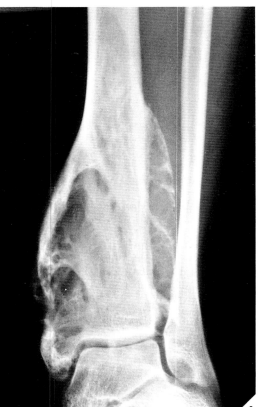 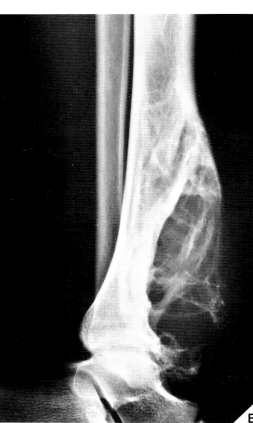

Figure 17.10 Oblique (A) and lateral (B) views of the left leg of a 32-year-old woman demonstrate a large, trabeculated radiolucent lesion in the distal tibia. Because of its aggressive features, it was thought to be a desmoplastic fibroma; however, biopsy proved it to be a fibrous dysplasia, a rare lesion at this site in adults.

weakened bone is the most frequent complication of monostotic fibrous dysplasia.

Histologically, fibrous dysplasia presents as an aggregate of moderately dense fibrous connective tissue containing bony trabeculae in haphazard distribution instead of the stress-oriented distribution expected in normal cancellous bone. The trabeculae are curved and branching, with sparse interconnections; low-power photomicrographs have been likened to "alphabet soup" or Chinese ideographs. They are composed of woven, immature bone and exhibit no evidence of osteoblastic activity ("naked trabeculae"). Occasionally, an area of cartilage formation may be present within the lesion.

Polyostotic Fibrous Dysplasia

Although radiographically similar to the monostotic form, polyostotic fibrous dysplasia is a more aggressive disorder. It also has a different distribution in the skeleton and a striking predilection for one side of the body (Fig. 17.12), a tendency that has been noted in over

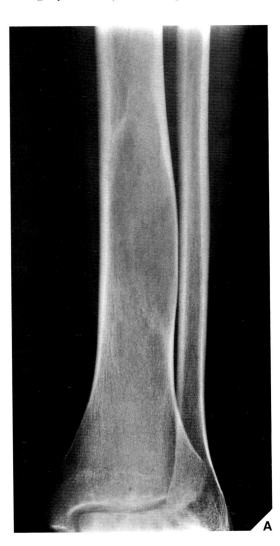
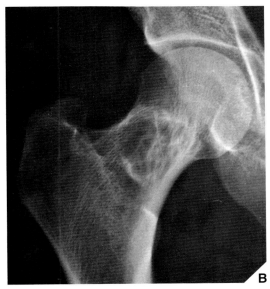

Figure 17.11 (A) Anteroposterior view of the distal leg of a 17-year-old girl shows a monostotic focus of fibrous dysplasia in the diaphysis of the tibia. Observe the slight expansion and thinning of the cortex and the partial loss of trabecular pattern in the cancellous bone, which gives the lesion a "ground-glass" or "smoky" appearance. (B) The focus of fibrous dysplasia in the femoral neck in this 25-year-old man exhibits a more sclerotic appearance than that seen in A.

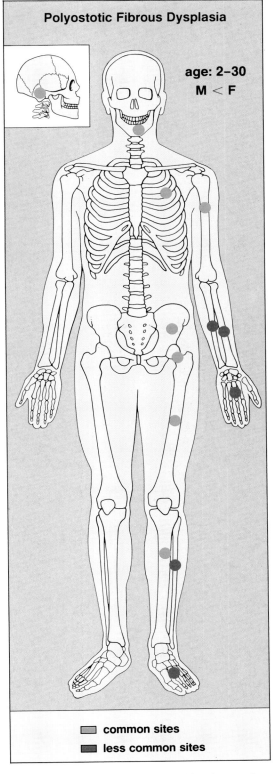

Figure 17.12 Skeletal sites of predilection, peak age range, and male-to-female ratio in polyostotic fibrous dysplasia, which is usually seen in only one side of the skeleton.

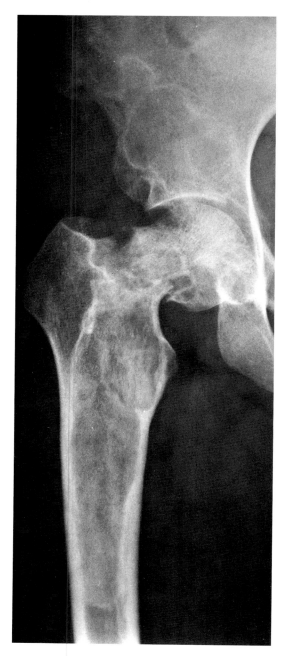

Figure 17.13 Anteroposterior view of the hip of an 18-year-old girl with polyostotic fibrous dysplasia shows unilateral involvement of the ilium and femur. There is a pathologic fracture of the femoral neck with a varus deformity.

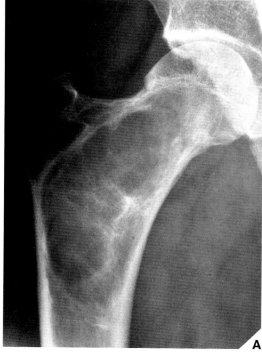

A

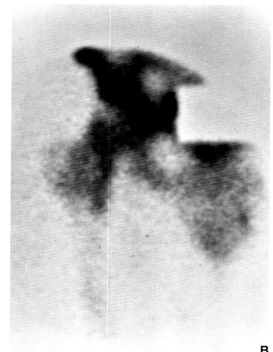

B

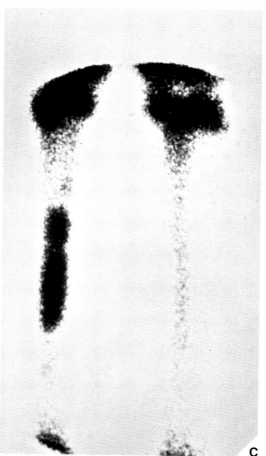

C

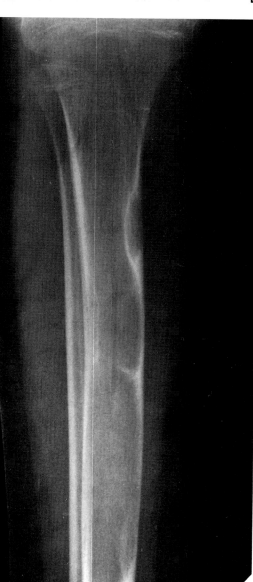

D

Figure 17.14 A 13-year-old girl injured her right hip. (A) A plain film of the hip, obtained to exclude a fracture, demonstrates a silent focus of fibrous dysplasia in the femoral neck. To determine other sites of involvement, a radionuclide bone scan was obtained. In addition to the focus in the femoral neck (B), increased uptake of isotope was demonstrated at various other sites, but predominantly the right leg (C). Subsequent plain film of the right lower leg in the anteroposterior projection (D) confirms the presence of multiple foci of polyostotic fibrous dysplasia.

90% of cases. The pelvis is frequently affected, followed by the long bones, skull, and ribs; the proximal end of the femur is a common site of involvement (Fig. 17.13). The lesions generally progress in number and size until the end of skeletal maturation, at which time they become quiescent. In only 5% of cases do they continue to enlarge.

Radiographically, the changes typical of fibrous dysplasia may occur in a limited segment or a major portion of the long bones affected by the polyostotic form of the disease, but as in the monostotic form, the articular ends are usually spared. The cortex, which is generally left intact, is often thinned by the expansile component of the lesion, and the inner cortical margins may show scalloping. The lesion has a well defined border. Occasionally, as in the monostotic form, the replacement of medullary bone by fibrous tissue leads to a loss of the trabecular pattern, giving the lesions a ground-glass, "milky," or "smoky" appearance (see Fig. 17.11); more osseous lesions appear dense. The quickest means of determining the distribution of the lesion in the skeleton is radionuclide bone scan, which often discloses unsuspected sites of skeletal involvement (Fig. 17.14).

COMPLICATIONS The most frequent complication of polyostotic fibrous dysplasia is pathologic fracture. If fracture occurs at the femoral neck, it commonly leads to a deformity called "shepherd's crook" (Fig. 17.15). Massive cartilage hyperplasia may also be seen in this disorder, resulting in the accumulation of cartilaginous masses in the medullary portion of the affected bone. Occasionally, accelerated growth of a bone or hypertrophy of a digit may be encountered (Fig. 17.16). The sarcomatous transformation of either

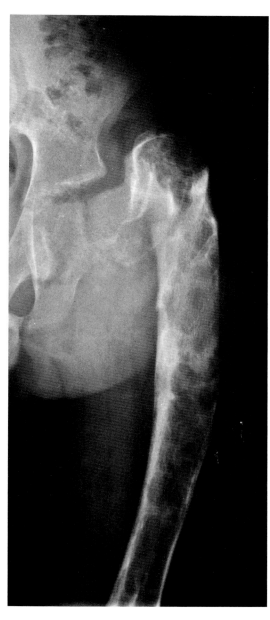

Figure 17.15 A "shepherd's-crook" deformity, seen here in the proximal femur in a 12-year-old boy with polyostotic fibrous dysplasia, is often the result of multiple pathologic fractures.

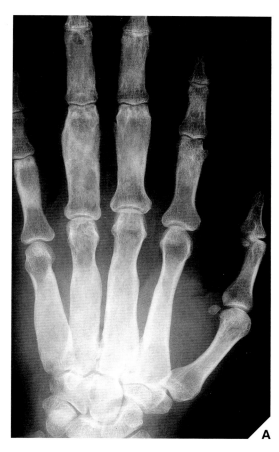

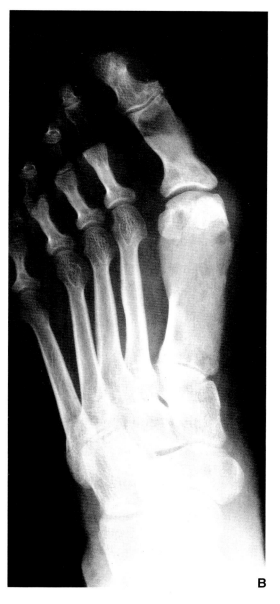

Figure 17.16 Posteroanterior view of the hand (A) and dorsoplantar view of the foot (B) of a 20-year-old man with polyostotic fibrous dysplasia demonstrate a frequent complication of this condition—accelerated growth of affected bones. In the hand observe the enlargement of the third and fourth rays, including the metacarpals and phalanges, and in the foot the hypertrophy of the first metatarsal.

form of fibrous dysplasia is extremely rare, but it may occur spontaneously (Fig. 17.17) or, more commonly, following radiation therapy (Fig. 17.18).

ASSOCIATED DISORDERS When polyostotic fibrous dysplasia is associated with endocrine disturbances (premature sexual development, hyperparathyroidism, and other endocrinopathies) and abnormal pigmentation marked by café au lait spots of the skin, the disorder is called Albright-McCune syndrome (Fig. 17.19). Overall this condition almost exclusively affects girls who present with true sexual precocity secondary to acceleration of the normal process of gonado-

tropin release by the anterior lobe of the pituitary gland. The café au lait spots seen in Albright-McCune syndrome have characteristically irregular ragged borders (commonly called "coast of Maine" borders), as opposed to the smoothly marginated ("coast of California") borders of the spots seen in neurofibromatosis.

Osteofibrous Dysplasia

Osteofibrous dysplasia (Kempson-Campanacci lesion), called in the past "ossifying fibroma," is a rare, benign fibro-osseus lesion that occurs predominantly in children, although it may not be discov-

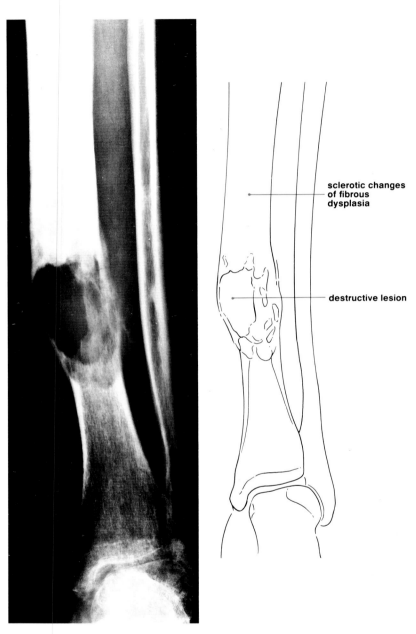

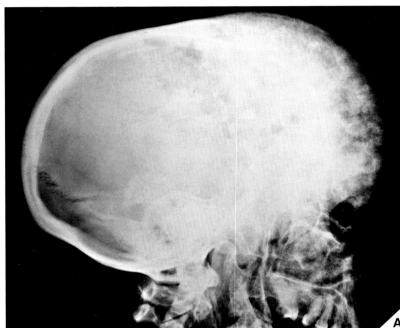

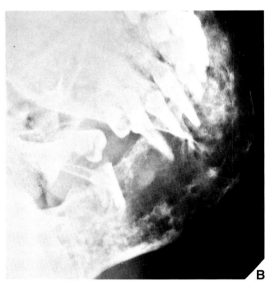

Figure 17.17 A 34-year-old man was noted to have a deformity of the left leg at age five. Radiographic examination at that time showed typical involvement of the tibia by fibrous dysplasia, which subsequently was confirmed by biopsy. No treatment was given and he was asymptomatic for 28 years until he developed acute pain in his left leg. Standard radiograph shows evidence of fibrous dysplasia affecting the proximal shaft of the tibia. A large osteolytic destructive lesion in the distal third of the tibia is also seen encroaching on the dense segment of bone and affecting the medullary portion and the cortex. There is a periosteal reaction and a soft tissue mass. Biopsy revealed transformation of fibrous dysplasia to undifferentiated spindle-cell sarcoma.

Figure 17.18 Eleven years prior to this examination, a 35-year-old woman with polyostotic fibrous dysplasia underwent radiation treatment of the mandible. (A) Lateral view of the skull demonstrates predominant involvement of the frontal bones with a characteristic expansion of the outer table. The base of the skull, a frequent site of polyostotic fibrous dysplasia, is typically thickened, and the frontal and ethmoid sinuses are obliterated. The maxilla and mandible are also affected. This advanced stage of involvement of the skull and facial bones by polyostotic fibrous dysplasia is frequently termed leontiasis ossea. (B) Oblique view of the mandible shows an expansile lytic lesion in the body of the left mandible, with partial destruction of the cortex. Biopsy revealed an osteosarcoma.

ered until adolescence. It has a decided preference for the tibia, being located with few exceptions in the proximal third or midsegment of the bone and often localized to its anterior cortex. In more than 80% of patients, there is some degree of anterior bowing. Larger lesions may destroy the cortex and invade the medullary cavity.

The Kempson-Campanacci lesion exhibits a lobulated sclerotic margin and a striking resemblance to nonossifying fibroma and fibrous dysplasia (Fig. 17.20). In particular, osteofibrous dysplasia and fibrous dysplasia, as the similarity in their names might suggest, display a remarkable histopathologic similarity. Like a lesion of fibrous dysplasia, osteofibrous dysplasia is composed of a

fibrous background containing deformed trabeculae. These trabeculae, however, unlike those of fibrous dysplasia, display woven bone only in the center, being surrounded by an outer zone of lamellar bone with prominent appositional osteoblastic activity ("dressed trabeculae").

This lesion should not be confused with the lesion, also called ossifying fibroma, that is seen almost exclusively in the jaw (mandible) of women in their third and fourth decades, although it is still uncertain whether some of the latter lesions represent an atypical form of fibrous dysplasia. Recently, Sissons and colleagues reported two cases of fibroosseous lesions that differed histologically from osteofibrous dysplasia and fibrous dysplasia. They proposed the term *ossifying fibroma* for

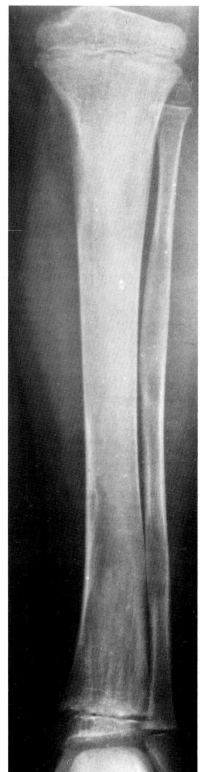

Figure 17.19 Polyostotic fibrous dysplasia typically affects one side of the skeleton, as seen here in a 5-year-old girl with precocious puberty whose left upper and lower extremities were affected (Albright-McCune syndrome). Plain film of the lower leg shows expansion of the tibia and fibula associated with thinning of the cortex. Note the ground-glass appearance of the medullary portion of these bones.

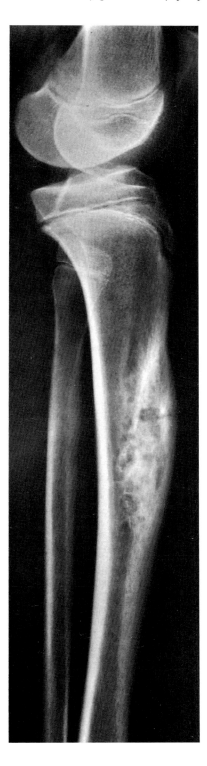

Figure 17.20 This lesion in the anterior aspect of the right tibia of a 14-year-old girl was originally thought to be a nonossifying fibroma. Although it is similar to a nonossifying fibroma and fibrous dysplasia, its site is typical of osteofibrous dysplasia, which was confirmed by biopsy. Note the characteristic anterior bowing of the tibia.

these, suggesting that the term *osteofibrous dysplasia* continue to be used for lesions of the tibia and fibula (Kempson-Campanacci lesions). To avoid confusion in terminology, the differential features of the various lesions are summarized in Figure 17.21.

COMPLICATIONS AND TREATMENT Osteofibrous dysplasia is known to be an aggressive lesion that frequently recurs after local excision. According to some researchers, it may coexist with another very aggressive lesion, adamantinoma (see Chapter 18).

Figure 17.21 Differential Features of Various Fibro-Osseus Lesions With Similar Radiographic Appearance

SEX	AGE	LOCATION	RADIOGRAPHIC APPEARANCE	HISTOPATHOLOGY
		Fibrous Dysplasia		
M/F	Any age (monostotic) First to third decades (polyostotic)	Femoral neck (frequent) Long bones Pelvis Ends of bones usually spared Polyostotic: unilateral in skeleton	Radiolucent, ground-glass, or smoky lesion Thinning of cortex with endosteal scalloping "Shepherd's crook" deformity Accelerated growth	Woven (nonlamellar) type of bone in loose to dense fibrous stroma; bony trabeculae lacking osteoblastic activity ("naked trabeculae")
		Nonossifying Fibroma		
M/F	First to third decades	Long bones (frequently posterior femur)	Radiolucent, eccentric lesion Scalloped, sclerotic border	Whorled pattern of fibrous tissue containing giant cells, hemosiderin, and lipid-filled histiocytes
		Osteofibrous Dysplasia (Kempson-Campanacci Lesion)		
M/F	First to second decades	Tibia (frequently anterior aspect) Fibula Intracortical (frequent)	Osteolytic, eccentric lesion Scalloped, sclerotic border Anterior bowing of long bone	Mature (lamellar) type of bone surrounded by cellular fibrous spindle-cell growth in whorled or matted pattern; bony trabeculae rimmed by osteoblasts ("dressed trabeculae")
		Ossifying Fibroma of Jaw		
F	Third to fourth decades	Mandible (90%) Maxilla	Expansile radiolucent lesion Sclerotic, well defined borders	Uniformly cellular fibrous spindle-cell growth with varying amounts of lamellar bone formation and small, round cementum-like bodies
		Ossifying Fibroma (Sissons Lesion)		
M/F	Second decade	Tibia Humerus	Radiolucent lesion Sclerotic border Similar to osteofibrous dysplasia	Fibrous tissue containing rounded and spindle-shaped cells with scant intercellular collegen and small, partially calcified spherules resembling cementum-like bodies of ossifying fibroma of jaw

Desmoplastic Fibroma

Desmoplastic fibroma (also called intraosseous desmoid tumor) is a rare lesion that occurs in individuals under 40 years of age, with 50% of all cases occurring in the patient's second decade. Pain and local swelling are the most common symptoms. The long bones (femur, humerus, and radius), the pelvis, and the mandible are frequent sites of involvement (Fig. 17.22). In the long bones, the lesion occurs in the diaphysis but often extends into the metaphysis. Although the epiphysis is spared, the lesion may extend into the articular end of the bone after closure of the growth plate.

Desmoplastic fibroma has no characteristic radiographic features. The lesion is generally expansile and radiolucent, with sharply defined borders; the cortex of the bone may be thickened or thinned, with no significant periosteal response (Fig. 17.23).

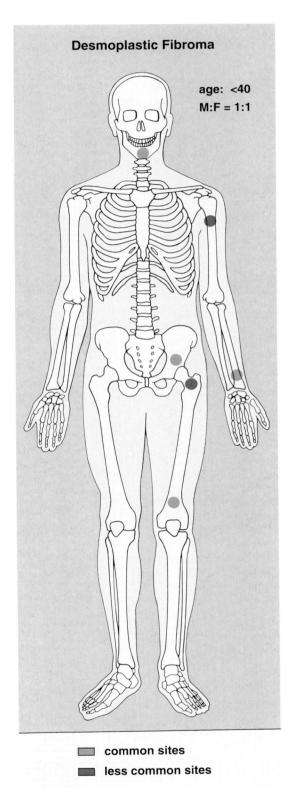

Figure 17.22 Skeletal sites of predilection, peak age range, and male-to-female ratio in desmoplastic fibroma.

Aggressive lesions of this type are marked by bone destruction and invasion of the soft tissues and may simulate malignant bone tumors. Pathologic fractures through the tumor are rare (9%).

Usually a geographic pattern of bone destruction is noted, with narrow zones of transition and nonsclerotic margins (76%). Internal pseudotrabeculation is present in 90% of cases.

Histologically, the lesion is composed of spindle-shaped and occasionally stellate fibroblasts associated with a densely collagenized matrix. Cells are almost always in a smaller proportion to the matrix. The stroma usually contains large, thin-walled vessels similar to those seen in desmoid tumors of soft tissues. Desmoplastic fibroma may be difficult to distinguish from other fibrous tumors, particularly low-grade fibrosarcoma.

Wide excision is the treatment of choice, although the recurrence rate is high even after complete excision of the tumor. Despite this aggressiveness, metastases have never been reported.

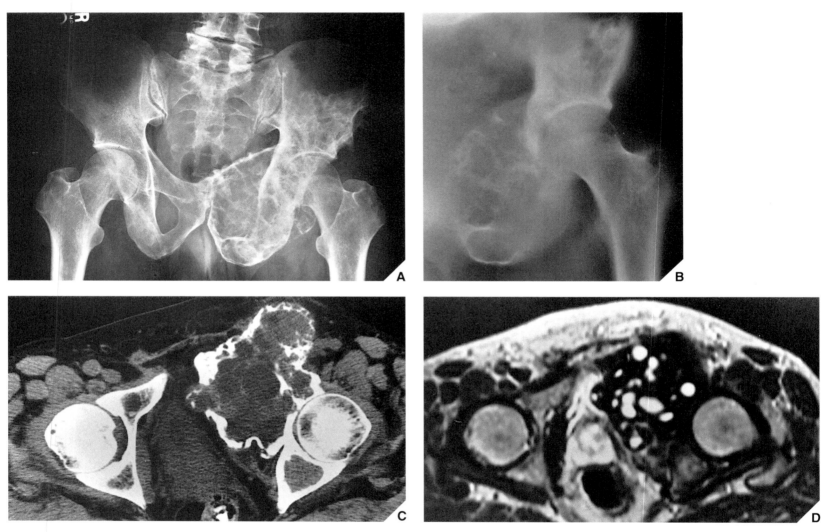

Figure 17.23 A 67-year-old man presented with a large pelvic mass. (A) Anteroposterior radiograph of the pelvis demonstrates an expansile, trabeculated lytic lesion that involves ischeim and pubis and extends into the supra-acetabular portion of the ilium. (B) Conventional tomography shows the lytic nature of the tumor and its expansile character. The involvement of ilium is better demonstrated. (C) CT section of the tumor through the hip joint shows a lobulated appearance and a thick, sclerotic margin.

This lesion extends into the pelvic cavity, displacing the urinary bladder. (D) Axial spin-echo T2-weighted MR image (TR 2000/TE 80) demonstrates nonhomogeneity of the signal from tumor: The bulk of the lesion displays low-to-intermediate signal intensity with central areas of high signal intensity. An incisional biopsy revealed desmoplastic fibroma. (Reprinted with permission from Greenspan A, et al., 1992)

OTHER BENIGN TUMORS AND TUMOR-LIKE LESIONS
Simple Bone Cyst

The simple bone cyst, also called a unicameral bone cyst, is a tumor-like lesion of unknown etiology; it has been attributed to a local disturbance of bone growth. More common in males than females, it is ordinarily seen during the first two decades of life. The vast majority of simple bone cysts are located in the proximal diaphysis of the humerus and femur, especially in patients under the age of 17 years (Fig. 17.24). In older patients, the incidence of bone cysts in atypical sites such as the calcaneus (Fig. 17.25), talus, and ilium rises significantly. Radiographically, a simple bone cyst appears as a radiolucent, centrally located, well circumscribed lesion with sclerotic margins (Fig. 17.26). There is no periosteal reaction, a feature distinguishing a simple bone cyst from an aneurysmal bone cyst, which invariably shows some degree of periosteal response; however, in the presence of pathologic fracture, there is periosteal reaction. Plain-film radiography usually suffices to make a diagnosis; tomography is necessary only in equivocal cases.

Histologically, a simple bone cyst is a diagnosis of exclusion. A sur-

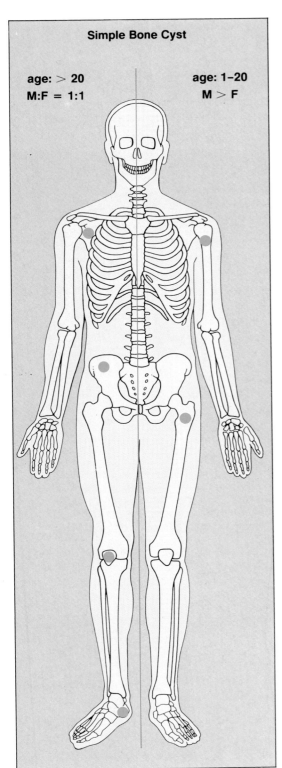

Figure 17.24 Skeletal sites of predilection, peak age range, and male-to-female ratio in simple bone cyst. The left half of the skeleton shows unusual sites of occurrence seen in an older patient population.

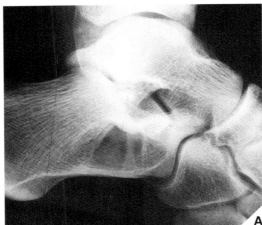

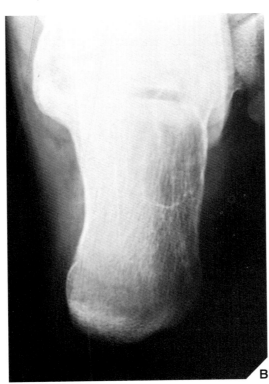

Figure 17.25 Lateral (A) and Harris-Beath (B) views of the ankle in a 32-year-old man show a simple bone cyst in the os calcis. Typically, bone cysts occurring at this site are located in the anterolateral aspect of the bone, as shown here.

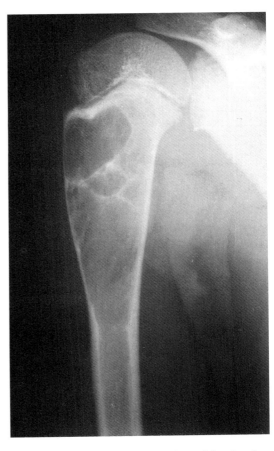

Figure 17.26 Anteroposterior view of the shoulder demonstrates the typical appearance of a simple bone cyst in a 6-year-old boy. Its location in the metaphysis and the proximal diaphysis of the humerus is also characteristic. The radiolucent lesion is centrally located and shows pseudosepta. Note the slight thinning of the cortex and lack of periosteal reaction.

gical curettage yields almost no solid tissue, but the walls of the cavity may show remnants of fibrous tissue or a flattened single-cell lining. The fluid content of the cyst contains elevated levels of alkaline phosphatase.

COMPLICATIONS AND DIFFERENTIAL DIAGNOSIS The most common complication of a simple bone cyst is pathologic fracture, which occurs in about 66% of cases (Fig. 17.27). Occasionally, one can identify a piece of fractured cortex in the interior of the lesion—the "fallen-fragment" sign—indicating that the lesion is either hollow or fluid-filled, as most simple bone cysts are. This sign permits the differentiation of a bone cyst, particularly in a slender bone such as the fibula (Fig. 17.28), from other radiolucent, radiographically similar lesions containing solid fibrous or cartilaginous tissue, such as fibrous dysplasia, nonossifying fibroma, or enchondroma. A bone abscess may occasionally mimic a simple bone cyst, particularly if located in the upper humerus or upper femur, the sites of predilection for simple bone cysts. In such cases, the presence of a periosteal reaction and extension beyond the growth plate are important differentiating features favoring a bone abscess (Fig. 17.29).

TREATMENT The treatment of simple bone cysts is based on the premise that the induction of osteogenesis results in complete healing of the lesion. The simplest inducement for bone repair is fracture, but this alone is insufficient to completely obliterate the lesion. Nor do simple bone cysts usually disappear following spontaneous fracture. The most common treatment is curettage followed by grafting with small pieces of cancellous bone. With this procedure, however, there is a higher rate of recurrence in patients under 10 years of age. Moreover, this approach may lead to damage to the growth plate, since most solitary bone cysts abut the physis. Recently, Scaglietti reported treating bone cysts with simple injection of methylprednisolone acetate. In younger patients so treated, complete bone repair occurred more rapidly than in older patients, who sometimes had to be given several injections.

Aneurysmal Bone Cyst

Aneurysmal bone cysts are seen predominantly in children; 90% of these lesions occur in patients under 20 years old. The metaphysis of long bones is a frequent site of predilection, although aneurysmal bone cysts may sometimes be seen in the diaphysis of a long bone, as

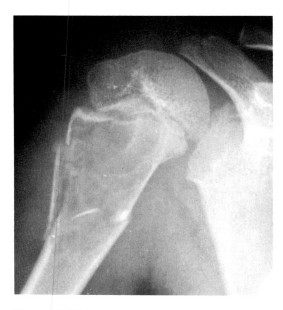

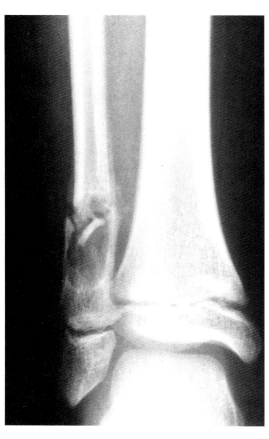

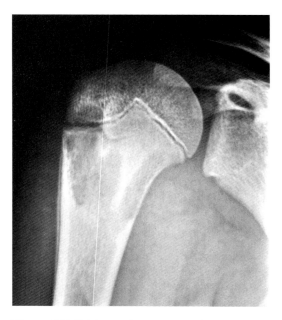

Figure 17.27 One of the most common complications of simple bone cyst is pathologic fracture, as seen here in the proximal humeral diaphysis in a 6-year-old boy. The presence of the "fallen-fragment" sign is characteristic of a simple bone cyst.

Figure 17.29 A bone abscess may mimic a simple bone cyst, as seen here in the proximal humerus of a 12-year-old boy. The periosteal reaction in the absence of pathologic fracture and the extension of the lesion into the epiphysis favors the diagnosis of bone abscess.

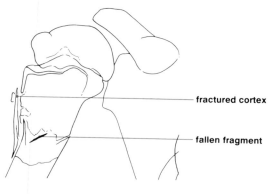

fractured cortex

fallen fragment

Figure 17.28 Anteroposterior view demonstrates a radiolucent lesion in the distal diaphysis of the right fibula of a 5-year-old boy who sustained mild injury to the lower leg. Note the pathologic fracture through the lesion and the associated periosteal reaction. A radiodense cortical fragment in the center of the lesion represents the "fallen-fragment" sign, identifying this lesion as a simple bone cyst.

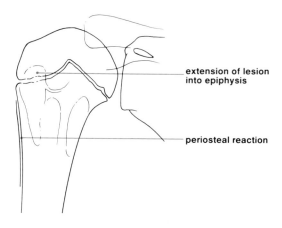

extension of lesion into epiphysis

periosteal reaction

well as in flat bones such as the scapula or pelvis and even in the vertebrae (Fig. 17.30). These lesions can develop de novo or as a result of cystic changes in a pre-existing lesion such as a chondroblastoma, osteoblastoma, giant cell tumor, or fibrous dysplasia (Fig. 17.31).

The radiographic hallmark of an aneurysmal bone cyst is multicystic eccentric expansion ("blow-out") of the bone, with a buttress or thin shell of periosteal response (Fig. 17.32). Although plain radiographs usually suffice for evaluating the lesion, conventional tomography,

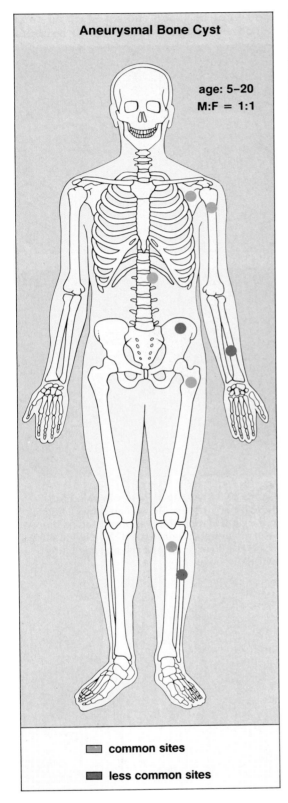

Figure 17.30 Skeletal sites of predilection, peak age range, and male-to-female ratio in aneurysmal bone cyst.

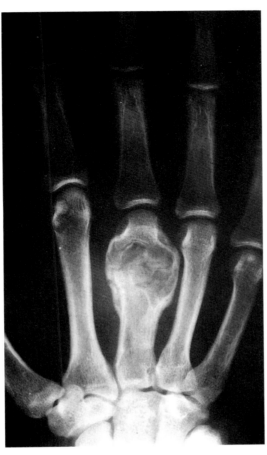

Figure 17.31 A 14-year-old boy had a painless swelling on the dorsum of the left hand. Dorsovolar film of the hand shows an expansile lesion in the distal segment of the third metacarpal. The lesion exhibits a well organized periosteal reaction; the articular end of the bone is spared. Biopsy revealed an aneurysmal bone cyst engrafted on a monostotic focus of fibrous dysplasia.

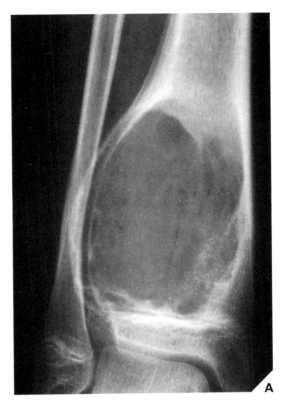

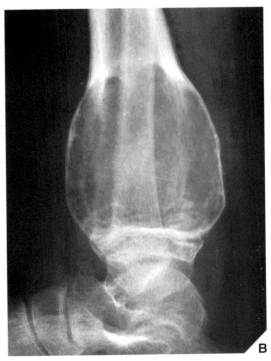

Figure 17.32 Anteroposterior (A) and lateral (B) views of the lower leg in an 8-year-old girl with a history of lower-leg pain demonstrate an expansile radiolucent lesion in the metaphysis of the distal tibia, extending into the diaphysis. Note its eccentric location in the bone and the buttress of periosteal response at the proximal aspect of the lesion. Biopsy revealed an aneurysmal bone cyst.

Histologically, a giant cell tumor is composed of a related dual population of mononuclear stromal cells and multinucleated giant cells. The tumor background contains varying amounts of collagen. Morphologically, the giant cells bear some resmblance to osteoclasts and they display increased acid phosphatase activity.

DIFFERENTIAL DIAGNOSIS When occurring in unusual locations in elderly individuals, giant cell tumor may easily be confused with metastatic disease, plasmacytoma, malignant fibrous histiocytoma, fibrosarcoma, or chondrosarcoma.

TREATMENT AND COMPLICATIONS The treatment of benign giant cell tumors consists either of surgical curettage and bone grafting (Fig. 17.41) or wide resection with secondary implantation of an allograft (Fig. 17.42) or an endoprosthesis (see Fig. 17.40). Marcove recommends cryosurgery using liquid nitrogen, while

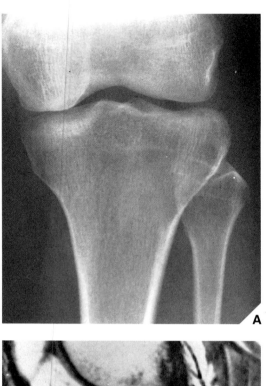

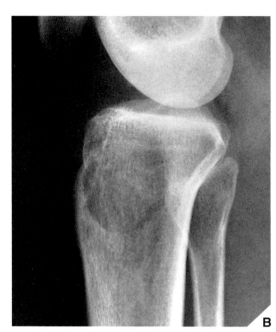

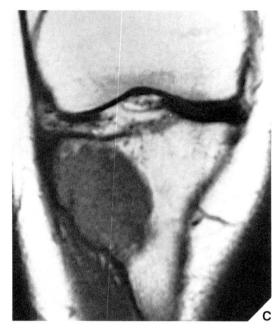

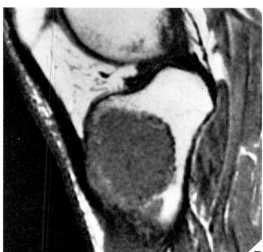

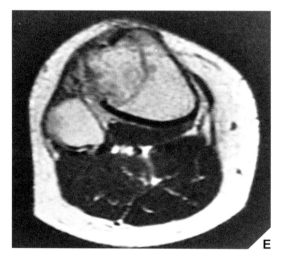

Figure 17.38 A 45-year-old woman presented with pain in the right knee of six months duration. Anteroposterior (A) and lateral (B) views demonstrate a radiolucent lesion in the proximal tibia, extending into the articular end of the bone. Coronal (C) and sagittal (D) spin-echo T1-weighted MR images (TR 600/TE 20) outline the lesion, which displays intermediate signal intensity, to the better advantage. Axial (E) T2-weighted image (TR 2000/TE 80) reveals that the lesion penetrates the cortex and extends into the soft tissues. On this image the lesion displays a nonhomogenous signal varying from intermediate to high intensity.

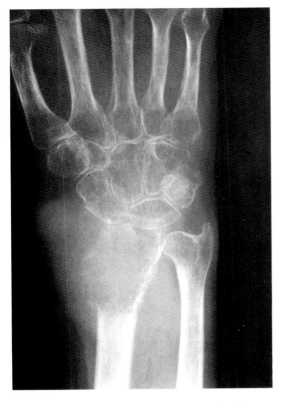

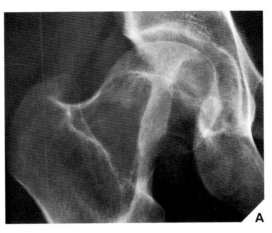

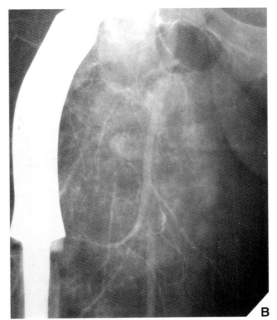

Figure 17.39 Dorsovolar view of the wrist of a 56-year-old woman shows a giant cell tumor of the distal radius that has destroyed the cortex and that extends into the soft tissues. Despite this aggressive radiographic presentation, on histopathologic examination the tumor had a typically benign appearance, without malignant features. After wide resection, a five-year follow-up showed no evidence of recurrence or of distant metastases.

Figure 17.40 A 28-year-old man had a 4-month history of right hip pain. (A) Anteroposterior view of the hip shows a destructive radiolucent lesion involving the medial aspect of the femoral head and extending into the femoral neck. Biopsy revealed an aneurysmal bone cyst. Five months after curettage and packing of the cavity with cancellous bone chips, the lesion recurred. This time the histopathologic examination revealed a benign giant cell tumor with an engrafted aneurysmal bone cyst. The proximal femur was resected and an endoprosthesis was implanted. Eight months after this procedure the patient was readmitted to the hospital with increased pain and a significant increase in the circumference of the thigh. (B) A femoral arteriogram demonstrates multiple soft tissue nodules, which on biopsy proved to be metastases from the giant cell tumor. The patient also developed pulmonary metastases.

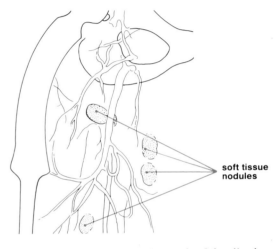

soft tissue nodules

Figure 17.41 (A) Plain radiograph of the distal forearm of a 32-year-old woman shows a giant cell tumor in the distal radius. (B) After extensive curettage, postoperative film shows the cavity of the lesion packed with bone chips.

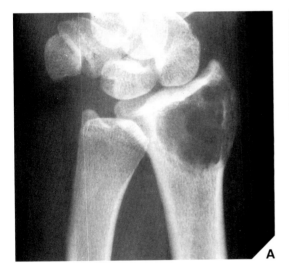

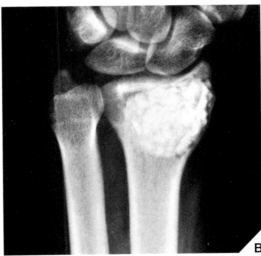

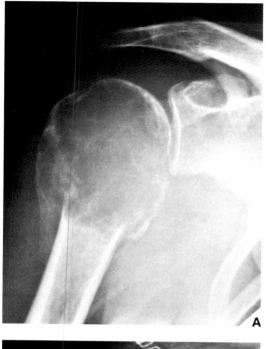

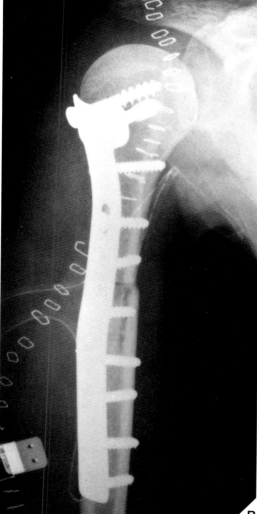

Figure 17.42 Plain film of the shoulder of a 27-year-old woman shows a giant cell tumor affecting almost the entire proximal end of the humerus. (B) Wide resection was performed and the humerus was reconstructed by means of allograft.

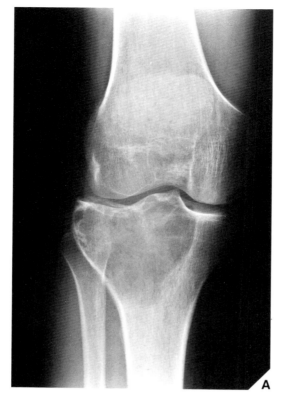

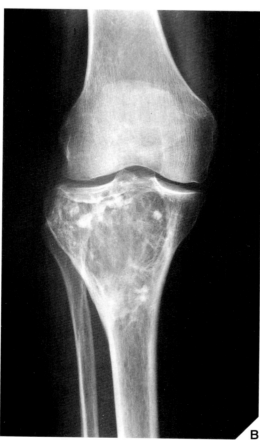

Figure 17.43 A 30-year-old woman was diagnosed as having a giant cell tumor of the proximal end of the right tibia (A) and was subsequently treated with curettage and application of cancellous bone chips. Twenty months after surgery, she began to experience progressive knee pain. (B) Follow-up film shows that most of the bone chips have been resorbed; the osteolytic foci indicate recurrence of the tumor.

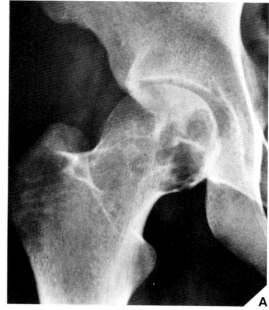

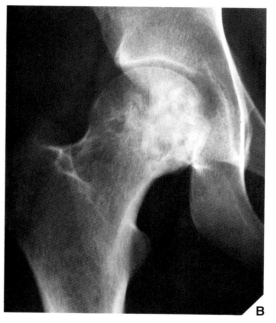

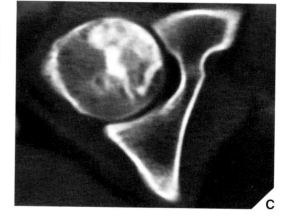

Figure 17.44 A 27-year-old woman had a giant cell tumor in the femoral head (A). (B) Two years following curettage and application of allograft there was no recurrence of the lesion. (C) CT demonstrates good incorporation of the graft into the normal bone (compare with Figure 17.43).

other authorities recommend heat using methylmethacrylate to pack the tumor bed following intralesional excision. Recurrences are often encountered and are recognized radiographically by resorption of the bone graft and the appearance of radiolucent areas like those in the original tumor (Fig. 17.43). Good healing and lack of recurrence are recognized by incorporation of the bone graft into the normal bone (Fig. 17.44). Especially following radiation therapy, recurrent lesions may exhibit malignant transformation to fibrosarcoma, malignant fibrous histiocytoma, or osteosarcoma. Occasionally, even histologically benign lesions produce distant (to the lung) metastases.

Hemangioma

A hemangioma is a benign bone lesion arising from newly formed blood vessels. Some investigators consider these lesions benign neoplasms; others put them into the category of congenital vascular malformations. They are classified, according to the type of vessels in the lesion, as capillary, cavernous, venous, or mixed. The incidence of hemangiomas seems to increase with age and is most frequent after middle age. Women are affected twice as often as men. The most common sites are the spine, particularly the thoracic segment, and the skull (Fig. 17.45). In the spine, the lesion typically involves a vertebral body, although it may extend into the pedicle or lamina

Figure 17.45 Skeletal sites of predilection, peak age range, and male-to-female ratio in hemangioma.

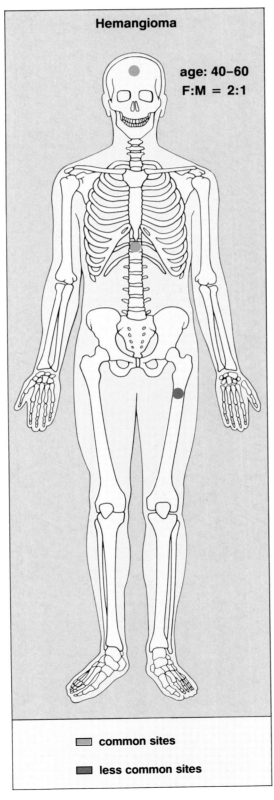

Hemangioma

age: 40–60
F:M = 2:1

☐ common sites

☐ less common sites

and, rarely, to the spinous process. Occasionally, multiple vertebrae may be affected. Most hemangiomas of the vertebral column are asymptomatic and discovered incidentally. Symptoms occur when the lesion in an affected vertebra compresses the nerve roots or spinal cord secondary to epidural extension. This neurologic complication is more commonly associated with lesions in the midthoracic spine (Fig. 17.46). Another mechanism considered responsible for compression of the cord, although seen less frequently, is fracture of the involved vertebral body with formation of an associated soft tissue mass or hematoma.

Hemangioma is typified radiographically by the presence of coarse vertical striations. In a vertebral body, this pattern is referred to as a "honeycomb" or "corduroy cloth" pattern (Fig. 17.47), and in the skull as a "spoke-wheel" configuration. When seen in the spine, this pattern is considered virtually pathognomonic for hemangioma; CT examination characteristically shows the pattern as multiple dots, which represent a cross-section of reinforced trabeculae (Fig. 17.48). In the long and short tubular bones, hemangiomas are recognized by a typical lace-like pattern and honeycombing (Fig. 17.49).

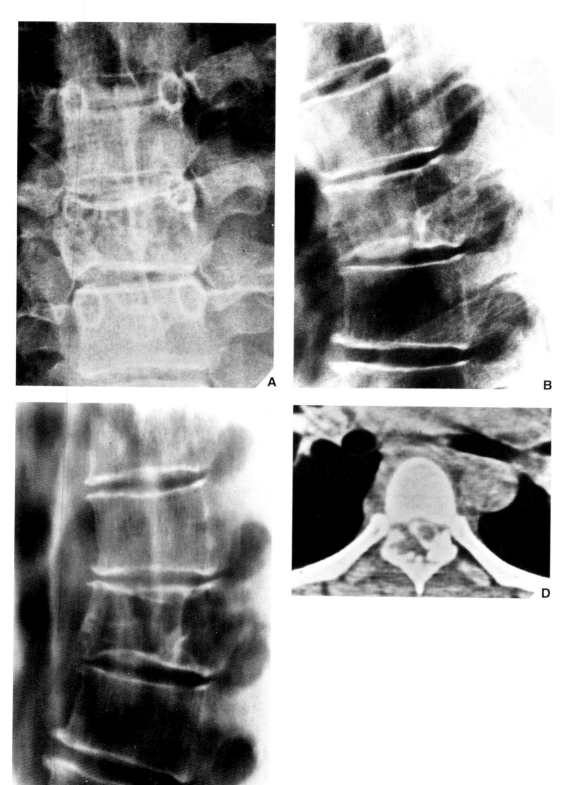

A

B

C

D

Figure 17.46 A 39-year-old woman presented with back pain and decreased sensation and strength in the right upper extremity. Anteroposterior (A) and lateral (B) radiographs of the thoracic spine show a radiolucent lesion involving the body of T-6 and extending into the pedicle. (C) Lateral tomographic cut demonstrates ballooning of the posterior cortex of the vertebra and extension of the lesion into the posterior elements. (D) CT shows a soft tissue mass encroaching on the spinal canal and displacing the spinal cord. Biopsy revealed a hemangioma. (Reprinted with permission from Greenspan A, et al., 1983)

Histologically, most hemangiomas consist of simple endothelium-lined channels, morphologically identical with capillary endothelium. Some or all of the vascular channels may be enlarged and have a sinusoid-like appearance, in which case the lesion is referred to as cavernous type.

DIFFERENTIAL DIAGNOSIS The differential diagnosis of hemangioma, particularly in the spine, should include Paget disease, eosinophilic granuloma, myeloma, and metastatic lesions. The characteristic "picture-frame" appearance of a vertebra affected by Paget disease (see Fig. 24.5), as well as its larger than normal size, distinguishes it from hemangioma. Myeloma in a vertebra, unlike hemangioma, is purely radiolucent—as are most metastatic lesions—and shows no vertical striations.

TREATMENT Asymptomatic hemangiomas do not require treatment. Symptomatic lesions are usually treated with radiation therapy to ablate the venous channels forming the lesions. Embolization, laminectomy, spinal fusion, or a combination of these are also used in treatment (see Fig. 14.15).

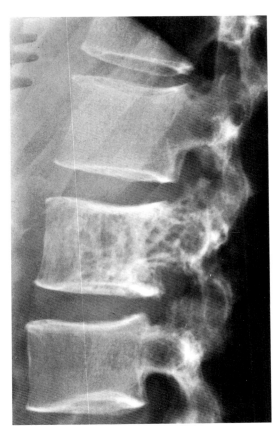

Figure 17.47 A 42-year-old man was injured in a car accident. Lateral view of the spine shows a hemangioma in the L-1 vertebra extending into the pedicle. Note the characteristic coarse, vertical striations, referred to as a "corduroy cloth" or "honeycomb" pattern.

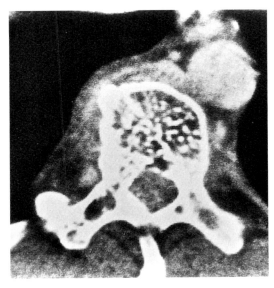

Figure 17.48 CT section of a T-10 vertebra demonstrates coarse dots that indicate reinforced vertical trabeculae of the cancellous bone, characteristic of hemangioma.

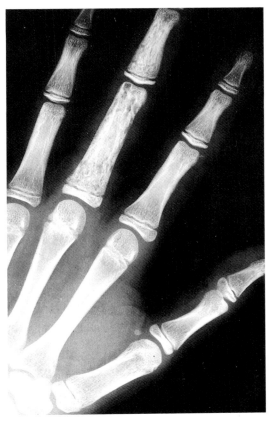

Figure 17.49 Dorsovolar view of the hand of an 11-year-old girl with hemangioma involving the middle finger shows the lace-like pattern and honeycombing characteristic of this lesion. Overgrowth of the digit, as seen here, is a frequent complication of hemangioma.

Non-Neoplastic Lesions Simulating Tumors

Some non-neoplastic conditions that may mimic bone tumors include intraosseous ganglion, a "brown tumor" of hyperparathyroidism, eosinophilic granuloma, encystified bone infarct, and myositis ossificans.

INTRAOSSEOUS GANGLION This lesion of unknown etiology is frequently encountered in adults between 20 and 60 years of age. It has a predilection for the articular ends of the long bones, usually the nonweight-bearing segment. Radiographically, it exhibits the characteristic picture of a round or oval radiolucent area located eccentri-

cally in the bone and rimmed by a sclerotic margin (Fig. 17.50). Its appearance is very similar to that of a degenerative cyst, but the adjacent joint does not show any degenerative changes; in most cases the ganglion, in contrast to a degenerative cyst, does not communicate with the joint cavity. An intraosseous ganglion may also mimic chondroblastoma, osteoblastoma, enchondroma, pigmented villonodular synovitis, or bone abscess (Fig. 17.51).

BROWN TUMOR OF HYPERPARATHYROIDISM Hyperparathyroidism is a condition resulting from the excess secretion of parathormone by overactive parathyroid glands (see Chapter 23). Not infrequently,

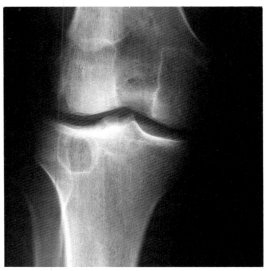

Figure 17.50
A 28-year-old man sustained an injury to the right knee that tore the medial meniscus. Anteroposterior view of the knee discloses a radiolucent lesion in the articular end of the proximal tibia. During surgery to remove the meniscus, the lesion was biopsied and histopathologic examination revealed it to be an intraosseous ganglion.

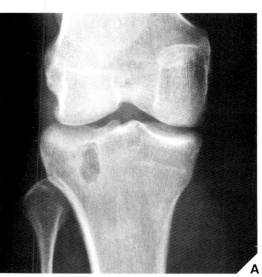

Figure 17.51
A 24-year-old man presented with an 8-week history of pain in the knee. Anteroposterior view of the knee (A) and CT section (B) demonstrate an oval radiolucent lesion eccentrically located in the proximal tibia with ramifications, rimmed by a zone of reactive sclerosis. The differential diagnosis included a bone abscess, osteoblastoma, chondroblastoma, and an intraosseous ganglion. Biopsy confirmed an intraosseous ganglion.

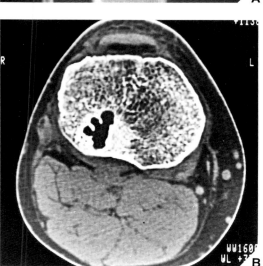

Figure 17.52 Plain film of the lower legs of a 28-year-old woman with hyperparathyroidism shows multiple brown tumors involving both tibiae. This condition can easily be misdiagnosed as multiple myeloma or metastatic disease.

patients with this disorder present with solitary or multiple lytic lesions, most commonly in the long and short tubular bones; on radiographic examination the lesions may resemble a tumor (Fig. 17.52). This lesion is called a brown tumor because in addition to fibrous tissue it contains decomposing blood, which gives specimens obtained for pathologic examination a brown coloration. The correct diagnosis can be made on plain films by observing associated abnormalities, including a decrease in bone density (osteopenia); subperiosteal bone resorption, which is best seen on the radial aspect of the proximal and middle phalanges of the second and third fingers; a granular, "salt-and-pepper" appearance of the cranial vault; resorption of the acromial ends of the clavicles; and soft tissue calcifications. Because of disturbed calcium and phosphorus metabolism, the serum calcium concentration is usually high (hypercalcemia) and the serum phosphorus concentration low (hypophosphatemia), laboratory findings that usually confirm the diagnosis.

EOSINOPHILIC GRANULOMA A non-neoplastic condition, eosinophilic granuloma belongs to the group of disorders known as reticuloendothelioses (or histocytoses X, according to Lichtenstein's proposed name), a group that includes two other conditions, Hand-Schüller-Christian disease (xanthomatosis) and Letterer-Siwe disease (nonlipid reticulosis). The grouping has gained wide acceptance with the recognition that all three entities represent different clinical manifestations of a single pathologic disorder, characterized by granulomatous proliferation of the reticulum cell.

Eosinophilic granuloma may manifest with solitary or with multiple lesions. It is usually seen in children, the common age of occurrence ranging from 1 to 15 years, with a peak incidence from 5 to 10 years. The most frequently affected sites are the skull, ribs, pelvis, spine, and long bones (Fig. 17.53). In the skull, the lytic lesions have a characteristic "punched-out" appearance, with sharply defined borders (Fig. 17.54). In the mandible or maxilla, the radiolucent lesions have the appearance of "floating teeth" (Fig. 17.55). In the spine,

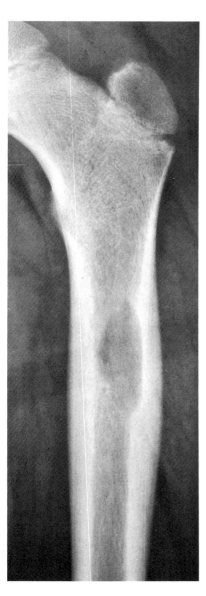

Figure 17.53 Radiograph of the proximal femur of a 3-year-old boy with a limp and tenderness localized to the upper thigh shows an osteolytic lesion in the medullary portion of the bone, without sclerotic changes. There is fusiform thickening of the cortex and a solid periosteal reaction. The patient's age, the location of the lesion, and its radiographic appearance are typical of eosinophilic granuloma.

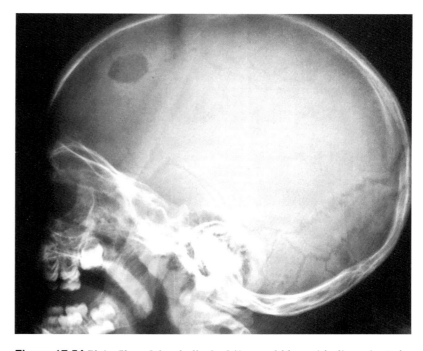

Figure 17.54 Plain film of the skull of a 2 ½-year-old boy with disseminated eosinophilic granuloma shows an osteolytic lesion in the frontal bone with a sharply outlined margin, giving it a punched-out appearance. Uneven involvement of the inner and outer tables results in its beveled appearance.

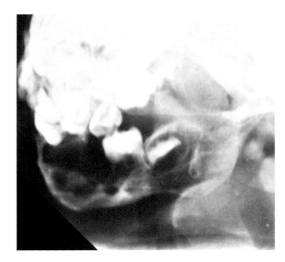

Figure 17.55 A 3-year-old girl with extensive skeletal involvement of eosinophilic granuloma had in addition a large destructive lesion in the mandible. Note the characteristic appearance of a floating tooth, which results from destruction of supportive alveolar bone.

collapse of a vertebral body, the so-called vertebra plana, is a characteristic manifestation of the disease (Fig. 17.56). This finding was for a long time mistakenly interpreted as representing osteochondrosis of the vertebra and was called "Calvé disease."

In the long bones, eosinophilic granuloma presents as a destructive radiolucent lesion commonly associated with a lamellated periosteal reaction. It may mimic a malignant round cell tumor such as lymphoma or Ewing sarcoma (Fig. 17.57). In its later stages, the lesion becomes more sclerotic, with dispersed radiolucencies (Fig. 17.58). The distribution of the lesion and the detection of silent sites in the skeleton are best ascertained by a radionuclide bone scan; this may also be helpful in differentiating eosinophilic granuloma from Ewing sarcoma, which rarely presents with multiple foci.

Histologically, eosinophilic granuloma is composed of a variable admixture of two types of cells: eosinophilic leukocytes possessing bilobate nuclei and coarse eosinophilic cytoplasmic granules, and histiocytes, identical with the Langerhans histiocytes seen in the skin.

MEDULLARY BONE INFARCT Radiographically, a medullary bone infarct presents with calcifications in the marrow cavity, usually surrounded by a well defined, hyalinized fibrotic or sclerotic border (see Fig. 15.32); occasionally, this presentation may be mistaken for a cartilage tumor such as an enchondroma. In the rare instances when a cyst develops in an infarcted segment of a long or flat bone—i.e., an encystified bone infarct—it is visualized radiographically as an expanding radiolucent lesion associated with thinning of the surrounding cortex. Usually, the cyst cavity is sharply outlined and the lesion is demarcated by a thin shell of reactive bone (Fig. 17.59). This encystification of a bone infarct can resemble an intraosseous lipoma or even a chondrosarcoma.

MYOSITIS OSSIFICANS Myositis ossificans is a localized formation of heterotopic bone in the soft tissues that is initiated by trauma. Two types of these lesions have been identified. The first is a well circumscribed lesion frequently seen adjacent to the cortex of a long tubular or flat bone; the other is a veil-like lesion that is less delineated. Radiographically, myositis ossificans circumscripta is characterized by a zonal phenomenon—dense, well organized bone at the periphery of the lesion and less organized, immature bone at the center—and a radiolucent cleft that separates the lesion from the cortex of the adjacent bone (see Figs. 2.47, 2.57A). The appearance of this lesion may mimic a malignant bone tumor such as parosteal or periosteal osteosarcoma (see Figs. 18.14, 18.16). Most errors in diagnosis occur when a biopsy of the lesion is obtained too early in onset, when its histologic appearance may resemble sarcomatous tissue.

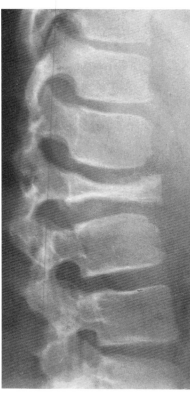

Figure 17.56 Vertebra plana in eosinophilic granuloma represents collapse of a vertebral body secondary to the destruction of bone by a granulomatous lesion. Note the preservation of the intervertebral disk spaces.

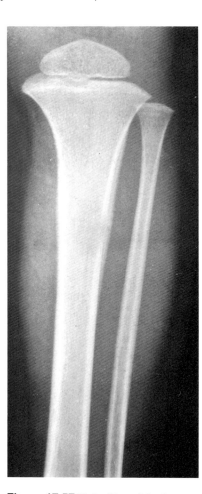

Figure 17.57 Plain film of the lower leg of a 4-year-old boy demonstrates a lesion in the diaphysis of the left tibia exhibiting a permeative type of bone destruction and a lamellated (onion-skin) type of periosteal response not infrequently seen in osteomyelitis or Ewing sarcoma. The duration of the patient's symptoms (fever and pain for ten days), however, favored an eosinophilic granuloma.

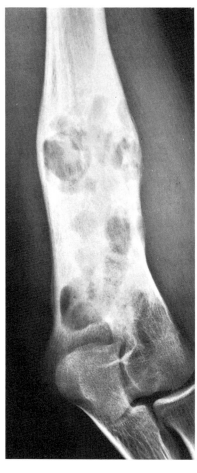

Figure 17.58 The healing stage of an eosinophilic granuloma, seen here in the distal humerus of a 16-year-old girl, exhibits predominantly sclerotic changes with interspersed radiolucent foci, thickening of the cortex, and a well organized periosteal reaction. In this stage, the lesion mimics chronic osteomyelitis.

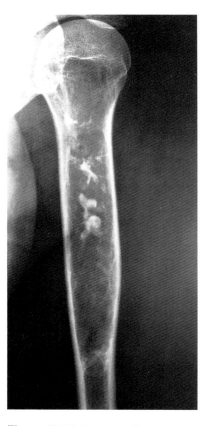

Figure 17.59 An expanding, radiolucent lesion in the proximal shaft of the left humerus was an incidental finding in a 31-year-old woman. The lesion exhibits the classic features of an encystified bone infarct: its location in the medullary portion of the bone with central calcifications and a thin rim of reactive sclerosis. Note that although the cortex is thinned and expanded, there is no evidence of a periosteal reaction or soft tissue mass. (Courtesy of Dr. A. Norman, New York, NY)

PRACTICAL POINTS TO REMEMBER

Benign Fibrous and Fibro-Osseous Lesions

[1] A fibrous cortical defect (metaphyseal fibrous defect) and nonossifying fibroma are closely related lesions of similar histopathologic structure. They differ radiologically only in their size.

[2] Periosteal desmoid has a characteristic predilection for the posteromedial cortex of the medial femoral condyle. It should not be mistaken for a malignant bone tumor.

[3] Fibrous dysplasia may be monostotic or polyostotic, with the latter having a decided preference for one side of the skeleton. The polyostotic form, if accompanied by precocious puberty and café au lait spots (with irregular, ragged, or "coast of Maine" borders) is called Albright-McCune syndrome, and is seen predominantly in girls.

[4] The best radiologic technique for evaluating the distribution of fibrous dysplasia is radionuclide bone scan.

[5] Osteofibrous dysplasia, a benign fibro-osseous lesion seen in children and adolescents, has a decided predilection for the anterior aspect of the tibia. This lesion may be associated with adamantinoma.

Other Benign Tumors and Tumor-Like Lesions

[1] Simple bone cysts have a predilection for:
- the proximal diaphysis of the humerus and femur in children and adolescents
- the pelvis and os calcis in adults.

[2] A simple bone cyst is characterized by:
- its central location in a long bone
- lack of periosteal reaction in the absence of fracture.

It may be complicated by pathologic fracture, in which case the "fallen-fragment" sign is often present and may help in the differential diagnosis.

[3] An aneurysmal bone cyst, seen almost exclusively in children and adolescents below age 20, is characterized by:
- its eccentric location in a bone
- a buttress of periosteal reaction
- its usual containment by a thin shell of periosteum.

[4] Giant cell tumors, seen characteristically at the articular ends of long bones, most often present as purely radiolucent lesions without any sclerotic reaction at their periphery. It is impossible to determine radiographically whether a giant cell tumor is benign or malignant.

[5] Hemangiomas are commonly seen in a vertebral body. Although most frequently asymptomatic, they may produce symptoms if they expand into the spinal canal.

[6] Non-neoplastic conditions frequently mistaken for tumors include:
- an intraosseous ganglion
- the brown tumor of hyperparathyroidism
- eosinophilic granuloma
- an encystified medullary bone infarct
- posttraumatic myositis ossificans.

[7] Intraosseous ganglion resembles a degenerative cyst and has a predilection for the nonweight-bearing segments of the articular end of the long bones.

[8] Eosinophilic granuloma is seen predominantly in children and may be mistaken for Ewing sarcoma.

[9] Myositis ossificans is characterized by a zonal phenomenon (well-organized bone at the periphery of the lesion and immature bone at the center), and a radiolucent cleft that separates the lesion from the cortex of adjacent bone

References

Albright F, Butler AM, Hampton AO, Smith P: Syndrome characterized by osteitis fibrosa disseminata, areas of pigmentation and endocrine dysfunction with precocious puberty in females. *N Engl J Med* 216:727, 1937.

Arata MA, Peterson HA, Dahlin DC: Pathological fractures through nonossifying fibromas—review of the Mayo Clinic experience. *J Bone Joint Surg* 63A:980, 1981.

Baker ND, Greenspan A, Klein MJ, Neuwirth M: Symptomatic vertebral hemangiomas: A report of four cases. *Skeletal Radiol* 15:458, 1986.

Barnes GR, Gwinn JL: Distal irregularities of the femur simulating malignancy. *Am J Roentgenol* 122:180, 1974.

Brower AC, Culver JC, Keats TE: Histological nature of medial posterior distal femoral metaphysis in children. *Radiology* 99:389, 1971.

Campanacci M: Osteofibrous dysplasia of the long bones. A new clinical entity. *Ital J Orthop Traumatol* 2:221, 1976.

Campanacci M, Laus M: Osteofibrous dysplasia of the tibia and fibula. *J Bone Joint Surg* 63A:367, 1981.

Carrasco CH, Murray JA: Giant cell tumors. *Orthop Clin North Am* 20:395, 1989.

Clarke BE, Xipell JM, Thomas DP: Benign fibrous histiocytoma of bone. *Am J Surg Pathol* 9:806, 1985.

Crim JR, Gold RH, Mirra JM, Eckardt JJ, Bassett LW: Desmoplastic fibroma of bone: Radiographic analysis. *Radiology* 172:827, 1989.

Gebhardt MC, Campbell CJ, Schiller AL, Mankin HJ: Desmoplastic fibroma of bone. A report of eight cases and review of the literature. *J Bone Joint Surg* 67A:732, 1985.

Greenspan A, Klein MJ, Bennett AJ, et al: Hemangioma of the T6 vertebra with a compression fracture, extradural block and spinal cord compression. Case report #242. *Skeletal Radiol* 10:183, 1983.

Greenspan A, Unni KK: Desmoplastic fibroma of the pelvis. *Skeletal Radiol* 1992. In press.

Hudson TM, Schiebler M, Springfield DS, Enneking WF, Hawkins IF, Spanier SS: Radiology of giant cell tumors of bone: Computed tomography, arthro-tomography, and scintigraphy. *Skeletal Radiol* 11:85, 1984.

Huvos AG, Higinbotham NL, Miller TR: Bone sarcomas arising in fibrous dysplasia. *J Bone Joint Surg* 54A:1047, 1972.

Jaffe HL: Aneurysmal bone cyst. *Bull Hosp Jt Dis Orthop Inst* 11:3, 1950.

Jaffe HL, Lichtenstein L: Non-osteogenic fibroma of bone. *Am J Pathol* 18:205, 1942.

Jaffe HL, Lichtenstein L: Solitary unicameral bone cyst with emphasis on the roentgen picture, pathologic appearance and pathogenesis. *Arch Surg* 44:1004, 1942.

Kempson RL: Ossifying fibroma of the long bones. A light and electron microscopic study. *Arch Pathol* 82:218, 1966.

Kenney PJ, Gilula LA, Murphy WA: The use of computed tomography to distinguish osteochondroma and chondrosarcoma. *Radiology* 139:129, 1981.

Laredo JD, Reizine D, Bard M, Merland JJ: Vertebral hemangioma: Radiologic evaluation. *Radiology* 161:183, 1986.

Lichtenstein L, Jaffe HL: Fibrous dysplasia of bone. *Arch Pathol* 33:777, 1942.

Marks KE, Bauer TW: Fibrous tumors of bone. *Orthop Clin North Am* 20:377, 1989.

Norman A: Myositis ossificans and fibrodysplasia ossificans progressiva. In: Taveras JM, Ferrucci JT (eds): *Radiology—Diagnosis, Imaging, Intervention, Vol 5.* ch 132. Philadelphia, Lippincott, 1986.

Norman A, Schiffman M: Simple bone cysts: Factors of age dependency. *Radiology* 124:779, 1977.

Norman A, Steiner GC: Radiographic and morphological features of cyst formation in idiopathic bone infarction. *Radiology* 146:335, 1983.

Parker BR, Pinckney L, Etcubanas E: Relative efficacy of radiographic and radionuclide bone surveys in the detection of the skeletal lesions of histiocytosis X. *Radiology* 134:377, 1980.

Reynolds J: The "fallen fragment sign" in the diagnosis of unicameral bone cyst. *Radiology* 92:949, 1969.

Scaglietti O, Marchetti PG, Bartolozzi P: The effects of methylprednisolone acetate in the treatment of bone cysts. Results of three years follow-up. *J Bone Joint Surg* 61B:200, 1979.

Schmaman A, Smith I, Ackerman LV: Benign fibro-osseous lesions of the mandible and maxilla. A review of 35 cases. *Cancer* 26:303, 1970.

Sissons HA, Kancherla PL, Lehman WB: Ossifying fibroma of bone. Report of two cases. *Bull Hosp Jt Dis Orthop Inst* 43:1, 1983.

Malignant Bone Tumors

OSTEOSARCOMA

OSTEOSARCOMA (osteogenic sarcoma) is one of the most common primary malignant bone tumors. There are several types of osteosarcoma (Fig. 18.1), each having distinctive clinical, radiographic, and histologic characteristics. The common feature of all types is that the osteoid and bone matrix are formed by malignant cells of connective tissue.

The vast majority of osteosarcomas are of unknown cause and can therefore be referred to as idiopathic, or *primary*. A smaller number of tumors can be related to known factors predisposing to malignancy, such as Paget disease, fibrous dysplasia, external ionizing irradiation, or ingestion of radioactive substances. These lesions are referred to as *secondary* osteosarcomas. All types of osteosarcomas may be further subdivided by anatomic site into lesions of the appendicular skeleton and axial skeleton. Furthermore, they may be classified on the basis of their location in the bone as central and juxtacortical. A separate group consists of primary osteosarcoma originating in the soft tissues (so-called extraskeletal or soft tissue osteosarcomas).

Histopathologically, osteosarcomas can be graded on the basis of their cellularity, nuclear pleomorphism, and degree of mitotic activity. Generally speaking, central osteosarcomas are much more frequent than juxtacortical tumors, and they tend to have a higher histologic grade. Although pulmonary metastasis is the most common and most significant complication in high-grade osteosarcoma, it is rare in two subtypes: osteosarcoma of the jaw and multicentric osteosarcoma.

Primary Osteosarcoma

Conventional Osteosarcoma

Conventional osteosarcoma is the most frequent type of osteosarcoma, having its highest incidence in patients in their second decade and affecting males slightly more often than females. It has a predilection for the knee region (distal femur and proximal tibia), while the second most common site is the proximal humerus (Fig. 18.2). Patients usually present with bone pain, occasionally accompanied by a soft tissue mass or swelling. At times the first symptoms are related to pathologic fracture.

The distinctive radiologic features of conventional osteosarcoma, as demonstrated by plain-film radiography, are medullary and cortical bone destruction, an aggressive periosteal reaction, a soft tissue mass, and tumor bone either within the destructive lesion or at its periphery, including the soft tissue mass (Fig. 18.3). In some instances, the type of bone destruction may not be obvious, but patchy densities representing tumor bone and an aggressive periosteal reaction on the conventional studies are clues to the diagnosis (Fig. 18.4). The most common types of periosteal response encountered with this tumor are the "sunburst" type and a Codman triangle; the lamellated

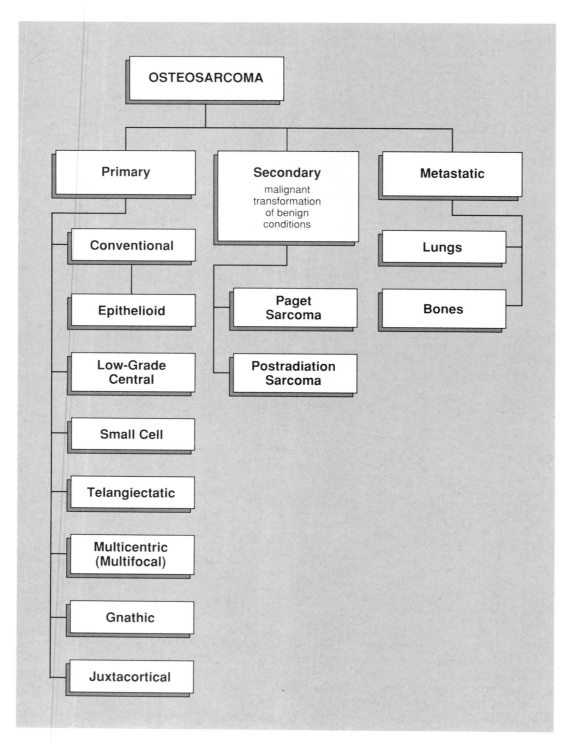

Figure 18.1 Classification of the types of osteosarcoma.

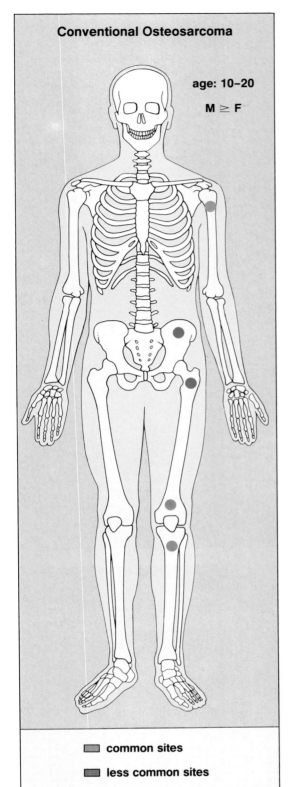

Conventional Osteosarcoma

age: 10–20

M ≥ F

☐ common sites

☐ less common sites

Figure 18.2 Skeletal sites of predilection, peak age range, and male-to-female ratio in conventional osteosarcoma.

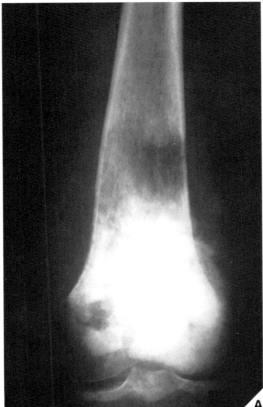

A

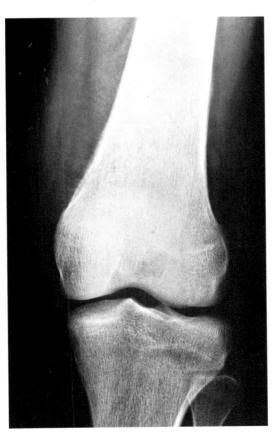

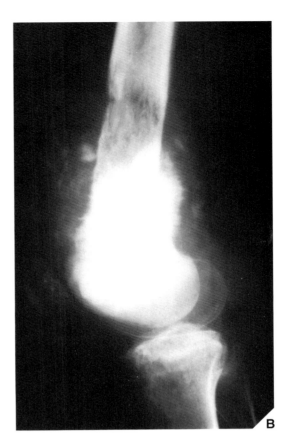

B

Figure 18.3 Anteroposterior (A) and lateral (B) plain films demonstrate the typical features of osteosarcoma in the femur of a 19-year-old female. Medullary and cortical bone destruction can be seen in association with an aggressive periosteal response of the velvet and sunburst types, as well as with a soft tissue mass containing tumor bone.

Figure 18.4 Although there is no gross bone destruction evident in the distal femur of this 16-year-old girl, the patchy densities in the medullary portion of the femur and the sunburst appearance of the periosteal response are clues to the diagnosis of osteosarcoma. Note also the presence of a Codman triangle.

osteosarcoma is sometimes referred to as epithelioid osteosarcoma. The diagnosis usually becomes evident from the patient's age, the production of obvious tumor matrix, and a radiographic appearance typical of osteosarcoma.

COMPLICATIONS AND TREATMENT The most frequent complications of conventional osteosarcoma are pathologic fracture and the development of pulmonary metastases.

If a limb-salvage procedure is feasible, a course of multidrug chemotherapy is employed, followed by wide resection of the bone and insertion of an endoprosthesis (Fig. 18.9). Less frequently, amputation is performed, followed by chemotherapy. Currently, the five-year survival rate after adequate therapy exceeds 50%.

Low-Grade Central Osteosarcoma

This rare form of osteosarcoma (1% of all osteosarcomas) has only recently been recognized. It usually occurs in patients older than those presenting with conventional osteosarcoma, although the sites of predilection are similar. Radiographically, it may be indistinguishable from conventional osteosarcoma, but it grows more slowly and

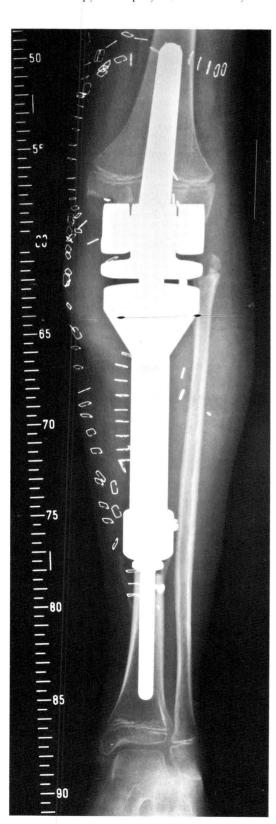

Figure 18.9 An 8-year-old boy underwent a limb-salvage procedure for osteosarcoma in the left tibia. After a full course of chemotherapy, consisting of a combination of methotrexate, doxorubicin hydrochloride, and cisplatin, a wide resection of the proximal tibia was done and a LEAP metallic spacer inserted. This expandable prosthesis can be adjusted to maintain limb length with the normal contralateral limb as the child grows. (Courtesy of Dr. MM Lewis, New York, NY)

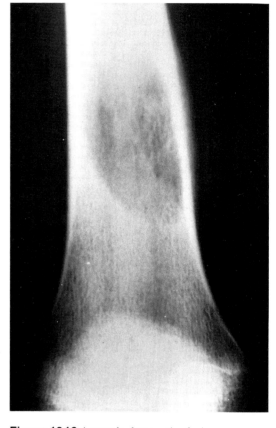

Figure 18.10 A purely destructive lesion can be seen in the diaphysis of the femur of this 17-year-old girl. Note the velvet type of periosteal reaction. The sclerotic changes usually seen in osteosarcomas are absent, and there is no radiographic evidence of tumor bone. Biopsy revealed a telangiectatic osteosarcoma, one of the most aggressive types of this tumor. (Courtesy of Dr. MJ Klein, New York, NY)

has a better prognosis. At times its radiographic presentation clearly mimics fibrous dysplasia.

Telangiectatic Osteosarcoma

A very aggressive type of osteosarcoma, the telangiectatic variant is twice as common in males as in females and is seen predominantly in patients in their second and third decades of life. It is rare, comprising approximately 3% of all malignant bone tumors. It is characterized by a high degree of vascularity and large cystic spaces filled with blood, which account for its atypical radiographic presentation. It is an osteolytic destructive lesion with an almost complete absence of sclerotic changes; a soft tissue mass may also be present (Fig. 18.10). Grossly, the tumor resembles a "bag" of blood and is characterized by blood-filled spaces, necrosis, and hemorrhage. Histologically, it is composed of loculated blood-filled spaces, partially lined by malignant cells producing sparse osteoid tissue. It resembles an aneurysmal bone cyst.

Small Cell Osteosarcoma

Described by Sim and associates, small cell osteosarcoma usually occurs as a radiolucent lesion with permeative borders and a large soft tissue mass. Its radiographic appearance thus mimics that of a round cell bone sarcoma. These lesions usually exhibit small round cells in many histologic fields, much like Ewing sarcoma. The presence, however, of spindled tumor cells, as well as the focal production of osteoid or bone, helps to make a histologic diagnosis of osteosarcoma. The distal femur, proximal humerus, and proximal tibia are predilected sites.

Multicentric Osteosarcoma

The simultaneous development of foci of osteosarcoma in multiple bones is a very rare occurrence (Fig. 18.11). Whether this entity is truly separate, or represents multiple bone metastases from a primary conventional osteosarcoma, remains a controversy. This type of osteosarcoma is currently recognized as having two variants: syn-

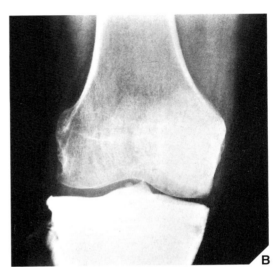

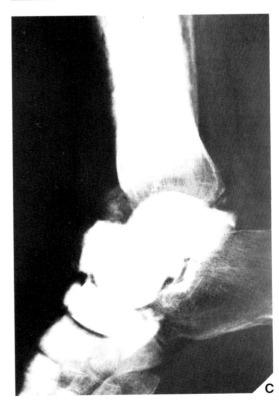

Figure 18.11
Multicentric osteosarcoma, a very rare bone tumor, is demonstrated here in the right hemipelvis (A), right tibia (B), and several bones of the right foot (C).

chronous and metachronous. Multifocal osteosarcoma must be differentiated from osteosarcoma metastasized to other bones.

Juxtacortical Osteosarcomas
The term *juxtacortical* is a general designation for a group of osteosarcomas that arise on the bone surface (Fig. 18.12).

Usually, these lesions are much rarer and occur a decade later than their intraosseous counterparts. The great majority of juxtacortical osteosarcomas are low-grade tumors, although there are moderately and even highly malignant variants.

PAROSTEAL OSTEOSARCOMA Parosteal tumors are seen largely in patients in their third and fourth decades, with a characteristic site of predilection in the posterior aspect of the distal femur (Fig. 18.13).

Conventional radiography is usually adequate for making a diagnosis of parosteal osteosarcoma. The lesion presents as a dense oval or spherical mass attached to the cortical surface of the bone and sharply demarcated from the surrounding soft tissues (Fig. 18.14A). CT (Fig. 18.14B) or MRI (see Fig. 15.18) are often necessary to determine whether the lesion has penetrated the cortex and invaded the medullary region of the bone.

Histologically, the lesion consists of fibrous stroma, probably derived from the outer fibrous periosteal layer. The bony component is often trabeculated but at least partially immature, particularly at the periphery of the tumor. This is an important point in differentiating it from the sometimes similar appearing myositis ossificans, which, however, matures in a centripetal fashion, with its most mature portion outermost.

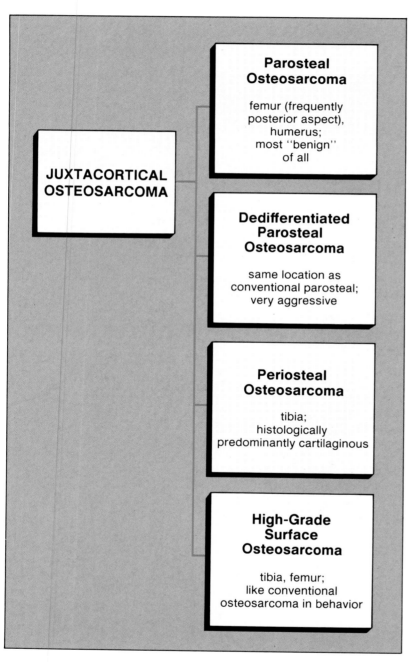

Figure **18.12** Variants of juxtacortical osteosarcoma.

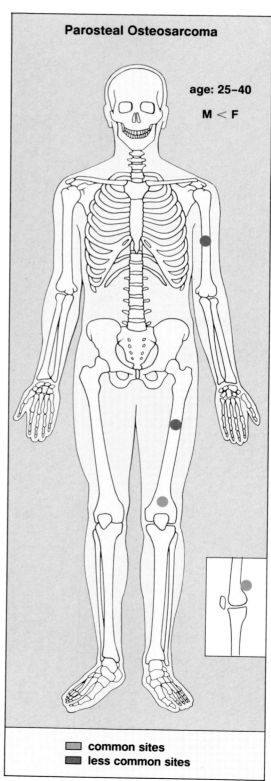

Figure **18.13** Skeletal sites of predilection, peak age range, and male-to-female ratio in parosteal osteosarcoma.

DIFFERENTIAL DIAGNOSIS Parosteal osteosarcoma must be differentiated from myositis ossificans, soft tissue osteosarcoma, parosteal liposarcoma with ossifications, and osteochondroma. Differentiation from myositis ossificans and osteochondroma is the most frequent source of confusion. Myositis ossificans is distinguished by a zonal phenomenon and by a cleft separating the ossific mass from the cortex (Fig. 18.15; see also Figs. 4.49, 4.60, 16.41). In osteochondroma, on the other hand, the cortex of the lesion merges without interruption into the cortex of the host bone (see Figs. 16.40, 16.41), a feature not seen in parosteal osteosarcoma. Because the lesion is relatively slow-growing and most often involves only the surface of the bone, the prognosis for patients with parosteal osteosarcoma is much better than for those with other types of osteosarcoma. Simple wide resection of the lesion often constitutes sufficient treatment.

DEDIFFERENTIATED PAROSTEAL OSTEOSARCOMA A rare and unusual bone tumor, dedifferentiated parosteal osteosarcoma was recently identified by a group from the Mayo Clinic. Most cases reportedly originate as conventional parosteal osteosarcomas that, following resection and multiple local recurrences, have undergone transformation to histologically high-grade sarcomas. Some cases, however, have presented as primary tumors arising on the cortical surface of a

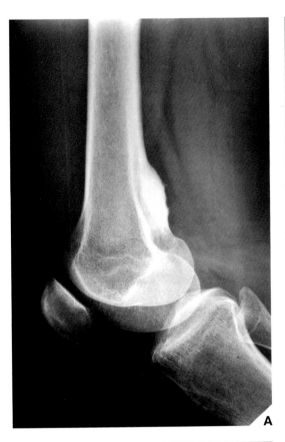

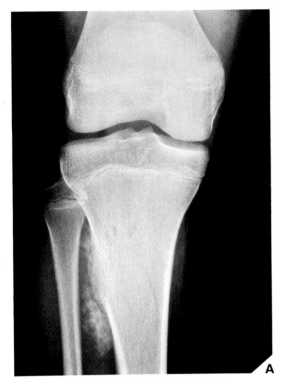

Figure 18.15 Juxtacortical myositis ossificans, seen here near the medial cortex of the femoral neck, typically presents as a more mature lesion at its periphery, with a center less dense than in parosteal osteosarcoma, and a clear zone representing complete separation of the lesion from the cortex.

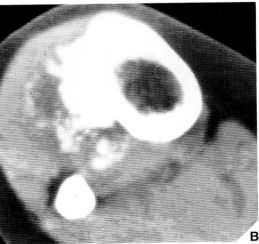

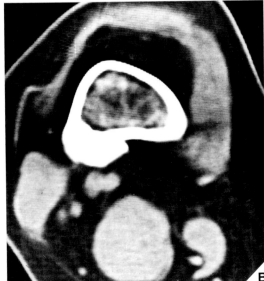

Figure 18.14 (A) Lateral radiograph of the knee of a 37-year-old woman shows an ossific mass attached to the posterior cortex of the distal femur. Its location and appearance are typical of parosteal osteosarcoma. (B) Contrast-enhanced CT section demonstrates that the medullary portion of the bone has not been invaded.

Figure 18.16 (A) Anteroposterior view of the right knee of a 12-year-old girl with "discomfort" in the upper leg for two months demonstrates poorly defined calcifications and ossifications in a mass attached to the surface of the lateral tibial cortex. There appears to be no bone destruction. (B) CT section shows the extent of the soft tissue mass. Note that the tumor, a periosteal osteosarcoma, is intimately attached to the cortex, a factor that virtually excludes myositis ossificans.

bone de novo. Radiographically and histologically, dedifferentiated parosteal osteosarcoma mimics the features of conventional parosteal osteosarcoma. There are, however, some traits of a high-grade sarcoma, such as radiographically identifiable cortical destruction and histologically identifiable pleomorphic tumor cells with hyperchromatic nuclei and a high mitotic rate. Hence, the prognosis is much worse than that of parosteal osteosarcoma.

PERIOSTEAL OSTEOSARCOMA Most often occurring in adolescence, periosteal osteosarcoma is a very rare tumor that grows on the bone surface, usually at the midshaft of a long bone such as the tibia. The characteristic feature of this tumor, which radiographically may resemble myositis ossificans, is a predominance of cartilaginous tissue (Fig. 18.16); this may lead to an erroneous diagnosis of periosteal chondrosarcoma. Periosteal osteosarcoma is marked by a better prognosis than the conventional type but a worse one than the parosteal variant.

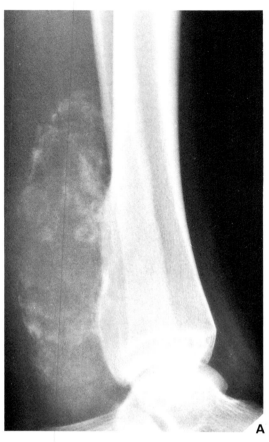

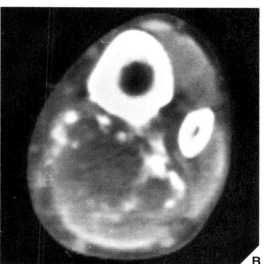

Figure 18.17 (A) Lateral view of the knee demonstrates a high-grade surface osteosarcoma attached to the posterior cortex of distal tibia in a 24-year-old man. Poorly defined ossific foci are seen within a large soft tissue mass. Note the similarity of the tumor to periosteal osteosarcoma (see Fig. 18.16). (B) CT section demonstrates the extent of the lesion. Characteristically, the marrow cavity is not affected.

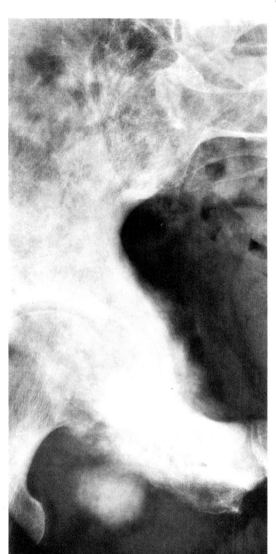

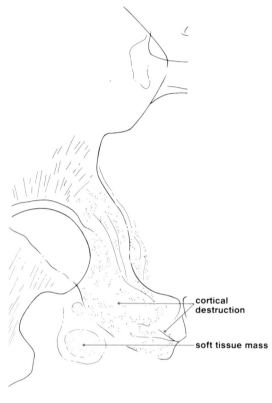

Figure 18.18 Plain film in a 66-year-old man who had extensive skeletal involvement by Paget disease and who developed pain in the right hip shows the typical features of osteitis deformans in the right ilium and ischium. There is also destruction of the cortex associated with a soft tissue mass containing tumor bone—characteristic features of malignant transformation to osteosarcoma.

HIGH-GRADE SURFACE OSTEOSARCOMA High-grade surface osteosarcoma may exhibit radiographic features similar to those of parosteal or periosteal osteosarcoma (Fig. 18.17). Histologically, this lesion shows elements identical to those of conventional osteosarcoma. It also carries a high potential for metastasis.

Secondary Osteosarcomas

In contrast to primary osteosarcomas, secondary lesions occur in an older population. A large proportion of these tumors is responsible for the complications of Paget disease (osteitis deformans) and, characteristically, develop in pagetic bone (Fig. 18.18). The typical radiographic changes in malignant transformation of Paget disease include a destructive lesion in the affected bone, the presence of tumor bone in the lesion, and an associated soft tissue mass. Osteosarcoma in these patients must be differentiated from metastases to pagetic bone from primary carcinomas elsewhere in the body (most commonly the prostate, breast, and kidney). Secondary osteosarcoma may also develop spontaneously in fibrous dysplasia or following radiation therapy for benign bone lesions such as fibrous

dysplasia and giant cell tumor, as well as following irradiation of malignant processes in the soft tissues such as breast carcinoma and lymphoma. (For further discussion of malignant transformation, see the sections below on Paget disease and radiation-induced sarcoma under the heading Benign Conditions with Malignant Potential.)

CHONDROSARCOMA

Chondrosarcoma is a malignant bone tumor characterized by the formation of cartilage by tumor cells. As in osteosarcoma, there are several types of this tumor (Fig. 18.19), each with characteristic clinical, radiographic, and pathologic features.

Primary Chondrosarcomas

Conventional Chondrosarcoma

Also known as central or medullary chondrosarcoma, this tumor is seen twice as frequently in males as in females and more commonly in adults, usually in those past their third decade. The most frequent locations are the pelvis and long bones, particularly the femur and

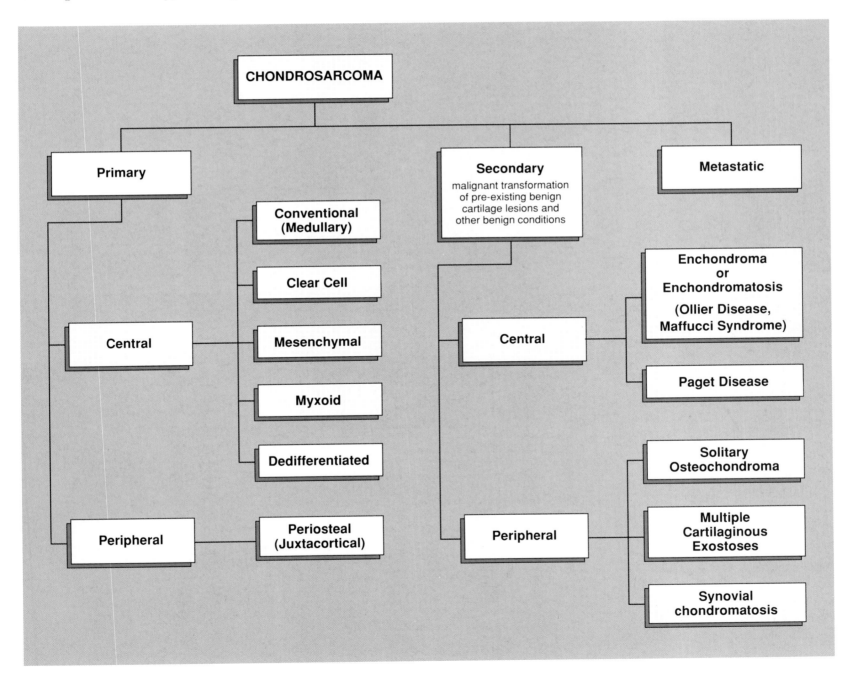

Figure 18.19 Classification of the types of chondrosarcoma.

humerus (Fig. 18.20). Most conventional chondrosarcomas are slow-growing tumors, often discovered incidentally. Occasionally, local pain and tenderness may be present.

Radiographically, conventional chondrosarcoma appears as an expansile lesion in the medulla with thickening of the cortex and characteristic endosteal scalloping; popcorn-like, annular, or comma-shaped calcifications are seen in the medullary portion of the bone. A soft tissue mass may sometimes be present. In typical cases, plain-film radiography is sufficient to make a diagnosis (Fig. 18.21). CT and MRI help delineate the extent of intraosseous and soft tissue involvement (Fig. 18.22).

Histologically, chondrosarcoma is typified by the formation of cartilage by tumor cells. It is more cellular and pleomorphic in appearance than enchondroma and contains an appreciable number of plump cells, with large or double nuclei. Mitotic cells are infrequent. The histologic distinction among low-grade, intermediate,

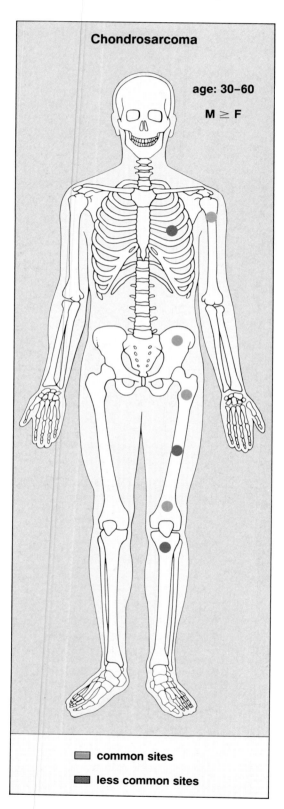

Figure 18.20 Skeletal sites of predilection, peak age range, and male-to-female ratio in conventional chondrosarcoma.

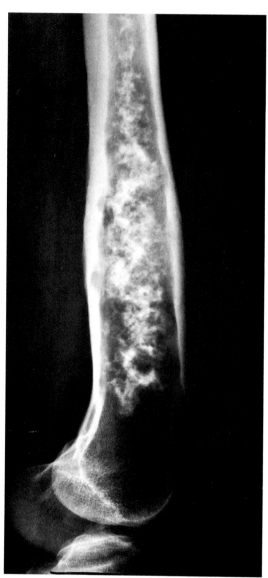

Figure 18.21 Oblique plain film in a 46-year-old man shows the characteristic features of a central chondrosarcoma of the right femur. Within the destructive lesion in the medullary portion of the bone are annular and comma-shaped calcifications. The thickened cortex, which is due to periosteal new bone formation in response to destruction of the cortex by the chondroblastic tumor, shows the typical endosteal scalloping.

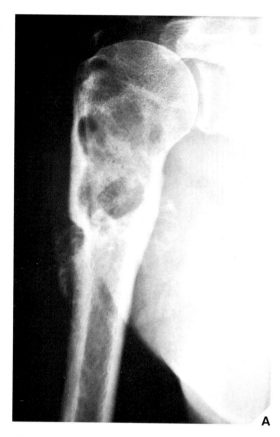

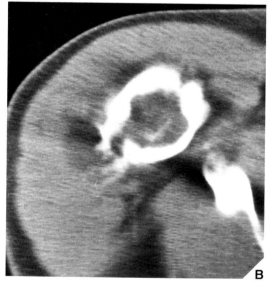

Figure 18.22 (A) Anteroposterior plain film of the right shoulder of a 62-year-old man is not adequate for demonstrating the soft tissue extension of the chondrosarcoma in the proximal humerus. (B) CT section through the lesion demonstrates cortical destruction and an extensive soft tissue mass.

and high-grade lesions is based on the cellularity of the tumor tissue, the degree of pleomorphism of the cells and nuclei, and the number of mitoses present. Some investigators (e.g., Unni) disregard the last feature in grading these tumors.

DIFFERENTIAL DIAGNOSIS In exceptional cases, particularly in the early stage of development, this lesion can be indistinguishable from an enchondroma. For this reason, all centrally located cartilage tumors in long bones, particularly in adult patients, should be regarded as malignant until proven otherwise. At the articular ends of the bone, chondrosarcomas frequently lack characteristic calcifications and may mimic giant cell tumor.

COMPLICATIONS AND TREATMENT Pathologic fractures through conventional chondrosarcomas are rare (Fig. 18.23). Moreover, conventional chondrosarcomas are slow-growing tumors, and only in rare cases do they metastasize to distant areas. Since they are not radiosensitive, surgical resection is the major means of therapy.

Clear Cell Chondrosarcoma

Clear cell chondrosarcoma is a rare (less than 4% of all chondrosarcomas in the Mayo Clinic series) and recently recognized variant of chondrosarcoma. It occurs twice as often in males as in females, and usually in their third to fifth decades. It is predominantly a lytic lesion with a sclerotic border, which occasionally may contain calcifications. Many of these lesions resemble chondroblastomas, and many involve the proximal end of the humerus and femur (Fig. 18.24).

Histologically, the clear cell variant exhibits larger and more rounded tumor cells than other chondrosarcomas with clear or vacuolated cytoplasm. A chondroid matrix, trabeculae of reactive bone, and numerous osteoclast-like giant cells are distinctive features of this tumor.

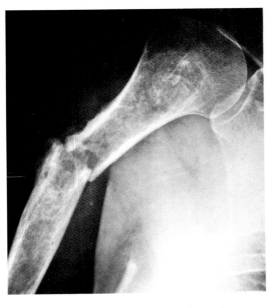

Figure 18.23 Pathologic fracture through a chondrosarcoma, as seen here in the right humerus in a 60-year-old man, is a rare complication of this lesion.

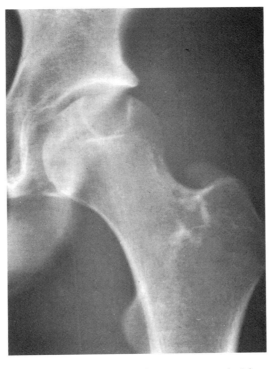

Figure 18.24 A 22-year-old man presented with left hip pain for three months. Anteroposterior radiograph demonstrates an osteolytic lesion located in the superolateral aspect of the femoral head and extending into the articular surface. The lesion, which is demarcated by a thin sclerotic border, closely resembles a chondroblastoma. On biopsy, however, it proved to be a clear cell chondrosarcoma.

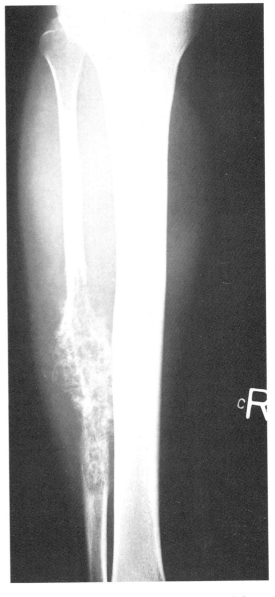

Figure 18.25 Anteroposterior film of the right lower leg of a 43-year-old woman with a six-month history of intermittent pain in the right calf shows a destructive lesion at the midportion of the fibula associated with a large soft tissue mass. The central portion of the lesion exhibits annular and comma-shaped calcifications typical of a cartilage tumor, but its periphery shows a permeative type of bone destruction characteristic of round cell tumors. Biopsy revealed mesenchymal chondrosarcoma.

TREATMENT Clear cell chondrosarcoma is considered a low-grade malignancy. It has been managed in a variety of ways, from simple observation or curettage to wide resection and even amputation. Although it is a less aggressive tumor than conventional chondrosarcoma, inadequate treatment may lead to recurrence. Therefore, en bloc resection with wide surgical margins of bone and soft tissue is the current treatment of choice.

Mesenchymal Chondrosarcoma

Mesenchymal chondrosarcoma is very uncommon (less than 1% of all malignant bone tumors) and tends to occur in the patient's second or third decade. It presents radiographically with the permeative type of bone destruction seen in round cell tumors, and calcifications in the cartilaginous portion of the tumor (Fig. 18.25). It may be indistinguishable from conventional chondrosar-

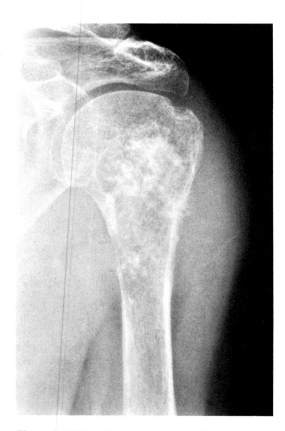

Figure 18.26 A 70-year-old woman developed a destructive lesion in the medullary cavity of the proximal shaft of the left humerus with calcifications typical of a cartilage tumor; there was also a soft tissue mass. But while the lesion seen on this plain film exhibits features typical of medullary chondrosarcoma, biopsy revealed, in addition to typical chondrosarcomatous tissue, elements of a giant cell tumor and malignant fibrous histiocytoma, leading to a diagnosis of dedifferentiated chondrosarcoma—the most aggressive of all such tumors.

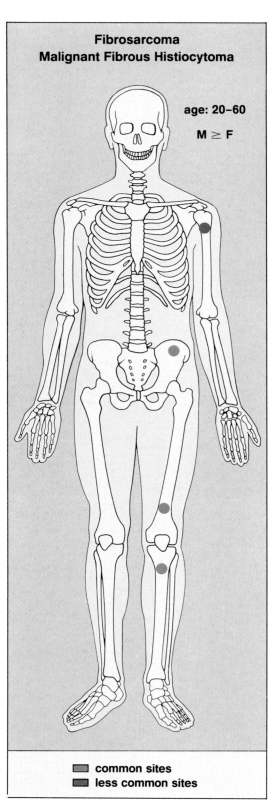

Figure 18.27 Skeletal sites of predilection, peak age range, and male-to-female ratio in fibrosarcoma and malignant fibrous histiocytoma.

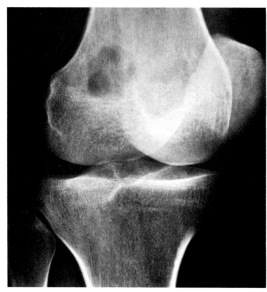

Figure 18.28 Oblique view of the right knee of a 28-year-old woman shows a purely destructive osteolytic lesion in the intercondylar fossa of the distal femur. Note the absence of reactive sclerosis and periosteal response. Biopsy proved it to be a fibrosarcoma.

coma and is a highly malignant lesion with a strong capacity to metastasize.

Histologically, the mesenchymal variant demonstrates a high degree of malignancy, typified by areas of more or less differentiated cartilage, together with highly vascular stroma of mesenchymal tissue containing spindle-cells and round cells.

Dedifferentiated Chondrosarcoma
Dedifferentiated chondrosarcoma is the most malignant of all chondrosarcomas and consequently carries a very poor prognosis; most patients succumb to the disease within two years of diagnosis. The patient typically has pain of long duration, followed by a more recent onset of rapid swelling and local tenderness. The prolonged pain probably reflects a slow-growing lesion, and the swelling and tenderness may be related to the development of a rapidly growing, more malignant component. The hallmark of this lesions is the appearance of an aggressive sarcoma engrafted on a benign-appearing low-grade chondrosarcoma. Although it may radiographically resemble a conventional chondrosarcoma, its histologic composition differs. The dedifferentiated tissue may appear to be a fibrosarcoma, a malignant fibrous histiocytoma, or an osteosarcoma. Radiographically, dedifferentiated chondrosarcomas exhibit calcific foci with aggressive bone destruction, and are often accompanied by a large soft tissue mass (Fig. 18.26).

Histologically, dedifferentiated chondrosacroma often shows a cartilaginous component of low-grade malignancy combined with highly cellular sarcomatous tissue.

Recently, the validity of the term "dedifferentiation" has been challenged. Studies using electron microscopy and immunohistochemistry indicate that sarcomatous dedifferentiation represents, in fact, the synchronous differentiation of separate clones of cells from a primitive spindle-cell sarcoma to various types of sarcoma.

Periosteal Chondrosarcoma
Generally, periosteal chondrosarcoma has the same radiographic and pathologic features as central chondrosarcoma. Because the lesion appears on the bone surface, it must be distinguished from periosteal osteosarcoma. The differentiation of this lesion may create problems for the radiologist and pathologist alike.

Secondary Chondrosarcomas
The most common types of secondary chondrosarcomas are tumors developing in pre-existing enchondromas (see Fig. 16.35) or in multiple cartilaginous exostoses (see Figs. 16.45, 16.46). These tumors develop in a slightly younger age group (20 to 40 years of age) than primary chondrosarcomas and run a more benign course. Because they are usually of low-grade malignancy, the prognosis is more favorable than in conventional chondrosarcoma. Total excision is the treatment of choice. (For further discussion of malignant transformation, see the sections below under the heading Benign Conditions with Malignant Potential.)

FIBROSARCOMA AND MALIGNANT FIBROUS HISTIOCYTOMA
Fibrosarcoma and malignant fibrous histiocytoma are malignant fibrogenic tumors that have very similar radiographic presentations and histologic patterns. Both typically occur in the patient's third to sixth decades, and both have a predilection for the femur, humerus, and tibia (Fig. 18.27).

Histologically, fibrosarcoma and malignant fibrous histiocytoma are characterized by tumor cells that produce collagen fibers. In fibrosarcoma, however, there is a herring-bone pattern of fibrous growth with mild cellular pleomorphism, while histiocytic features of a characteristic storiform or pinwheel arrangement of fibrogenic tissue typify malignant fibrous histiocytoma. Neither tumor is capable of producing osteoid matrix or bone, a factor distinguishing them from osteosarcoma.

Radiographically, both fibrosarcoma and malignant fibrous histiocytoma are recognized by an osteolytic area of bone destruction and a wide zone of transition; the lesions are usually eccentrically located close to or in the articular end of the bone. They exhibit little or no reactive sclerosis and in most cases no periosteal reaction (Fig. 18.28); a soft tissue mass, however, is frequently present.

DIFFERENTIAL DIAGNOSIS Both tumors may resemble a giant cell tumor (Fig. 18.29) or telangiectatic osteosarcoma (see Fig. 18.10). They are also often mistaken for metastatic lesions (Fig. 18.30).

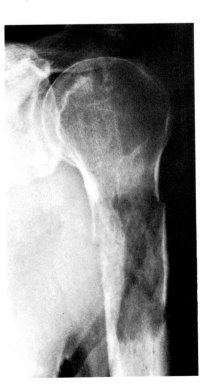

Figure 18.30 A 62-year-old man sustained a pathologic fracture through an osteolytic lesion in the proximal shaft of the left humerus. A metastatic lesion was suspected, but biopsy revealed a primary fibrosarcoma of the bone.

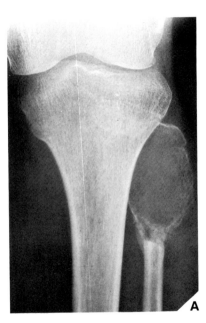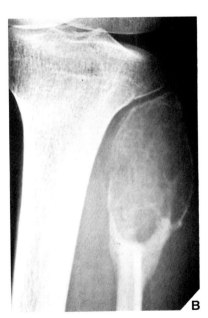

Figure 18.29 Anteroposterior view of the left knee (A) and a magnification study in the oblique projection (B) demonstrate an expanding, lytic lesion in the proximal end of the fibula in a 13-year-old girl. The cortex has been partially destroyed, and there is a buttress of periosteal new bone formation secondary to pathologic fracture. Biopsy revealed a malignant fibrous histiocytoma. The differential diagnosis of this malignancy at this site should include giant cell tumor and aneurysmal bone cyst.

Some authorities believe that an almost pathognomonic sign of fibrosarcoma is small sequestrum-like fragments of cortical bone and spongy trabeculae, which may be demonstrated on conventional radiography or CT scan.

Immunohistochemical studies have been helpful in the diagnosis of malignant fibrous histiocytoma by demonstrating certain non-specific markers of histiocytic enzymes such as lysozyme and α_1-antitrypsin in the tumor.

COMPLICATIONS AND TREATMENT Since these tumors do not respond satisfactorily to radiation or chemotherapy, surgical resec-tion is the treatment of choice. Pathologic fracture may occur, and, as a palliative measure, internal splinting with a metallic implant may be justified. The tumor has been reported to recur after local excision and may spread to regional lymph nodes. Both fibrosar-coma and malignant fibrous histiocytoma may complicate benign conditions such as fibrous dysplasia, Paget disease, bone infarction, or chronic draining sinuses of osteomyelitis. They may also arise in bones that were previously irradiated (see the discussion under the heading Benign Conditions with Malignant Potential). The five-year survival rate following treatment varies according to different studies from 29% to 67%.

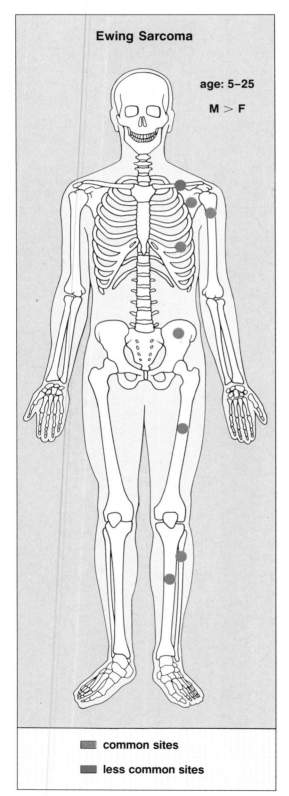

Figure 18.31 Skeletal sites of predilection, peak age range, and male-to-female ratio in Ewing sarcoma.

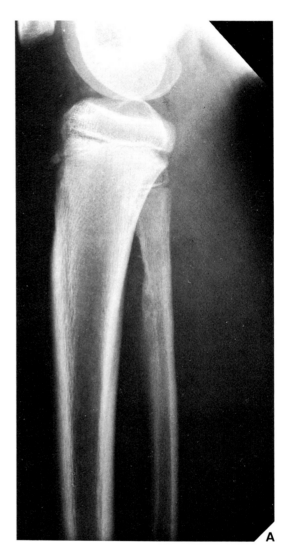

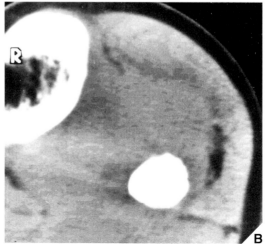

Figure 18.32 (A) Lateral film in a 12-year-old boy shows the typical appearance of Ewing sarcoma in the fibula. The poorly defined lesion exhibits a per-meative bone destruc-tion associated with an aggressive periosteal reaction. (B) CT sec-tion through the lesion demonstrates a large soft tissue mass, not clear on the routine study. Note the com-plete obliteration of the marrow cavity by tumor.

phoma from the other round cell tumors is the stain for leukocyte-common antigen because lymphoid cells are the only cells that stain positively.

DIFFERENTIAL DIAGNOSIS Histiocytic lymphoma must be distinguished from secondary involvement of the skeleton by systemic lymphoma. It may resemble Ewing sarcoma, particularly in younger patients (Fig. 18.39), or Paget disease if the articular end of a bone is involved and there is a mixed sclerotic and osteolytic pattern (Fig. 18.40).

TREATMENT The treatment for primary bone lymphoma consists of radiotherapy since this tumor is radiosensitive. Some cases may also require chemotherapy.

Myeloma

Myeloma, also known as "multiple myeloma" or "plasma cell myeloma," is a tumor originating in the bone marrow and is the most common primary malignant bone tumor. It is usually seen between the patient's fifth and seventh decades, and more frequently in men than women. The axial skeleton (skull, spine, ribs, and pelvis) are the most commonly affected sites, but no bone is exempt from involvement (Fig. 18.41). Rarely, the presentation can be that of a solitary lesion, in which case it is called a *solitary myeloma* or *plasmacytoma*; far more commonly, however, it presents with widespread involvement, in which case the name *multiple myeloma* is applied. Mild and transient pain exacerbated by heavy lifting or other activity is present in about 75% of cases and may be the initial

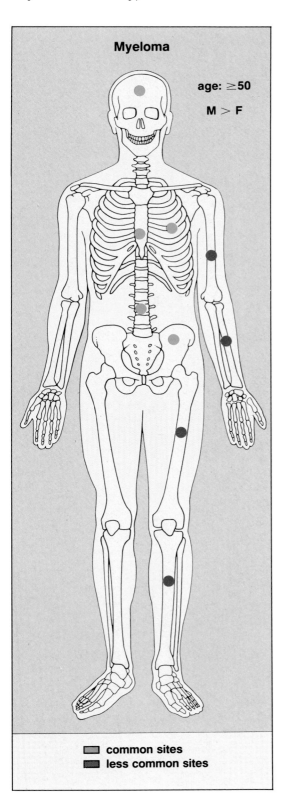

Figure 18.41 Skeletal sites of predilection, peak age range, and male-to-female ratio in myeloma.

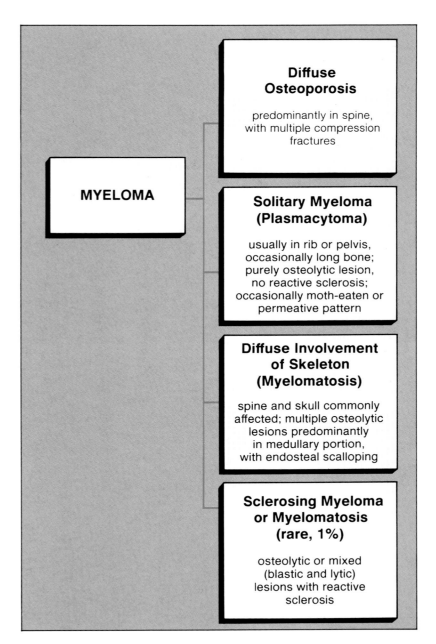

Figure 18.42 Variants in the radiographic presentation of myeloma.

complaint. Because of this, in its early course and before diagnosis, the disease may resemble sciatica or intercostal neuralgia. Rarely, a pathologic fracture through the lesion is the first sign of disease. The patient's urine in cases of myeloma contains Bence-Jones protein; the serum albumin-to-globulin ratio is reversed and the total serum protein is elevated. There is also the presence of monoclonal gamma-globulin with IgG and IgA peaks demonstrated on serum electrophoresis.

Histologically, the diagnosis is made by finding sheets of atypical plasmacytoid cells replacing the normal marrow spaces. The plasma cell is recognized by the presence of eccentrically situated nucleus within a large amount of cytoplasm that stains either light blue or pink. The neoplastic cells contain double or even multiple nuclei, usually hyperchromatic and enlarged, with prominent nucleoli.

Multiple myeloma may present in a variety of radiographic patterns (Fig. 18.42). Particularly in the spine, it may be seen only as diffuse osteoporosis with no clearly identifiable lesion; multiple compression fractures of the vertebral bodies may also be evident. More commonly, it exhibits multiple lytic lesions scattered throughout the skeleton. In the skull, characteristic "punched-out" areas of bone destruction, usually of uniform size, are noted (Fig. 18.43), while the ribs may contain lace-like areas of bone destruction and small osteolytic lesions, sometimes accompanied by adjacent soft tissue masses. Areas of medullary bone destruction are noted in the flat

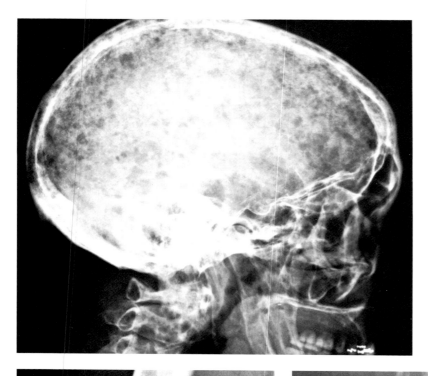

Figure 18.43 Involvement of the skull is prominent in this 60-year-old woman with multiple myeloma. Note the characteristic "punched-out," lytic lesions, most of which are uniform in size and lack sclerotic borders. Occasionally, this pattern may be seen in metastatic disease.

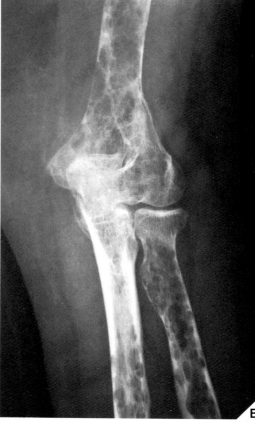

Figure 18.44 Lateral radiograph of the distal femur (A) and anteroposterior view of the elbow (B) in a 65-year-old woman show endosteal scalloping of the cortex typical of diffuse myelomatosis.

and long bones, and if these abut the cortex, they are accompanied by scalloping of the inner cortical margin (Fig. 18.44). Ordinarily, there is no evidence of sclerosis and no periosteal reaction. Fewer than 1% of myelomas may be of a sclerosing type, called sclerosing myelomatosis.

Whereas in osteolytic myeloma only 3% of patients have polyneuropathy, the incidence of polyneuropathy in the osteosclerotic variant has been reported as 30% to 50%. Compared to classic myeloma, this variant usually occurs in younger individuals and shows fewer plasma cells in the bone marrow, lower levels of monoclonal protein, and a better prognosis.

An interesting variant of sclerosing myeloma is the so-called POEMS syndrome, first described in 1968 but gaining wide acceptance only more recently. It consists of polyneuropathy (P), organomegaly (O), particularly of the liver and the spleen, endocrine disturbances (E) such as amenorrhea and gynecomastia, monoclonal gammopathy (M), and skin changes (S) such as hyperpigmentation and hirsutism.

DIFFERENTIAL DIAGNOSIS If the spine is involved, as is frequently the case, multiple myeloma must be differentiated from metastatic carcinoma. In this respect, the "vertebral-pedicle" sign identified by Jacobson and colleagues may be helpful. They contend that in the early stages of myeloma, the pedicle (which does not contain as much red marrow as the vertebral body) is not involved, whereas even in an early stage of metastatic cancer the pedicle and vertebral body are both affected (Fig. 18.45). In the late stages of multiple myeloma, however, both the pedicle and vertebral body may be destroyed. Radionuclide bone scan can more reliably distinguish these two malignancies at this stage. It is invariably positive in cases

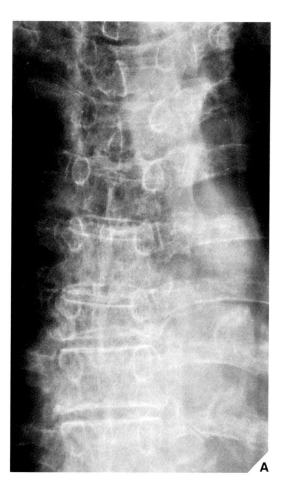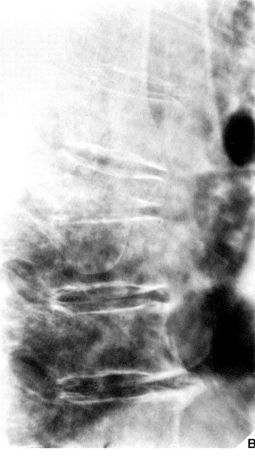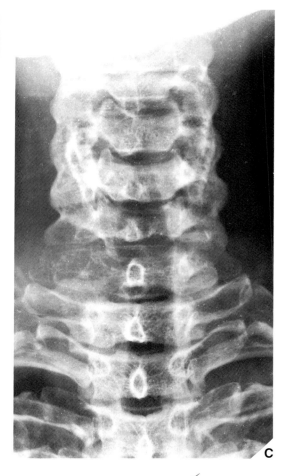

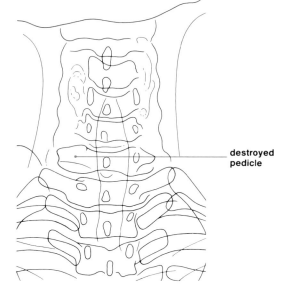

Figure 18.45 Anteroposterior (A) and lateral (B) views of the spine in a 70-year-old man with multiple myeloma involving both the spine and appendicular skeleton show a compression fracture of the body of T-8; several other vertebrae show only osteoporosis. The pedicles are preserved in contrast to metastatic disease of the spine (which usually also affects the pedicles), as seen on this anteroposterior view of the cervical spine (C) in a 65-year-old man with colon carcinoma and multiple lytic metastases. Note the involvement of the right pedicle of C-7.

of metastatic carcinoma, while in most cases of multiple myeloma there is no increased uptake of radiopharmaceutical. This phenomenon appears to reflect the purely lytic nature of most myelomatous lesions and the absence of significant reactive new bone formation in response to the tumor.

A solitary myeloma may create even greater diagnostic difficulty. As a purely osteolytic lesion, it may mimic such other purely destruc-

tive processes as the brown tumor of hyperparathyroidism, giant cell tumor, fibrosarcoma, malignant fibrous histiocytoma, or a solitary metastatic focus of carcinoma from the kidney, thyroid, gastrointestinal tract, or lung.

COMPLICATIONS AND TREATMENT A common complication of bone myelomas is pathologic fracture, especially in lesions of the long

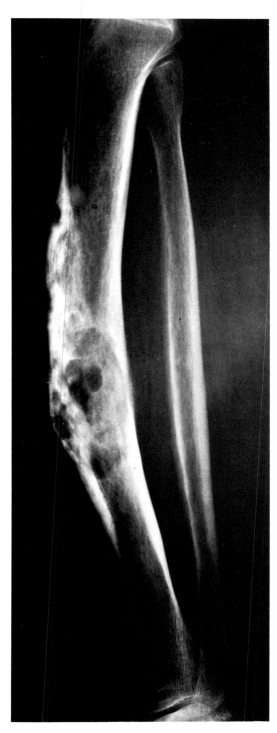

Figure 18.46 Lateral view of the left tibia in a 64-year-old woman shows a lesion in the midshaft, which proved on biopsy to be an adamantinoma. The destructive lesion is multicystic and slightly expansile, with mixed osteolytic and sclerotic areas creating a "soap bubble" appearance resembling that of osteofibrous dysplasia (see Fig. 17.20).

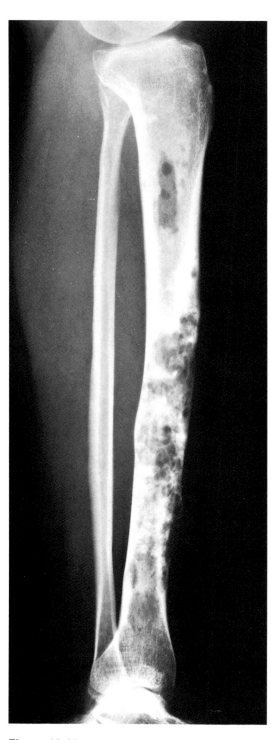

Figure 18.47 Lateral view of the right tibia of a 28-year-old woman shows multiple, confluent lytic lesions of adamantinoma involving almost the entire bone; only the articular ends are spared. The anterior cortex exhibits a predominantly saw-tooth type of destruction.

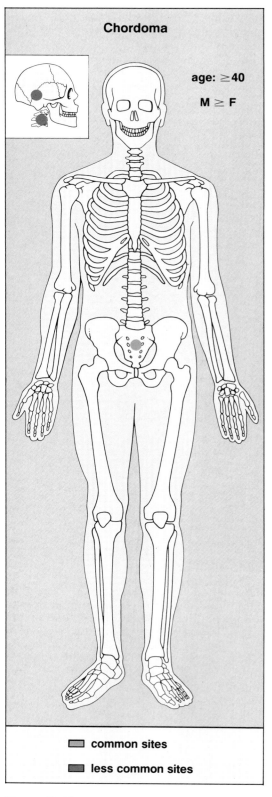

Figure 18.48 Skeletal sites of predilection, peak age range, and male-to-female ratio in chordoma.

bones, ribs, sternum, and vertebrae. The development of amyloidosis has also been reported in approximately 15% of patients.

Treatment consists of radiotherapy and systemic chemotherapy. The five-year survival rate is approximately 10%.

OTHER MALIGNANT BONE TUMORS
Adamantinoma

Adamantinoma is a rare malignant tumor occurring equally in males and females between their second and fifth decades of life; 90% of cases involve the tibia. Radiographically, the disease is marked by well defined and elongated osteolytic defects of varying size, separated by areas of sclerotic bone, which occasionally give the lesion a "soap bubble" appearance; ordinarily there is no periosteal reaction (Fig. 18.46). At times, adamantinoma may affect an entire bone with multiple satellite lesions (Fig. 18.47); "saw-tooth" areas of cortical destruction in the tibia are quite distinctive of this tumor.

Histologically, the tumor is biphasic and consists of an epithelial component intimately admixed in varying proportions with a fibrous component. Although it has been speculated that adamantinoma represents a form of vascular neoplasm, ultrastructural and immunohistochemical evidence points toward an epithelial derivation.

A relationship of adamantinoma with osteofibrous dysplasia and fibrous dysplasia has been postulated, and its coexistence with either

of these lesions has been suggested. However, this is still controversial, with some investigators maintaining that the lesions of adamantinoma may contain a fibro-osseous component that can resemble a Kempson-Campanacci lesion or fibrous dysplasia on histopathologic examination.

TREATMENT Since adamantinoma is insensitive to radiotherapy, the treatment of choice is en bloc surgical resection with application of bone graft. Recurrences have been reported.

Chordoma

A chordoma is a malignant bone tumor arising from developmental remnants of the notochord. Consequently, these tumors occur almost exclusively in the midline of the axial skeleton. Chordomas represent from 1% to 4% of all primary malignant bone tumors. They arise between the patient's fourth and seventh decades and affect men slightly more often than women. The three most common sites for a chordoma are the sacrococcygeal area, the spheno-occipital area, and the C-2 vertebra (Fig. 18.48).

The radiographic appearance is that of a highly destructive lesion with irregular scalloped borders; it is sometimes accompanied by calcifications in the matrix, probably as a result of extensive tumor necrosis (Fig. 18.49). Bone sclerosis has been reported in 64% of cases. Soft tissue masses are commonly associated with the lesion. Conventional radiography, including tomography, usually suffices to

Figure 18.49 This destructive lesion in the sacrum of a 60-year-old woman proved to be a chordoma. Note its scalloped borders and the amorphous calcifications in the tumor matrix.

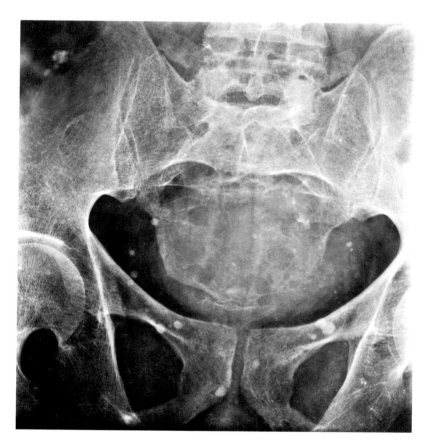

rarely is a metastasis seen distal to the elbows or knees (Fig. 18.56). These lesions result from the hematogenous spread of a malignancy, the usual mechanism by which a primary neoplasm erodes regional blood vessels, seeding malignant cells to the capillary beds of the lung and liver. Tumor emboli become lodged in the axial skeleton through communication with the vertebral venous plexus.

The incidence of metastases to bone varies with the type of primary neoplasm and the duration of disease. Some malignant tumors have a far greater propensity for osseous metastatic involvement than do others. Because of their frequency, cancers of the breast, lung, and prostate are responsible for the majority of bone metastases, although primary tumors of the kidney, small and large intestines, stomach, and thyroid may also metastasize to bone.

Carcinoma of the prostate has been reported to underlie nearly 60% of all bone metastases in men, while in women carcinoma of the breast is responsible for nearly 70% of all metastatic skeletal lesions.

Most skeletal metastases are asymptomatic. In those that are symptomatic, pain is the major clinical symptom, with a pathologic fracture through a lesion only occasionally calling attention to the disease. Metastasis to bone can be solitary or multiple and can be further divided into purely lytic, purely blastic, and mixed lesions. The primary tumors that give rise to purely osteolytic metastases are usually those of the kidney, lung, breast, thyroid, and gastrointestinal tract, although purely lytic lesions may become sclerotic after radiation therapy, chemotherapy, or hormonal therapy. Primary

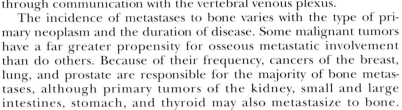

Figure 18.56 Skeletal sites of predilection and peak age range of metastatic lesions. The occurrence of such lesions distal to the elbow and knee is very uncommon, and in those sites a primary malignancy of the breast or lung is usually the origin.

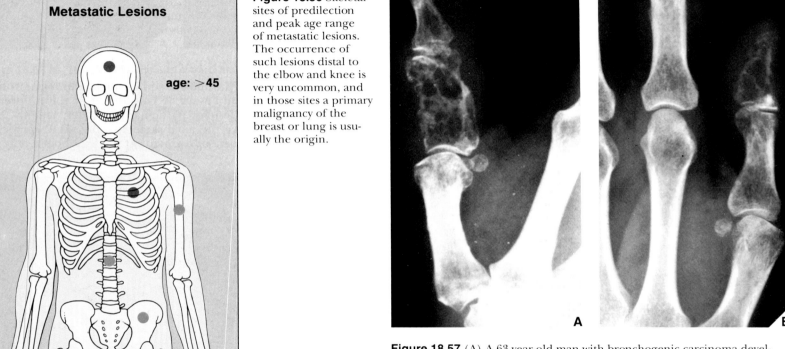

Figure 18.57 (A) A 63-year-old man with bronchogenic carcinoma developed a single metastatic lesion in the proximal phalanx of the left thumb. (B) A 50-year-old woman with breast carcinoma had a solitary metastatic lesion in the distal phalanx of the right thumb.

tumors responsible for purely osteoblastic metastases are generally those of the prostate gland.

The detection of skeletal metastases is not always possible on routine radiography, since destruction of the bone may not be visible with this technique. Radionuclide bone scan is the best means of screening for early metastatic lesions, whether they are lytic or blastic, although recently several investigators have pointed out the usefulness of MRI in detecting metastases, particularly in the spine. The accuracy of MRI in identifying intramedullary lesions and assessing spinal cord and soft tissue involvement has been demonstrated.

In general terms, skeletal metastases may appear highly similar, irrespective of their primary source. However, there are instances in which the morphologic appearance, location, and distribution of metastatic lesions may suggest their site of origin. Thus, for instance, 50% of skeletal metastases distal to the elbows and knees—rare sites for metastases—are secondary to breast or bronchogenic carcinomas (Fig. 18.57). Lesions that have an expanded, "blown-out" appearance on plain films and are highly vascular on arteriography are characteristic of metastatic renal carcinoma (Fig. 18.58). Multiple round dense foci or diffuse bone density is often seen in metastatic carcinoma of the prostate (Fig. 18.59); in females, sclerotic metastases are usually from breast carcinoma.

Recently, characteristic cortical metastases have been described as originating from bronchogenic carcinoma; these metastases cause

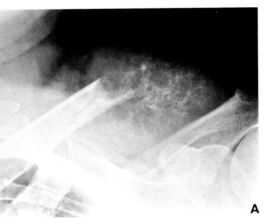

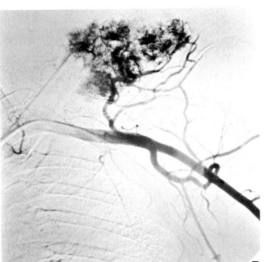

A

B

Figure 18.58
A 52-year-old man with renal cell carcinoma (hypernephroma) developed a solitary metastatic lesion in the acromial end of the left clavicle.
(A) Plain film shows an expanding "blown-out" lesion associated with a soft tissue mass destroying the acromial end of the clavicle. (B) Subtraction study of a selective left subclavian arteriogram demonstrates hypervascularity of the tumor, a characteristic feature of metastatic hypernephroma.

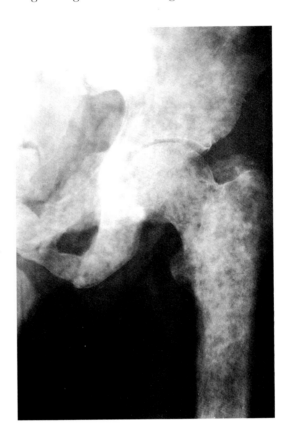

Figure 18.59
Anteroposterior view of the left hemipelvis and femur of a 55-year-old man with carcinoma of the prostate shows extensive blastic skeletal metastases. Multiple sclerotic foci are scattered through the ilium, pubis, ischium, and proximal femur.

what Resnick has called "cookie-bite" or "cookie-cutter" lesions of the cortices of the long bones (Fig. 18.60). Because the bulk of metastases that reach the skeleton via hematogenous spread lodge in the bone marrow and in spongy bone, the initial radiographic appearance of metastatic lesions in the skeleton is that of destruction of cancellous bone; only with further growth do such lesions affect the cortex. The anastomosing vascular systems of the cortex, originating in the overlying periosteum, probably serve as the pathway by which malignant cells from the lung reach the compact bone to produce destruction of the cortex. Occasionally other primary tumors (for example, breast and kidney) may also metastasize to the cortex.

Single metastatic lesions in a bone must be distinguished from primary malignant and benign bone tumors. A few characteristic features of metastatic lesions may be helpful in making the distinction: 1) metastatic lesions usually present without or with only a small adjacent soft tissue mass, and 2) they usually lack a periosteal reaction unless they have broken through the cortex. The latter feature, however, is not invariably reliable, since in some series more than 30% of metastatic lesions—particularly metastases from carcinoma of the prostate—have been accompanied by a periosteal response. Metastatic lesions to the spine usually destroy the pedicle, a useful feature for distinguishing them from myeloma or neurofibroma invading the vertebra (Fig. 18.61).

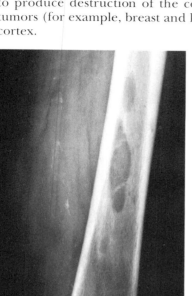
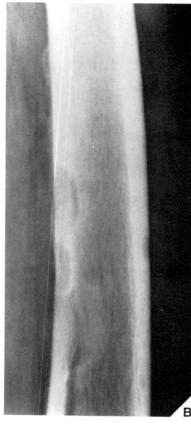

Figure 18.60 Anteroposterior (A) and lateral magnification (B) views of the left femur in an 82-year-old man with progressive femoral pain demonstrate multiple sharply marginated osteolytic areas of bone destruction, predominantly affecting the cortical bone. There is no evidence of periosteal reaction. Note the characteristic "cookie-bite" appearance of the lesion on the lateral radiograph. On the basis of this feature, attention was focused on the chest, where tomographic examination demonstrated bronchogenic carcinoma. (Reproduced with permission from Greenspan A, et al., 1984)

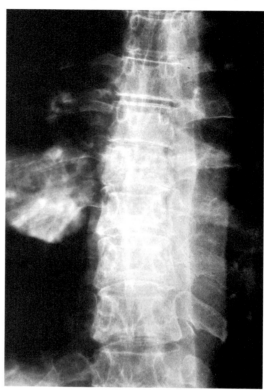

Figure 18.61
Anteroposterior view of the thoracolumbar spine in a 59-year-old woman with bronchogenic carcinoma shows a metastatic lesion in the body of T-7. Note the destroyed left pedicle and associated paraspinal mass, features helpful in distinguishing this lesion from myeloma or neurofibroma. The lung tumor is obvious.

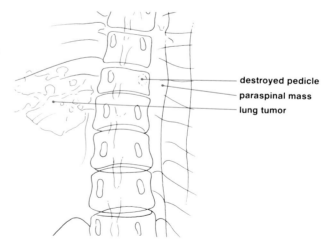

destroyed pedicle
paraspinal mass
lung tumor

Histologically, metastatic tumors are easier to diagnose than many primary tumors because of their essential epithelial pattern. Although biopsies of suspected metastases are useful for diagnosis in patients with unknown primary tumors, these procedures are seldom helpful in specifying an exact site of an unknown primary tumor. Occasionally, if gland formation is present, a specific diagnosis of metastatic adenocarcinoma can be made, but rarely will a specific type of the tumor be detected. On occasion, a metastatic lesion may demonstrate a morphologic pattern that strongly suggests the site of a primary tumor, such as the clear cells of renal carcinoma or the pigment production of melanoma.

COMPLICATIONS Although metastases are themselves complications of a primary malignant process, it must be emphasized that they can cause secondary complications such as pathologic fracture (Fig. 18.62), or, when occurring in the spine, compression of the thecal sac and spinal cord, producing neurologic symptoms (Fig. 18.63).

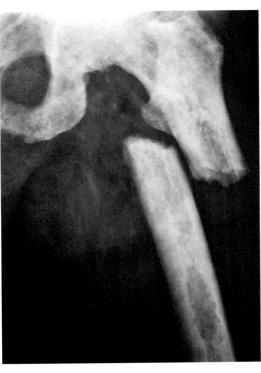

Figure 18.62 Pathologic fracture may complicate metastatic disease of the skeleton, as seen here in the proximal shaft of the left femur in a 74-year-old man with multiple skeletal metastases from a prostatic carcinoma.

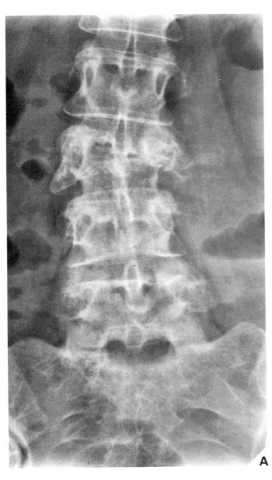

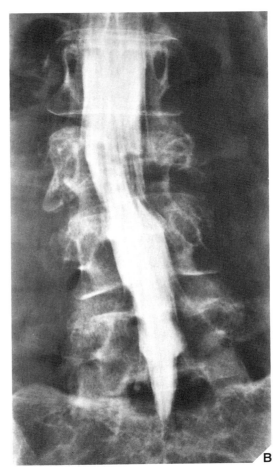

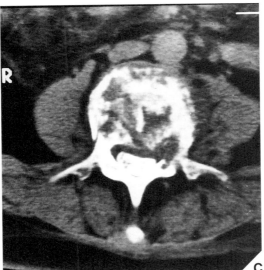

Figure 18.63 (A) Anteroposterior view of the lumbar spine in a 47-year-old woman with breast carcinoma shows destruction of the body of L-3 with a pathologic fracture. Note the involvement of the left pedicle. (B) A myelogram demonstrates compression of the thecal sac. (C) On CT section compression fracture of the vertebral body and involvement of the left pedicle are evident; the tumor extends into the soft tissue and compresses the ventral aspect of the thecal sac.

PRACTICAL POINTS TO REMEMBER

Osteosarcoma

[1] Osteosarcoma has the ability to produce osteoid tissue or bone. Its most characteristic radiographic features are:
- the presence of tumor bone in the lesion—the hallmark of this malignancy
- destruction of the medullary portion of the bone or cortex
- an aggressive periosteal reaction—sunburst, lamellated, or Codman triangle
- the presence of a soft tissue mass.

[2] In the radiologic evaluation of the different types of osteosarcoma—conventional, telangiectatic, multifocal, and juxtacortical:
- plain-film radiography is usually sufficient to identify the radiographic characteristics of each type and make a definitive diagnosis
- CT and MRI are invaluable for defining the extent of the tumor in the bone and soft tissues, and for monitoring the results of presurgical chemotherapy and radiation therapy.

[3] Telangiectatic osteosarcoma, among the most aggressive of osteosarcomas, may present radiographically as a purely osteolytic lesion. It may resemble an aneurysmal bone cyst.

[4] Parosteal osteosarcoma, the least malignant type of osteosarcoma:
- has a predilection for the posterior aspect of the distal femur
- is usually seen attached to the cortex, without invasion of the medullary cavity.

[5] Periosteal osteosarcoma, like parosteal osteosarcoma, is a "surface" lesion. It is, however, more aggressive and contains an excessive amount of cartilaginous tissue. It may resemble periosteal chondrosarcoma and myositis ossificans.

[6] The most common form of secondary osteosarcoma is that complicating Paget disease. It is an extremely aggressive lesion; patients usually do not survive beyond eight months after diagnosis.

Chondrosarcoma

[1] Chondrosarcoma is a malignant bone tumor capable of forming cartilage. Its most characteristic radiographic features are:
- an expansile, destructive lesion in the medullary portion of the bone
- the presence of annular and comma-shaped calcifications within the tumor matrix
- thickening of the cortex and endosteal scalloping
- the presence of a soft tissue mass.

[2] Dedifferentiated chondrosarcoma, the most aggressive type of all cartilage tumors, carries a poor prognosis. In addition to chondrogenic tissue, it can contain elements of fibrosarcoma, malignant fibrous histiocytoma, or osteosarcoma.

[3] Secondary chondrosarcoma usually develops in a pre-existing benign lesion such as an enchondromatosis or multiple cartilaginous exostoses.

Other Malignant Bone Tumors

[1] Fibrosarcoma and malignant fibrous histiocytoma:
- characteristically present as purely osteolytic lesions, frequently in the long bones
- may resemble giant cell tumor, lymphoma, or telangiectatic osteosarcoma
- may develop in certain benign conditions, such as fibrous dysplasia and bone infarct.

[2] Ewing sarcoma, a round cell tumor, usually presents with characteristic radiographic features including:
- a permeative type of bone destruction
- cortical saucerization
- an aggressive periosteal reaction
- a soft tissue mass.

The diaphysis of long bones, and the pelvis, ribs, and scapula are the most common sites of involvement.

[3] In the differential diagnosis of Ewing sarcoma, osteomyelitis and eosinophilic granuloma should always be considered, as well as metastatic neuroblastoma, particularly in patients in their first decade. The most important distinguishing feature is the duration of symptoms. The amount of bone destruction seen radiographically in patients with Ewing sarcoma reporting symptoms for four to six months is usually the same as that:
- in patients with osteomyelitis reporting symptoms for four to six weeks
- and in patients with eosinophilic granuloma reporting symptoms for one to two weeks.

[4] Myeloma, the most common primary malignant bone tumor, has a predilection for the axial skeleton. Four distinctive forms of this lesion can be distinguished radiographically:
- a solitary lesion (plasmacytoma), usually affecting the pelvis or ribs
- diffuse myelomatosis
- diffuse osteoporosis, usually seen in the vertebral column
- sclerosing myeloma, the rarest manifestion of this tumor.

[5] Primary myeloma of the spine can usually be distinguished from radiographically similar metastatic disease by the preservation of the pedicles (vertebral-pedicle sign) in the early stages of the disease.

[6] In myeloma, radionuclide bone scan usually shows no increase in uptake of radiopharmaceutical.

[7] Adamantinoma, a malignant tumor with a strong predilection for the tibia, is characterized radiographically by:
- a "soap bubble" appearance of the lesion due to lytic and sclerotic areas
- a "saw-tooth" appearance of cortical destruction.

[8] Chordoma, which arises from the remnants of the notochord, is located almost exclusively in the midline of the axial skeleton. It tends to arise in the spheno-occipital and sacrococcygeal areas and in the body of C-2.

[9] Benign conditions with malignant potential include medullary bone infarct, the chronic draining sinus tract of osteomyelitis, plexiform neurofibromatosis, Paget disease, normal tissue undergoing radiation, enchondroma, osteochondroma, synovial chondromatosis, and fibrous dysplasia.

Skeletal Metastases

[1] Prostatic carcinoma is the primary tumor most often responsible for blastic metastases to bone. The primary tumors most often responsible for osteolytic skeletal metastases are carcinomas of the kidney, lung, breast, thyroid, and gastrointestinal tract.

[2] Bronchogenic carcinoma frequently produces cortical metastases ("cookie-bite" lesions) and is responsible for metastases in sites distal to the elbow, including lesions of the phalanges.

[3] Carcinoma of the kidney usually produces lytic, "blown-out," hypervascular metastatic lesions.

[4] The best technique for mapping metastatic lesions in the skeleton is radionuclide bone scan.

References

Abrams HL: Skeletal metastases in carcinoma. *Radiology* 55:534, 1950.

Amstutz HC: Multiple osteogenic sarcomata—metastatic or multicentric? *Cancer* 24:923, 1969.

Baker ND, Greenspan A: Pleomorphic liposarcoma of the soft tissue, arising in generalized plexiform neurofibromatosis. *Skeletal Radiol* 7:150, 1981.

Barnes R, Catto M: Chondrosarcoma of bone. *J Bone Joint Surg* 45B:729, 1966.

Bayrd ED, Bennett WA: Amyloidosis complicating myeloma. *Med Clin North Am* 34:1151, 1950.

Beltran J, Chandnani V, McGhee RA Jr, Kursunoglu-Brahme S: Gadopentate dimeglumine-enhanced MR imaging of the musculoskeletal system. *Am J Roentgenol* 156:457, 1991.

Bergsagel DE: Plasma cell myeloma. *Cancer* 30:1588, 1972.

Bitter MA, Komaiko W, Franklin WA: Giant lymphnode hyperplasia with osteoblastic bone lesions and the POEMS (Takatsuki) syndrome. *Cancer* 56:188, 1985.

Boston HC Jr, Dahlin DC, Ivins JC, Cupps RE: Malignant lymphoma (so-called) reticulum cell sarcoma of bone. *Cancer* 34:1131, 1974.

Brown TS, Paterson CR: Osteosclerosis in myeloma. *J Bone Joint Surg* 55B:621, 1973.

Campanacci M, Guernelli N, Leonessa C, Boni A: Chondrosarcoma: A study of 133 cases. *Ital J Orthop Traumatol* 1:387, 1975.

Castellino RA: The non-Hodgkin lymphomas: Practical concepts for the diagnostic radiologist. *Radiology* 178:315, 1991.

Daffner RH, Lupetin AR, Dash N, et al: MRI in the detection of malignant infiltration of bone marrow. *Am J Roentgenol* 146:353, 1986.

Dahlin DC, Coventry MB: Osteogenic sarcoma: A study of six hundred cases. *J Bone Joint Surg* 49A:101, 1967.

Dahlin DC, Ivins JC: Fibrosarcoma of bone: A study of 114 cases. *Cancer* 23:35, 1969.

Dahlin DC, Beabout JW: Dedifferentiation of low-grade chondrosarcomas. *Cancer* 28:461, 1971.

Dahlin DC, Unni KK: Osteosarcoma of bone and its important recognizable varieties. *Am J Surg Pathol* 1:61, 1977.

Dahlin DC, Unni KK, Matsuno T: Malignant (fibrous) histiocytoma of bone—fact or fancy? *Cancer* 39:1508, 1977.

deLange EE, Pope TL Jr, Fechner RE: Dedifferentiated chondrosarcoma: Radiographic features. *Radiology* 160:489, 1986.

Deutsch A, Resnick D: Eccentric cortical metastases to the skeleton from bronchogenic carcinoma. *Radiology* 137:49, 1980.

Dorfman HD, Norman A, Wolff H: Fibrosarcoma complicating bone infarction in a caisson worker. A case report. *J Bone Joint Surg* 48A:528, 1966.

Edeiken J, Raymond AK, Ayala AG, Benjamin RS, Murray JA, Carrasco HC: Small-cell osteosarcoma. *Skeletal Radiol* 16:621, 1987.

Feldman F, Lattes R: Primary malignant fibrous histiocytoma (fibrous xanthoma) of bone. *Skeletal Radiol* 1:145, 1977.

Frassica FJ, Unni KK, Beabout JW, et al: Dedifferentiated chondromsarcoma: A report of the clinico-pathological features and treatments of seventy-eight cases. *J Bone Joint Surg* 68A: 1197, 1986.

Frouge C, Vanel D, Coffre C, Covanet D, Contesso G, Sarrazin D: The role of magnetic resonance imaging in the evaluation of Ewing sarcoma. *Skeletal Radiol* 17:387, 1988.

Glicksman AS, Toker C: Osteogenic sarcoma following radiotherapy for bursitis. *Mt Sinai J Med* 43:163, 1976.

Greenspan A, Klein MJ: Osteosarcoma: Radiologic imaging, differential diagnosis, and pathologic considerations. *Semin Orthop* 6:156, 1991.

Greenspan A, Klein MJ, Lewis MM: Skeletal cortical metastases in the left femur arising from bronchogenic carcinoma. *Skeletal Radiol* 11:297, 1984.

Greenspan A, Klein MJ, Lewis MM: Osteolytic cortical metastasis in the femur from bronchogenic carcinoma. *Skeletal Radiol* 12:146, 1984.

Greenspan A, Norman A, Steiner G: Squamous cell carcinoma arising in chronic draining sinus tract secondary to osteomyelitis of right tibia. *Skeletal Radiol* 6:149, 1981.

Greenspan A, Steiner G, Norman A, Lewis MM, Matlen J: Osteosarcoma of the soft tissues of the distal end of the thigh. *Skeletal Radiol* 16:489, 1987.

Hall FM, Gore SM: Osteosclerotic myeloma variants. *Skeletal Radiol* 17:101, 1988.

Healey JH, Lane JM: Chordoma: A critical review of diagnosis and treatment. *Orthop Clin North Am* 20:417, 1989.

Hermann G, Leviton M, Mendelson D, Norton K, Harris M, Weiner M, Lewis MM: Osteosarcoma: Relation between extent of marrow infiltration on CT and frequency of lung metastases. *Am J Roentgenol* 149:1203, 1987.

Hopper KD, Moser RP, Haseman DB, Sweet DE, Madewell JE, Kransdorf MJ: Osteosarcomatosis. *Radiology* 175:233, 1990.

Huvos AG, Higinbotham NL: Primary fibrosarcoma of bone. A clinicopathologic study of 130 patients. *Cancer* 35:837, 1975.

Jacobson HG, Poppel MH, Shapiro JH, et al: The vertebral pedicle sign. A roentgen finding to differentiate metastatic carcinoma from multiple myeloma. *Am J Roentgenol* 80:817, 1958.

Kim JH, Chu FCH, Pope RA, et al: Radiation induced soft tissue and bone sarcoma. *Radiology* 129:501, 1978.

Klein MJ, Kenan S, Lewis MM: Osteosarcoma. Clinical and pathological considerations. *Orthop Clin North Am* 20:327, 1989.

Krishnamurthy GT, Tubis M, Hiss J, Blahd WM: Distribution pattern of metastatic bone disease. A need for total body skeletal image. *JAMA* 237:2504, 1977.

Kumar R, David R, Cierney G III: Clear cell chondrosarcoma. *Radiology* 154:45, 1985.

Levine E, De Smet AA, Huntrakoon M: Juxtacortical osteosarcoma: A radiologic and histologic spectrum. *Skeletal Radiol* 14:38, 1985.

Lewis MM: Current concept: The expandable prosthesis. *Bull Hosp Jt Dis Orthop Inst* 45:29, 1985.

Lichtenstein L, Jaffe HL: Ewing's sarcoma of bone. *Am J Pathol* 23:43, 1947.

Lindell MM Jr, Shirkhoda A, Raymond AK, Murray JA, Harle TS: Parosteal osteosarcoma: Radiologic-pathologic correlation with emphasis on CT. *Am J Roentgenol* 148:323, 1987.

Malcolm AJ: Osteosarcoma: Classification, pathology, and differential diagnosis. *Semin Orthop* 3:1, 1988.

Markel SF: Ossifying fibroma of long bone. Its distinction from fibrous dysplasia and its association with adamantinoma of long bone. *Am J Clin Pathol* 69:91, 1978.

Matsuno T, Unni KK, McLeod RA, Dahlin DC: Telangiectatic osteogenic sarcoma. *Cancer* 38:2538, 1976.

McKenna RJ, Schwinn CP, Soong KY, Higinbotham NL: Osteogenic sarcoma arising in Paget's disease. *Cancer* 17:42, 1964.

Mirra JM, Gold RH, Marafiote R: Malignant (fibrous) histiocytoma arising in association with a bone infarct in sickle-cell disease: Coincidence or cause-and-effect? *Cancer* 39:186, 1977.

Mulvey RB: Peripheral bone metastases. *Am J Roentgenol* 91:155, 1964.

Norman A, Ulin R: A comparative study of periosteal new-bone response in metastatic bone tumors (solitary) and primary bone sarcomas. *Radiology* 92:705, 1969.

Pan G, Raymond AK, Carrasco CH, et al: Osteosarcoma: MR imaging after preoperative chemotherapy. *Radiology* 174:517, 1990.

Pear BL: Skeletal manifestations of the lymphomas and leukemias. *Semin Roentgenol* 9:229, 1974.

Reiter FB, Ackerman LV, Staple TW: Central chondrosarcoma of the appendicular skeleton. *Radiology* 105:525, 1972.

Schajowicz F: Ewing's sarcoma and reticulum cell sarcoma of bone: With special reference to the histochemical demonstration of glycogen as an aid to differential diagnosis. *J Bone Joint Surg* 41A:394, 1959.

Schreiman JS, Crass JR, Wick MR, Maile CW, Thompson RC Jr: Osteosarcoma: Role of CT in limb-sparing treatment. *Radiology* 161:485, 1986.

Sim FH, Unni KK, Beabout JW, et al: Osteosarcoma with small cells simulating Ewing's tumor. *J Bone Joint Surg* 61A:207, 1979.

Smith J, Ludwig RL, Marcove RC: Sacrococcygeal chordoma. A clinicoradiological study of 60 patients. *Skeletal Radiol* 16:37, 1987.

Sundaram M, McGuire MH, Herbold DR: Magnetic resonance imaging of osteosarcoma. *Skeletal Radiol* 16:23, 1987.

Tanaka O, Ohsawa T: The POEMS syndrome: Report of three cases with radiographic abnormalities. *Radiology* 24:472, 1984.

Thrall JH, Ellis BI: Skeletal metastases. *Radiol Clin North Am* 25:1155, 1987.

Triche TJ, Cavazzana A: Round cell tumors of bone. In: Unni KK (ed). *Bone Tumors*. New York, Churchill Livingstone, 1988, pp 199–223.

Unni KK: Osteosarcoma of bone. In: Unni KK (ed): *Bone Tumors*. New York, Churchill Livingstone, 1988, p. 107.

Unni KK, Dahlin DC, Beabout JW, Ivins JC: Parosteal osteogenic sarcoma. *Cancer* 37:2466, 1976.

Unni KK, Dahlin DC, Beabout JW: Periosteal osteogenic sarcoma. *Cancer* 37:2476, 1976.

Unni KK, Dahlin DC, Beabout JW, Sim JH: Chondrosarcoma: Clear-cell variant: A report of sixteen cases. *J Bone Joint Surg* 58A:676, 1976.

Van Der Heul RO, Von Ronnen JR: Juxtacortical osteosarcoma: Diagnosis, differential diagnosis, treatment, and an analysis of eighty cases. *J Bone Joint Surg* 49A:415, 1967.

Wetzel LH, Levine E, Murphey MD: A comparison of MR imaging and CT in the evaluation of musculoskeletal masses. *RadioGraphics* 7:851, 1987.

Wold LE, Unni KK, Beabout JW, Pritchard DJ: High-grade surface osteosarcoma. *Am J Surg Pathol* 8:181, 1984.

Wold LE, Unni KK, Beabout JW, Sim FH, Dahlin DC: Dedifferentiated parosteal osteosarcoma. *J Bone Joint Surg* 66A:53, 1984.

PART V

Infections

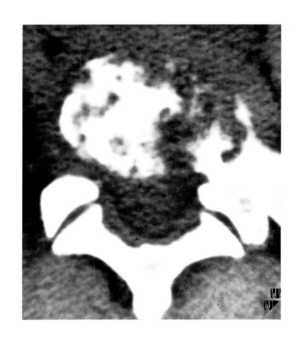

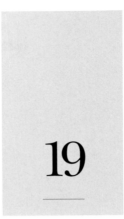

19

Radiologic Evaluation of Musculoskeletal Infections

MUSCULOSKELETAL INFECTIONS

INFECTIONS OF THE MUSCULOSKELETAL system can be subdivided into three categories: 1) those involving bones (osteomyelitis); 2) those involving joints (infectious arthritis); and 3) those involving soft tissues (cellulitis). Because of the complexity of the vertebrae and their soft tissue structures, infectious processes of the spine are considered under a separate heading.

Osteomyelitis

Three basic mechanisms allow an infectious organism—whether bacterium, virus, mycoplasma, rickettsia, or fungus—to reach the bone: 1) *hematogenous spread* via the bloodstream from a remote site of infection, such as the skin, tonsils, gallbladder, or urinary tract; 2) spread from a *contiguous source* of infection, as from the soft tissues, teeth, or sinuses; and 3) *direct implantation*, such as through a puncture or missile wound or an operative procedure (Fig. 19.1).

Figure 19.1 Infectious agents may gain entry to a bone through hematogenous spread, a source of infection in the contiguous soft tissues, or through direct implantation secondary to trauma or surgery.

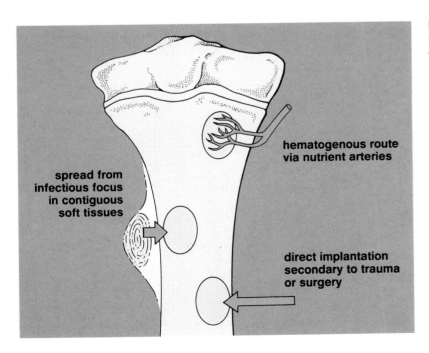

Hematogenous spread is common in children, and the usual focus of infection develops in the metaphysis. The metaphyseal location of infection in children is related to an osseous-vascular anatomy that differs in the infant, child, and adult (Fig. 19.2). In the child (ages 1 to 16 years), there is separation of the blood supply to the metaphysis and epiphysis, each having its own source. Moreover, the arteries and capillaries of the metaphysis turn sharply without penetrating the open growth plate, and in the region where capillaries become venules the rate of blood flow is sluggish. Also contributing to the greater incidence of metaphyseal osteomyelitis in children is secondary thrombosis of end-arteries with bacteria during transient bacteremia. In the infant (up to 1 year), on the other hand, osteomyelitis may sometimes have its focus in the epiphysis, since some metaphyseal vessels may penetrate the growth plate and reach the epiphysis (see Fig. 19.2). With obliteration of the growth plate in the adult (above 16 years), there is vascular continuity between the shaft and the articular ends of the bone; hence, the focus of osteomyelitis can develop in any part of a bone.

Contiguous spread and direct implantation are more common in adults. The sites of bone infection via either of these routes are directly related to the focus of soft tissue infection or the location of the wound.

Infectious Arthritis

An infectious agent may enter the joint by the same basic routes as in osteomyelitis: by direct invasion of the synovial membrane, either secondary to a penetrating wound or following a joint-replacement procedure; from an infection of the adjacent soft tissues; or indirectly via a blood-borne infection. Infectious arthritis may also occur secondary to a focus of osteomyelitis in the adjacent bone (Fig. 19.3).

Cellulitis

Soft tissue infections most commonly result from a break in the skin leading to direct introduction of an infectious agent. Some patients, such as those with diabetes, are particularly prone to cellulitis due to a combination of factors, including skin breakdown and local ischemia.

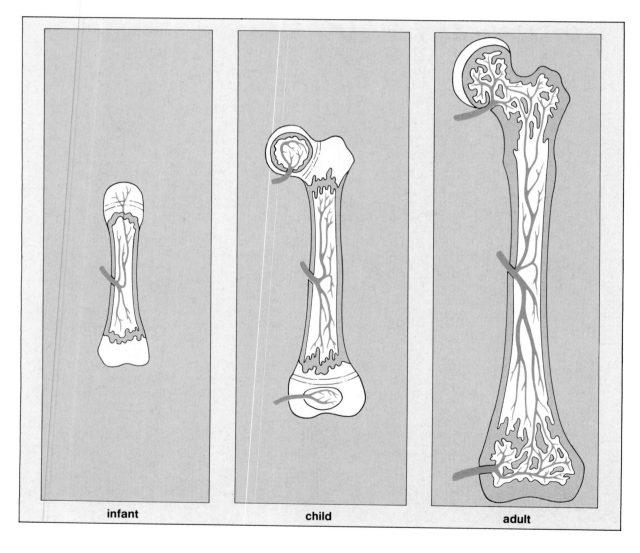

infant   child   adult

Figure 19.2 The vascular anatomy of a long bone differs in an infant, a child, and an adult. These differences account for the various locations of infection in each age group. In an infant, nutrient, transphyseal, and foveal arteries are abundant. In a child, the physis becomes avascular when the foveal and transphyseal arteries recede. After the growth plate closes, the foveal arteries and periarticular arteries again become prominent.

Infections of the Spine

Infections in the spine may be located in a vertebral body, an intervertebral disk, the paravertebral soft tissues, or the epidural compartment; very rarely an infection may involve the contents of the spinal canal or the spinal cord. The mechanisms of infection are the same as those of osteomyelitis and infectious arthritis. An intervertebral disk infection, for example, may result from a puncture of the canal or of the disk itself during a procedure, as well as from a penetrating injury; it can also spread from a contiguous source of infection such as a paraspinal abscess. Most common, however, is hematogenous spread following surgical procedures such as laminectomy or spinal fusion, or during generalized bacteremia or sepsis (Fig. 19.4). Regardless of the primary location of the infectious process, *Staphylococcus aureus* is responsible for over 90% of all infections of the spine.

RADIOLOGIC EVALUATION OF INFECTIONS

The radiologic modalities used to evaluate infections of the musculoskeletal system include:

1. Plain-film radiography (including magnification studies)
2. Conventional tomography
3. Computed tomography (CT)
4. Arthrography
5. Myelography and diskography
6. Fistulography (sinogram)
7. Arteriography
8. Radionuclide imaging (scintigraphy, bone scan)
9. Magnetic resonance imaging (MRI)
10. Percutaneous aspiration and biopsy (fluoroscopy- or CT-guided)

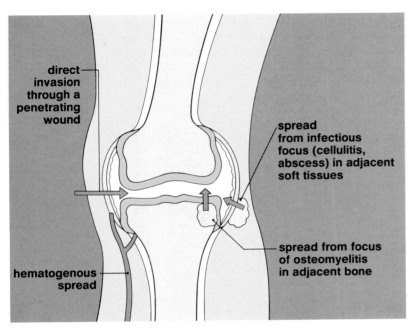

Figure 19.3 The routes of infection in infectious arthritis are similar to those of osteomyelitis, which itself may be a source of spread.

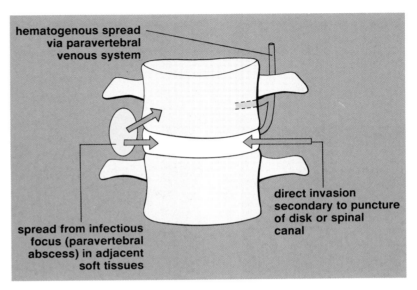

Figure 19.4 The potential routes of infection of a vertebra or an intervertebral disk are direct invasion, hematogenous spread, and extension from a focus of infection in the adjacent soft tissues.

In most instances, plain-film radiography is sufficient to demonstrate the pertinent features of a bone or joint infection (Fig. 19.5; see also Figs. 4.43, 4.44A). Magnification radiography is helpful in delineating subtle changes representing cortical destruction or periosteal new bone formation (Fig. 19.6) and is occasionally required for differentiating osteoporosis from the early stages of infection, which may appear radiographically similar. Conventional tomography using multidirectional motion (trispiral tomography) is particularly effective in demonstrating sequestra or subtle sinus tracts in the bone (Fig. 19.7; see also Fig. 4.44B). CT plays a determining role in demonstrating the extent of infection in bones and soft tissues, and at times may be very helpful in making a specific diagnosis (Fig. 19.8).

Arthrography has rather limited application in the diagnosis of joint infections (see Fig. 20.16B). Scintigraphy, on the other hand, has a much more prominent role. In suspected osteomyelitis, radionuclide bone scan using technetium-99m-labeled phosphonates is routinely used, since there is an accumulation of tracer in the infected areas. A three-phase technique is particularly useful for distinguishing infected joint tissues from infected periarticular soft tissues if the plain films are not diagnostic (Fig. 19.9).

However, once the bone sustains an injury such as surgery, fracture, or neuropathic osteoarthropathy that causes increased bone turnover, the routine scintigraphy with technetium-labeled phosphonates becomes less specific for infection. On the other hand, radionuclide studies using gallium (a ferric analogue) and indium are more specific in these instances. There is still no general agreement on the exact mechanism of gallium localization in infected tissues. After intravenous injections of gallium, more than 99% is bound to various plasma proteins, including transferrin, haptoglobin, lactoferrin, albumin, and ferritin. At least five mechanisms of gallium transfer from the plasma into inflammatory exudates and cells have been suggested. These include direct leukocyte uptake, direct bacteria uptake, the protein-bound tissue uptake, increased vascularity, and increased bone turnover. Since gallium binds to the iron-binding molecule transferrin, the mechanism of gallium uptake in infectious processes is best explained by hyperemia and elevated permeability that increase delivery of the protein-bound tracer transferrin into the area of inflammation. Cells associated with the inflammatory response, particularly polymorphonuclear white cells in which lactoferrin is carried within intracytoplasmic granules, deposit iron-binding proteins extracellularly at the site of inflammation, serving to combat the infection by sequestering needed iron from bacteria. Lactoferrin, which has a high binding affinity for iron, takes the gallium away from the transferrin.

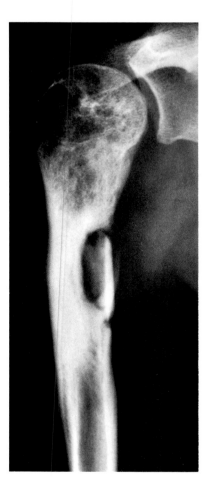

Figure 19.5 Anteroposterior view of the right humerus demonstrates the classic features of chronic active osteomyelitis. There is destruction of the medullary portion of the bone, reactive sclerosis, and periosteal new bone formation. Note also a large sequestrum on the medial aspect of the humerus, the hallmark of an active infectious process.

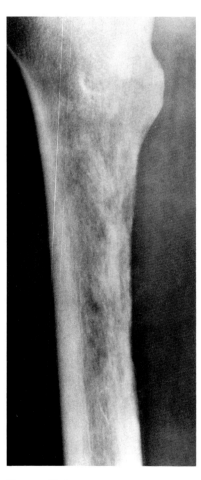

Figure 19.6 Magnification study of the right femur demonstrates subtle changes representative of cortical destruction and formation of periosteal new bone in an early stage of osteomyelitis. These findings were not well delineated on the standard radiographs.

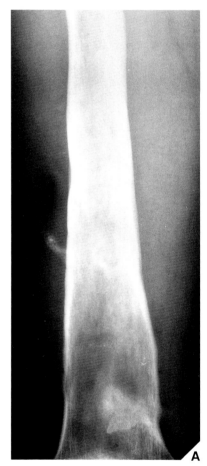

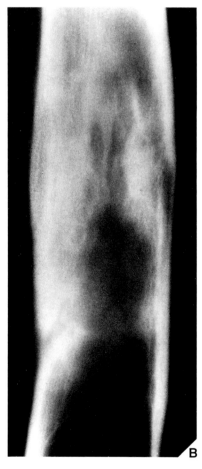

Figure 19.7 (A) Plain film of the left femur shows thickening of the cortex, reactive sclerosis, and foci of destruction in the medullary cavity. Faint calcifications in the soft tissue suggest the presence of a fistula. (B) Conventional tomogram enhanced by magnification clearly demonstrates a sequestrum and a sinus tract in the cortex, the characteristic features of active osteomyelitis.

Gallium can also be used to assess the patient's response to therapy. Particularly in osteomyelitis, gallium concentrations enhance the specificity of an abnormal bone scan, and decreased gallium uptake closely follows a good response to therapy.

The other tracer used in infections is indium. Since indium-labeled white blood cells are usually not incorporated into areas of increased bone turnover, scintigraphy with indium-111 oxine-labeled leukocytes is used as a sensitive and specific test in the general diagnosis of infection

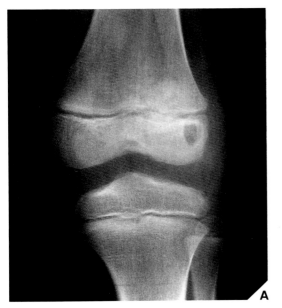

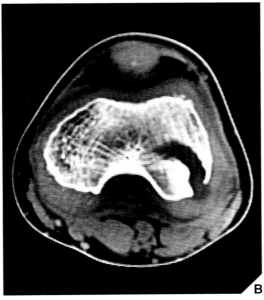

Figure 19.8 A 7-year-old boy had intermittent pain in the left knee for three weeks; the pain was worse at night and was promptly relieved by salicylates. (A) Initial anteroposterior radiograph of the left knee demonstrates a radiolucent lesion with a well defined, partly sclerotic border in the lateral portion of the distal femoral epiphysis. Osteoid osteoma and chondroblastoma were considered in the differential diagnosis. (B) CT examination, however, reveals cortical disruption at the posterolateral aspect of the lateral femoral condyle, a finding not seen on the standard radiographs. The serpentine configuration of the radiolucent tract and its extension into the cartilage prompted a diagnosis of epiphyseal bone abscess, which was confirmed on bone biopsy.

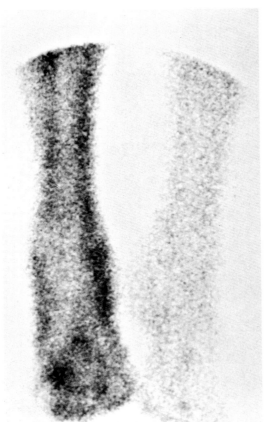

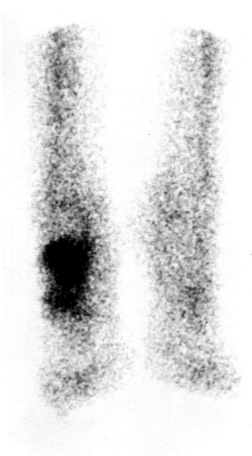

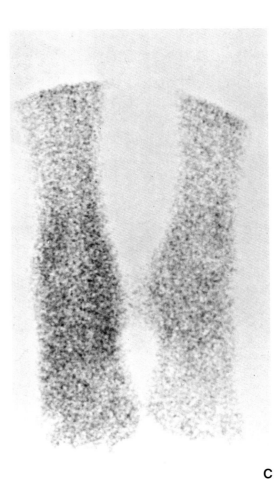

A   B   C

Figure 19.9 A 52-year-old woman with pain in her right ankle had cellulitis around the ankle joint. Although plain radiographs did not reveal changes in the joint suggestive of infectious arthritis, this possibility could not be ruled out clinically since early changes of infection may not be detected on standard radiographs. A three-phase radionuclide bone scan was performed. (A) In the first phase, one minute after intravenous injection of a 15 mCi (555 MBq) bolus of technetium-99m-labeled methylene diphosphonate, there is increased activity in the major vessels of the right leg. (B) In the second phase, three minutes after injection, a blood pool scan demonstrates increased uptake in the area of the infected soft tissues. (C) In the third phase, two hours after injection, almost complete washout of the radiopharmaceutical, with no evidence of localization in the bones on both sides of the joint, excludes the diagnosis of infectious arthritis. (Courtesy of Dr. R Goldfarb, New York, NY)

of the musculoskeletal system, and in specific instances when infection complicates previous fracture or surgery. Like other imaging procedures in nuclear medicine, this test monitors the internal distribution of a tracer agent to provide diagnostic information. The inherent ability of white blood cells to localize at sites of inflammation makes their use in this test particularly effective in the diagnosis of infections. Merkel reported the sensitivity of indium scintigraphy in detecting infections to be 83%, with a specificity of 94% and an accuracy of 88%.

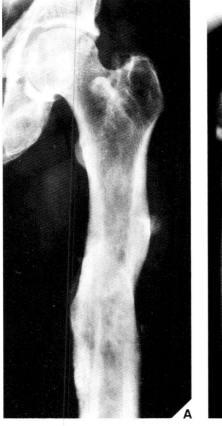
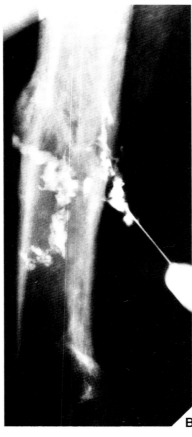

A   B

Figure 19.10 A 48-year-old man who had sustained a fracture of the femur was treated with open reduction and internal fixation using an intramedullary rod. He developed chronic osteomyelitis postoperatively. The rod was removed and the infection was treated with antibiotics. He subsequently developed a draining sinus. (A) Plain film of the left femur demonstrates changes typical of chronic osteomyelitis. There is focal destruction of the medullary portion of the bone, reactive sclerosis, and a periosteal reaction. (B) A sinogram performed to evaluate the extent of the draining fistula demonstrates a sinus tract with multiple ramifications.

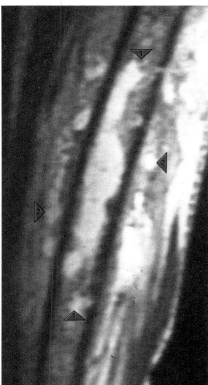

Figure 19.11 Sagittal T2-weighted MR image (SE, TR 2000/TE 80) shows a well defined area of increased signal intensity in the medullary space of the midshaft of the femur indicating acute hematogenous osteomyelitis in this intravenous drug user. There are soft tissue inflammatory changes with multiple small abscesses adjacent to the femur. (From Beltran J, 1990)

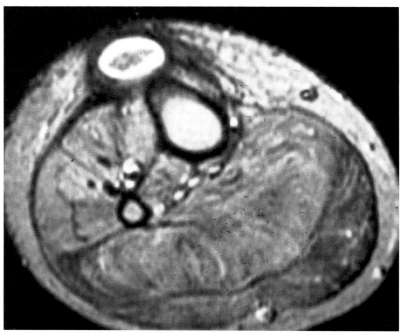

Figure 19.12 Axial T2-weighted MR image (SE, TR 2000/TE 80) shows a high signal intensity of soft tissue fluid collection anterior to the tibia, with a focus of lower signal intensity in the center, representing the soft tissue abscess. The abscess is surrounded by a thick, low signal intensity capsule. Note the high signal intensity edema involving diffusely the subcutaneous fat and muscles. (From Beltran J, 1990)

Indium-111-labeled leukocyte scintigraphy has also been reported to be highly specific and sensitive in the detection of soft tissue abscesses. The study is limited, however, by poor spatial resolution. It may be difficult to differentiate between bone and soft tissue activity when the two are close together. In these instances the study may be enhanced by sequential use of technetium-99m-labeled phosphonates and indium.

Arteriography is important in the evaluation of the patient's vascular supply, particularly if a reconstructive procedure is planned. Myelography is still useful in evaluating infections within the spinal canal, as well as in vertebral osteomyelitis and disk infection (see Fig. 20.29). Fistulography (sinogram) is an important examination for outlining sinus tracts in the soft tissues and evaluating their extension into the bone (Fig. 19.10).

Recently MRI established its place in the evaluation of bone and soft tissue infections. As several studies have indicated, osteomyelitis, soft tissue abscesses, joint and tendon sheath effusions, and various forms of cellulitis are well depicted by this modality. MRI is as sensitive as technetium-99m methylene diphosphonate (MDP) in demonstrating osteomyelitis and more sensitive and more specific than other scintigraphic techniques in demonstrating soft tissue infections, primarily because of its superior spatial resolution. The proper evaluation of musculoskeletal infections with MRI requires both T1- and T2-weighted images in at least two imaging planes. In anatomically complex areas such as the pelvis, spine, foot and hand, three planes may be necessary. Diagnostic criteria for MRI in diagnosing osteomyelitis are findings of decreased signal intensity in the bone marrow cavity on short spin echo TR/TE sequences (T1-weighting) along with increased signal intensity in the bone marrow cavity on long TR/TE sequences (T2-weighting) (Fig. 19.11). Increased signal intensity of the soft tissues on long TR/TE sequences with poorly defined margins is considered indicative of edema and/or nonspecific inflammatory changes. Well demarcated collections of decreased signal intensity on T1-weighted sequences and increased signal intensity surrounded by zones of decreased signal intensity on T2-weighted images are considered indicative of soft tissue abscesses (Fig. 19.12). Decreased signal intensity on short TR/TE sequences and increased signal intensity on long TR/TE sequences in the area of the joint capsule or tendon sheath are consistent with synovial effusions and fluid in the tendon sheath.

Percutaneous aspiration and CT- or fluoroscopy-guided biopsy of a suspected focus of infection may be done in the radiology suite; it can rapidly confirm a suspected diagnosis of infection as well as reveal the causative organism.

MONITORING THE TREATMENT AND COMPLICATIONS OF INFECTIONS

Radiology plays an indispensable role in monitoring the treatment of infectious disorders of bone and associated soft tissues (Fig. 19.13). Follow-up radiographs and radionuclide bone scans should be obtained at regular intervals to evaluate the disease state (acute, sub-

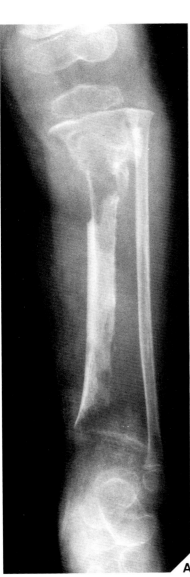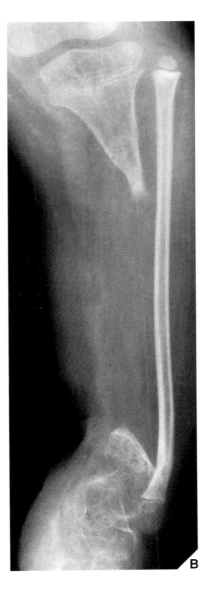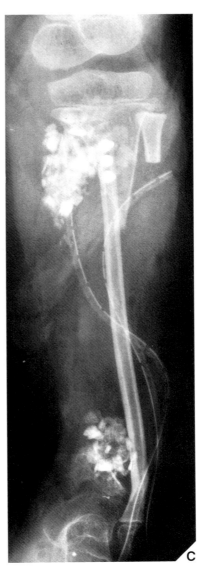

Figure 19.13 A 3-year-old girl developed osteomyelitis of the left tibia following chronic tonsillitis.
(A) Anteroposterior view of the left leg shows extensive destruction of the tibia with sequestration of the diaphysis. Extensive and longstanding conservative treatment using broad-spectrum antibiotics failed to produce any improvement. (B) One year later, the dead sequestered segment of the tibial diaphysis was resected as a first stage in reconstruction of the limb. (C) Two months later, a fibular graft was attached to the proximal stump of the tibial diaphysis, and bone chips were applied proximally and distally to assure bony union and stability.

acute, chronic, or inactive) (Fig. 19.14) and any complications that may arise (Fig. 19.15). The differentiation of active from inactive osteomyelitis may, however, be extremely difficult by radiologic techniques. The extensive osteosclerotic changes in inactive infection may obscure small foci of osteolytic change signifying reactivation. Tomography may at times be helpful in delineating fluffy periostitis, poorly marginated areas of osteolysis, or sequestra.

The main complication of osteomyelitis in infants and children is growth disturbance if the focus of infection is in the vicinity of the growth plate (Fig. 19.16). Pathologic fracture is another frequent complication of osteomyelitis (Fig. 19.17). In adults, the most serious complication is the development of a malignant neoplasm in a chronically draining sinus tract (see Fig. 18.52).

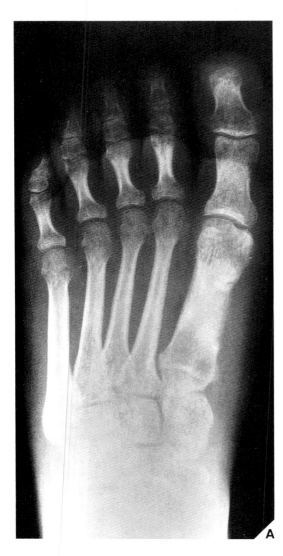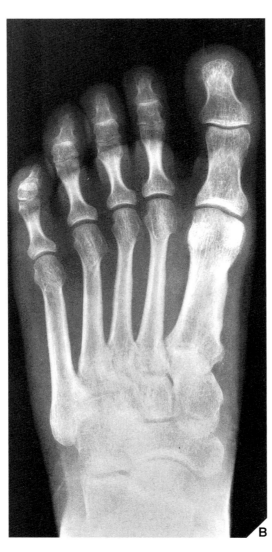

Figure 19.14 A 17-year-old girl developed an acute pyogenic infection of the first metatarsal bone after a puncture injury of her right foot. (A) Anteroposterior projection demonstrates changes typical of active osteomyelitis: cortical and medullary bone destruction, a periosteal reaction, and diffuse soft tissue swelling. Note also the significant periarticular osteoporosis. After extensive treatment with antibiotics, a plain film of the foot (B) shows complete healing of the infection, which is in an inactive phase. There is residual endosteal sclerosis, but no destructive changes are evident and the soft tissue planes are normal.

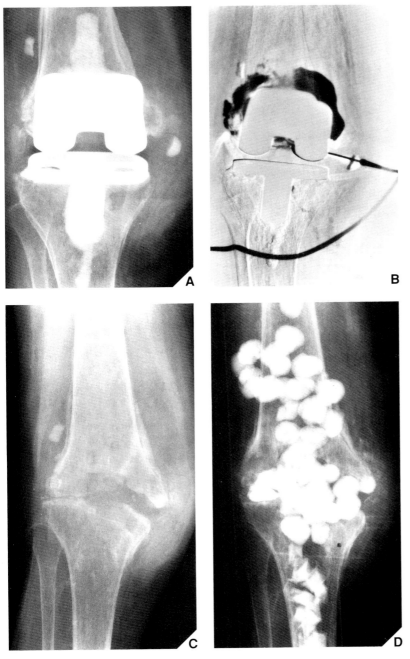

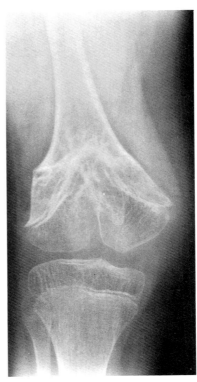

Figure 19.16 Anteroposterior view of the right knee of an 8-year-old girl shows a growth disturbance as a sequela of metaphyseal osteomyelitis. Note the hypoplasia of the femur secondary to disuse of the limb and the deformity of the distal epiphysis. The cone-shaped growth plate shows almost complete fusion.

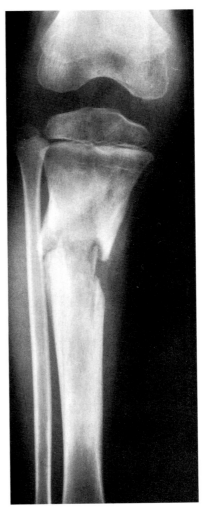

Figure 19.17 Plain film of the lower leg of a 6-year-old boy with chronic active osteomyelitis shows a pathologic fracture, a complication of the infectious process.

Figure 19.15 A 62-year-old woman developed an infection of the right knee joint following total knee arthroplasty. (A) Anteroposterior film shows the joint replacement with a condylar-type prosthesis. Active infection is still evident, as demonstrated by the soft tissue swelling, joint effusion, and periosteal reaction. Small foci of bone destruction are seen in the proximal tibia. (B) An aspiration arthrogram (subtraction study) demonstrates abnormal extension of contrast medium into osteolytic areas of the tibia. The irregular outline on the lateral aspect of the joint is due to synovitis. Bacteriologic examination of the aspirated material yielded *Staphylococcus aureus*. (C) After unsuccessful treatment of the infection with broad-spectrum antibiotics, the prosthesis had to be removed. Note the typical appearance of active osteomyelitis. (D) The treatment at this stage consisted of methylmethacrylate cement balls soaked with antibiotics and applied to the infected joint and medullary cavity of the femur and tibia.

PRACTICAL POINTS TO REMEMBER

[1] Three basic mechanisms allow an infectious organism to reach a bone or joint:
- hematogenous spread
- spread from a contiguous source
- direct implantation.

[2] The metaphysis is the most common site of an infectious focus in children, primarily due to the nature of the osseous-vascular anatomy at this stage of development, while the shaft of a long bone is a common site of infection in adult patients.

[3] Radionuclide bone scan using technetium-99m-labeled phosphonates is a very useful radiologic modality for distinguishing a joint infection from cellulitis of the periarticular soft tissues.

[4] The radiopharmaceuticals most specific for detection of musculoskeletal infection are gallium-67 citrate and indium-111 oxine.

[5] Magnetic resonance imaging is more specific and more sensitive than scintigraphic techniques in demonstrating bone and soft tissue infections primarily because of its superior spatial resolution. Both T1- and T2-weighted sequences in at least two imaging planes should be obtained.

[6] Percutaneous aspiration biopsy of a suspected focus of infection is the most direct route for confirming a diagnosis, as well as identifying the causative organism.

References

Al-Sheikh W, Sfakianakis GN, Mnaymneh W, et al: Subacute and chronic bone infections: Diagnosis using In-111, Ga-67 and Tc-99m MDP bone scintigraphy, and radiography. *Radiology* 155:501, 1985.

Bassett LW, Gold RH, Webber MM: Radionuclide bone imaging. *Radiol Clin North Am* 19: 675, 1981.

Beltran J: *MRI: Musculoskeletal System.* Philadelphia, Lippincott, 1990.

Beltran J, Noto AM, McGhee RB, Freedy RM, McCalla MS: Infections of the musculoskeletal system: High field-strength MR imaging. *Radiology* 164:449, 1987.

Butt WP: The radiology of infection. *Clin Orthop* 96:20, 1973.

Capitanio MA, Kirkpatrick JA: Early roentgen observations in acute osteomyelitis. *Am J Roentgenol* 108:488, 1970.

Hoffer P: Gallium: Mechanisms. *J Nucl Med* 21:282, 1980.

Israel O, Gips S, Jerushalmi J, Frenkel A, Front D: Osteomyelitis and soft-tissue infection: Differential diagnosis with 24 hour/4 hour ratios of Tc-99m MDP uptake. *Radiology* 163:724, 1987.

Lewin JS, Rosenfield NS, Hoffer PB, Downing D: Acute osteomyelitis in children: Combined Tc-99m and Ga-67 imaging. *Radiology* 158:795, 1986.

Lisbona R, Rosenthal L: Observations on the sequential use of 99m Tc-phosphate complex and 67 Ga in osteomyelitis, cellulitis and septic arthritis. *Radiology* 123:123, 1977.

Mason MD, Zlatkin MB, Esterhai JL, Dalinka MK, Velchik MG, Kressel HY: Chronic complicated osteomyelitis of the lower extremity: Evaluation with MR imaging. *Radiology* 173:355, 1989.

Merkel KD, Brown ML, Dewanjee MK, Fitzgerald RH Jr: Comparison of indium-labeled-leukocyte imaging with sequential technetium-gallium scanning in the diagnosis of low-grade musculoskeletal sepsis. A prospective study. *J Bone Joint Surg* 67A:465, 1985.

Modic MT, Pflanze W, Feiglin DHI, Belhobek G: Magnetic resonance imaging of musculoskeletal infections. *Radiol Clin North Am* 24:247, 1986.

Schauwecker DS: Osteomyelitis: diagnosis with In-111-labeled leukocytes. *Radiology* 171:141, 1989.

Tang JSH, Gold RH, Bassett LW, Seeger LL: Musculoskeletal infection of the extremities: Evaluation with MR imaging. *Radiology* 166:205, 1988.

Tsan M: Mechanism of gallium-67 accumulation in inflammatory lesions. *J Nucl Med* 26:88, 1985.

Tumeh SS, Aliabadi PA, Weissmann BN, McNeil BJ: Chronic osteomyelitis: Bone and gallium scan patterns associated with active disease. *Radiology* 158:685, 1986.

Wukich DK, Abreu SH, Callaghan JJ, et al: Diagnosis of infection by preoperative scintigraphy with indium-labeled white blood cells. *J Bone Joint Surg* 69A:1353, 1987.

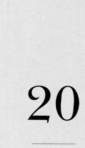

20

Osteomyelitis, Infectious Arthritis, and Soft Tissue Infections

OSTEOMYELITIS

OSTEOMYELITIS CAN GENERALLY be divided into pyogenic and nonpyogenic types. The former may be further classified, on the basis of clinical findings, as subacute, acute, or chronic (active and inactive), depending on the intensity of the infectious process and its associated symptoms. From the viewpoint of anatomic pathology, osteomyelitis can be divided into diffuse and localized (focal) forms, with the latter referred to as bone abscesses.

Pyogenic Bone Infections
Acute and Chronic Osteomyelitis

The earliest radiographic signs of bone infection are soft tissue edema and loss of fascial planes. These are usually encountered within 24 to 48 hours of the onset of infection. The earliest changes in the bone are evidence of a destructive lytic lesion, usually within seven to ten days after the onset of infection (Fig. 20.1), and a positive radionuclide bone scan. Within two to six weeks, there is progres-

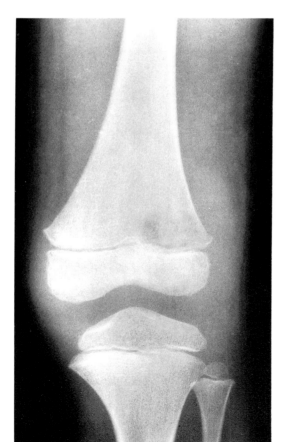

Figure 20.1 A 7-year-old boy had a fever and a painful knee for one week. Anteroposterior view of the knee demonstrates the earliest radiographic signs of bone infection: a poorly defined osteolytic area of destruction in the metaphyseal segment of the distal femur and soft tissue swelling.

sive destruction of cortical and medullary bone, an increased endosteal sclerosis indicating reactive new bone formation, and a periosteal reaction (Fig. 20.2). In six to eight weeks, sequestra indicating areas of necrotic bone usually become apparent; they are surrounded by a dense involucrum, representing a sheath of periosteal new bone (Fig. 20.3). The sequestra and involucra develop as the result of an accumulation of inflammatory exudate (pus), which penetrates the cortex and strips it of periosteum, thus stimulating the inner layer to form new bone. The newly formed bone is in turn infected, and the resultant barrier causes the cortex and spongiosa to be deprived of a blood supply and become necrotic. At this stage, termed *chronic osteomyelitis*, a draining sinus tract often forms (Fig. 20.4; see also Figs. 19.7, 19.10B). Small sequestra are gradually resorbed, or they may be extruded through the sinus tract.

Subacute Osteomyelitis

BRODIE ABSCESS This lesion, originally described by Brodie in 1832, represents a subacute localized form of osteomyelitis. Its onset is

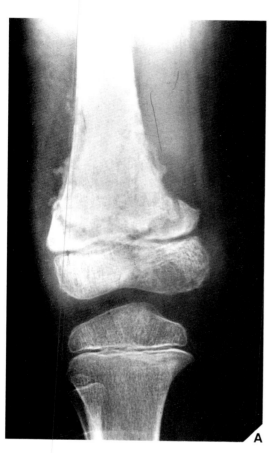

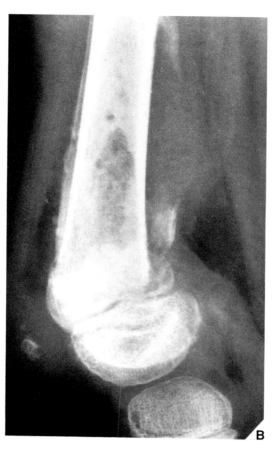

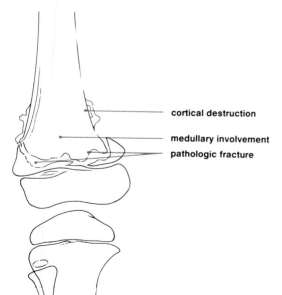

Figure 20.2 Anteroposterior (A) and lateral (B) views of the knee of an 8-year-old boy with acute osteomyelitis show widespread destruction of the cortical and medullary portions of the metaphysis and diaphysis of the distal femur, together with periosteal new bone formation. Note the pathologic fracture. On the lateral view, a large subperiosteal abscess is evident.

cortical destruction
medullary involvement
pathologic fracture

subperiosteal abscess

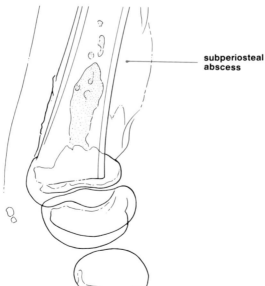

Figure 20.3 Sequestra surrounded by involucrum, as seen here in the left leg of a 2-year-old child, is a feature of advanced osteomyelitis, usually apparent after six to eight weeks of active infection. (Courtesy of Dr. RH Gold, Los Angeles, Ca)

often insidious, and systemic manifestations are generally mild or absent. The abscess, which is usually localized in the metaphysis of the tibia or femur, is typically elongated with a well demarcated margin and surrounded by reactive sclerosis. As a rule, sequestra are absent, but a radiolucent tract may be seen extending from the lesion into the growth plate (Fig. 20.5). A bone abscess may often cross the epiphyseal plate, but seldom does an abscess develop in and remain localized to the epiphysis (Fig. 20.6; see also Fig. 19.8).

Nonpyogenic Bone Infections

The most common nonpyogenic bone infections are tuberculosis, syphilis, and fungal infections.

Tuberculous Bone Infections

Tuberculous infection usually occurs secondarily as a result of hematogenous spread from a primary focus of infection such as the lung or genitourinary tract. Skeletal tuberculosis represents about 3% of all cases of tuberculosis and about 30% of all extrapulmonary tuberculous infections. In 10% to 15% of cases, bone involvement without articular disease is encountered. In children, tuberculous osteomyelitis has a predilection for the metaphyseal segment of the long bones; in adults, the joints are more often affected.

In both the long and short bones, progressive destruction of the medullary region with abscess formation is apparent on plain-film studies. Typically, there is evidence of osteoporosis, but at least in the early stage of the disease little or no reactive sclerosis is usually

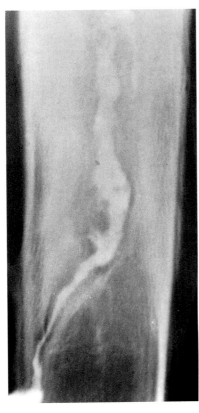

Figure 20.4 A 28-year-old man with sickle-cell disease developed osteomyelitis, a frequent complication of this condition. A sinogram enhanced by magnification shows a draining sinus typical of chronic osteomyelitis. Note the extent of the serpentine tract in the medullary portion of the bone.

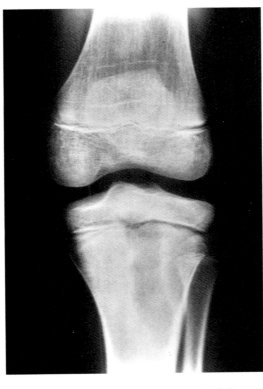

Figure 20.5 Anteroposterior view of the left knee of an 11-year-old boy with a subacute Brodie abscess in the proximal diaphysis of the tibia shows a radiolucent tract extending into the growth plate.

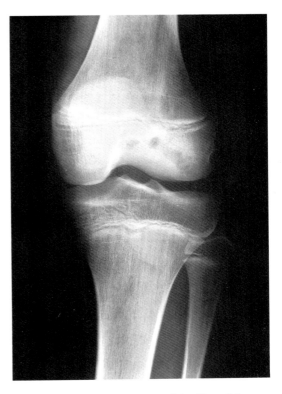

Figure 20.6 Anteroposterior plain film of the left knee of a 13-year-old boy demonstrates a well defined osteolytic lesion surrounded by reactive sclerosis in the distal epiphysis of the femur. This is a rare site for a bone abscess.

present (Fig. 20.7). Occasionally, destruction in the mid-diaphysis of a short tubular bone of the hand or foot *(tuberculous dactylitis)* may produce a fusiform enlargement of the entire diaphysis, a condition known as spina ventosa (Fig. 20.8). The appearance of multiple disseminated lytic lesions in short tubular bones is termed cystic tuberculosis, a form of skeletal tuberculosis seen particularly in children.

Fungal Infections

Fungal bone infections are infrequent, the most common being coccidioidomycosis, blastomycosis, actinomycosis, and nocardiosis. The infection is usually low-grade, with the formation of an abscess and a draining sinus. The lesion may resemble a tuberculous skeletal infection, since the abscess is usually found in cancellous bone with little or no reactive sclerosis or periosteal response (Fig. 20.9). The location of a lesion at a point of bony prominence—such as along the edges of the patella, the ends of the clavicles, or in the acromion, coracoid process, olecranon, or styloid process of the radius or ulna—may also suggest a fungal infection. Solitary marginal lesions of the ribs and lesions involving the vertebrae in an indiscriminate fashion, including the body, neural arch, and spinous and transverse processes, also favor fungal infectious process.

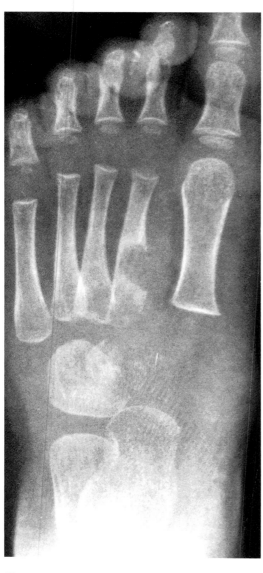

Figure 20.7 A 20-month-old girl had progressive swelling of the right foot. Anteroposterior view of the foot shows a well defined lytic defect in the medial aspect of the second metatarsal; there is no evidence of reactive sclerosis or periosteal new bone formation, but soft tissue swelling is apparent. Aspiration of a mass yielded 1 mL of pus-like fluid, which on bacteriologic examination revealed acid-fast bacteria. The causative agent proved to be *Mycobacterium tuberculosis*.

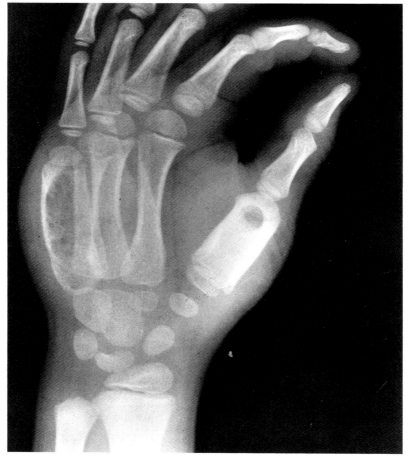

Figure 20.8 Oblique film of the hand of a 7-year-old boy with skeletal tuberculosis shows expansile fusiform lesions of the first and fifth metacarpals associated with soft tissue swelling; there is no evidence of a periosteal reaction. Such diaphyseal enlargement secondary to tuberculosis is known as spina ventosa.

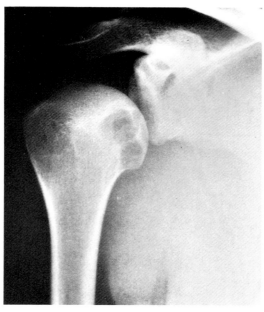

Figure 20.9 Anteroposterior view of the right shoulder of an 18-year-old male demonstrates a destructive osteolytic lesion in the medial aspect of the humeral head, with minimal sclerosis and no periosteal reaction—the typical appearance of a fungal infection. Aspiration biopsy showed the abscess to be due to a cryptococcal infection.

Syphilitic Infection

Syphilis is a chronic systemic infectious disease caused by a spirochete, *Treponema pallidum. Congenital syphilis,* which is transmitted from mother to fetus, may manifest as a chronic osteochondritis, periostitis, or osteitis. The lesions, which most frequently involve the tibia, are characteristically widespread and symmetric in appearance; destructive changes are usually seen in the metaphysis at the junction with the growth plate, producing what is called the Wimberger sign (Fig. 20.10). In the later stages of disease, involvement of the tibia results in a characteristic anterior bowing known as "saber-shin" deformity.

Acquired syphilis may manifest either as a chronic osteitis exhibiting irregular sclerosis of the medullary cavity or as syphilitic abscesses known as gumma (Fig. 20.11). The latter form of the dis-

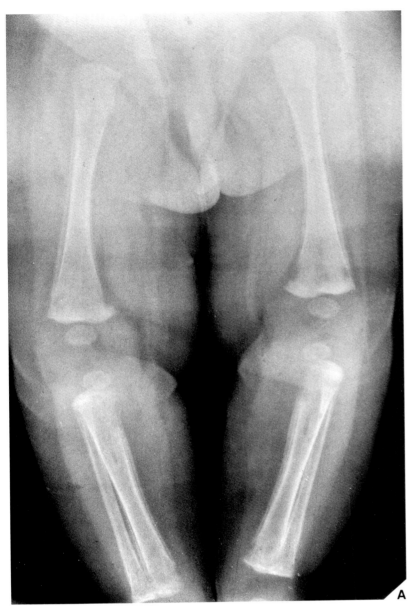

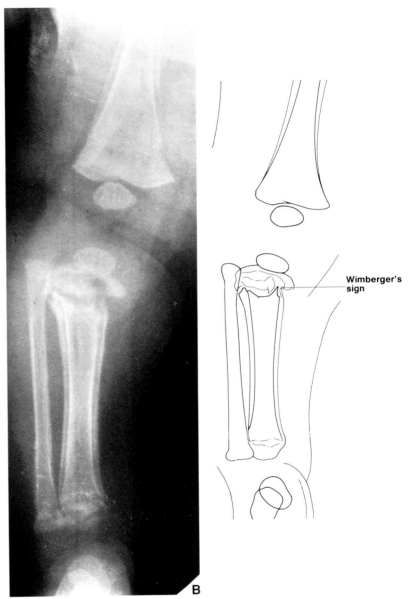

Figure 20.10 (A) Anteroposterior view of the lower legs of a 7-week-old infant with congenital syphilis demonstrates characteristic periostitis affecting the femora and tibiae. In addition, destructive changes are evident in the medullary portion of the proximal tibiae. (B) Two months later, the infectious process has progressed, with destruction of the tibial metaphysis and marked periostitis. The characteristic erosion of the medial surface of the proximal tibial metaphysis is termed the Wimberger sign.

ease may simulate pyogenic osteomyelitis, but the absence of sequestra typically found in bacterial osteomyelitis allows the distinction to be made.

Differential Diagnosis of Osteomyelitis

Usually, the radiographic appearance of osteomyelitis is so characteristic that the diagnosis is easily made with the patient's clinical history and ancillary radiologic examinations such as tomography, computed tomography, and scintigraphy. Nevertheless, osteomyelitis may at times mimic other conditions. Particularly in its acute form, it may resemble eosinophilic granuloma or Ewing sarcoma (Fig. 20.12). The soft tissue changes in each of these conditions, however, are characteristic and different. In osteomyelitis, soft tissue swelling is diffuse, with obliteration of the fascial planes, whereas eosinophilic granuloma as a rule is not accompanied by soft tissue swelling or a mass. The extension of a Ewing sarcoma into the soft tissues presents as a well defined soft tissue mass with preservation of the fascial planes. The duration of a patient's symptoms also plays an important diagnostic role. It takes a tumor such as a Ewing sarcoma from four to six months to destroy the bone to the same extent that osteomyelitis does in four to six weeks and eosinophilic granuloma in only seven to ten days. Despite these differentiating features, however, the radiographic pattern of bone destruction, periosteal reaction, and location in the bone may be very similar in all three conditions (see Fig. 18.34).

A bone abscess, particularly in the cortex, may closely simulate an osteoid osteoma (see Fig. 16.13). In the medullary region, however, the presence of a serpentine tract favors the diagnosis of bone abscess over osteoid osteoma (Fig. 20.13).

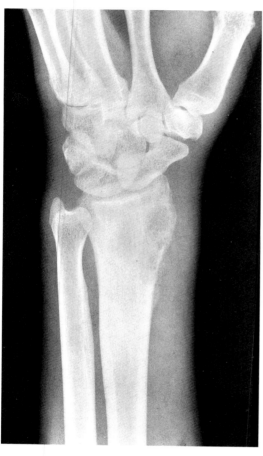

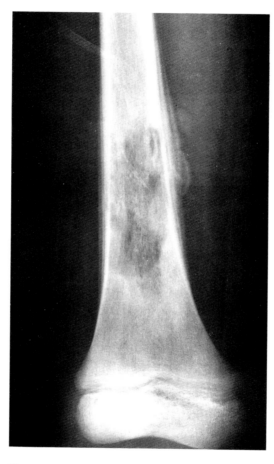

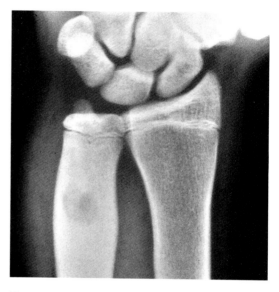

Figure 20.13 A 17-year-old boy had a typical history of osteoid osteoma: nocturnal bone pain relieved promptly by salicylates. Posteroanterior view of the distal forearm demonstrates a radiolucent lesion in the distal ulnar diaphysis. The presence of a serpentine tract extending from the radiolucent focus into the growth plate indicates a diagnosis of bone abscess.

Figure 20.11 Oblique view of the distal forearm of a 51-year-old man with acquired syphilis shows a lytic abscess (gumma) in the lateral aspect of the distal radius.

Figure 20.12 A 7-year-old boy presented with pain in his right leg for three weeks. Anteroposterior radiograph demonstrates a lesion in the medullary portion of the distal femoral diaphysis with a moth-eaten type of bone destruction, associated with a lamellated periosteal reaction and a small soft tissue prominence. These radiographic features suggest a diagnosis of Ewing sarcoma. The absence of a definite soft tissue mass and the short symptomatic period, however, point to the correct diagnosis of osteomyelitis, which was confirmed by biopsy.

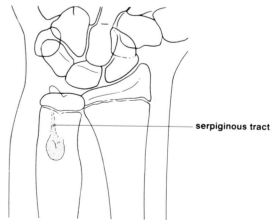

— serpiginous tract

INFECTIOUS ARTHRITIS

Most infectious arthritides demonstrate a positive radionuclide bone scan and a very similar radiographic picture, including joint effusion and destruction of cartilage and subchondral bone with consequent joint space narrowing (see Figs. 11.21, 11.23). However, certain clinical and radiographic features are characteristic of individual infectious processes as demonstrated at various target sites (Fig. 20.14).

Pyogenic Joint Infections

The clinical signs and symptoms of pyogenic (septic) arthritis depend on the site and extent of involvement as well as the specific infectious organism. Although the majority of cases of septic arthri-

tis are caused by *Staphylococcus aureus* and *Neisseria gonorrhoeae*, other pathogens—including *Pseudomonas aeruginosa*, *Enterobacter cloacae*, *Klebsiella pneumoniae*, *Candida albicans*, and *Serratia marcescens*—are being encountered with increasing frequency in joint infections in drug users due to the contamination of injected drugs or needles.

Any small or large joint can be affected by septic arthritis, and hematogenous spread in drug addicts is characterized by unusual locations of the lesion, such as the spine (vertebrae and intervertebral disks), sacroiliac joints, sternoclavicular and acromioclavicular articulations, and pubic symphysis.

Standard radiography usually suffices to demonstrate septic arthritis. Certain characteristic radiographic features may be helpful in arriving at the correct diagnosis. Generally, a single joint is affected, most commonly a weight-bearing joint like the knee or hip.

Figure 20.14 Clinical and Radiographic Hallmarks of Infectious Arthritis at Various Target Sites

TYPE	SITE	CRUCIAL ABNORMALITIES	TECHNIQUES/PROJECTIONS
Pyogenic Infections*	Peripheral joints	Periarticular osteoporosis Joint effusion Destruction of subchondral bone (on both sides of joint)	Radionuclide bone scan (early) Standard views specific for site of involvement Aspiration and arthrography
	Spine	Narrowing of disk space Loss of definition of vertebral end plate Paraspinal mass Partial or complete obstruction of intrathecal contrast flow Destruction of disk	Anteroposterior and lateral views CT, MRI Myelogram Diskogram and aspiration
Nonpyogenic Infections Tuberculosis	Large joints	Monoarticular involvement (similar to rheumatoid arthritis) "Kissing" sequestra (knee) Sclerotic changes in subchondral bone	Radionuclide bone scan Standard views Tomography
	Spine	Gibbous formation Lytic lesion in vertebral body Destruction of disk Paraspinal mass Soft tissue abscess ("cold" abscess) Obstruction of intrathecal contrast flow	Anteroposterior and lateral views Diskogram and aspiration CT, MRI Myelogram
Lyme disease	Knee	Narrowing of femoropatellar compartment Edematous changes in infrapatellar fat pad	Lateral view CT, MRI

*In IV drug users, unusual sites of infection are encountered, including the vertebra; the sacroiliac, sternoclavicular, and acromioclavicular joints; and the pubic symphysis. The radiologic techniques used to evaluate infections at these sites, as well as the crucial radiographic abnormalities, are the same as those for the more common sites.

The early stage of joint infection may be seen simply as joint effusion, soft tissue swelling, and periarticular osteoporosis (Fig. 20.15).

In the later phase of pyogenic arthritis, articular cartilage is destroyed, and characteristically both subarticular plates are involved and the joint space narrows (Fig. 20.16A). Arthrography, which is often performed following aspiration of the joint to obtain a fluid specimen for bacteriologic examination, helps determine the extent of joint destruction and demonstrate the presence of synovitis (Fig.

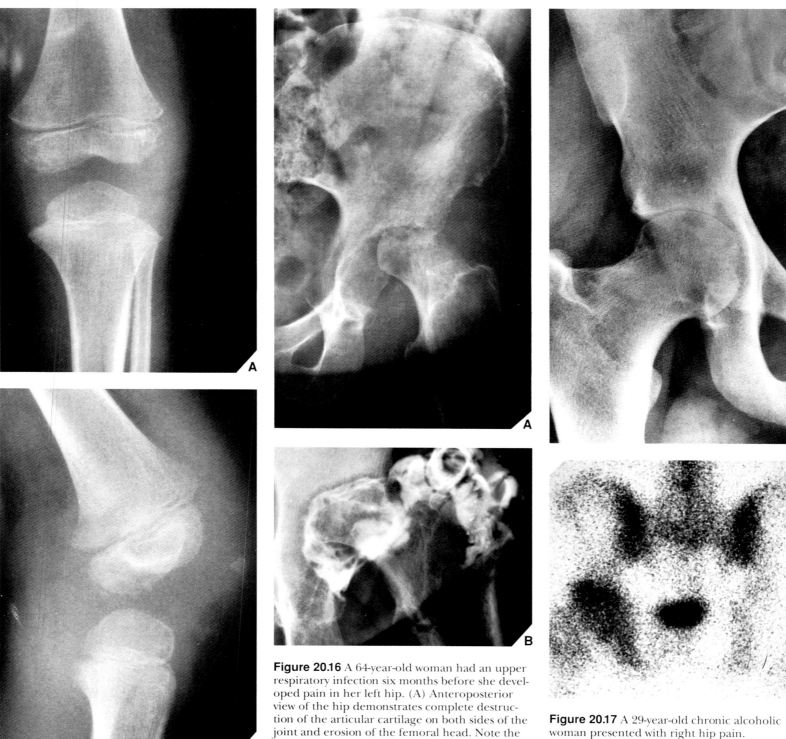

Figure 20.15 Anteroposterior (A) and lateral (B) views of the left knee of a 4-year-old child demonstrate a significant degree of periarticular osteoporosis and a large joint effusion. Note the small erosions of the distal epiphysis of the femur and the preservation of the joint space. Aspiration revealed hematogenous spread of a staphylococcal urinary tract infection.

Figure 20.16 A 64-year-old woman had an upper respiratory infection six months before she developed pain in her left hip. (A) Anteroposterior view of the hip demonstrates complete destruction of the articular cartilage on both sides of the joint and erosion of the femoral head. Note the significant degree of osteoporosis. (B) Contrast arthrography was performed primarily to obtain joint fluid for bacteriologic examination, which yielded *Staphylococcus aureus*. The contrast medium outlines the destroyed joint, showing a synovial irregularity consistent with chronic synovitis.

Figure 20.17 A 29-year-old chronic alcoholic woman presented with right hip pain. (A) Anteroposterior view of the hip demonstrates diminution of the joint space, particularly in the weight-bearing region, as well as periarticular osteoporosis. (B) Radionuclide bone scan using technetium-99m-labeled diphosphonate demonstrates increased isotope uptake only in the right hip. The increased activity at both sacroiliac joints is a normal finding. The diagnosis of tuberculous arthritis was confirmed by joint aspiration.

20.16B). Radionuclide bone scan is often effective in distinguishing a joint infection from a periarticular soft tissue infection (see Fig. 19.9). It is also useful in monitoring the progress of treatment, although several weeks may be required before the scan demonstrates a completely normal appearance.

COMPLICATIONS Infectious arthritis of peripheral joints in children may lead to the destruction of the growth plate with resulting growth arrest (see Fig. 19.16). The infection may also spread to an adjacent bone, causing osteomyelitis. Degenerative arthritis and intra-articular bony ankylosis may also occur.

Nonpyogenic Joint Infections

Tuberculous Arthritis

Tuberculous arthritis represents 1% of all forms of extrapulmonary tuberculosis, although the number of cases has recently been on the rise. The acid-fast tubercle bacilli *Mycobacterium tuberculosis* and *Mycobacterium bovi* are the causative organisms. The infection may be found in all groups, but more frequently in children and young adults. Predisposing factors such as trauma, alcoholism, drug abuse, intra-articular injection of steroids, or prolonged systemic illness are found in most patients with tuberculous arthritis. The joint infection usually is caused by either direct invasion from an adjacent focus of osteomyelitis or by hematogenous dissemination of the tubercle bacillus. Large weight-bearing joints such as the hip or knee are most often affected, and monoarticular involvement is the rule.

Plain-film radiography is usually sufficient to demonstrate the identifying features of tuberculous arthritis, although its early radiographic appearance is often indistinguishable from that of monoarticular rheumatoid arthritis. However, the involvement of only one joint, as demonstrated by scintigraphy, favors an infectious process (Fig. 20.17). A triad of radiographic abnormalities (Phemister triad), comprised of periarticular osteoporosis, peripherally located osseous erosions, and gradual diminution of the joint space, should suggest the correct diagnosis; CT examination, however, can be helpful in delineating subtle features (Fig. 20.18). Occasionally, wedge-shaped necrotic foci, so-called kissing sequestra, may be present on both sides of the affected joint, especially in the knee. At a later stage of the disease, there may be complete destruction of the joint, and sclerotic changes in adjacent bones are more frequently encountered (Fig. 20.19).

Other Infectious Arthritides

Less frequently encountered than pyogenic or tuberculous arthritis are joint infections caused by fungi (actinomycosis, cryptococcosis, coccidioidomycosis, histoplasmosis, sporotrichosis, candidiasis), viruses (smallpox), and spirochetes (syphilis, yaws).

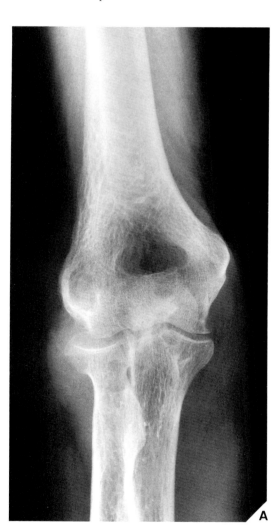
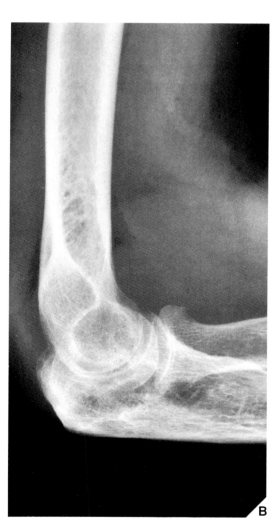
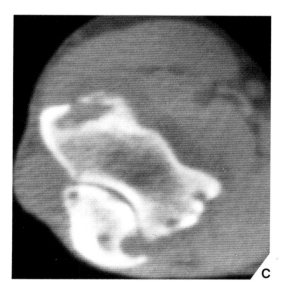

Figure 20.18 A 70-year-old man from India had pain in the left elbow for four months. According to his daughter, he had been treated for chronic lung disease. Anteroposterior (A) and lateral (B) views of the elbow demonstrate a large joint effusion, as indicated by positive anterior and posterior fat pad signs on the lateral projection. Small periarticular erosions are not clear on these views. (C) CT section shows narrowing of the joint and peripheral erosions typical of tuberculous infection.

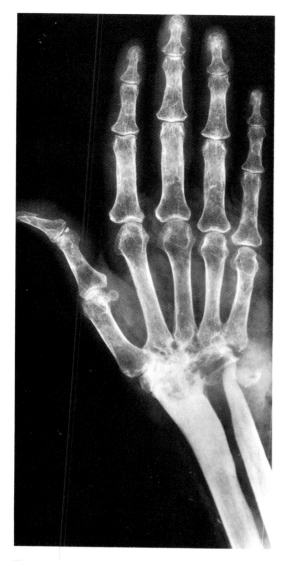

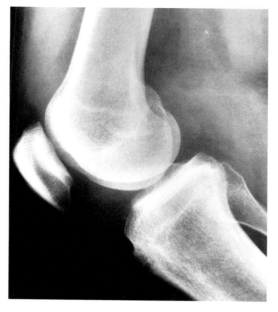

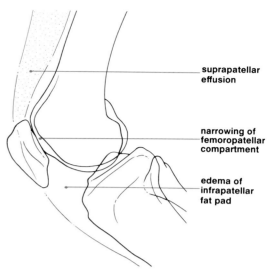

Figure 20.20 A 28-year-old man presented with a 10-month history of arthritis in the right knee. Lateral radiograph demonstrates a suprapatellar joint effusion and edematous changes in the infrapatellar fat pad. Note the minimal narrow- ing of the femoropatellar joint compartment. There are no articular erosions present. Bacteriologic studies confirmed a diagnosis of Lyme arthritis.

Figure 20.19 Posteroanterior view of the left forearm of a 52-year-old woman with pulmonary tuberculosis shows advanced tuberculous arthritis involving the left wrist. There is com- plete destruction of the radiocarpal, midcarpal, and carpometacarpal articulations, as well as whit- tling and sclerotic changes in the distal radius and ulna. Note the osteoporosis distal to the affected joints and the soft tissue swelling.

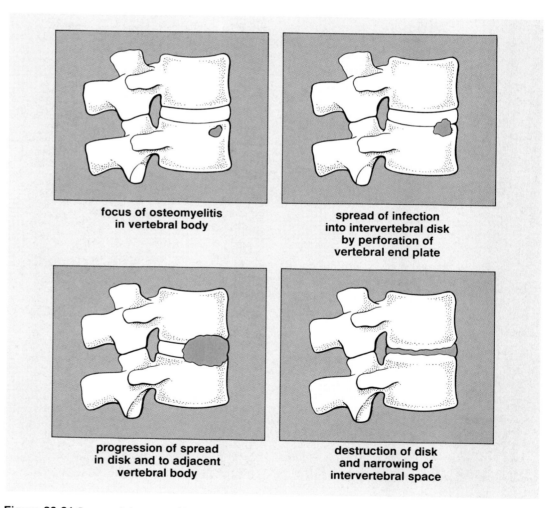

focus of osteomyelitis
in vertebral body

spread of infection
into intervertebral disk
by perforation of
vertebral end plate

progression of spread
in disk and to adjacent
vertebral body

destruction of disk
and narrowing of
intervertebral space

Figure 20.21 Sequential stages of involvement of a vertebral body and disk by an infectious process.

Of interest is *Lyme arthritis*, an infectious articular condition caused by the spirochete *Borrelia burgdorfesi*, which is transmitted by the tick *Ixodes dammini* or related ticks. The illness usually begins in the summer with a characteristic skin lesion and flu-like symptoms; within weeks to months a chronic arthritis develops that is characterized by erosions of cartilage and bone. The joint involvement has some similarities to juvenile rheumatoid arthritis and Reiter syndrome. A joint effusion may be present in the early stages of the disease, and characteristic edematous changes of the infrapatellar fat pad may be noted in the knee (Fig. 20.20).

INFECTIONS OF THE SPINE

Pyogenic Infections

Infectious organisms may reach the spine by several routes. Hematogenous spread occurs by way of arterial and venous routes (the Batson paravertebral venous system), and the organism lodges in the vertebral body, commonly in the anterior subchondral region. This osteomyelitic focus can spread to the intervertebral disk through perforation of the vertebral endplate, causing disk space infection (diskitis) (Fig. 20.21). Disk space infection can also be induced directly by the implantation of an organism through puncture of the spinal canal, either during spinal surgery or, rarely, by spread from a contiguous site of infection such as a paravertebral abscess (see Fig. 19.4). Disk infection may also occur in children via a hematogenous route because there is still a blood supply to the disk.

Radiographically, disk infection is characterized by narrowing of the disk space, destruction of the adjacent vertebral end plates, and a paraspinal mass. Although most cases are obvious on standard anteroposterior and lateral films of the spine (Fig. 20.22), conventional and computed tomography may yield additional information (Fig. 20.23). Radionuclide bone scan can detect early infection, prior to any changes noticed radiographically (Fig. 20.24). Occasionally, diskography is performed, but as in the use of arthrography in joint infections, the primary objective is obtaining a specimen for bacteri-

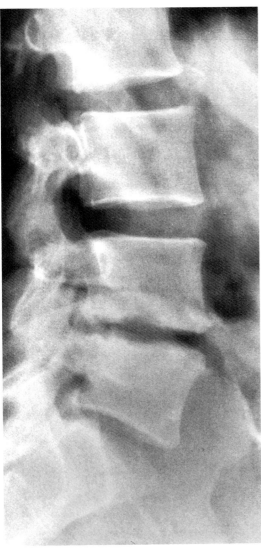

Figure 20.22 Lateral view of the lumbar spine in a 32-year-old man demonstrates the typical radiographic changes of disk infection. There is narrowing of the disk space at L4–5, and the inferior end plate of L-4 and superior end plate of L-5 are indistinctly outlined. Note the normal end plates at the L3–4 disk space.

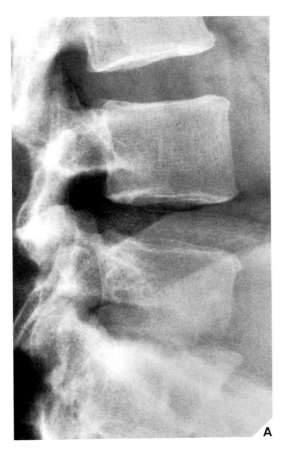

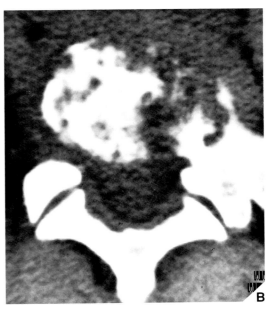

Figure 20.23 A 40-year-old man presented with lower-back pain for eight weeks, which he attributed to lifting a heavy object. (A) Lateral view of the lumbosacral spine shows narrowing of the L5–S1 disk space and suggests some fuzziness of the adjacent vertebral end plates. (B) CT section through the disk space clearly shows destructive changes of the disk and vertebral end plate characteristic of infection.

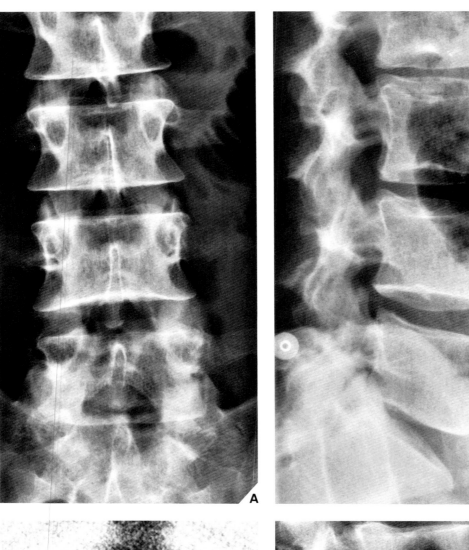

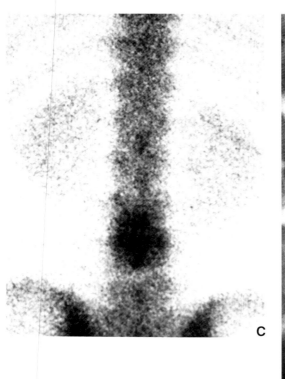

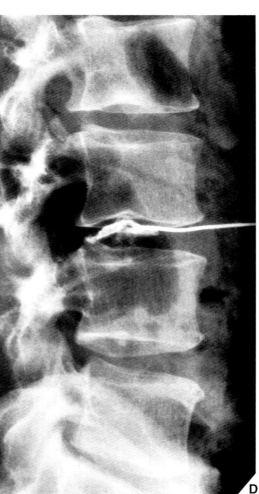

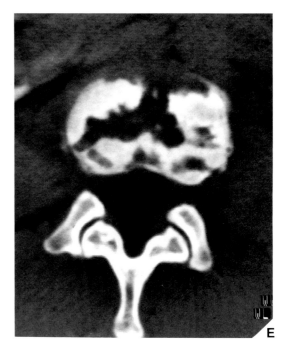

Figure 20.24 Standard anteroposterior (A) and lateral (B) radiographs of the lumbar spine of a 40-year-old man who had back pain for four weeks show no definite abnormalities. (C) Radionuclide bone scan, however, reveals increased uptake of radiopharmaceutical at the L3–4 level. (D) On a subsequent diskogram, using the oblique approach, partial disk destruction is evident. (E) The extent of destruction is revealed by CT. Bacteriologic examination of aspirated fluid yielded *Escherichia coli.*

ologic examination. A contrast study, however, may outline the extent of a disk infection (Fig. 20.25).

Magnetic resonance imaging (MRI) has become the modality of choice in diagnosing and evaluating infections of the spine. Characteristic findings of disk space narrowing, disk destruction, paraspinal soft tissue thickening, and edematous changes in the paraspinal musculature are well demonstrated by this technique (Fig. 20.26).

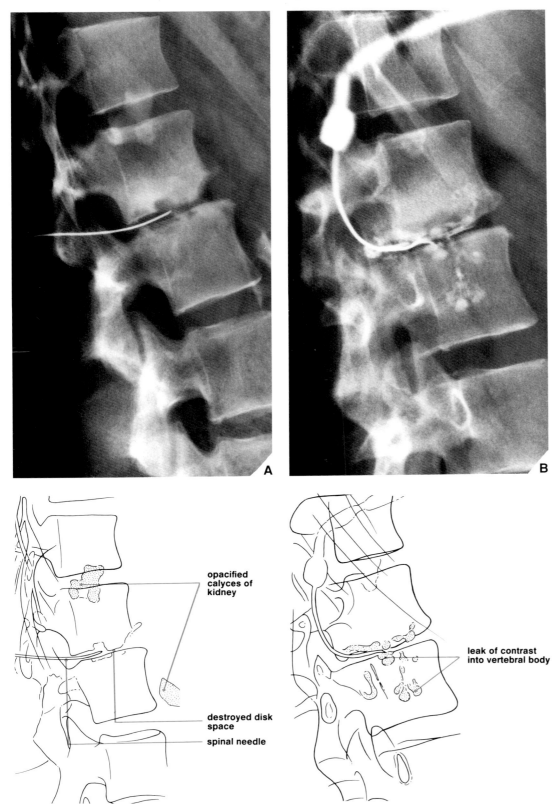

Figure 20.25 A 22-year-old IV drug user with back pain for two months developed an intervertebral disk infection. A diskogram was performed primarily to aspirate fluid for bacteriologic examination, which revealed *Pseudomonas aeruginosa*. Prior to the puncture, the patient received an intravenous injection of iodine contrast medium to visualize the kidneys, as a precautionary step before spine biopsy at that level. (A) Lateral view of the lumbar spine shows narrowing of the disk space at L1–2 and destruction of the adjacent vertebral end plates. The spinal needle is located in the center of the disk. (B) Lateral radiograph obtained during the injection of metrizamide demonstrates extension of the contrast medium into the body of L-2, indicating the presence of vertebral osteomyelitis.

opacified
calyces of
kidney

destroyed disk
space

spinal needle

leak of contrast
into vertebral body

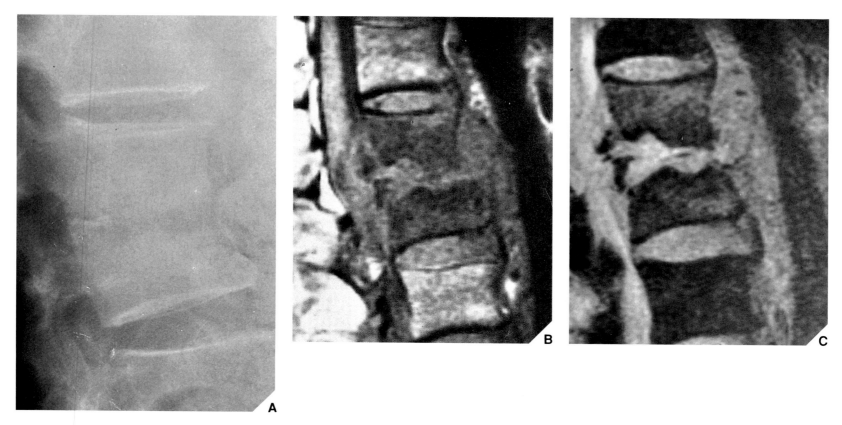

Figure 20.26 A 48-year-old male IV drug user developed disk infection at L1–2. (A) Plain lateral radiograph demonstrates classic changes of disk space infection: narrowing of the disk space and destruction of the vertebral end plates. (B) Sagittal spin-echo T1-weighted MR image (TR 600/TE 20) demonstrates, in addition to the destruction of the disk, a large inflamma- tory mass extending anteriorly, destroying anterior longitudinal ligament and infiltrating paraspinal soft tissues. Posteriorly, it invades the content of spinal canal. (C) Sagittal T2*-weighted gradient (MPGR) MR image shows more clearly the fragmentation of the posterior aspect of adjacent vertebral bodies and compression of the thecal sac by a large abscess.

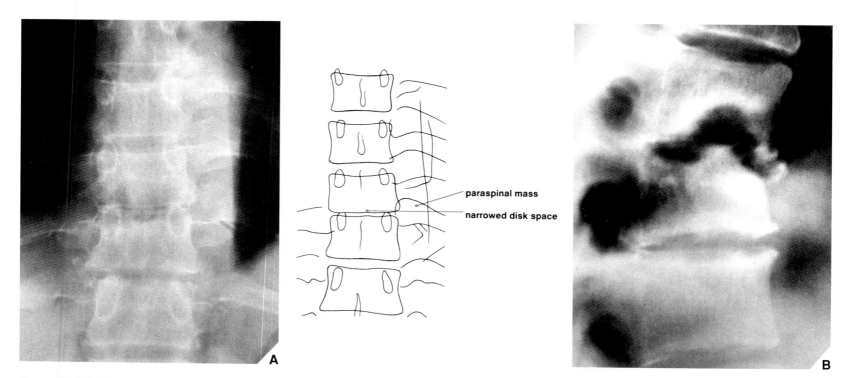

Figure 20.27 (A) Anteroposterior view of the thoracic spine in a 50-year-old man with tuberculous spondylitis shows narrowing of the T8–9 disk space, associated with a paraspinal mass on the left side. (B) Lateral tomogram shows destruction of the disk and extensive erosion of the inferior aspect of the body of T-8.

Nonpyogenic Infections

Tuberculosis of the Spine

Infection of the spine by the tubercle bacillus is known as *tuberculous spondylitis* or *Pott disease*. The vertebral body or intervertebral disk may be involved, with the lower thoracic and upper lumbar vertebrae being the preferred sites of infection. The disease constitutes 25% to 50% of all cases of skeletal tuberculosis.

The radiographic features of tuberculous infection of the spine are similar to those seen in pyogenic infections. There is disk space narrowing, and the vertebral end plates adjacent to the involved disk show evidence of destruction. A paraspinal mass is common (Fig. 20.27). Rarely, the infectious process may destroy a single vertebra or part of a vertebra (pedicle) without invasion of the disk.

COMPLICATIONS Tuberculosis of the spine may cause collapse of a partially or completely destroyed vertebra, leading to kyphosis and a gibbous formation. Extension of infection to the adjacent ligaments and soft tissues is also rather frequent; the psoas muscles are often the site of secondary tuberculous infections, commonly called "cold" abscesses (Fig. 20.28). The most common complication of tuberculous spondylitis, however, is compression of the thecal sac and spinal

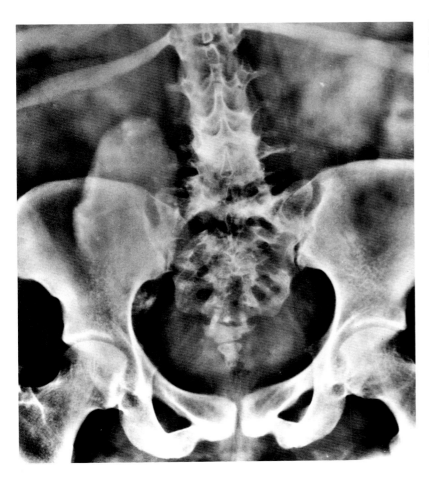

Figure 20.28 Anteroposterior view of the pelvis in a 35-year-old woman with spinal tuberculosis shows an oval radiodense mass with spotted calcifications overlapping the medial part of the ilium and right sacroiliac joint (right psoas muscle). This is the typical appearance of a "cold" abscess.

cord with resulting paraplegia. Myelography and MRI are very helpful diagnostically if compression is suspected (Fig. 20.29).

SOFT TISSUE INFECTIONS

Soft tissue infections (cellulitis) usually result from direct introduction of organisms through a skin puncture; they are also seen as a complication of systemic disorders such as diabetes. The most frequently encountered organisms are *Clostridium novyi* and *Clostridium perfringens*. These gas-forming organisms may cause an accumulation of gas in the soft tissues that can easily be recognized on plain films as radiolucent bubbles or streaks in the subcutaneous tissues or muscles. This finding usually indicates gangrene caused by anaerobic bacteria. Soft tissue edema and obliteration of

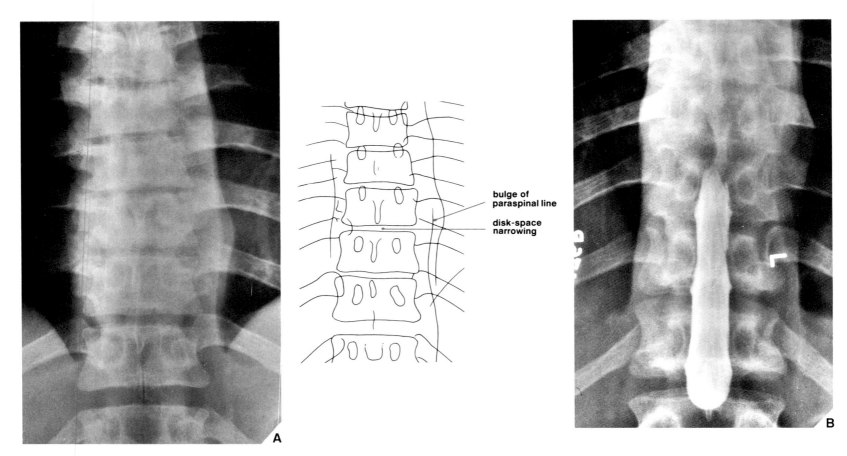

Figure 20.29 A 39-year-old man with a history of pulmonary tuberculosis developed neurologic symptoms of spinal cord compression. (A) Anteroposterior view of the thoracic spine shows minimal disk space narrowing at T9–10 and a large left paraspinal mass. (B) A myelogram shows complete obstruction of the flow of contrast in the subarachnoid space at the level of the disk infection.

fat and fascial planes are also evident on the standard examination (Fig. 20.30).

Recently, MRI has been used to evaluate soft tissue infection. In particular, soft tissue abscesses as well as involvement of tendon sheaths and muscles, are accurately depicted with this modality. Soft tissue abscesses appear as rounded or elongated—but always well demarcated—areas of decreased signal intensity on T1-weighted images, changing to increased signal intensity on T2-weighted images (Fig. 20.31). Occasionally a peripheral band of decreased signal intensity is seen that represents the fibrous capsule surrounding the abscess (see Fig. 19.12). Infected fluid collection within the tendon sheath is always hyperintense on T2-weighting and hypointense on T1-weighting, but this cannot be differentiated from noninfected fluid.

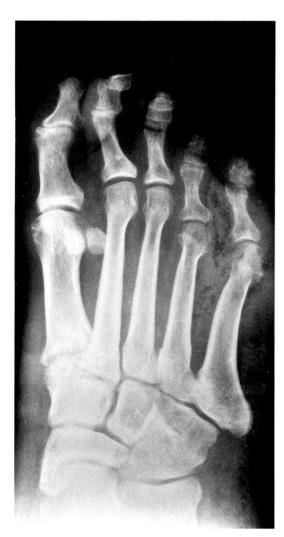

Figure 20.30
Anteroposterior plain film of the foot of a 59-year-old man with longstanding diabetes mellitus shows marked soft tissue swelling and edema, particularly in the region of the fourth and fifth digits. Radiolucent streaks of gas are typical of gangrenous infection.

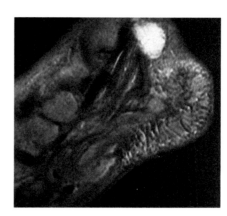

Figure 20.31 Sagittal spin-echo T2-weighted MR image (TR 2000/TE 80) of a soft tissue abscess. There is a high signal intensity fluid collection adjacent to the medial malleolus in this diabetic patient with a foot infection. (From Beltran J, 1990)

PRACTICAL POINTS TO REMEMBER

Osteomyelitis

[1] The radiographic hallmarks of osteomyelitis include:
- cortical and medullary bone destruction
- reactive sclerosis and a periosteal reaction
- the presence of sequestra and involucra.

[2] The metaphysis is a characteristic site of osteomyelitis in children.

[3] Acute osteomyelitis of a long bone frequently mimics Ewing sarcoma and eosinophilic granuloma. The clinical history, especially the duration of symptoms prior to the discovery of bone changes, usually serves as a clue to the correct diagnosis.

[4] A destructive metaphyseal lesion extending into the epiphysis usually indicates a bone abscess.

[5] A Brodie abscess may clinically and radiographically mimic an osteoid osteoma. In the differential diagnosis, the presence of a radiolucent tract extending from the lesion into the growth plate favors an infectious process.

[6] In congenital syphilis:
- osteochondritis, periostitis, and osteitis are typical features
- destruction at the medial aspect of the metaphysis of a long bone (Wimberger sign) is characteristic.

Infectious Arthritis

[1] The characteristic radiographic features of septic arthritis of the peripheral joints include:
- periarticular osteoporosis, joint effusion, and soft tissue swelling (early phase)
- destruction of cartilage and the subchondral plates on both sides of the joint (late phase).

[2] In tuberculosis of a peripheral joint, which usually manifests as a monoarticular disease (strongly resembling rheumatoid arthritis), the Phemister triad of radiographic abnormalities is characteristic, and includes:
- periarticular osteoporosis
- peripheral osseous erosions
- gradual narrowing of the joint space.

Infections of the Spine

[1] Pyogenic infection of the spine is recognized radiographically by:
- narrowing of the disk space
- destruction of both vertebral end plates adjacent to the involved disk
- a paraspinal mass.

[2] The radiographic hallmarks of tuberculous infection of an intervertebral disk are:
- narrowing of the disk space
- loss of the sharp outline of the adjacent vertebral end plates.

[3] Tuberculous infection of the spine may:
- destroy the disk and vertebra, leading to kyphosis and a gibbus formation
- extend into the soft tissues, forming a "cold" abscess.

[4] In the radiologic evaluation of spine infections:
- radionuclide bone scan can detect disk infection prior to the appearance of any radiographic signs
- the diskogram is a valid examination performed primarily to obtain aspirate fluid for bacteriologic study
- MRI is the modality of choice to diagnose and evaluate spine infection.

Soft Tissue Infections

[1] Cellulitis due to gas-forming bacteria in soft tissues (gangrene) is recognized radiographically by:
- soft tissue edema and swelling
- radiolucent bubbles or streaks representing accumulations of gas.

[2] Diabetics are particularly prone to developing soft tissue infections, the feet being common sites.

[3] Scintigraphy using indium-111-labelled white cells is useful in detecting and localizing the site of infection, while MRI is ideal in evaluating the extent of infection in the soft tissues.

References

Abdelwahab IF, Present DA, Zwass A, Klein MJ, Mazzara J: Tumorlike tuberculous granulomas of bone. *Am J Roentgenol* 149:1207, 1987.

Alexander GM, Mansuy MM: Disseminated bone tuberculosis (so-called multiple cystic tuberculosis). *Radiology* 55:839, 1950.

Beltran J: *MRI: Musculoskeletal System.* Philadelpha, Lippincott, 1990.

Brodie BC: An account of some cases of chronic abscess of the tibia. *Trans Med Chir Soc* 17:238, 1832.

Bruno MS, Silverberg TN, Goldstein DH: Embolic osteomyelitis of the spine as a complication of infection of the urinary tract. *Am J Med* 29:865, 1960.

Cremin BJ, Fisher RM: The lesions of congenital syphilis. *Br J Radiol* 43:333, 1970.

David R, Barron BJ, Madewell JE: Osteomyelitis, acute and chronic. *Radiol Clin North Am* 25:1171, 1987.

Erlich I, Kricun ME: Radiographic findings in early acquired syphilis: Case report and critical review. *Am J Roentgenol* 127:789, 1976.

Fletcher BD, Scoles PV, Nelson AD: Osteomyelitis in children: Detection by magnetic resonance. *Radiology* 150:57, 1984.

Gilmour WM: Acute haematogenous osteomyelitis. *J Bone Joint Surg* 44B:841, 1962.

Graves VB, Schreiber MN: Tuberculous psoas muscle abscess. *J Can Assoc Radiol* 24:268, 1973.

Guyot DR, Manoli A II, Kling GA: Pyogenic sacroiliitis in IV drug users. *Am J Roentgenol* 149:1209, 1987.

Kido D, Bryan D, Halpern M: Hematogenous osteomyelitis in drug addicts. *Am J Roentgenol* 118:356, 1973.

Modic MT, Feiglin DH, Piraino DW, Boumphrey F, Weinstein MA, Duchesneau PM, Rehm S: Vertebral osteomyelitis: Assessment using MR. *Radiology* 157:157, 1985.

Paterson DC: Acute suppurative arthritis in infancy and childhood. *J Bone Joint Surg* 52B:474, 1970.

Phemister DB, Hatcher CM: Correlation of pathological and roentgenological findings in the diagnosis of tuberculous arthritis. *Am J Roentgenol* 29:736, 1933.

Resnik CS, Resnick D: Pyogenic osteomyelitis and septic arthritis. In: Taveras JM, Ferrucci JT (eds): *Radiology—Diagnosis, Imaging, Intervention.* Philadelphia, Lippincott, 1986.

Resnik CS, Ammann AM, Walsh JW: Chronic septic arthritis of the adult hip: Computed tomographic features. *Skeletal Radiol* 16:513, 1987.

Ruppert D, Barron BJ, Madewell JE: Osteomyelitis, acute and chronic. *Radiol Clin North Am* 25:1171, 1987.

Trueta J: The three types of acute, haematogenous osteomyelitis. *J Bone Joint Surg* 41B:671, 1959.

Waldvogel FA, Vasey MD: Osteomyelitis: The past decade. *N Engl J Med* 303:360, 1980.

Wolfgang GL: Tuberculous joint infection. *Clin Orthop* 136:225, 1978.

Young LW: Neonatal and infantile osteomyelitis and septic arthritis. In: Taveras JM, Ferrucci JT (eds): *Radiology—Diagnosis, Imaging, Intervention.* Philadelphia, Lippincott, 1986.

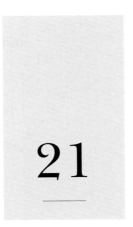

21

Radiologic Evaluation of Metabolic and Endocrine Disorders

COMPOSITION AND PRODUCTION OF BONE

BONE TISSUE CONSISTS of two types of material: 1) an extracellular material, which includes *organic matrix* or *osteoid tissue* (collagen fibrils within a mucopolysaccharide ground substance) and an *inorganic crystalline component* (calcium phosphate or hydroxyapatite);

and 2) a cellular material, which includes *osteoblasts* (cells that induce bone formation), *osteoclasts* (cells that induce bone resorption), and *osteocytes* (inactive cells).

Bone is a living, dynamic tissue; old bone is constantly being removed and replaced with new bone. Normally, this continuous process of bone resorption and formation is in balance (Fig. 21.1A),

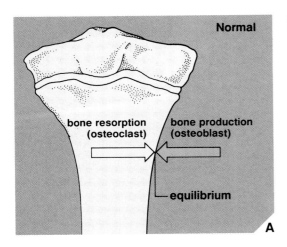

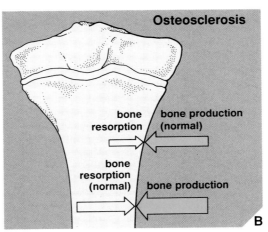

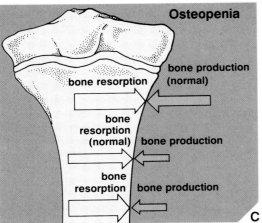

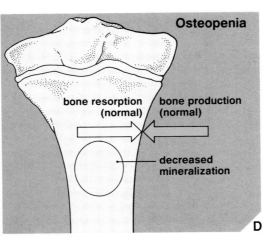

Figure 21.1 (A) In normal bone, the relationship between bone resorption and bone production is in balance. (B) One abnormal state ("too much bone") is characterized by decreased bone resorption and normal bone production, or by normal bone resorption and increased bone production. (C) The other abnormal state ("too little bone") is characterized by increased bone resorption and normal bone production, by normal bone resorption and decreased bone production, or by increased bone resorption and decreased bone production. (D) Too little bone may also be due to a decrease in bone mineralization, with bone resorption and production in balance.

and the mineral content of the bones remains relatively constant. In some abnormal circumstances, however, when the metabolism of the bone is disturbed, this balance may be upset. If, for example, osteoblasts are more active than usual, or osteoclasts are less active, more bone is produced (a state known as "too much bone") (Fig. 21.1B). If, on the other hand, osteoclasts are normal or overactive and osteoblasts underactive, less bone is produced ("too little bone") (Fig. 21.1C). A generalized reduction in bone mass may also be caused by decreased mineralization of osteoid, with equilibrium in the rate of bone resorption and production (Fig. 21.1D).

The growth and mineralization of bone are influenced by a variety of factors, the most important of which are the levels of growth hormone produced by the pituitary gland, of calcitonin produced by the thyroid gland, and of parathormone produced by the parathyroid glands, along with the dietary intake, intestinal absorption, and urinary excretion of vitamin D, calcium, and phosphorus.

It should be remembered, however, that normal bone density changes with age, increasing from infancy until age 35 to 40, and then progressively decreasing at the rate of 8% per decade in women and 3% in men.

EVALUATION OF METABOLIC AND ENDOCRINE DISORDERS

Most metabolic and endocrine disorders are characterized radiographically by abnormalities in bone density that are generally related to increased bone production, increased bone resorption, or inadequate bone mineralization. The bones affected by these conditions appear abnormally radiolucent (osteopenia) or abnormally radiodense (osteosclerosis) (Fig. 21.2).

Radiologic Imaging Modalities

The radiologic modalities most often used to evaluate metabolic and endocrine bone disorders are:

1. Plain-film radiography
2. Magnification radiography
3. Conventional tomography
4. Computed tomography (CT)
5. Radionuclide imaging (scintigraphy, bone scan).

Plain-Film and Magnification Radiography

Plain-film radiography is the simplest and most widely used method of evaluating bone density. This technique can easily detect even very small increases in bone density; however, it generally fails to detect decreases in overall skeletal mineralization unless the reduction reaches at least 30%. It must be pointed out that normal bone can easily acquire an abnormal radiographic appearance as a result of technical errors, such as improper settings for kilovoltage and milliamperage. Overexposure, for instance, creates the appearance of increased bone radiolucency, whereas underexposure creates an artificially increased bone radiodensity.

For these reasons, inspection of a standard radiograph should focus less on apparent increases or decreases in bone density than on the thickness of the bone cortex. Cortical thickness is directly correlated with skeletal mineralization; it can be objectively measured and compared either with a normal standard or with subsequent studies in the same patient. The cortical thickness measurement is obtained by adding the width of the two cortices in the midpoint of a given bone, a sum that should be roughly one-half the overall diameter of the bone; it may also be expressed as an index of bony mass, derived by dividing the combined cortical thickness by the total diameter of the bone (Fig. 21.3). The second or third metacarpal bone is frequently used to obtain these measurements (Fig. 21.4).

A related method for assessing bone density that also uses plain radiographs is the photodensitometry technique. This technique is based on the observation that the photographic density of a bone on a radiographic film is proportional to its mass. Through use of a

---

Figure 21.2 Metabolic and Endocrine Disorders Characterized by Abnormalities in Bone Density

INCREASED RADIODENSITY	INCREASED RADIOLUCENCY
Secondary hyperparathyroidism	Osteoporosis
Renal osteodystrophy	Osteomalacia
Hyperphosphatasia	Rickets
Idiopathic hypercalcemia	Scurvy
Paget disease	Primary hyperparathyroidism
Osteopetrosis*	Hypophosphatasia
Pycnodysostosis*	Acromegaly
Melorheostosis*	Gaucher disease
Hypothyroidism	Homocystinuria
Mastocytosis	Osteogenesis imperfecta*
Myelofibrosis	Fibrogenesis imperfecta
Gaucher disease (reparative stage)	Cushing syndrome
Fluorine poisoning	Ochronosis (alkaptonuria)
Intoxication with lead, bismuth, or phosphorus	Wilson disease (hepatolenticular degeneration)

*These conditions are discussed in Part VII: Congenital and Developmental Anomalies.

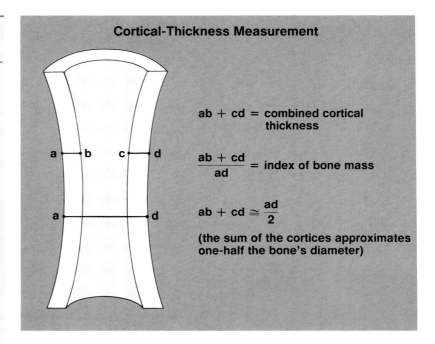

Cortical-Thickness Measurement

$ab + cd$ = combined cortical thickness

$$\dfrac{ab + cd}{ad} = \text{index of bone mass}$$

$$ab + cd \cong \dfrac{ad}{2}$$

(the sum of the cortices approximates one-half the bone's diameter)

Figure 21.3 Determination of cortical thickness is based on the measurement of the cortices of the metacarpals (usually the second or third). It may be expressed either as the simple sum of the two cortices or as that sum divided by the total thickness of the bone, in which case it is considered an index of bony mass. Normally, the sum of the cortices should be roughly one-half the overall diameter of the metacarpal bone.

photodensitometer, the photographic density of a given bone can be compared with that of known standard wedges, giving an accurate assessment of the degree of bone density.

The appearance of relative increased bone radiolucency on standard radiographs should not be called osteoporosis, since such a finding is not specific for either osteoporosis, osteomalacia, or hyperparathyroidism. Most authorities agree that increased radiolucency is best termed *osteopenia* (poverty of bone). *Osteoporosis* refers specifically to a reduction in the amount of bone tissue (deficient bone matrix) and *osteomalacia* to a reduction in the amount of mineral in the matrix (deficient mineralization); both conditions are characterized by increased bone radiolucency (Fig. 21.5). As Resnick has pointed out, any condition in which bone resorption exceeds bone formation results in osteopenia, regardless of the specific pathogenesis of the condition. In fact, diffuse osteopenia is found in osteoporosis, osteomalacia, hyperparathyroidism,

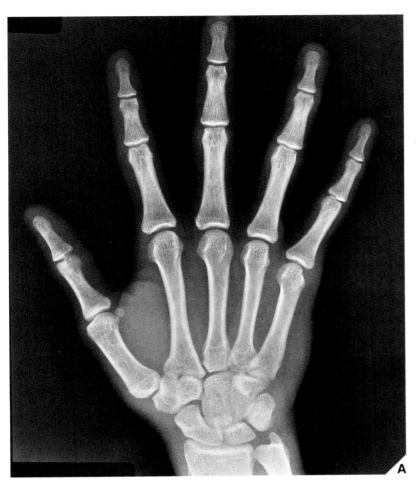
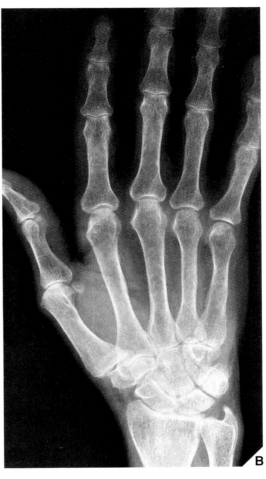

Figure 21.4 Dorso-volar views of the hand show normal (A) and abnormal (B) thickness of the cortex of the second and third metacarpal bones.

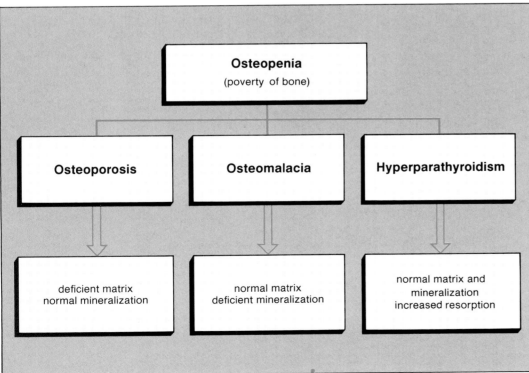

Figure 21.5 Increased radiolucency of bone on a standard radiograph is best termed osteopenia or bone rarefaction rather than osteoporosis, and it is a typical feature not only of osteoporosis but also of osteomalacia and hyperparathyroidism, which are clinically distinct conditions.

neoplastic conditions such as multiple myeloma, and a wide variety of other disorders.

Although osteopenia is a nonspecific finding, plain-film radiography can help detect other important radiographic features leading to a specific diagnosis. Among these are: Looser zones, representing pseudofractures that are characteristic of osteomalacia (Fig. 21.6); widening of the growth plate and flaring of the metaphysis, which are typical findings in rickets (Fig. 21.7); subperiosteal bone resorption, an identifying feature of hyperparathyroidism (Fig. 21.8); and focal areas of osteolytic destruction and endosteal scalloping, which are characteristic of multiple myeloma (Fig. 21.9).

Magnification radiography is useful in metabolic disorders for demonstrating the details of bone structure. The subperiosteal bone resorption characteristic of hyperparathyroidism, or cortical tunnel-

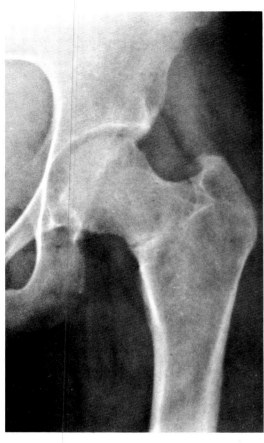

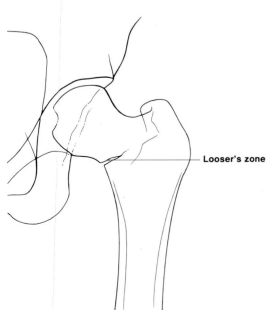

Figure 21.6 Looser zone or Pseudofracture, seen here in the femoral neck, is represented by a radiolucent defect in the cortical bone that reflects accumulation of nonmineralized osteoid tissue and is a characteristic finding in osteomalacia.

Looser's zone

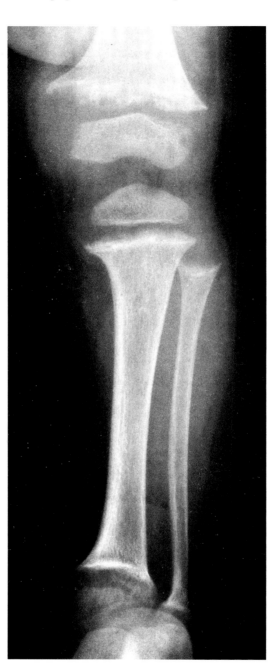

Figure 21.7 Plain film of the lower leg of a 2½-year-old child with rickets shows the characteristic widening of the growth plate, specifically the zone of provisional calcification, and "cupping" of the metaphysis.

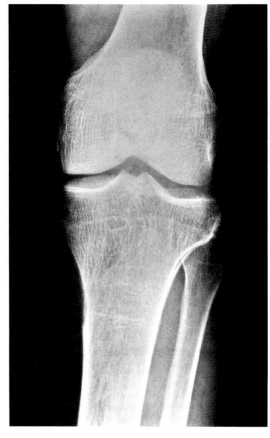

Figure 21.8 Anteroposterior view of the left knee of a 42-year-old woman with primary hyperparathyroidism due to hyperplasia of the parathyroid glands. This demonstrates increased bone radiolucency and areas of subperiosteal bone resorption on the medial aspect of the upper tibia, characteristic of the condition.

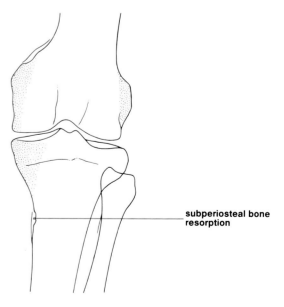

subperiosteal bone resorption

ing (Fig. 21.10), which may be seen in any process that causes increased bone resorption, can be well delineated on magnification studies. Cortical tunneling occurs very early in a pathologic process and may be found even in the absence of other radiographic abnormalities.

Conventional and Computed Tomography

While conventional tomography is occasionally useful for demonstrating lesions that are not well visualized on conventional radiographs, CT plays an important role in the evaluation of metabolic and endocrine disorders. The ability of CT to define a specific volume and to accurately measure the density of that volume makes it possible to perform quantitative analysis of bone mineral content. As Genant has pointed out, CT also has the unique ability to measure the cancellous bone of the axial skeleton, particularly that of the vertebrae, a site that is especially sensitive to metabolic stimuli.

Several methods have been developed for assessing mineral content in the spine, including single-photon absorptiometry (SPA), dual-photon absorptiometry (DPA), dual-x-ray absorptiometry (DXA), and probably the most widely used, quantitative computed tomography (QCT). SPA is used to assess the status of peripheral long bones (distal radius, distal femur), and it measures primarily cortical bone. These measurements are relatively insensitive to metabolic stimuli and therefore are of limited value for monitoring changes in the individual patient. DPA and DXA are radiologic projection methods for measuring the bone mineral content of different skeletal areas, usually the lumbar spine and the proximal femur.

In dual-photon absorptiometry, a radioisotope is used that emits photons at two different energy levels and allows differentiation of yellow and red marrow from the mineral component of the trabecular bone. DPA is based on the contrast difference between low-energy and high-energy beam attenuation in both bone and soft

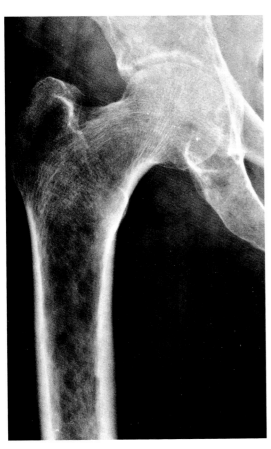

Figure 21.9 Radiograph of the hip of a 58-year-old woman with multiple myeloma shows increased radiolucency of the bones. Focal radiolucencies and endosteal scalloping can also be seen in the femur.

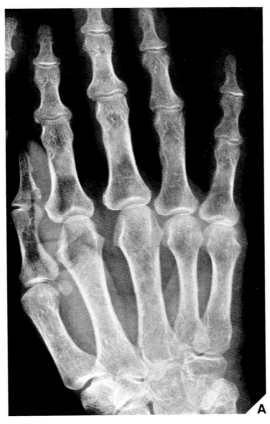

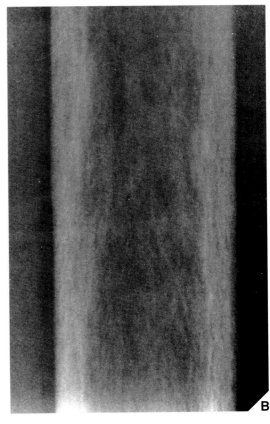

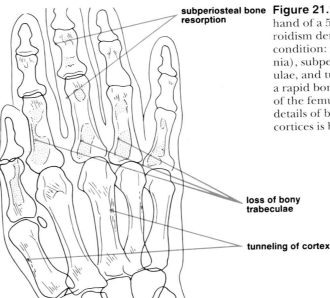

subperiosteal bone resorption

loss of bony trabeculae

tunneling of cortex

Figure 21.10 (A) Dorsovolar radiograph of the hand of a 52-year-old man with hyperparathyroidism demonstrates the typical changes of this condition: increased bone radiolucency (osteopenia), subperiosteal resorption, loss of bony trabeculae, and tunneling of the cortices, which reflects a rapid bone turnover. (B) Magnification study of the femur of the same patient shows the fine details of bone structure. The tunneling of the cortices is better appreciated.

tissue (bone yields a higher contrast at low energies than at high energies). QCT is a method for measuring the lumbar spine mineral content in which the average density values of a region of intrest are referenced to that of a calibration material scanned at the same time as the patient. Measurements are performed on CT scanner and use a mineral standard for simultaneous calibration, a computed radiograph (scout view) for localization, and either single-energy or dual-energy techniques. In quantitative CT scanning, a cross-sectional image of the vertebral body is obtained, allowing differentiation of cortical and trabecular bone. The attenuation, referenced to a mineral equivalent phantom, is expressed as a trabecular bone density in mg/cm^3 of calcium hydroxyapatite. The usual examination procedure consists of taking CT scans through the midplane line of three or four adjacent vertebral bodies, (usually from T-12 to L-3 or L-1 to L-4). Axial images of the vertebral bodies are obtained by scanning the midplane of vertebral bodies while the patient is supine on a standard phantom. The average density from all vertebrae is calculated. The patient's values are compared with the values of bone density calibrated in the phantom (Fig. 21.11). For measuring the spine, QCT has advantages over other methods because of its great sensitivity and precise three-dimensional anatomic localization, its ability to distinguish cancellous bone from cortical bone, and its ability to exclude extraosseous minerals from the measurement.

All these methods are used in clinical practice to assess patients with metabolic disease affecting the skeleton, to establish a diagnosis of osteoporosis or assess its severity, and to monitor response to

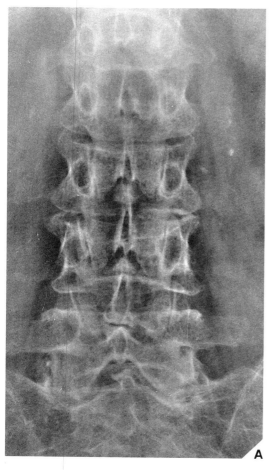

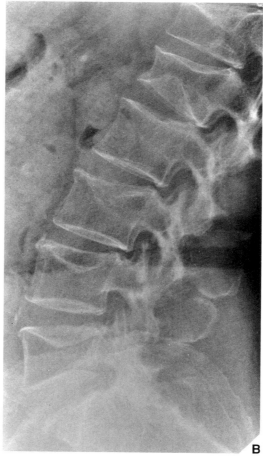

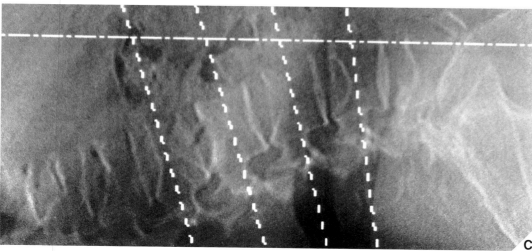

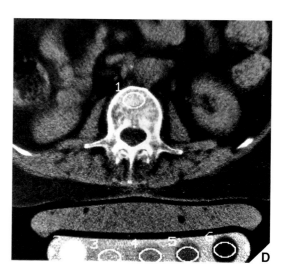

Figure 21.11 A 62-year-old woman was evaluated for degree of osteoporosis. The anteroposterior (A) and lateral (B) views of the lumbar spine show diffuse osteopenia with multiple compression fractures. Quantitative computed tomography (QCT) measurements were obtained in the following fashion: The patient was supine on a standard bone mineral calibration phantom. Values were referenced to a translucent calibration phantom scanned with the patient, which contains tubes filled with standard solutions of potassium phosphate (representing minerals) ethanol (representing fat), and water (representing soft tissue). For each axial image, the regions of interest were positioned over the center portion of the phantom calibration compartments, as well as over the central portion of the vertebral body. Transverse (axial) CT scans were made through L-1, L-2, L-3, and L-4, with phantom included. Bone density values in mg/cm^3 were calculated for each vertebral body using the CT numbers (Hounsfield units) obtained from the calibrated density phantom (C,D). Readings are averaged and compared with normal values for given age and sex. Average of readings for vertebral mineral content is also expressed in mg/cm^3. In this particular case, the average values of 77.4 mg of mineral/cm^3 are below the average values for the patient's age (97.5 mg/cm^3) as well as below the levels of fracture threshold (110 mg/cm^3).

therapy. In general, the usefulness of CT for measurement of bone mineral lies in its ability to provide a measurement of trabecular, cortical, or integral bone, in either the axial or appendicular skeleton. In particular, these methods are useful for measurement of spinal bone mineral density in postmenopausal women, in patients with existing osteoporosis, and in patients being treated with corticosteroids.

Scintigraphy

Radionuclide imaging is a nonspecific modality, but it is a very sensitive detector of active bone turnover. For this reason, it is frequently effective in the evaluation of various metabolic diseases. It is particu-

larly valuable in screening patients with Paget disease to determine the distribution of the lesion and activity of the disease (Fig. 21.12). Insufficiency type stress fractures frequently seen in osteomalacia may be identified by this modality. In renal osteodystrophy, radionuclide bone scan may reveal the absence of renal images, confirming poor renal function. In hyperparathyroidism, it may detect silent sites of brown tumors. In the reflex sympathetic dystrophy syndrome, it may reveal abnormalities in the affected bone even prior to positive changes seen on standard radiography. Similarly, in regional migratory osteoporosis focal abnormalities may be present on the radionuclide bone scan long before radiographic changes become prominent.

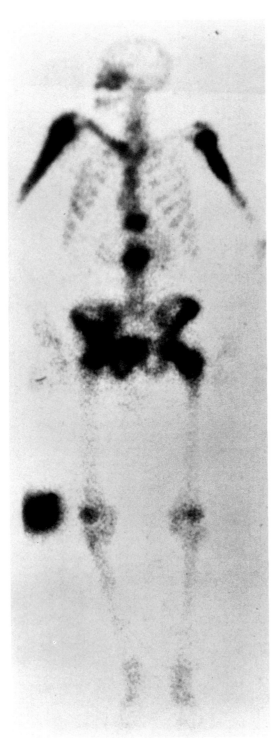

Figure 21.12 Radionuclide bone scan in this 72-year-old man with obvious clinical and radiographic evidence of Paget disease in the pelvis and proximal femora shows additional, silent sites of involvement in both patellae and humeri, as well as in several thoracic and lumbar vertebrae.

PRACTICAL POINTS TO REMEMBER

[1] On a standard radiograph increased bone radiolucency (osteopenia) or increased bone density (osteosclerosis) is related to the process of bone formation and resorption, which under normal circumstances is in equilibrium.
  • If bone resorption exceeds bone production, either because of an increase in osteoclast activity or a decrease in osteoblast activity, or if there is insufficient mineral deposition in the matrix, the result is increased radiolucency of the bone.
  • If bone production surpasses bone resorption, either because of an increase in osteoblast activity or a decrease in osteoclast activity, the result is increased radiodensity of the bone.

[2] Instead of the specific term *osteoporosis*, the nonspecific descriptive term *osteopenia* is used to refer to any generalized or regional rarefaction of the skeleton, expressed radiographically as increased bone radiolucency, regardless of the specific pathogenesis. The main reason for this usage is that it is usually impossible to distinguish between the various causes of increased bone radiolucency. The term *osteosclerosis* refers to any increase in bone density, again regardless of the etiology of the condition.

[3] Osteoporosis is a specific term defining a state in which bone tissue (bone matrix) is reduced but mineralization of the organic matrix is normal. Osteomalacia is a specific term defining a state in which there is insufficient mineralization of osteoid tissue.

[4] The important radiologic modalities used in evaluation of various metabolic and endocrine conditions include:
  • plain-film radiography
  • magnification radiography
  • conventional tomography
  • computed tomography
  • radionuclide imaging (scintigraphy, bone scan).

[5] Several methods have been developed for accurate assessment of mineral content of the bone, including single-photon absorptiometry (SPA), dual-photon absorptiometry (DPA), dual-x-ray absorptiometry (DXA), and quantitative computed tomography (QCT).

[6] QCT is an accurate method for measuring mineral content of cancellous (trabecular) bone of the vertebrae. In this method, the average density of a measured region is referenced to that of a calibration phantom exposed simultaneously with a patient undergoing examination.

[7] Scintigraphy is a nonspecific but very sensitive modality to detect bone turnover in various metabolic and endocrine disorders.

References

Cann CE: Quantitative CT for determination of bone mineral density: A review. *Radiology* 166:509, 1988.

Cann CE, Genant HK: Precise measurement of vertebral mineral content using computed tomography. *J Comput Assist Tomogr* 4:493, 1980.

Garn SM, Poznanski AK, Nagy JM: Bone measurement in the differential diagnosis of osteopenia and osteoporosis. *Radiology* 100:509, 1971.

Genant HK, Block JE, Steiger P, Glueer CC, Ettinger B, Harris ST: Appropriate use of bone densitometry. *Radiology* 170:817, 1989.

Genant HK, Cann CE, Ettinger B, et al: Quantitative computed tomography for spinal mineral assessment: Current status. *J Comput Assist Tomogr* 9:602, 1985.

Griffith HJ, Zimmerman R, Bailey G, Snider R: The use of photon absorptiometry in the diagnosis of renal osteodystrophy. *Radiology* 109:277, 1973.

Jensen PS, Orphanoudakis SC, Baron R, Lang R, Rauschkolb EN, Rasmussen H: Determination of bone mass by CT and correlation with quantitative histomorphometric analysis. *J Comput Assist Tomogr* 3:847, 1979.

Krolner B, Nielsen SP: Bone mineral content of the lumbar spine in normal and osteoporotic women: Cross-sectional and longitudinal studies. *Clin Sci* 62:329, 1982.

Krolner B, Nielsen SP: Measurement of bone mineral contents (BMC) of the lumbar spine, part I: Theory and application of a new two-dimensional dual photon attenuation method. *Scand J Clin Lab Invest* 40:485, 1980.

Lang P, Steiger P, Faulkner K, Glüer C, Genant HK: Osteoporosis. Current techniques and recent developments in quantitative bone densitometry. *Radiol Clin North Am* 29:49, 1991.

Mazess, RB: Bone densitometry of the axial skeleton. *Orthop Clin North Am* 21:51, 1990.

Mazess RB, Barden HS: Measurement of bone by dual-photon absorptiometry (DPA) and dual-energy x-ray absorptiometry (DEXA). *Ann Chir Gynaecol* 77:197, 1988.

Pullan BR, Roberts TE: Bone mineral measurement using an EMI scanner and standard methods: A comparative study. *Br J Radiol* 51:24, 1978.

Resnick D, Niwayama G: Osteoporosis. In: *Diagnosis of Bone and Joint Disorders, vol 2.* Philadelphia, Saunders, 1981, p 1638.

Reynolds WA, Karo JJ: Radiographic diagnosis of metabolic bone disease. *Orthop Clin North Am* 3:521, 1972.

Rupich R, Pacifici R, Delabar C, et al: Lateral dual energy radiography: New technique for the measurement of L3 bone mineral density. *J Bone Miner Res* 4:S194, 1989.

Sartoris DJ, Resnick D: Dual energy radiographic absorptiometry for bone densitometry: Current status and prospective. *Am J Roentgenol* 152:241, 1989.

Virtama P, Helela T: Radiographic measurements of corti bone. *Acta Radiol* (suppl) 293:7, 1969.

Virtama P, Helala T: Radiographic measurements of cortical bone: Variations in a normal population between 1 and 90 years of age. *Acta Radiol* (suppl) 293:1, 1969.

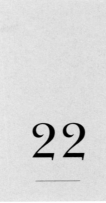

22

Osteoporosis, Rickets, and Osteomalacia

OSTEOPOROSIS

OSTEOPOROSIS IS A GENERALIZED metabolic bone disease characterized by insufficient formation or increased resorption of bone matrix that results in decreased bone mass. Although there is a reduction in the amount of bone tissue, the tissue present is still fully mineralized. In other words, the bone is quantitatively deficient but qualitatively normal.

Osteoporosis has a variety of possible causes and consequently manifests in a number of different forms (Fig. 22.1). The basic distinction in osteoporosis is between those types that are *generalized* or *diffuse*, involving the entire skeleton, and those that are *localized* to a single region or bone (*regional*) (Fig. 22.2). The basic distinction between possible causes is between those that are *congenital* and those that are *acquired*.

Figure 22.1 Causes of Osteoporosis

GENERALIZED (DIFFUSE)

Genetic (Congenital)
Osteogenesis imperfecta
Gonadal dysgenesis:
  Turner syndrome (XO)
  Klinefelter syndrome (XXY)
Hypophosphatasia
Homocystinuria
Mucopolysaccharidosis
Gaucher disease
Anemias:
  Sickle-cell syndromes
  Thalassemia
  Hemophilia
  Christmas disease

Endocrine
Hyperthyroidism
Hyperparathyroidism
Cushing syndrome
Acromegaly
Estrogen deficiency
Hypogonadism
Diabetes mellitus
Pregnancy

Deficiency States
Scurvy
Malnutrition
Anorexia nervosa
Protein deficiency
Alcoholism
Liver disease

Neoplastic
Myeloma
Leukemia
Lymphoma
Metastatic disease

Iatrogenic
Heparin-induced
Dilantin-induced
Steroid-induced

Miscellaneous
Involutional (senescent/postmenopausal)
Amyloidosis
Ochronosis
Paraplegia
Weightlessness
Idiopathic

LOCALIZED (REGIONAL)

Immobilization (cast)
Disuse
Pain
Infection
Reflex sympathetic dystrophy syndrome
    (Sudeck atrophy)
Transient regional osteoporosis:
  Transient osteoporosis of the hip
  Regional migratory osteoporosis
  Idiopathic juvenile osteoporosis
Paget disease (hot phase)

Generalized Osteoporosis

Certain radiographic features are common to virtually all forms of osteoporosis, regardless of their specific cause. There is always some diminution of cortical thickness and decrease in the number and thickness of the spongy bone trabeculae. These changes are more prominent in nonweight-bearing segments and those not subject to stress. The first sites affected by osteoporosis, as well as the ones that are best demonstrated on radiographic study, are the periarticular regions, where the cortex is anatomically thinner. In the long bones, the thickness of the cortices decreases, the bones become brittle, and there is increased clinical incidence of fractures, particularly of the proximal femur (Fig. 22.3), the proximal humerus, the distal radius, and the ribs.

Besides quantitative computed tomography (QCT) and other methods of evaluating osteoporosis (discussed in detail in Chapter 21), some simple methods using plain film radiography have been developed.

The analysis of the trabecular pattern of the bones has been emphasized as an effective method to evaluate osteoporosis, since patterns of trabecular loss correlate well with increasing severity of osteoporosis.

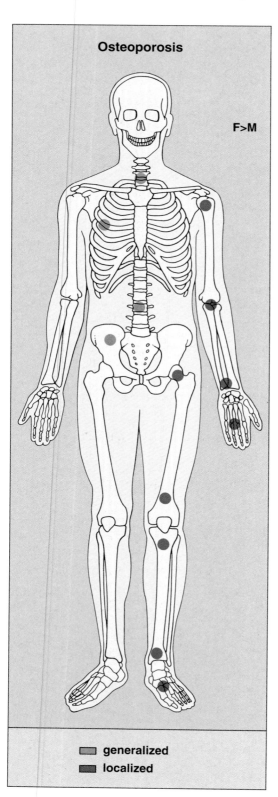

Osteoporosis

F>M

☐ generalized
☐ localized

Figure 22.2 Target sites of osteoporosis.

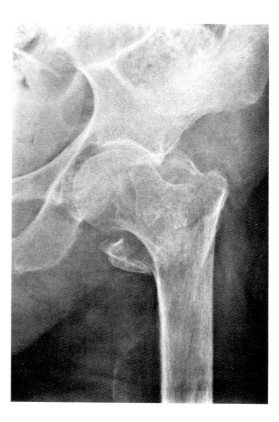

Figure 22.3
An 85-year-old woman with advanced post-menopausal osteoporosis sustained an intertrochanteric fracture of the left femur, as seen on this antero-posterior view. Note the thinning of the cortex and the increased radio-lucency of the bones.

In the femur, these changes may be evaluated using Singh index, which is based on the trabecular architecture of the proximal femur—namely, the pattern of the principal compressive group of trabeculae, the secondary compressive group of trabeculae, and the principal tensile group of trabeculae (Fig. 22.4). The trabecular pattern of the proximal end of the femur is an excellent indicator of the severity of the osteoporosis. Singh has shown that trabecular loss occurs in a predictable sequence that can be used to grade the severity of osteopenia. He recognized that the compressive trabeculae were more essential than the tensile trabeculae, and that the peripherally located trabeculae were more vital than central ones.

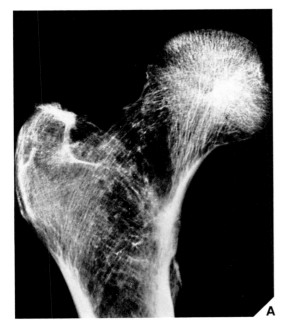

Figure 22.4 (A) The trabecular pattern of the proximal end of the femur is an excellent indicator of the severity of the osteoporosis. (B) The most readily visible trabeculae belong to one of five groups. (C) The trabecular arcades important to the Singh trabecular index. Confluence of principal tensile, principal compressive, and secondary compressive trabeculae in the femoral neck forms a triangular region of radio-lucency, Ward triangle. The principal tensile trabeculae are more important than the secondary trabeculae, the compressive trabeculae more important than the tensile trabeculae.
Bone loss occurs in order of increasing importance. (Modified from Singh M, et al., 1970)

Figure 22.4B The Five Major Groups of Trabeculae

1. Principal Compressive Group
   - Extend from medial cortex of femoral neck to superior part of femoral head
   - Major weight-bearing trabeculae
   - In normal femur are the thickest and most densely packed
   - Appear accentuated in osteoporosis
   - Last to be obliterated

2. Secondary Compressive Group
   - Originate at the cortex, near the lesser trochanter
   - Curve upwards and laterally toward the greater trochanter and upper femoral neck
   - Characteristically thin and widely separated

3. Principal Tensile Group
   - Originate from the lateral cortex, inferior to the greater trochanter
   - Extend in an arch-like configuration medially, terminating in the inferior portion of the femoral head

4. Secondary Tensile Group
   - Arise from the lateral cortex below the principal tensile group
   - Extend superiorly and medially to terminate after crossing the middle of the femoral neck

5. Greater Trochanter Group
   - Composed of slender and poorly defined tensile trabeculae
   - Arise laterally below the greater trochanter
   - Extend upward to terminate near the greater trochanter's superior surface

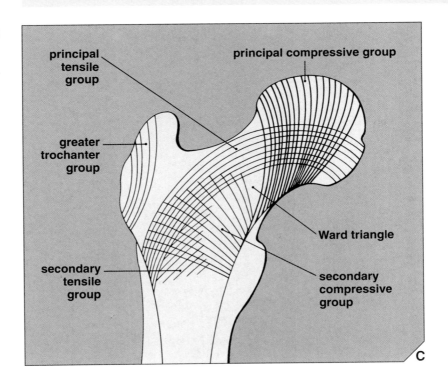

Six radiologic grades have been defined according to the trabecular pattern (Fig. 22.5).

In early osteoporosis, both the compressive and tensile trabeculae are accentuated because of initial resorption of the randomly oriented trabeculae, and thus the radiolucency of the Ward triangle becomes more prominent. With increasing severity of osteoporosis, the tensile trabeculae are reduced in number and regress from the medial femoral border to the lateral. When trabecular resorption increases, the outer portion of the principal tensile trabeculae opposite the greater trochanter disappear, opening the Ward triangle laterally. As osteoporosis increases in severity, resorption of all trabeculae occur, with the exception of those in the principal compressive group. In advanced osteoporosis, the principal compressive component is the last to be involved, a process manifested by a decrease in the number and length of individual trabeculae. Eventually, the upper femur may be completely devoid of all trabecular markings.

The other major area in which osteoporotic changes are evaluated is the axial skeleton, particularly the spine. This is especially true in osteoporosis associated with aging—i.e., *involutional* (senescent and postmenopausal) *osteoporosis*—in which the vertebral bodies are particularly vulnerable. Initially, there is a relative increase in the density of the vertebral end plates due to resorption of the spongy bone, causing what is called an "empty box" appearance (Fig. 22.6). Later, there is an overall decrease in density with a loss of any trabecular pattern, creating a "ground glass" appearance. A typical

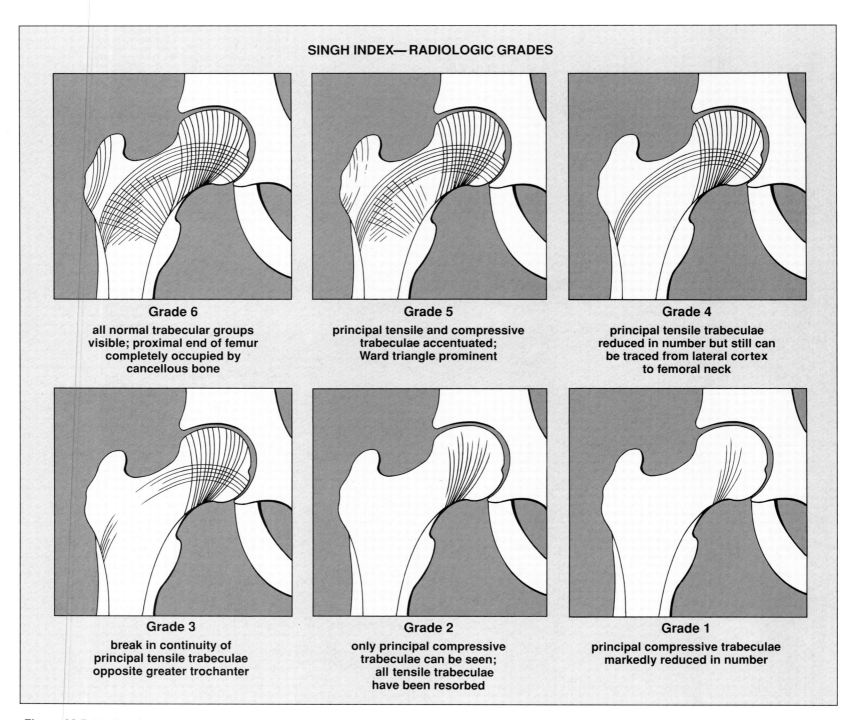

SINGH INDEX— RADIOLOGIC GRADES

Grade 6
all normal trabecular groups visible; proximal end of femur completely occupied by cancellous bone

Grade 5
principal tensile and compressive trabeculae accentuated; Ward triangle prominent

Grade 4
principal tensile trabeculae reduced in number but still can be traced from lateral cortex to femoral neck

Grade 3
break in continuity of principal tensile trabeculae opposite greater trochanter

Grade 2
only principal compressive trabeculae can be seen; all tensile trabeculae have been resorbed

Grade 1
principal compressive trabeculae markedly reduced in number

Figure 22.5 Singh Index—radiologic grades. (Modified from Singh M, et al., 1970)

feature of vertebral involvement in osteoporosis is biconcavity of the body, which exhibits a "fish mouth" appearance ("codfish vertebrae") (Fig. 22.7). This presentation results from expansion of the disks, leading to arch-like indentations on both superior and inferior margins of the weakened vertebral bodies. In advanced stages, there is complete collapse of the vertebral body associated with a wedge-shaped deformity. In the thoracic spine this leads to increased kyphosis.

Of special interest in generalized osteoporosis are the three major varieties of *iatrogenic osteoporosis. Heparin-induced osteoporosis* may develop after long-term, high-dose daily heparin treatment (more than 10,000 units). Precisely how this type of osteoporosis is initiated and develops is not clearly understood, although osteoclastic stimulation and osteoblastic inhibition with suppressed endochondral ossification have been implicated as potential causes. Spontaneous fractures of the vertebrae, ribs, and femoral neck are noted on radiographic studies. *Dilantin-induced osteoporosis* occasionally develops after prolonged use of phenytoin (Dilantin). The vertebral column and ribs are usually affected, and fractures are a common complication.

Steroid-induced osteoporosis, occurring either during the course of Cushing syndrome or iatrogenically during treatment with various corticosteroids, is characterized by decreased bone formation and increased bone resorption. Although the axial skeleton is most often affected, the appendicular skeleton may also be involved. In the spine, considerable thickening and sclerosis of the vertebral end plates occur without a concomitant change in the anterior and posterior vertebral margins.

Osteoporosis associated with neoplastic processes is discussed in Chapters 15 and 18.

Localized Osteoporosis

Transient regional osteoporosis is a collective term for a group of conditions that have one feature in common: rapidly developing osteoporosis that usually affects the periarticular regions and has no definite etiology like trauma or immobilization. It is a self-limiting and reversible disorder, of which three subtypes have been described. *Transient osteoporosis of the hip* is seen predominantly in pregnant women and in young and middle-aged men. Its primary manifestation is local osteoporosis involving the femoral head and neck and the acetabulum. *Regional migratory osteoporosis,* which affects the knee, the ankle, and the foot, is mainly seen in men in their fourth and fifth decades. This migratory condition is characterized by pain and swelling around the affected joints. It develops rapidly and subsides in about six to nine months; there may be subsequent recurrence and involvement of other joints. *Idiopathic juvenile osteoporosis* is commonly seen during or just before puberty, and typically regresses spontaneously. Skeletal involvement is often symmetrical and is generally juxta-articular in location. It is frequently associated with pain and the presence of vertebral body compression fractures.

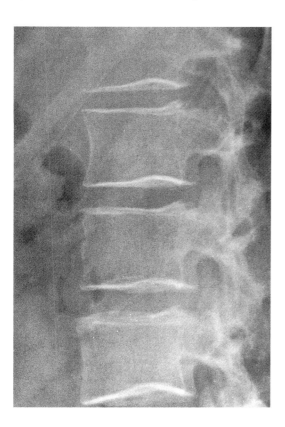

Figure 22.6 Lateral radiograph of the lumbar spine of an 89-year-old woman demonstrates a relative increase in the density of the vertebral end plates and resorption of the trabeculae of spongy bone, creating an "empty box" appearance. This is commonly seen in involutional osteoporosis.

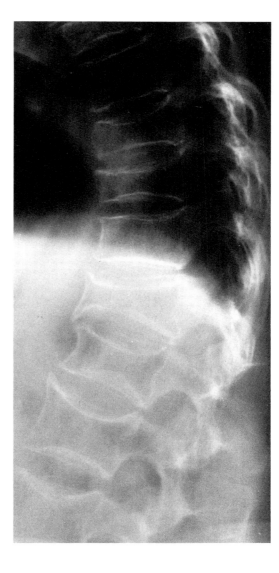

Figure 22.7 Biconcavity or "codfish vertebrae," seen here on the lateral view of the thoracolumbar spine in an 80-year-old woman with osteoporosis, results from weakness of the vertebral end plates and intravertebral expansion of nuclei pulposi.

Localized osteoporosis secondary to immobilization in a cast or due to disuse of a painful limb is discussed in Chapter 4. Sudeck atrophy (reflex sympathetic dystrophy syndrome) may also occur as a complication of fractures (see Fig. 4.47).

RICKETS AND OSTEOMALACIA

Whereas in osteoporosis the fundamental change is decreased bone mass, in rickets (which occurs in children) and osteomalacia (which occurs in adults) the essential bone abnormality is faulty mineralization (calcification) of the bone matrix. If adequate amounts of calcium and phosphorus are not available, proper calcification of osteoid tissue cannot occur.

In the past, the most common cause of rickets and osteomalacia was *deficient intake* of vitamin D, which is responsible for calcium and phosphorus homeostasis and for maintenance of proper bone mineralization. Now, however, the major causes include *inadequate intestinal absorption*, resulting in loss of calcium and phosphorus through the gastrointestinal tract in patients who have gastric, biliary, or enteric abnormalities or have undergone gastrectomy or other gastric surgery; *renal tubular disorders* (proximal and/or distal tubular lesions frequently leading to renal tubular acidosis); and *renal osteodystrophy* secondary to renal failure, which results in loss of calcium through the kidneys. Several other conditions associated with osteomalacia have been identified, such as neurofibromatosis, fibrous dysplasia, and Wilson disease, but the exact relationship between the underlying disorder and osteomalacia is still unclear (Fig. 22.8).

Rickets

Infantile Rickets

Found mainly in infants between 6 and 18 months of age, infantile rickets is characterized by generalized demineralization of the skeleton, which leads to bowing deformities in weight-bearing bones when infants begin to stand and walk. Infants with early rickets are

---

Figure 22.8 Etiology of Rickets and Osteomalacia

Nutritional Deficiency
Vitamin D:
  Dietary
  Insufficient sunlight
  Impaired synthesis
Calcium
Phosphorus

Absorption Abnormalities
Gastric surgery
Intestinal surgery (bypass)
Gastric disorders (obstruction)
Intestinal disorders (sprue)
Biliary diseases

Renal Disorders
Renal tubular disorders:
  Proximal tubular lesions (failure of absorption of inorganic
    phosphate, glucose, amino acids)
  Distal tubular lesions (renal tubular acidosis)
  Combined proximal and distal tubular lesions
Renal osteodystrophy

Miscellaneous
Associated with:
  Wilson disease
  Fibrogenesis imperfecta
  Fibrous dysplasia
  Neurofibromatosis
  Hypophosphatasia
  Neoplasm

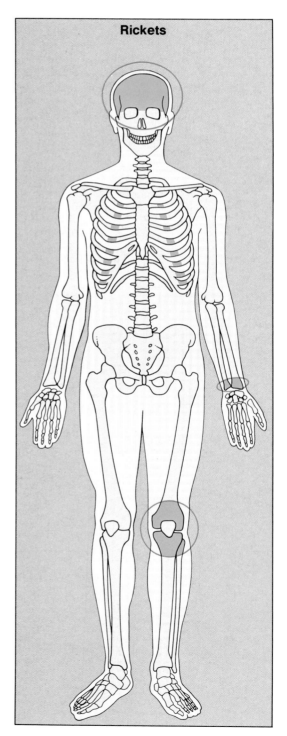

Rickets

Figure 22.9 Target sites of rickets.

restless and sleep poorly. Closing of the fontanelles is delayed. The earliest physical sign is softening of the cranial vault (craniotabes). Enlargement of the cartilage at the costochondral junction produces a prominence known as "rachitic rosary." The serum values of calcium and phosphorus are low, and that of alkaline phosphatase is increased.

The key radiographic features are observed in the metaphysis and the epiphysis—the regions where growth is most active—particularly at the distal ends of the radius, ulna, and femur, as well as at the proximal ends of the tibia and fibula (Fig. 22.9). Deficient mineralization in the provisional zone of calcification is reflected in widening of the growth plate and cupping and flaring of the metaphysis, which appears disorganized and "frayed" (Fig. 22.10; see also Fig. 21.7). In the secondary ossification centers of the epiphysis, similar changes are seen; the bone becomes radiolucent, with loss of sharpness at the periphery, and bowing deformities frequently occur (Fig. 22.11).

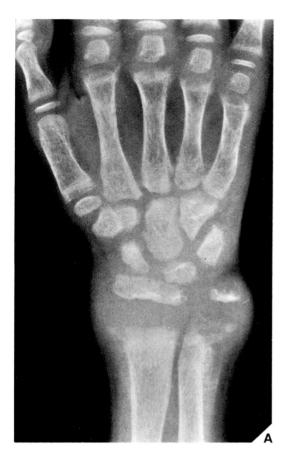
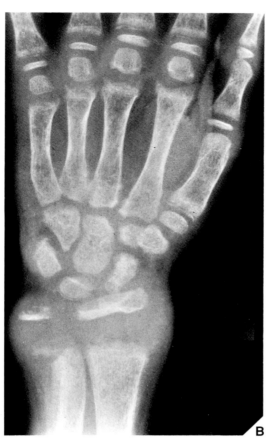

Figure 22.10 (A, B) Dorsovolar view of both hands of an 8-year-old boy with untreated dietary rickets shows osteopenia of the bones, widening of the growth plates of the distal radius and ulna, and flaring of the metaphyses, all typical features of this condition.

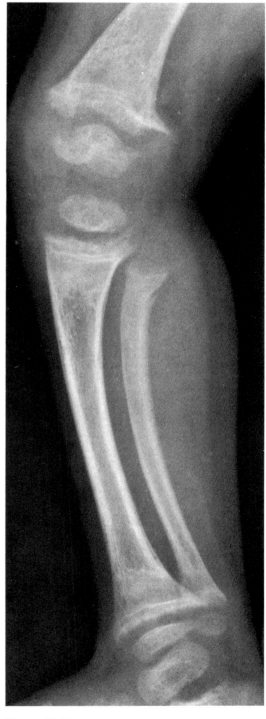

Figure 22.11 Lateral radiograph of the lower leg of a 3-year-old girl with vitamin D-deficiency rickets shows increased bone radiolucency, widening of the growth plates, cupping and flaring of the metaphyses, and blurring of the outline of the secondary ossification centers, all radiographic hallmarks of this condition. Note also bowing of both the tibia and fibula, a frequent feature of rickets.

Vitamin D-Resistant Rickets

This condition is found in older children (those above 30 months of age), and four distinct types have been reported. *Classic vitamin D-resistant* (or *hypophosphatemic*) *rickets*, also known as *familial vitamin D-resistant rickets*, is a congenital disorder that is transmitted as a sex-linked dominant trait. It is characterized by hypophosphatemia and normal levels of serum calcium. Patients are short, stocky, and bow-legged. Ectopic calcifications and ossifications in the axial and the appendicular skeleton, along with occasional sclerotic changes, are among the identifying radiographic findings. *Vitamin D-resistant rickets with glycosuria* is characterized by an abnormal resorptive mechanism for glucose and inorganic phosphate. *Fanconi syndrome* is characterized by a defect in the proximal renal tubules and deficient resorption of phosphate, glucose, and several amino acids. *Acquired hypophosphatemic syndrome* manifests in late adolescence or early adulthood; it is probably of toxic etiology.

The radiographic findings in all four types of vitamin D-resistant rickets are similar to those in infantile rickets. Bowing of the legs and shortening of the long bones, however, are more pronounced, and occasionally the bones appear sclerotic (Fig. 22.12).

Osteomalacia

Osteomalacia, which results from the same pathomechanism as rickets, occurs only after bone growth has ceased, and hence the term refers to changes in the cortical and trabecular bone of the axial and appendicular skeleton. It is most often caused by faulty absorption of fat-soluble vitamin D from the gastrointestinal tract secondary to malabsorption syndrome. It may also result from dysfunction of the proximal renal tubules, resulting in so-called renal osteomalacia. The most common clinical presentation of this condition is bone pain and muscle weakness.

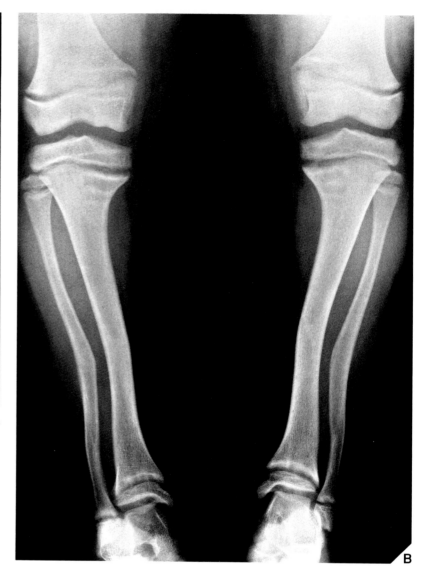

Figure 22.12 A) Anteroposterior view of the femora of a 9-year-old girl with vitamin D-resistant (hypophosphatemic) rickets shows lateral bowing and shortening of both bones. There is also evidence of sclerotic changes, which are occasionally seen in this condition. (B) The knees and lower legs of the same patient show a bowing deformity of the tibiae and fibulae, as well as widening and deformity of the growth plates about the knee and the distal femora and tibiae.

Histologically, osteomalacia is characterized by excessive quantities of inadequately mineralized bone matrix (osteoid) coating the surfaces of trabeculae in spongy bone and lining the haversian canals in the cortex.

Radiographically, osteomalacia presents with generalized osteopenia, and multiple, bilateral, and often symmetrical radiolucent lines are seen in the cortex perpendicular to the long axis of the bone; they are referred to as "pseudofractures" or Looser zones (Fig. 22.13, see also Fig. 21.6). These defects, which represent cortical stress fractures filled with poorly mineralized callus, osteoid, and fibrous tissue, are common along the axillary margins of the scapulae, the inner margin of the femoral neck, the proximal dorsal aspect of the ulnae, the ribs, and the pubic and ischial rami (Fig. 22.14). The condition, described by Milkman and known as "Milkman syndrome," is a mild form of osteomalacia in which the pseudofractures are particularly numerous.

Renal Osteodystrophy

A skeletal response to longstanding renal disease, renal osteodystrophy (also referred to as "uremic osteopathy") is usually associated with chronic renal failure due to glomerulonephritis or pyelonephritis. The condition is also seen in patients who are on dialysis or who have undergone renal transplantation.

Two main mechanisms, acting in unison but varying in severity and proportion, are responsible for bony changes associated with this condition: secondary hyperparathyroidism and abnormal vitamin D metabolism. The secondary hyperparathyroidism is provoked by phosphate retention and leads to depression of serum calcium, which in turn stimulates release of parathormone from parathyroid glands. The abnormal vitamin D metabolism is affected by renal insufficiency, since the kidney is the source of an enzyme, 25-OH-D-1α-hydroxylase, which converts the inactive vitamin D from 25-hydroxyvitamin D (25-OH-D) to active 1,25-dihydroxyvitamin D

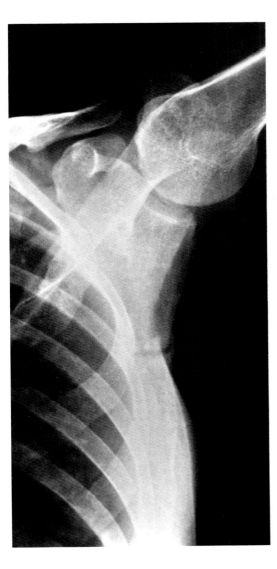

Figure 22.13 Anteroposterior radiograph of the shoulder of a 25-year-old woman with osteomalacia due to malabsorption syndrome shows a radiolucent cleft perpendicular to the cortex of the scapula. Such defects, known as pseudofractures (Looser zones), are almost pathognomonic for osteomalacia (see also Fig. 21.6).

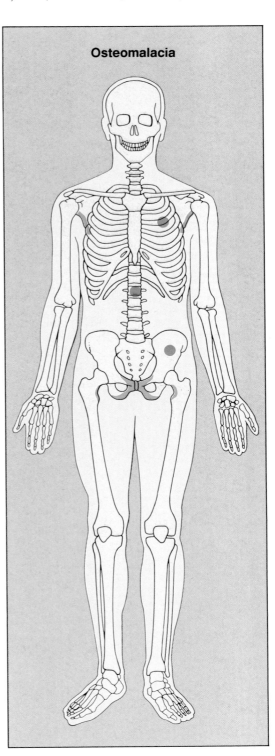

Osteomalacia

Figure 22.14 Target sites of osteomalacia.

(1,25 (OH)$_2$D). Only this most potent, physiologically active form of vitamin D is responsible for calcium and phosphorus homeostasis and for maintenance of proper bone mineralization.

The major radiographic manifestations of renal osteodystrophy are those associated with rickets, osteomalacia, and secondary hyperparathyroidism. Osteomalacia secondary to renal osteodystrophy is seldom seen in its pure form; usually there are superimposed changes typical of secondary hyperparathyroidism (Fig. 22.15). Increased bone radiolucency and cortical thinning may be present, but Looser zones are very uncommon. In most patients, some sclerotic changes develop in the bones. Slipped epiphyses may be seen in advanced uremic disease.

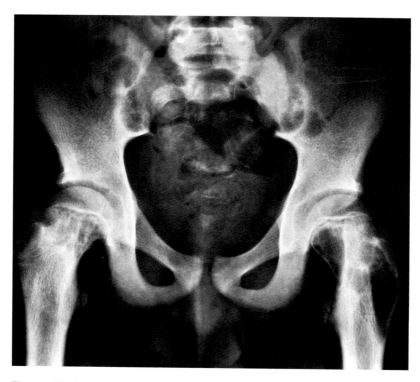

Figure 22.15 A 13-year-old boy with posterior urethral valves and secondary renal failure exhibited radiographic changes typical of renal osteodystrophy, encompassing a mixture of osteomalacia and secondary hyperparathyroidism. Anteroposterior view of the pelvis shows sclerotic changes in the bones and characteristic widening of the sacroiliac joints. The multiple cystic defects in the femora indicate secondary hyperparathyroidism.

PRACTICAL POINTS TO REMEMBER

Osteoporosis

[1] Osteoporosis is characterized by:
- insufficient formation or increased resorption of bone matrix, resulting in decreased bone mass
- increased radiolucency of bone and thinning of the cortices on standard radiography.

[2] The target sites of osteoporotic changes are:
- the axial skeleton (spine and pelvis)
- the periarticular regions of the appendicular skeleton.

[3] The analysis of the trabecular pattern in the proximal end of femur (Singh index) is an effective method of evaluating osteoporosis, since patterns of trabecular loss correlate well with increasing severity of osteoporosis.

[4] In the spine, characteristic radiographic features that indicate the severity of osteoporotic involvement are:
- "empty box" appearance (early stage)
- "codfish vertebrae"
- multiple wedge-shaped fractures (advanced stage).

[5] The most effective method of evaluating osteoporosis is quantitative computed tomography (QCT) for measuring the lumbar spine mineral content.

Rickets and Osteomalacia

[1] Rickets (in children) and osteomalacia (in adults) are the result of faulty mineralization (calcification) of the bone matrix.

[2] On radiographic examination, rickets is characterized by:
- generalized osteopenia
- bowing deformities of the long bones, particularly the femur and tibia
- widening of the growth plate (secondary to deficient mineralization in the provisional zone of calcification) and cupping or flaring of the metaphysis, particularly in the proximal humerus, distal radius and ulna, and distal femur.

[3] The radiographic findings in vitamin D-resistant rickets are similar to those in infantile rickets. Bowing deformities and shortening of the long bones are, however, more pronounced.

[4] Radiographically, osteomalacia is characterized by:
- generalized osteopenia
- symmetrical, radiolucent lines in the cortex (Looser zones or pseudofractures).

[5] Renal osteodystrophy, usually associated with chronic renal failure due to glomerulonephritis or pyelonephritis, represents a skeletal response to longstanding renal disease. The major radiographic manifestations are those associated with rickets, osteomalacia, and secondary hyperparathyroidism, with predominance of osteosclerosis, bone resorption, and bowing deformities.

References

Arnstein AR: Regional osteoporosis. *Orthop Clin North Am* 3:585, 1972.

Beaulieu JG, Razzano D, Levine RB: Transient osteoporosis of the hip in pregnancy. Review of the literature and a case report. *Clin Orthop* 115:165, 1976.

Cotton GE, Van Puffelen P: Hypophosphatemic osteomalacia secondary to neoplasia. *J Bone Joint Surg* 68:129, 1986.

Cumming WA: Idiopathic juvenile osteoporosis. *Can Assoc Radiol J* 21:19, 1970.

Dunn AW: Senile osteoporosis. *Geriatrics* 22:175, 1967.

Gillespie T III, Gillespy MP: Osteoporosis. *Radiol Clin North Am* 29:77, 1991.

Greenfield GB: Roentgen appearance of bone and soft tissue changes in chronic renal disease. *Am J Roentgenol* 116:749, 1972.

Griffith GC, Nichols G Jr, Asher JD, Flanagan B: Heparin osteoporosis. *JAMA* 193:91, 1965.

Houang MTW, Brenton DP, Renton P, Shaw DG: Idiopathic juvenile osteoporosis. *Skeletal Radiol* 3:17, 1978.

Hunder GG, Kelly PJ: Roentgenologic transient osteoporosis of the hip. A clinical syndrome? *Ann Intern Med* 68:539, 1968.

Jaworski AFG: Pathophysiology, diagnosis, and treatment of osteomalacia. *Orthop Clin North Am* 3:623, 1972.

Jones G: Radiological appearance of disuse osteoporosis. *Clin Radiol* 20:345, 1969.

Kaplan FS: Osteoporosis: Pathophysiology and prevention. *Clin Symposia* 39:2, 1987.

Mankin HJ: Rickets, osteomalacia, and renal osteodystrophy— Part I. *J Bone Joint Surg* 56A:101, 1974.

Mankin HJ: Rickets, osteomalacia, and renal osteodystrophy— Part II. *J Bone Joint Surg* 56A:352, 1974.

McCarthy JT, Kumar R: Behavior of the vitamin D endocrine system in the development of renal osteodystrophy. *Semin Nephrol* 6:21, 1986.

Milkman LA: Pseudofractures (hunger osteopathy, late rickets, osteomalacia). *Am J Roentgenol* 24:29, 1930.

Parfitt AM: Renal osteodystrophy. *Orthop Clin North Am* 3:681, 1972.

Parfitt AM, Chir B: Hypophosphatemic vitamin D refractory rickets and osteomalacia. *Orthop Clin North Am* 3:653, 1972.

Pitt MJ: Rachitic and osteomalacic syndromes. *Radiol Clin North Am* 19:581, 1981.

Pitt MJ: Rickets and osteomalacia. In: Resnick D (ed): *Bone and Joint Imaging*. Philadelphia, WB Saunders, 1989.

Pitt MJ: Rickets and osteomalacia are still around. *Radiol Clin North Am* 29:97, 1991.

Resnick DL: Fish vertebrae. *Arthritis Rheum* 25:1073, 1982.

Riggs BL, Melton JM: Involutional osteoporosis. *N Engl J Med* 306:446, 1986.

Sackler JP, Liu L: Case reports: Heparin-induced osteoporosis *Br J Radiol* 46:548, 1973.

Singh M, Nagrath AR, Maini PS: Changes in trabecular pattern of the upper end of the femur as an index of osteoporosis. *J Bone Joint Surg* 52A:457, 1970.

Singh M, Riggs BL, Beabout JW, et al: Femoral trabecular-pattern index for evaluation of spinal osteoporosis. *Ann Intern Med* 77:63, 1972.

Walton J: Familial hypophosphatemic rickets: A declination of its subdivisions and pathogenesis. *Clin Pediatr* 15:1007, 1976.

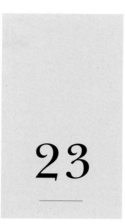

Hyperparathyroidism

HYPERPARATHYROIDISM

Pathophysiology

HYPERPARATHYROIDISM, ALSO known as generalized osteitis fibrosa cystica or Recklinghausen disease of bone, is the result of overactivity of the parathormone-producing parathyroid glands. Increased production of this hormone is secondary to either gland hyperplasia (9% of cases) or adenoma (90%); only in very rare instances (1%) does hyperparathyroidism occur secondary to parathyroid carcinoma. Excessive secretion of parathormone, which acts on the kidneys and on bone, leads to disturbances in calcium and phosphorus metabolism, resulting in hypercalcemia, hyperphosphaturia, and hypophosphatemia. Renal excretion of calcium and phosphate is increased, and serum levels of calcium are elevated, while those of phosphorus are reduced. Serum levels of alkaline phosphatase are also elevated.

Hyperparathyroidism can be divided into primary, secondary, and tertiary forms. The classic form of the disorder, *primary hyperparathyroidism,* is marked by increased secretion of parathormone resulting from hyperplasia, adenoma, or carcinoma of the parathyroid glands. Primary hyperparathyroidism is usually associated with hypercalcemia. Women are affected about three times as often as men, and the condition is most often seen in the patient's third to fifth decade. *Secondary hyperparathyroidism* is caused by increased secretion of parathyroid hormone in response to a sustained hypocalcemic state. Usually the fundamental cause of parathyroid gland hyperfunction is impaired renal function. Hyperphosphatemia due to renal failure results in chronic hypocalcemia, which in turn promotes increased parathyroid secretion. Although secondary hyperparathyroidism is usually hypocalcemic, it may be normocalcemic as an adaptive response to the hypocalcemic state. *Tertiary hyperparathyroidism* represents a transformation from a hypocalcemic to a hypercalcemic state. The parathyroid glands "escape" from the regulatory effect of serum calcium levels. Patients in whom this escape occurs are usually receiving kidney hemodialysis; they are considered to have autonomous hyperparathyroidism.

Although primary hyperparathyroidism is traditionally synonymous with the hypercalcemic form of the disorder, some patients nonetheless may have normal or even reduced serum calcium levels. For this reason, Reiss and Canterbury proposed an alternative method of classifying hyperparathyroidism based on serum calcium levels. In this system, hyperparathyroidism is considered either hypercalcemic, normocalcemic, or hypocalcemic.

In order to understand the clinical, pathologic, and radiologic manifestations of hyperparathyroidism, knowledge of the interrelated roles of parathyroid hormone and vitamin D in the metabolization of calcium is essential.

Physiology of Calcium Metabolism

Serum concentrations of calcium are maintained within a narrow normal physiologic range (2.20–2.65 mmol/L or 8.8–10.6 mg/dL) by the intestines and kidneys, the major sites of classic negative feedback mechanisms that balance calcium intake and excretion. The bones also contribute to preserving calcium homeostasis and, since they represent approximately 99% of elemental calcium in the human body, are considered to be a calcium reservoir. Essential to these mechanisms involving a variety of hormones is the action of parathyroid hormone (PTH), a polypeptide hormone whose secretion is induced by a decrease in the level of calcium in the extracellular fluid. In primary hyperparathyroidism, there is inappropriate oversecretion of PTH in the presence of elevated serum calcium levels, while secondary hyperparathyroidism is marked by appropriate PTH production in response to chronic hypocalcemia.

PTH works to increase serum calcium concentrations by several means. Predominant among these is conserving calcium in the kidneys by promoting both increased reabsorption of calcium and increased excretion of phosphates in the distal renal tubules. PTH also promotes release of calcium and phosphorus from bone by increasing the number and activity of osteoclasts, resulting in bone resorption, although the exact mechanism by which this occurs is not fully understood. Finally, although PTH has been shown to have no direct effect on intestinal calcium absorption, it plays a role in stimulating vitamin D metabolism, with subsequent increased absorption of calcium and phosphorus by the intestines.

Both of the forms of vitamin D in the human body—ergocalciferol (vitamin D_2), a synthetic compound and frequent food additive; and cholecalciferol (vitamin D_3), formed predominantly in the skin from

7-dehydrocholesterol by the action of ultraviolet light—are metabolized to 25-hydroxyvitamin D in the liver. The critical step in the metabolism of vitamin D occurs in the kidneys, where 25-hydroxyvitamin D undergoes hydroxylation to its most active form, 1,25-dihydroxyvitamin D, and an inactive metabolite, 24,25-dihydroxyvitamin D. This step is catalyzed by the renal enzyme 1-α-hydroxylase, which is synthesized in the kidneys under the stimulation of PTH in the presence of decreased serum calcium and phosphate levels. This gives the kidneys a unique central role in the metabolism of vitamin D. 1,25-dihydroxyvitamin D is the primary mediator of calcium and phosphorus absorption in the small intestine. The kidneys also have the ability to switch between producing the active and inactive forms of vitamin D, yielding a fine control of calcium metabolism.

The symptoms of hyperparathyroidism are related to hypercalcemia, skeletal abnormalities, and renal disease. Hypercalcemia produces weakness, muscular hypotonia, nausea, anorexia, constipation, polyuria, and thirst. The skeletal abnormalities most commonly seen are generalized osteopenia and foci of bone destruction, which are commonly referred to as brown tumors. These pseudotumors represent areas of fibrous scarring in which osteoclasts collect, blood decomposes, and cysts form (see Fig. 17.52). The most common sites of involvement are the mandible, clavicle, ribs, pelvis, and femur. Also,

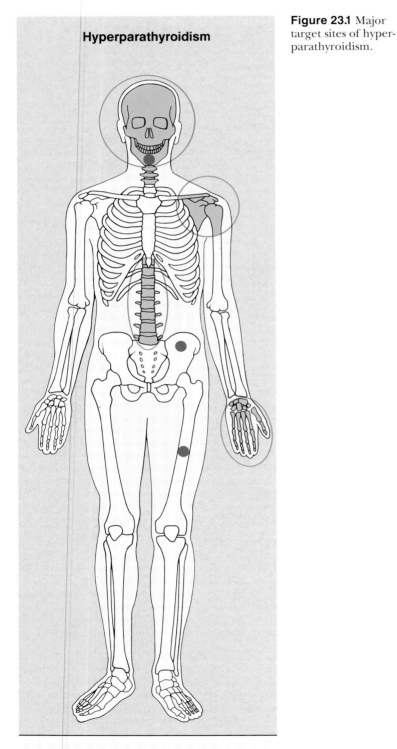

common sites of brown tumors

Figure 23.1 Major target sites of hyperparathyroidism.

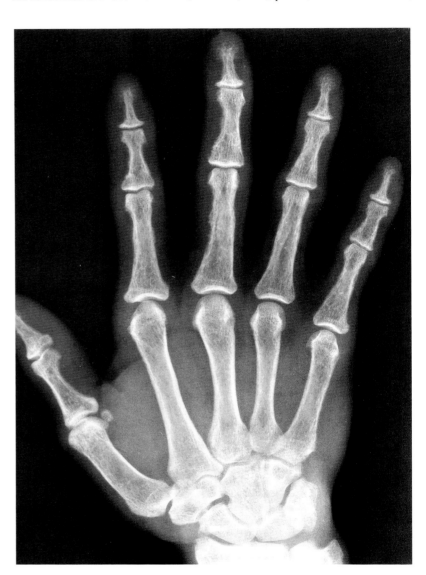

Figure 23.2 Dorsovolar view of the left hand of a 42-year-old man with primary hyperparathyroidism due to hypertrophy of the parathyroid glands shows typical subperiosteal resorption affecting primarily the radial aspects of the middle phalanges of the middle and index fingers.

subchondral and subperiosteal bone resorption is invariably present. Kidney involvement results in nephrocalcinosis, impairment of renal function, and uremia.

Radiographic Evaluation

The major target sites in the skeletal system for hyperparathyroidism are the shoulder, the hand, the vertebrae, and the skull (Fig. 23.1). Standard radiography is usually sufficient to demonstrate its characteristic features: generalized osteopenia; subperiosteal, subchondral, and cortical bone resorption; brown tumors; and soft tissue and cartilage calcifications. Subperiosteal resorption is particularly well demonstrated on plain films of the hands, where it usually affects the radial aspects of the middle phalanges of the middle and index fingers (Fig. 23.2; see also Fig. 21.8). Also characteristic of this condition is resorption of the acromial ends of the clavicle (Fig. 23.3). Intracortical resorption is manifested by longitudinal striations, a finding known as "tunneling," which can be most clearly appreciated on magnification studies (see Fig. 21.10). Another characteristic feature is loss of the lamina dura around the tooth socket, which normally is seen as a thin sharp white line surrounding the peridental membrane that attaches the tooth to bone (Fig. 23.4). In the skull, there is a characteristic mottling of the vault, which yields a "salt-and-pepper" appearance (Fig. 23.5). Localized destructive changes in bones affected by hyperparathyroidism take the form of cystlike lesions of various sizes, commonly referred to as brown

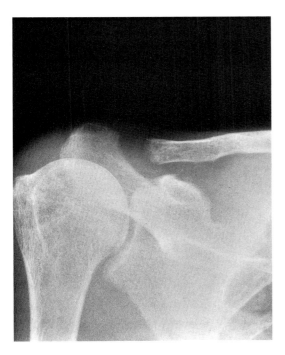

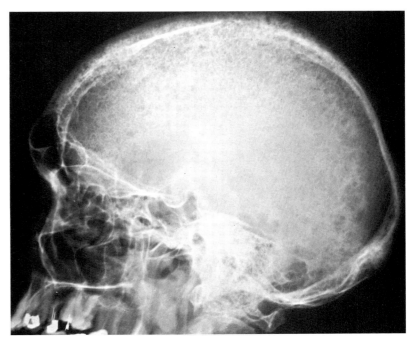

Figure 23.3 Anteroposterior radiograph of the shoulder of a 36-year-old woman with primary hyperparathyroidism shows resorption of the acromial end of the right clavicle.

Figure 23.5 Lateral radiograph of the skull of the patient seen in Figure 23.2 demonstrates a decrease in the overall density of the bone and a granular appearance of the vault—the so-called salt-and-pepper skull.

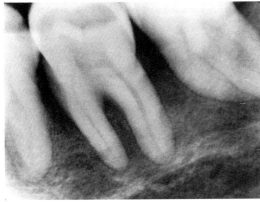

Figure 23.4 Radiograph of the lower second molar tooth in a patient with primary hyperparathyroidism shows loss of the lamina dura around the tooth socket.

tumors. The jaw, pelvis, and femora are the usual sites for these lesions, but they may be found in any part of the skeleton (Fig. 23.6).

In secondary hyperparathyroidism, other characteristic features may be present in addition to the radiographic abnormalities just discussed. A generalized increase in bone density occurs, particularly in younger patients. In the spine, this change is reflected in dense sclerotic bands seen adjacent to the vertebral end plates, giving the vertebrae a sandwich-like appearance. This phenomenon is termed "rugger-jersey" spine because the sclerotic bands form horizontal stripes resembling those of rugby shirts (Fig. 23.7). However, it must be kept in mind in the evaluation of hyperparathyroidism that osteosclerotic changes may also occur as a manifestation of healing, either spontaneously or as a result of treatment. Deposition of calcium in fibrocartilage, articular cartilage, and soft tissue is common, and vascular calcifications are much more frequent in patients with secondary hyperparathyroidism (Fig. 23.8).

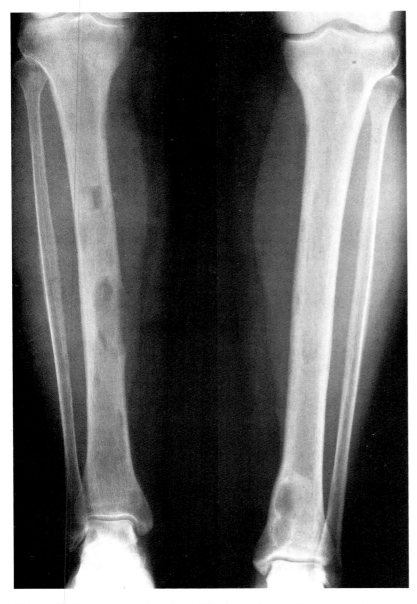

Figure 23.6 Anteroposterior view of the lower legs of the same patient seen in Figure 23.3 shows multiple lytic lesions (brown tumors) in both tibiae.

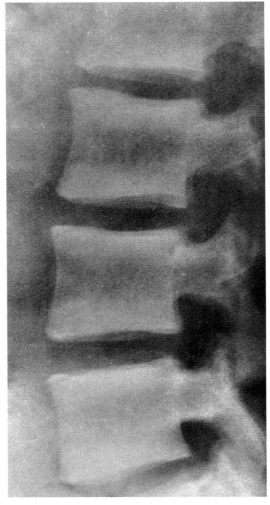

Figure 23.7 A 17-year-old boy with chronic renal failure developed secondary hyperparathyroidism. Lateral radiograph of the lumbar spine demonstrates sclerotic bands adjacent to the vertebral end plates—the so-called rugger-jersey spine.

Complications

Both primary and secondary hyperparathyroidism may be complicated by pathologic fractures, which usually occur in the ribs and vertebral bodies. Hyperparathyroidism arthropathy, another frequent complication, has been discussed in more detail in Chapter 14. Slipped capital femoral or humeral epiphysis may also be observed on occasion. The involvement of ligaments and tendons results in capsular and ligamentous laxity, which may lead to joint instability. Occasionally, spontaneous tendon avulsion has been observed, a phenomenon attributed to the direct effect of parathyroid hormone on connective tissue. Even less frequently intra-articular crystal deposition (calcium pyrophosphate dihydrate) in cartilage, capsule, and synovium may occur, which may lead to the pseudogout syndrome.

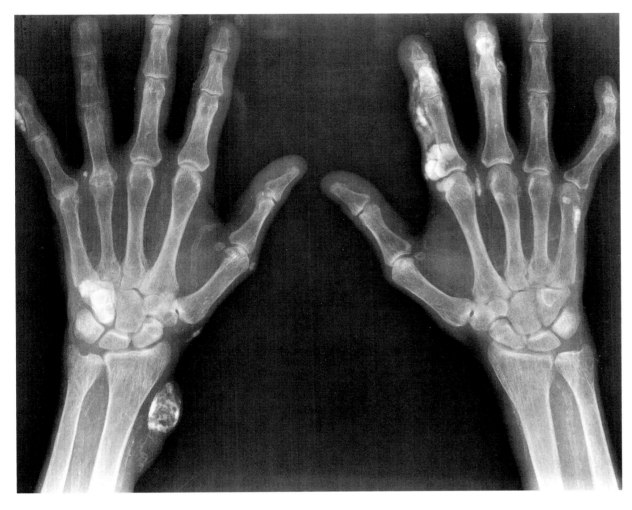

Figure 23.8 Posteroanterior view of the distal forearms and hands of a 48-year-old woman with secondary hyperparathyroidism shows evidence of soft tissue and vascular calcifications, characteristic findings in this condition. Note also diffuse osteopenia.

PRACTICAL POINTS TO REMEMBER

[1] The typical radiographic changes of primary (hypercalcemic) hyperparathyroidism include:
- generalized osteopenia
- subperiosteal, subchondral, and cortical resorption
- resorption of the acromial end of the clavicle
- a "salt-and-pepper" appearance of the skull
- cyst-like lesions (brown tumors) of varying sizes.

[2] Subperiosteal resorption of bone is best demonstrated on a dorsovolar radiograph of the hands, since these changes characteristically occur on the radial aspects of the middle phalanges of the middle and index fingers.

[3] Cortical resorption (tunneling) is best appreciated on magnification radiography of the hand or long bones.

[4] Secondary hyperparathyroidism (due to renal disease) is typified radiographically by:
- a generalized increase in bone density
- sclerotic bands adjacent to the vertebral end plates, known as "rugger-jersey" spine
- soft tissue calcifications.

[5] The most common complications of hyperparathyroidism include pathologic fractures (vertebral bodies, ribs), metabolic arthropathies, and slipped epiphyses (femoral and humeral).

References

Genant HK, Heck LL, Lanzl LH, Rossmann K, Vander Horst J, Paloyan E: Primary hyperparathyroidism: A comprehensive study of clinical, biochemical and radiographic manifestations. *Radiology* 109:513, 1973.

Greenfield GB: Roentgen appearance of bone and soft tissue changes in chronic renal disease. *Am J Roentgenol* 116:749, 1972.

Hayes CW, Convay WF: Hyperparathyroidism. *Radiol Clin North Am* 29:85, 1991.

Jensen PS, Kliger AS: Early radiographic manifestations of secondary hyperparathyroidism associated with chronic renal disease. *Radiology* 125:645, 1977.

Massry S, Ritz E: The pathogenesis of secondary hyperparathyroidism of renal failure. *Arch Intern Med* 138:853, 1978.

Reiss E, Canterbury JM: Spectrum of hyperparathyroidism. *Am J Med* 56: 794, 1974.

Resnick D: The "rugger jersey" vertebral body. *Arthritis Rheum* 24:1191, 1981.

Richardson ML, Pozzi-Mucelli RS, Kanter AS, et al: Bone mineral changes in primary hyperparathyroidism. *Skeletal Radiol* 15:85, 1986.

Rossi RL, ReMine SG, Clerkin EP: Hyperparathyroidism. *Surg Clin North Am* 65:187, 1985.

Shapiro R: Radiologic aspects of renal osteodystrophy. *Radiol Clin North Am* 10:557, 1972.

Weller M, Edeiken J, Hodes PJ: Renal osteodystrophy. *Am J Roentgenol* 104:354, 1968.

24

Paget Disease

PAGET DISEASE

Pathophysiology

PAGET DISEASE, A RELATIVELY common bone disorder, is a chronic, progressive disturbance in bone metabolism that primarily affects older persons. It is slightly more common in men than in women (3:2), with an average age of onset between 45 and 55 years, although the disease has been known to occur in young adults. The prevalence of Paget disease varies considerably in different parts of the world, reaching its greatest incidence in Great Britain, Australia, and New Zealand.

The precise nature of Paget disease and its etiology are still unknown. Sir James Paget named the disease *osteitis deformans* in the belief that the basic process was infectious in origin. Other etiologies have also been proposed, such as neoplastic, vascular, endocrinologic, immunologic, traumatic, and hereditary. Recent ultrastructural studies and the discovery of giant multinucleated osteoblasts containing microfilaments in the affected cytoplasm, as well as intranuclear inclusion bodies, suggest a viral etiology. Some investigators have obtained immunocytologic evidence identifying the particles as analogous to those from the measles group virus material. Other immunologic studies have demonstrated viral antigens in affected cells identical to those from the respiratory syncytial virus.

Whatever the fundamental cause of Paget disease, its basic pathologic process has to do with the balance between bone resorption and appositional new bone formation. There is disordered and extremely active bone remodeling, secondary to both osteoclastic bone resorption and osteoblastic bone formation in a characteristic mosaic pattern, which is the histologic hallmark of this condition. Biochemically, the increase in osteoblastic activity is reflected in elevated levels of serum alkaline phosphatase, which can rise to extremely high values. Similarly, the increase in osteoclastic bone resorption is reflected in high urinary levels of hydroxyproline, which is formed as a result of collagen breakdown.

The skeletal abnormalities seen in Paget disease are frequently asymptomatic and may be an incidental finding on radiographic examination or at autopsy. When the changes are symptomatic, clinical manifestations are often related to complications of the disease, such as deformity of the long bones, warmth in the involved extremity, periosteal tenderness and bone pain, fractures, secondary osteoarthritis, neural compression, and sarcomatous degeneration. The distribution of a lesion varies from monostotic involvement to widespread disease. The following bones, in order of decreasing frequency, are most often affected: the pelvis, femur, skull, tibia, vertebrae, clavicle, humerus, and ribs (Fig. 24.1). The fibula is involved only in exceptional cases.

Radiographic Evaluation

The radiographic features of Paget disease correspond to the pathologic processes in the bone and depend on the stage of the disorder. In the early phase, the *osteolytic* or *hot phase*, active bone resorption is evident as a radiolucent wedge or an elongated area with sharp borders that destroys both the cortex and cancellous bone as it advances along the shaft. The terms frequently used to describe this phenomenon are "advancing wedge," "candle flame," and "blade of grass" (Fig. 24.2). In flat bones such as the calvarium or the iliac bone, an area of active bone destruction known as osteoporosis circumscripta appears as a purely osteolytic lesion (Fig. 24.3).

In the *intermediate* or *mixed phase*, bone destruction is accompanied by new bone formation, with the latter process tending to predominate. Bone remodeling appears radiographically as thickening of the cortex and coarse trabeculation of cancellous bone (Fig. 24.4). In the spine, the thin cortex of the vertebral body, which disappears in the hot phase, is later replaced by broad, coarsely trabeculated bone,

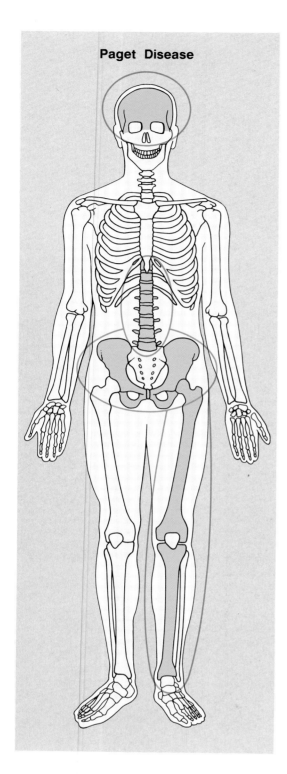

Paget Disease

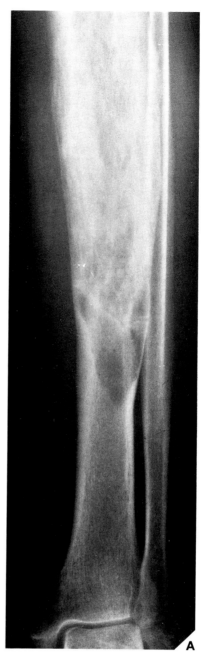

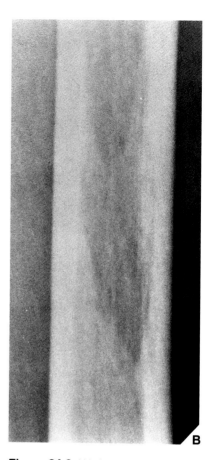

Figure 24.1 Major target sites of Paget disease.

Figure 24.2 (A) Anteroposterior view of the lower leg of a 68-year-old woman with Paget disease shows an advancing wedge of osteolytic destruction in the midportion of the tibia. (B) Magnification study of the mid-femur in another patient shows the purely osteolytic phase of Paget disease. In both examples, the lesion resembles a blade of grass or a candle flame. (A: reproduced with permission from Sissons HA, Greenspan A, 1986)

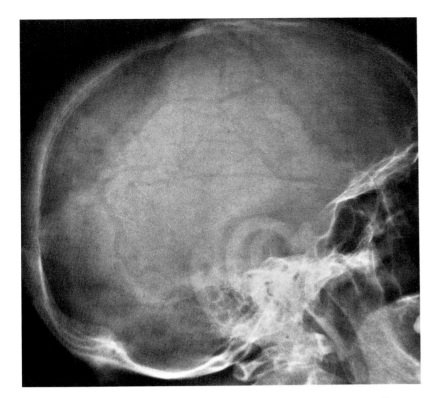

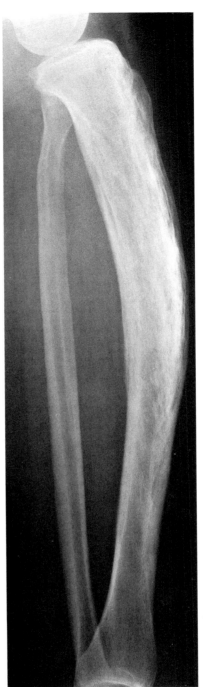

Figure 24.4 In the intermediate phase of Paget disease, seen here affecting the tibia in a 62-year-old woman, thickening of the cortex and a coarse trabecular pattern in the medullary portion of the bone are characteristic features. Note the anterior bowing.

Figure 24.3 Lateral view of the skull of a 60-year-old man with Paget disease shows an osteolytic lesion in the parieto-occipital area. This sharply demarcated defect, known as osteoporosis circumscripta, represents a hot phase of the disease.

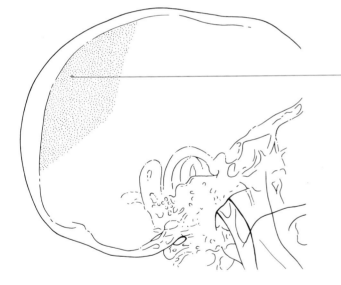

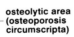

osteolytic area
(osteoporosis
circumscripta)

forming what appears to be a "picture frame" around the body (Fig. 24.5). In the skull, focal patchy densities with a "cotton-ball" appearance are characteristic (Fig. 24.6).

In the *cool phase*, a diffuse increase of bone density occurs together with enlargement and widening of the bone and marked cortical thickening, with blurring of the demarcation between cortex and spongiosa (Fig. 24.7). Bowing of long bones may become a striking feature (Fig. 24.8). Similar changes are observed in the skull, where obliteration of the diploic space is also a typical feature (Fig. 24.9).

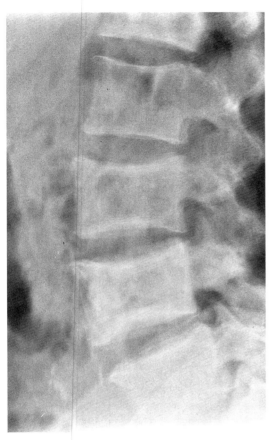

Figure 24.5
Involvement of the lumbar spine in the mixed phase of Paget disease can be recognized by the "picture-frame" appearance of the vertebral bodies created by dense sclerotic bone on the periphery and greater radiolucency in the center. Note the partial replacement of vertebral endplates by coarsely trabeculated bone. (Reproduced with permission from Sissons HA, Greenspan A, 1986)

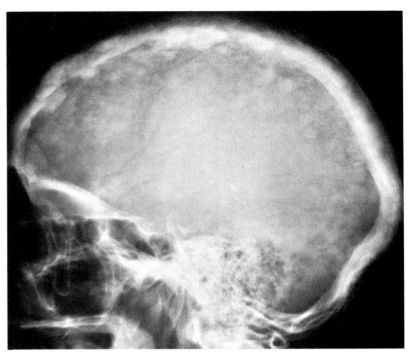

Figure 24.6 Focal patchy densities in the skull, having a "cotton-ball" appearance, are typical of the intermediate phase of Paget disease as seen in this radiograph of a 68-year-old woman.

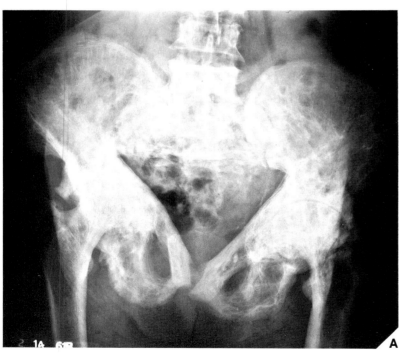

A

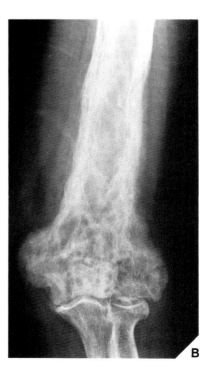

B

Figure 24.7 In the cool phase of Paget disease, there is considerable thickening of the cortex and bone deformity. (A) The pelvic cavity, seen here in an 80-year-old woman, may assume a triangular appearance. (B) Involvement of a long bone, in this case the distal humerus of a 60-year-old woman, exhibits marked cortical thickening, narrowing of the medullary cavity, and a coarse trabecular pattern. (Reproduced with permission from Sissons HA, Greenspan A, 1986)

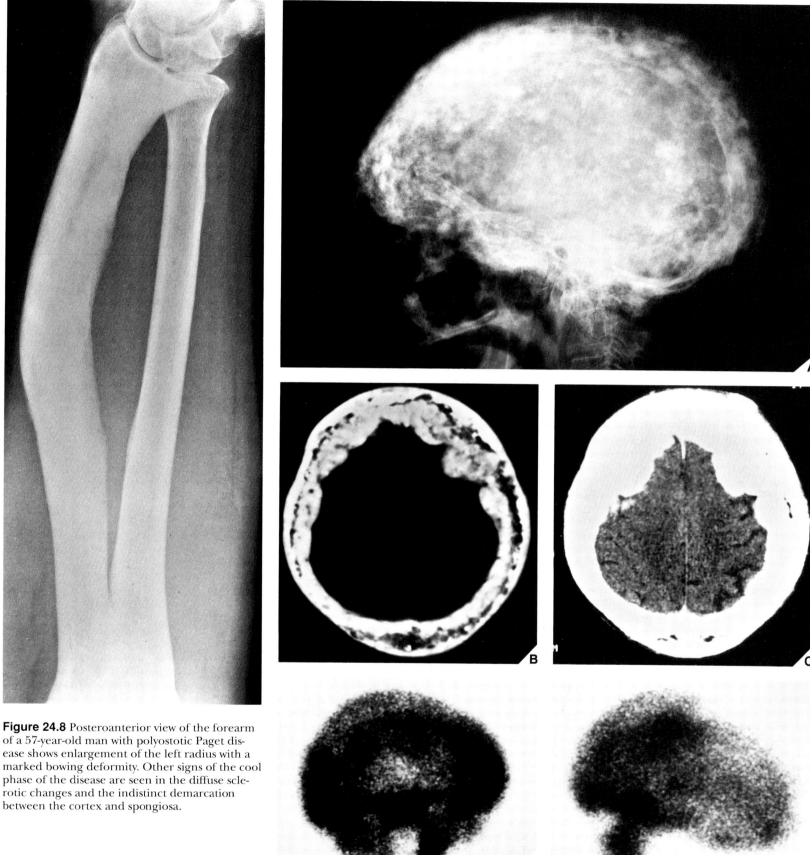

Figure 24.8 Posteroanterior view of the forearm of a 57-year-old man with polyostotic Paget disease shows enlargement of the left radius with a marked bowing deformity. Other signs of the cool phase of the disease are seen in the diffuse sclerotic changes and the indistinct demarcation between the cortex and spongiosa.

Figure 24.9 (A) Plain film of the skull of an 80-year-old woman with Paget disease in its cool phase demonstrates numerous coalescent densities associated with thickening and sclerosis of the cranial vault and base of the skull. CT sections clearly demonstrate predominant involvement of the inner table with marked diminution of the diploic space (B) and thickening of the cranial vault (C). (D,E) Scintigraphy demonstrates markedly increased uptake of radiopharmaceutical.

It is important to remember that, since in the long bones Paget disease starts at one articular end and advances to the other, all three phases of the disorder may coexist in the same bone (Fig. 24.10).

Differential Diagnosis

Several conditions may mimic Paget disease, while the disease itself may be mistaken for other pathologic processes; for example, involvement of a single bone can be mistaken for monostotic fibrous dysplasia, and a uniform increase in osseous density may mimic lymphoma or metastatic cancer. The rugger-jersey appearance of the spine in secondary hyperparathyroidism may resemble Paget vertebra (see Fig. 23.7). Vertebral hemangioma also looks very much like

Paget vertebra on a radiograph, except that the vertebral body is not enlarged and the vertebral end plates are well outlined (see Fig. 16.46). However, the condition that bears the most striking resemblance to Paget disease is familial idiopathic hyperphosphatasia, also called "juvenile Paget disease" (see Figs. 25.1, 25.2). In this condition, unlike Paget disease, the articular ends of the bone may not be affected.

Complications

PATHOLOGIC FRACTURES Of the numerous complications observed in patients with Paget disease, the most common are pathologic fractures in the long bones. They may resemble partial or incomplete

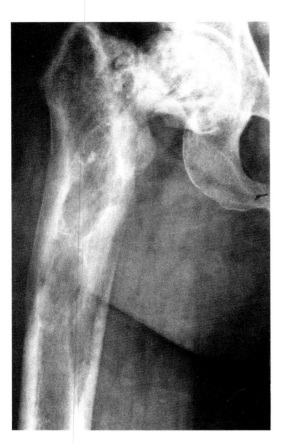

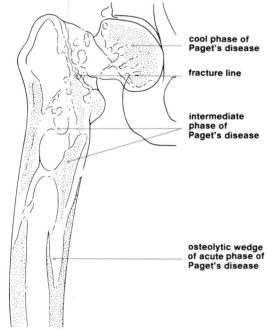

cool phase of Paget's disease

fracture line

intermediate phase of Paget's disease

osteolytic wedge of acute phase of Paget's disease

Figure 24.10
Anteroposterior view of the proximal half of the femur of a 77-year-old woman with Paget disease demonstrates all three phases of the disorder. The cool phase is seen in the femoral head, the intermediate phase in the proximal shaft, and the hot phase, represented by an osteolytic wedge of resorption, in the medial cortex more distally.

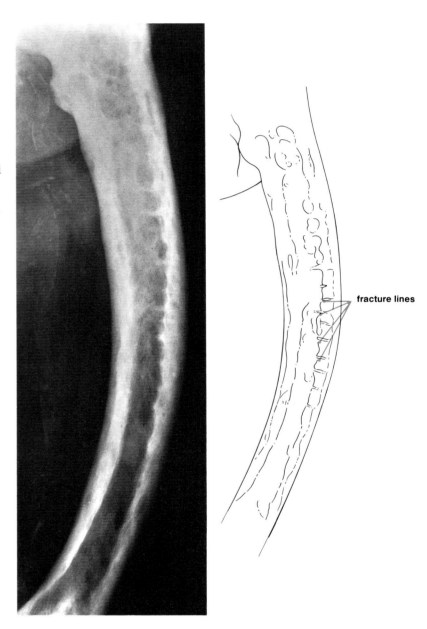

fracture lines

Figure 24.11 Numerous incomplete stress fractures, seen in the lateral cortex of the femur in an 80-year-old man with advanced Paget disease, are the most frequent complication of this condition.

stress fractures, appearing radiographically as multiple short horizontal radiolucent lines on the convex aspect of the cortex (Fig. 24.11). True complete fractures are referred to as "banana-type" because of the horizontal direction of the fracture line as it traverses the affected bone (Fig. 24.12), and they have also been compared with crushed rotten wood or chalk. Fractures are more likely to occur during the osteolytic or hot phase, and they are frequently the main presenting manifestation of Paget disease.

DEGENERATIVE JOINT DISEASE The development of degenerative joint disease is a common complication of Paget disease. This secondary form of osteoarthritis usually occurs in the knee and hip articulations, where the characteristic changes are present, including joint space narrowing and osteophyte formation. Involvement of the acetabulum may be complicated by acetabular protrusio (Fig. 24.13).

NEUROLOGIC COMPLICATIONS The neurologic complications of Paget disease are secondary to involvement of the vertebral column and skull. Collapse of a vertebral body, for example, causes extradural spinal canal block, which may lead to paraplegia (Fig. 24.14). Severe involvement of the bony spinal canal may lead to spinal stenosis, the presence of which can be effectively demonstrated by computed

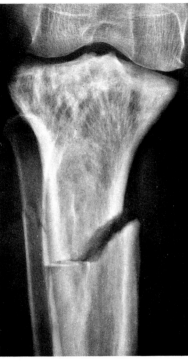

Figure 24.12 A 62-year-old man with monostotic Paget disease affecting the right tibia sustained a pathologic fracture. Note that the fracture line traverses the area of active, osteolytic bone destruction. (Reproduced with permission from Sissons HA, Greenspan A, 1986)

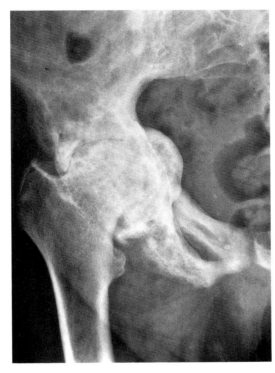

Figure 24.13 A 75-year-old woman with longstanding polyostotic Paget disease had been complaining for a year of progressive pain in her right hip. Anteroposterior view demonstrates advanced osteoarthritis and acetabular protrusio. (Reproduced with permission from Sissons HA, Greenspan A, 1986)

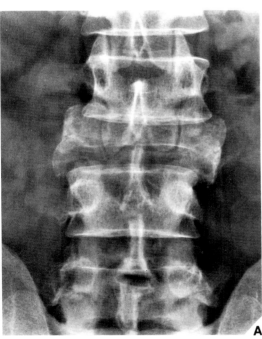

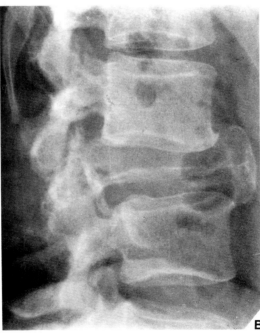

A   B

Figure 24.14 A 60-year-old man with Paget disease affecting the vertebrae presented with lower-back pain and neurologic symptoms. Anteroposterior (A) and lateral (B) views of the lumbar spine show a pathologic compression fracture of L-3 with encroachment on the spinal canal, which was the source of his symptoms. (Reproduced with permission from Sissons HA, Greenspan A, 1986)

tomography (Fig. 24.15). Basilar invagination due to softening of the skull may lead to encroachment on the foramen magnum and neurologic deficit.

NEOPLASTIC COMPLICATIONS Benign or malignant giant cell tumors, single or multiple, may complicate Paget disease. The usual sites of these tumors are the calvarium or the iliac bone.

The development of a bone sarcoma is a serious but rare complication of Paget disease; the incidence is less than 1%. Osteosarcoma is by far the most common histologic type (Fig. 24.16), followed by fibrosarcoma, malignant fibrous histiocytoma, and chondrosarcoma, with the pelvis, femur, and humerus at highest risk for development of malignant transformation. The main radiographic features of this complication are development of a lytic lesion at the site of Paget

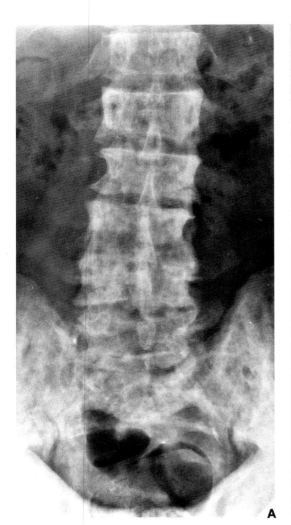

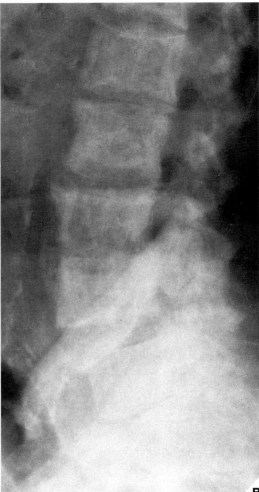

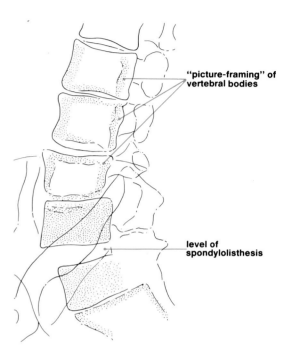

"picture-framing" of vertebral bodies

level of spondylolisthesis

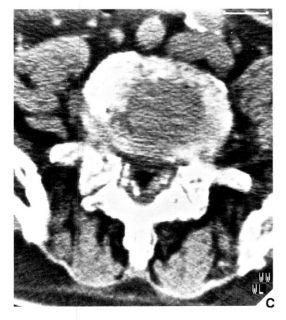

Figure 24.15 An 84-year-old man with extensive polyostotic Paget disease for many years developed degenerative spondylolisthesis and spinal stenosis. Anteroposterior (A) and lateral (B) views of the lumbar spine show Paget disease in the cool phase. Second-degree degenerative spondylolisthesis is seen at the L4-5 level. (C) CT section through L-5 demonstrates narrowing of the spinal canal characteristic of spinal stenosis, the major cause of most neurologic symptoms in Paget disease.

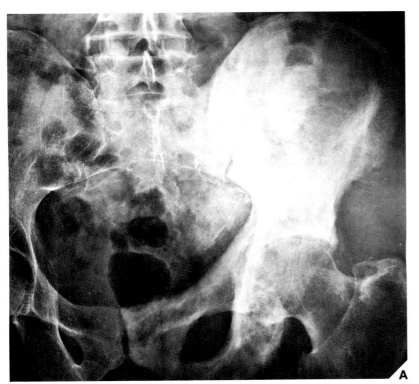

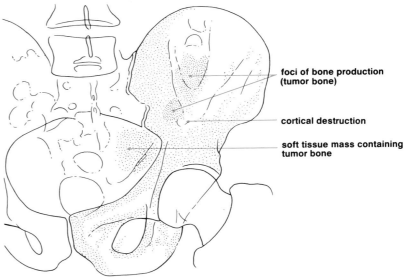

foci of bone production
(tumor bone)

cortical destruction

soft tissue mass containing
tumor bone

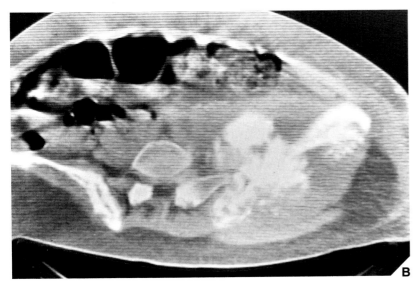

Figure 24.16 A 70-year-old woman with Paget disease affecting her left hemipelvis developed a rare complication, sarcomatous degeneration. (A) Plain film of the pelvis shows extensive involvement of the left ilium, pubis, and ischium by Paget disease. There is also destruction of the cortex and a large soft tissue mass accompanied by bone formation, typical findings for osteosarcoma. (B) CT scan demonstrates the soft tissue mass more clearly.

disease, cortical breakthrough, and formation of a soft tissue mass; a periosteal reaction is rare. There is often a pathologic fracture as well. The radiographic appearance of Paget sarcoma must be distinguished from that of metastases of a primary carcinoma of the kidney (Fig. 24.17), breast, or prostate. The metastatic deposit may be lodged in either unaffected or pagetic bone. The prognosis for patients with sarcomatous degeneration of Paget disease is poor; the mean survival time usually does not exceed six to eight months. Occasionally, an osteosarcoma in pagetic bone may metastasize to other bones and soft tissues, but metastases to the lung, liver, and adrenals are much more likely.

Orthopedic Management

Because of the variable clinical presentation of Paget disease, decisions regarding treatment must be based on the particular manifestations in each patient. The role of the orthopedic surgeon in the management of Paget disease is to evaluate and treat the cause of a patient's pain, to assess and manage any deformities, and to provide therapy for pathologic fractures and tumors developing in pagetic bone. The radiologist contributes to these aims by provid-

ing essential information. For instance, CT is useful for demonstrating spinal stenosis, which frequently leads to neurologic symptoms in patients with Paget disease (see Fig. 24.15). Radionuclide imaging is also a valuable technique, particularly for determining the skeletal distribution of the disease (see Fig. 21.12).

Treatment consists of inhibiting osteoclastic activity by calcitonin and oral administration of diphosphonates, which bind to areas of high bone turnover, decreasing bone resorption. Administration of mithramycin inhibits RNA synthesis and has a potent cytotoxic effect on osteoclasts. The serum alkaline phosphatase determination and the 24-hour urinary hydroxyproline measurement are the main indicators of the response of the disease to medical treatment.

Surgical intervention is indicated for treatment of pathologic fractures, advanced, disabling arthritis, and extreme bowing deformities of the long bones. Stress or pseudofractures, which occur most often in the tibia and proximal femur, are treated by bracing and protection from weight-bearing for a period of several months. Complete fractures are treated either with intramedullary rods or with compression plates and screws. For arthritic complications, which are particularly frequent in the hip and knee articulations, total joint replacement is usually performed.

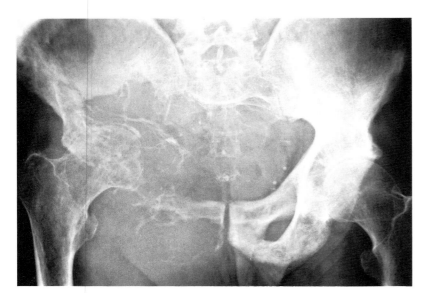

Figure 24.17 Anteroposterior radiograph of the pelvis of a 55-year-old woman with Paget disease for ten years shows extensive osteolytic destruction of the right ilium, ischium, and pubis secondary to metastatic renal cell carcinoma (hypernephroma). Note the typical involvement of the pelvis by Paget disease. This metastatic lesion should not be mistaken for Paget sarcoma.

PRACTICAL POINTS TO REMEMBER

[1] The histologic hallmark of Paget disease is a mosaic pattern of disorderly and active bone remodeling secondary to osteoclastic resorption and osteoblastic formation.

[2] The characteristic radiographic features of Paget disease of bone include:
- involvement of at least one articular end of a long bone
- thickening of the cortex and enlargement of the affected bone
- a coarse trabecular pattern to the spongiosa
- bowing deformities of the long bones
- a "picture-frame" appearance of a vertebral body.

[3] Particular radiographic changes in Paget disease are related to the stage of the disorder. In the acute (hot) phase, a radiolucent osteolytic area is seen
- in the calvarium or in a flat bone, where it is known as "osteoporosis circumscripta"
- in a long bone, where it appears as an advancing wedge of active disease, resembling a candle flame or a blade of grass.

[4] Radionuclide bone scan, which invariably shows increased uptake of the tracer in bones affected by Paget disease, is effective in determining the distribution of the lesion.

[5] The most frequent complication of Paget disease is pathologic fracture, either incomplete stress fractures or "banana-type" complete fractures.

[6] The most serious complication of Paget disease is sarcomatous degeneration. Radiographically, it can be recognized by:
- osteolytic bone destruction at the site of the pagetic lesion
- cortical breakthrough
- a soft tissue mass.

Malignant transformation must be distinguished from metastatic lesions to pagetic bone from a primary carcinoma of the lung, breast, kidney, GI tract, or prostate.

[7] Paget disease must be distinguished from:
- "juvenile Paget disease" (familial idiopathic hyperphosphatasia)
- van Buchem disease (hyperostosis corticalis generalisata)
- vertebral hemangioma
- rugger-jersey spine seen in secondary hyperparathyroidism
- lymphoma
- extensive osteoblastic metastases.

References

Barry HC: *Paget's Disease of Bone.* London, Livingstone, 1969.

Greenspan A, Norman A, Sterling AP: Precocious onset of Paget's disease—a report of three cases and review of the literature. *Can Assoc Radiol J* 28:69, 1977.

Hutter RVP, Foote FW Jr, Frazell EL, Francis KC: Giant cell tumors complicating Paget's disease of bone. *Cancer* 16:1044, 1963.

Krane SM: Paget's disease of bone. *Clin Orthop* 127:24, 1977.

Lander PH, Hadjipavlou AG: A dynamic classification of Paget's disease. *J Bone Joint Surg* 68B:431, 1986.

McKenna RJ, Schwinn CP, Soong KY, Higinbotham NI: Osteogenic sarcoma arising in Paget's disease. *Cancer* 17:42, 1964.

Milgram JW: Radiographical and pathological assessment of the activity of Paget's disease of bone. *Clin Orthop* 127:43, 1977.

Milgram JW: Orthopedic management of Paget's disease of bone. *Clin Orthop* 127:63, 1977.

Mirra JM: Pathogenesis of Paget's disease based on viral etiology. *Clin Orthop* 217:162, 1987.

Mirra JM, Gold RM: Giant cell tumor containing viral-like intranuclear inclusions, in association with Paget's disease. Case report. *Skeletal Radiol* 8:67, 1982.

Paget J: On a form of chronic inflammation of bones (osteitis deformans). *Med Chir Trans* 60:37, 1877.

Roberts MC, Kressel HY, Fallon MD, Zlatkin MB, Dalinka MK: Paget disease: MR imaging findings. *Radiology 173:341, 1989.*

Rosenbaum HD, Hanson DJ: Geographic variation in the prevalence of Paget's disease of bone. *Radiology* 92:959, 1969.

Sissons HA: Epidemiology of Paget's disease. *Clin Orthop* 45:73, 1966.

Sissons HA, Greenspan A: Paget's disease. In: Taveras JM, Ferrucci JT (eds): *Radiology—Imaging, Diagnosis, Intervention.* Philadelphia, Lippincott, 1986.

Smith J, Botet JF, Yeh SDJ: Bone sarcomas in Paget's disease: A study of 85 patients. *Radiology* 152:583, 1984.

Wellman HN, Schauwecker D, Robb JA, Khairi MR, Johnston CC: Skeletal scintimaging and radiography in the diagnosis and management of Paget's disease. *Clin Orthop* 127:55, 1977.

Miscellaneous Metabolic and Endocrine Disorders

FAMILIAL IDIOPATHIC HYPERPHOSPHATASIA

FAMILIAL IDIOPATHIC HYPERPHOSPHATASIA is a rare autosomal-recessive disorder affecting young children, generally within their first 18 months, and exhibiting a striking predilection for those of Puerto Rican descent. The condition is associated with progressive bone deformities. Clinically, it is characterized by painful bowing of the limbs, muscular weakness and abnormal gait, pathologic fractures, spinal deformities, loss of vision and hearing, elevation of serum alkaline phosphatase, and an increase in the amount of leucine aminopeptidase.

Radiographic Evaluation

Increased turnover of bone and skeletal collagen demonstrated by radionuclide bone scan is a characteristic finding in familial idiopathic hyperphosphatasia. Its radiographic features are typical. Although this disorder has no relationship to classic Paget disease, it is often referred to as "juvenile Paget disease," and it exhibits similar radiographic features. The long bones are increased in size, showing thickening of the cortex and a coarse trabecular pattern (Fig. 25.1). Likewise, bowing deformities are common, as are involvement of the pelvis and skull (Fig. 25.2). However, unlike Paget disease, the epiphyses are usually not affected.

Differential Diagnosis

There also exist a few conditions similar to familial idiopathic hyperphosphatasia that belong to the general group of endosteal hyperostoses, or hyperostosis corticalis generalisata. In particular an autosomal-recessive form of these disorders, van Buchem disease, although classified as chronic hyperphosphatasia tarda, is in fact a distinct dysplasia; its onset is later than that of congenital hyperphosphatasia and the age of patients ranges from 25 to 50 years. The major radiographic finding is a symmetrical thickening of the cortices of the long and short tubular bones. The femora are not bowed, and the articular ends are spared. The cranial bones show marked thickening of both the vault and the base. Serum alkaline phosphatase levels are elevated but calcium and phosphorus levels are normal.

ACROMEGALY

Increased secretion of growth hormone (somatotropin) by the eosinophilic cells of the anterior lobe of the pituitary gland, as a result of either hyperplasia of the gland or a tumor, leads to acceleration of bone growth. If this condition develops before skeletal maturity (i.e., while the growth plates are still open), it results in gigantism; development after skeletal maturity results in acromegaly. The onset of symptoms is usually insidious, and the involvement of certain target

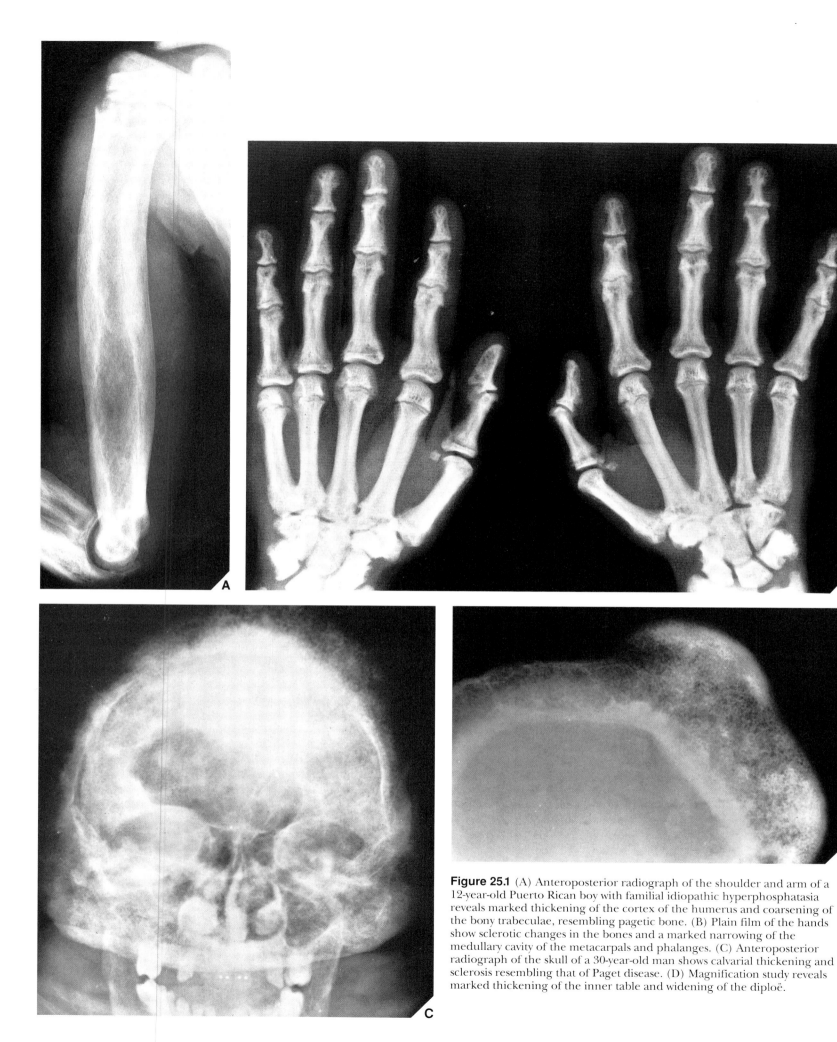

Figure 25.1 (A) Anteroposterior radiograph of the shoulder and arm of a 12-year-old Puerto Rican boy with familial idiopathic hyperphosphatasia reveals marked thickening of the cortex of the humerus and coarsening of the bony trabeculae, resembling pagetic bone. (B) Plain film of the hands show sclerotic changes in the bones and a marked narrowing of the medullary cavity of the metacarpals and phalanges. (C) Anteroposterior radiograph of the skull of a 30-year-old man shows calvarial thickening and sclerosis resembling that of Paget disease. (D) Magnification study reveals marked thickening of the inner table and widening of the diploë.

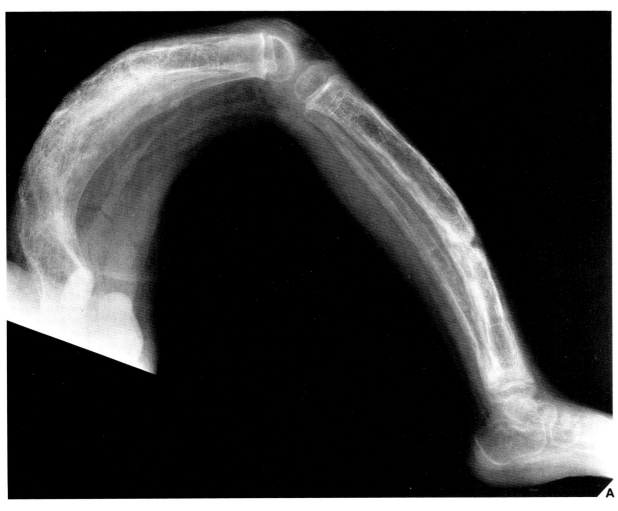

Figure 25.2 (A) Radiograph of a 4-year-old boy demonstrates marked bowing of the long bones of the lower extremity, a striking feature of familial idiopathic hyperphosphatasia. (B) Anteroposterior view of the pelvis shows the coarse trabecular pattern and cortical thickening typical of this condition. Note that the epiphyses are not affected. (C) Lateral view of the skull demonstrates thickening of the tables and a "cotton-ball" appearance of the cranial vault, similar to that of Paget disease. (B reproduced with permission from Sissons HA, Greenspan A, 1986)

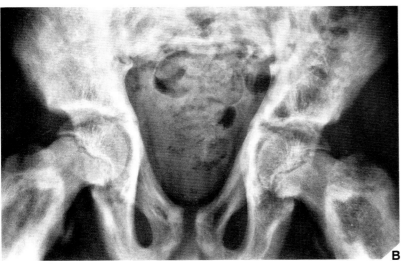

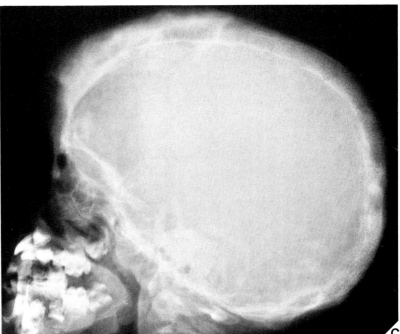

sites in the skeleton is typical (Fig. 25.3). Gradual enlargement of the hands and feet as well as exaggeration of facial features are the earliest manifestations. The characteristic facial changes result from overgrowth of the frontal sinuses, protrusion of the jaw (prognathism), accentuation of the orbital ridges, enlargement of the nose and lips, and thickening and coarsening of the soft tissues of the face.

Radiographic Evaluation

Radiographic examination reveals a number of characteristic features of this condition. A lateral view of the skull demonstrates thickening of the cranial bones and increased density; the diploë may be obliterated. The sella turcica, which houses the pituitary gland, may or may not be enlarged. The paranasal sinuses become enlarged (Fig. 25.4) and the mastoid cells overpneumatized. The prognathous jaw, one of the obvious clinical features of this condition, is apparent on the lateral view of the facial bones.

The hands also exhibit revealing radiographic changes. The heads of the metacarpals are enlarged, and irregular bony thickening along the margins, simulating osteophytes, may be seen. Increase in the size of the sesamoid at the metacarpophalangeal joint of the thumb may be helpful in evaluating acromegaly. Values of the sesamoid index (determined by the height and width of this ossicle measured in millimeters) greater than 30 in women and greater than 40 in men suggest acromegaly, but generally the dividing line between normal and abnormal values is not sharp enough

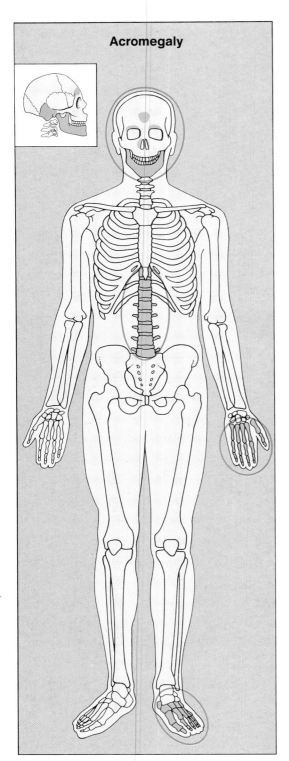

Figure 25.3 The most clearly revealing target sites of acromegaly.

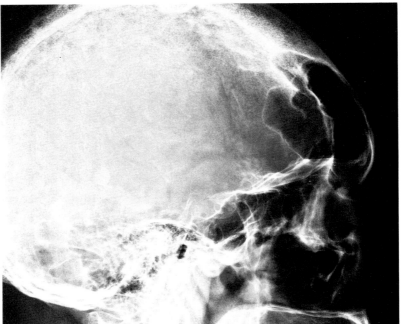

Figure 25.4 Lateral view of the skull of a 75-year-old woman with acromegaly shows marked enlargement of the frontal sinuses, prominent supraorbital ridges, and thickening of the frontal bones.

Figure 25.5 Dorsovolar view of the hand of a 38-year-old woman shows characteristic overgrowth of the terminal tufts and spur-like projections. The bases of the terminal phalanges are also enlarged, and the radiographic joint spaces are widened.

to allow individual borderline cases to be diagnosed on the basis of this index alone. Characteristic changes are also seen in the distal phalanges; their bases enlarge and the terminal tufts form spur-like projections. The joint spaces widen as a result of hypertrophy of articular cartilage (Fig. 25.5), and hypertrophy of the soft tissues may also occur, leading to the development of square, spade-shaped fingers.

Evaluation of the foot on the lateral view allows an important measurement to be made, the heel-pad thickness. This index is determined by the distance from the posteroinferior surface of the os calcis to the nearest skin surface. In a normal 150-pound subject, the heel-pad thickness should not exceed 22 mm. For each addi-

tional 25 pounds of body weight, 1 mm can be added to the basic value; thus 24 mm would be the highest normal value for a 200 pound person. If the heel-pad thickness is greater than the established normal value, acromegaly is a strong possibility (Fig. 25.6), and determination of growth hormone level by immunoassay is called for.

The spine in acromegaly may also reveal identifying features. A lateral view of the spine may disclose an increase in the anteroposterior diameter of a vertebral body, as well as scalloping or increased concavity of the posterior vertebral margin (Fig. 25.7). Although the exact mechanism of this phenomenon is not known, bone resorption has been implicated as a potential cause. Other conditions have

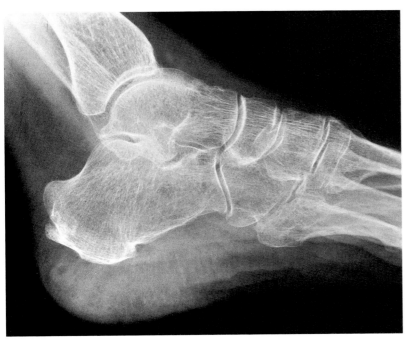

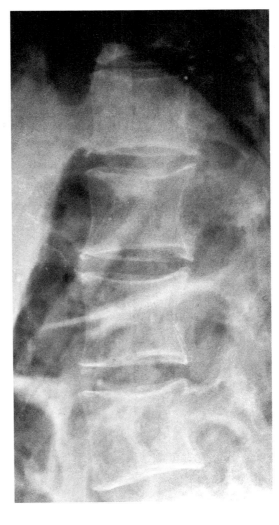

Figure 25.7 Lateral view of the thoracolumbar spine of a 49-year-old woman with acromegaly demonstrates posterior vertebral scalloping, a phenomenon apparently due to bone resorption.

Figure 25.6 Lateral view of the foot of a 58-year-old man shows a heel-pad thickness of 38 mm, far above normal for this patient, who weighs only 140 pounds. This measurement corresponds to the shortest distance between the calcaneus and the plantar aspect of the heel.

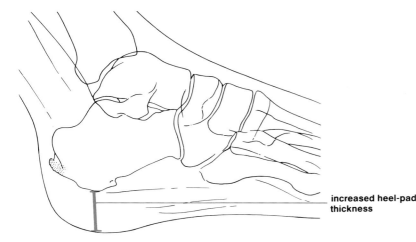

increased heel-pad thickness

also been associated with posterior vertebral scalloping (Fig. 25.8). In addition, thoracic kyposis is often increased in spinal acromegaly and lumbar lordosis accentuated. The invertebral disk space may be wider than normal due to overgrowth of the cartilaginous portion of the disk.

The articular abnormalities seen in acromegaly are the result of a frequent complication, degenerative joint disease (see Figs. 11.1 and 12.15), which is in turn the result of overgrowth of the articular cartilage and subsequent inadequate nourishment of abnormally thick cartilage. The combination of joint space narrowing, osteophytes, subchondral sclerosis, and formation of cyst-like lesions is similar to the primary osteoarthritic process.

GAUCHER DISEASE

Classification

Gaucher disease is a metabolic disorder characterized by the abnormal deposition of cerebrosides (glycolipids) in the reticuloendothelial cells of the spleen, liver, and bone marrow. These altered macrophages, called "Gaucher cells," are the histologic hallmark of the disease.

Gaucher disease is a familial inherited disturbance of unknown etiology, transmitted as an autosomal-recessive trait. It is classified into three distinct categories:

Type I   The *non-neuronopathic* or *adult type* is the most common form, occurring mainly in Ashkenazic Jews. Onset is in the patient's first or second decade, and the individuals affected usually live normal life spans. Bone abnormalities and hepatosplenomegaly characterize this form of the disease.

Type II   The *acute neuronopathic form* is lethal within the patient's first year. This type apparently has no predilection for any ethnic group.

Type III The *subacute juvenile neuronopathic form* begins in the latter part of the first year and follows a malignant course similar to that of type II. Patients suffer from mental retardation and seizures, and usually die by the end of their second decade of life.

Figure 25.8 Causes of Scalloping in Vertebral Bodies

Increased Intraspinal Pressure
Intradural neoplasms
Intraspinal cysts
Syringomyelia and hydromyelia
Communicating hydrocephalus

Dural Ectasia
Marfan syndrome
Ehlers-Danlos syndrome
Neurofibromatosis

Bone Resorption
Acromegaly

Congenital Disorders
Achondroplasia
Morquio disease
Hunter syndrome
Osteogenesis imperfecta (tarda)

Physiologic Scalloping

(From Mitchell GE, et al., 1967)

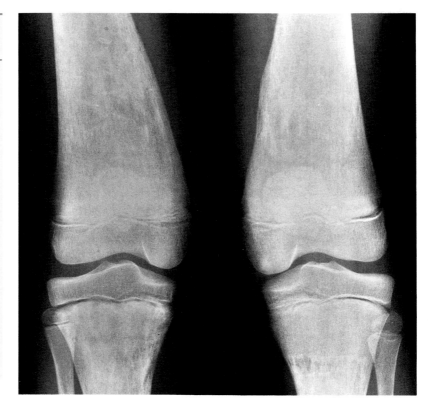

Figure 25.9
Anteroposterior radiograph of a 12-year-old boy with adult-type Gaucher disease shows the Erlenmeyer-flask deformity of both lower femora, secondary to medullary expansion. Note the thinning of the cortex due to diffuse osteoporosis.

The presenting clinical features of patients depend on the type of disease they have. The adult form of the disorder (type I) is the most common and typically presents with abdominal distention secondary to splenomegaly. Recurrent bone pain is a sign of skeletal involvement, and acute, severe bone pain, together with swelling and fever, suggests acute pyogenic osteomyelitis. This clinical complex, which is the result of ischemic necrosis of bone, has been called "aseptic osteomyelitis." Pingueculae may be present in the eyes, and the skin may acquire a brown pigmentation. Epistaxis or other hemorrhages due to thrombocytopenia may occur. The diagnosis is made by demonstrating characteristic Gaucher cells in bone-marrow aspirate or in a biopsy specimen from the liver.

Radiographic Evaluation

The radiographic examination in Gaucher disease reveals characteristic findings. There is a diffuse osteoporosis that is frequently associated with medullary expansion. In the ends of the long bones, this phenomenon is referred to as the "Erlenmeyer-flask" deformity (Fig. 25.9). Localized bone destruction assuming a honeycomb appearance is also typically seen (Fig. 25.10); gross osteolytic destruction is usually limited to the shafts of the long bones. Moreover, sclerotic changes are common, occurring secondary to a repair process or bone infarctions (Fig. 25.11). Medullary bone infarction and a periosteal reaction may lead to a bone-within-bone phenomenon, which may resemble osteomyelitis (Fig. 25.12).

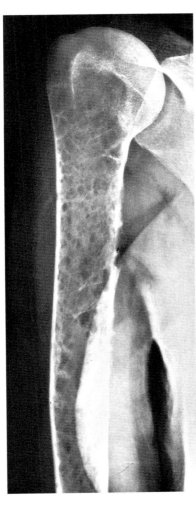

Figure 25.10 Destructive changes in Gaucher disease, seen here in the proximal right humerus of a 52-year-old woman with the adult form of the disease, may assume a honeycombed appearance.

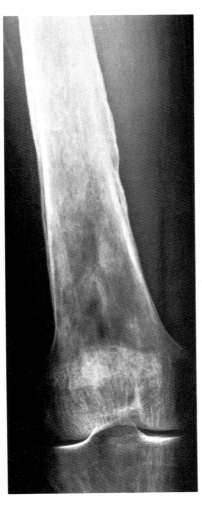

Figure 25.11 Anteroposterior radiograph of the right distal femur of a 29-year-old man with Gaucher disease demonstrates medullary infarction of the bone and endosteal and periosteal reactions secondary to reparative processes.

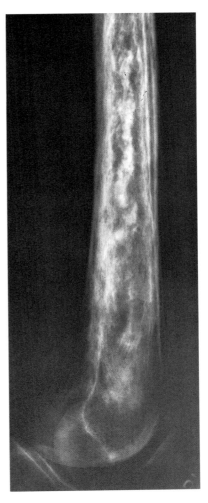

Figure 25.12 Lateral view of the distal femur in a 28-year-old woman with Gaucher disease shows extensive medullary infarction and periosteal new bone formation, producing a bone-within-bone appearance.

Complications

The most common complication of Gaucher disease is osteonecrosis of the femoral head and occasionally of the femoral condyles (Fig 25.13). Superimposition of degenerative changes is also a frequent finding, which necessitates surgery. Pathologic fractures are common, and they may involve the long bones as well as the spine. The most serious complication (although fortunately a rare one) is malignant transformation at the site of bone infarcts.

TUMORAL CALCINOSIS

Pathophysiology

First described by Inclan and co-workers in 1943, tumoral calcinosis is characterized by the presence of single or multiple periarticular lobulated cystic masses containing chalky material. Their formation is the result of the deposition of calcium salt in the soft tissues about the joints—the shoulders (particularly near the scapula), hips, and elbow joints—as well as on the extensile surfaces of the limbs. The masses are painless and usually occur in children and adolescents. Blacks are affected more frequently than other racial groups, with most cases of tumoral calcinosis reported from Africa and New Guinea. Since the etiology is unknown, the diagnosis is one of exclusion: Other causes of soft tissue calcifications, such as secondary hyperparathyroidism, hypervitaminosis D, gout and pseudogout, myositis ossificans, para-articular chondroma, and calcinosis circum-scripta must be excluded before the diagnosis of tumoral calcinosis can be made.

Radiographic Evaluation

Radiographic examination usually reveals well demarcated and lobulated calcific masses that are circular or oval in shape and located about the joints (Fig. 25.14). They vary in density; some are lacy and amorphous and others are almost bone-like in appearance. Only in very rare instances is the calcific deposit located within the joint capsule.

Treatment

Surgical excision of the calcified masses is the most effective form of treatment, although attempts to treat this disorder with low calcium and phosphate diets and phosphate-combining antacids have had some success.

HYPOTHYROIDISM

Pathophysiology

Hypothyroidism is a syndrome encountered in infants and children, resulting from a deficiency of the thyroid hormones, thyroxine and triiodothyronine, either during fetal life (cretinism) or

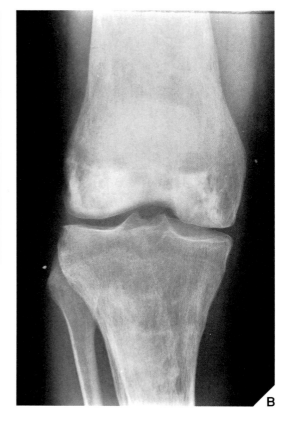

Figure 25.13 (A) Anteroposterior radiograph of the pelvis of an 11-year-old Ashkenazic Jew with non-neuronopathic Gaucher disease shows osteonecrosis of the left femoral head, a common complication of this disorder.
(B) Anteroposterior radiograph of the right knee of a 25-year-old man with Gaucher disease demonstrates osteonecrotic changes of the medial and lateral femoral condyles. Note also the extensive bone infarction of the proximal tibia.

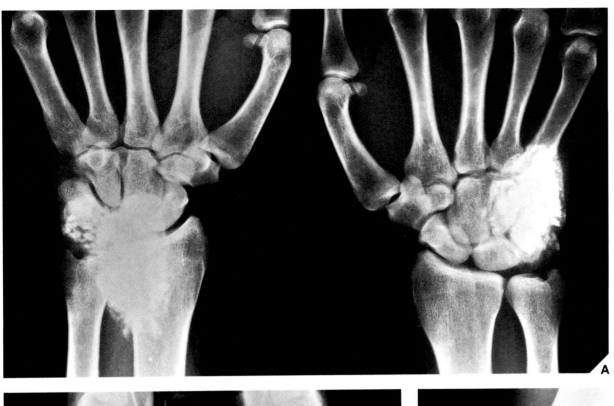

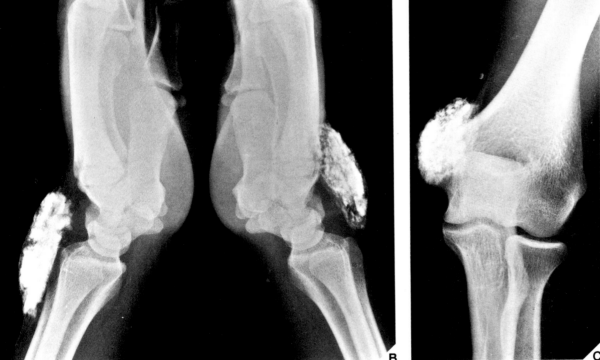

early childhood (juvenile myxedema or juvenile hypothyroidism). The deficiency may be primary, due to disease of the thyroid gland; or secondary, due to lack of thyroid-stimulating hormone (TSH) produced by the pituitary gland. The major target sites are the growth plates and epiphyses, best demonstrated in the hands and the hips (Fig. 25.15). The key symptoms and signs include lethargy, constipation, an enlarged tongue, abdominal distention, and dry skin. The manifestations are typically less severe when the deficiency occurs in early childhood as an acquired disease than when it is congenital.

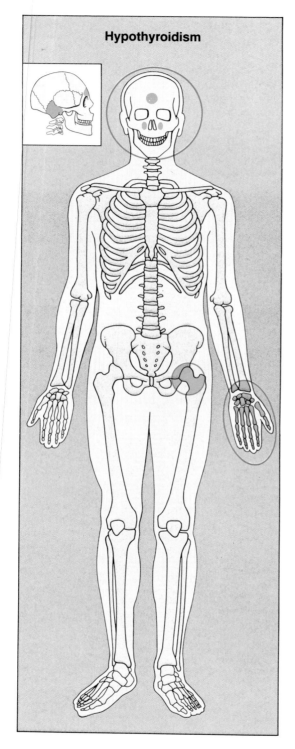

Hypothyroidism

Figure 25.15 Target sites of hypothyroidism.

Radiographic Evaluation

The fundamental radiographic feature in both forms of hypothyroidism is delayed skeletal maturation with stunting of bone growth leading to dwarfism. In particular, the appearance of the secondary ossification centers is greatly delayed, as a dorsovolar radiograph of the hand may demonstrate (Fig. 25.16). Epiphyses ossify from numerous ossification centers, thereby acquiring a fragmented appearance and on occasion appearing abnormally dense (Fig. 25.17). This process may be mistaken for osteonecrosis, as seen in Legg-Calvé-Perthes disease (see Figs. 27.23–27.26), or for certain dys-

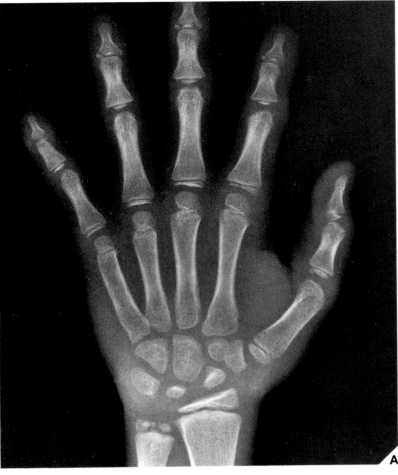

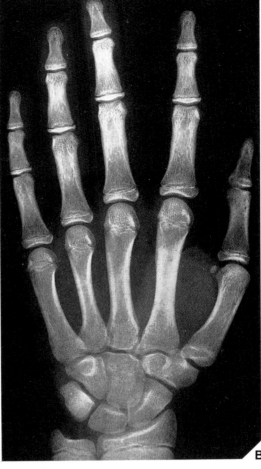

Figure 25.16 (A) Dorsovolar radiograph of the right hand of a 13-year-old boy with juvenile hypothyroidism demonstrates skeletal immaturity; the bone age is roughly eight years. Note the fragmented secondary ossification centers of the distal ulna and distal phalanges. In fact, they represent foci of ossification. (B) The hand of a normal boy of the same age is shown for comparison.

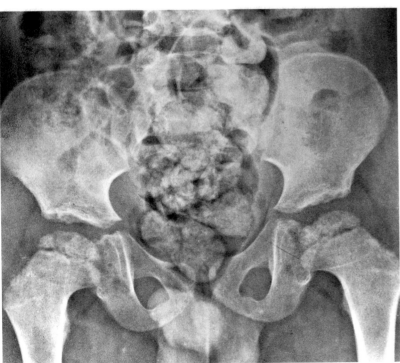

Figure 25.17 Anteroposterior radiograph of the pelvis of a 5-year-old girl with congenital hypothyroidism (cretinism) shows pseudofragmentation of both capital femoral epiphyses. This process may be mistaken for Legg-Calvé-Perthes disease.

plasias, such as dysplasia epiphysealis punctata, also known as Conradi disease. Underpneumatization of the sinuses and mastoids are also typical radiographic findings associated with hypothyroidism.

Complications

One of the common complications of hypothyroidism is the development of slipped femoral capital epiphysis. The radiographic findings of this condition are described in Chapter 27.

SCURVY

Pathophysiology

Barlow disease, as scurvy is also known, results from a deficiency of ascorbic acid (vitamin C). The function of vitamin C is to maintain intracellular substances of mesenchymal derivation, such as connective tissue, osteoid tissue in bones, and dentin in the teeth. In infants, primary deficiency is due most commonly to failure to supplement the diet with vitamin C, whereas in adults it is usually due to food idiosyncrasies or an insufficient diet. Deficiency of vitamin C causes a hemorrhagic tendency, leading to subperiosteal bleeding and abnormal function of osteoblasts and chondroblasts. The latter results in defective osteogenesis.

Radiographic Evaluation

The characteristic bone lesions of scurvy are caused by cessation of endochondral bone ossification due to failure of the osteoblasts to form osteoid tissue. Continuing osteoclastic resorption without adequate formation of new bone yields the appearance of osteoporosis, with generalized osteopenia and thinning of the cortices. Deposition of calcium phosphate continues in whatever osteoid tissue is formed, so that an area of increased density develops adjacent to the

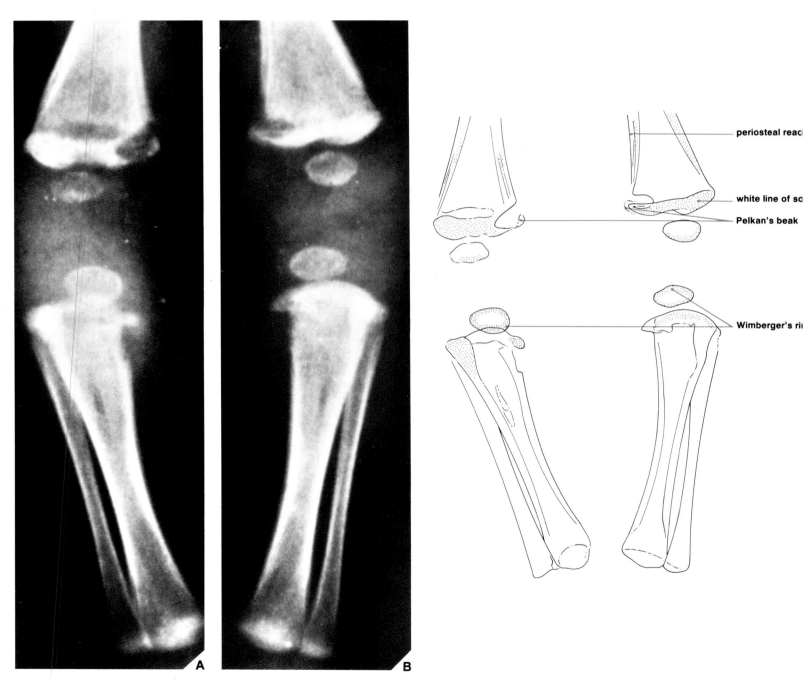

Figure 25.18 (A, B) Anteroposterior view of the lower legs of an 8-month-old infant shows the typical skeletal changes of scurvy. Note the dense segment adjacent to the growth plate ("white line of scurvy"), the ring of increased density around the secondary ossification centers of the distal femora and proximal tibiae (Wimberger ring sign), and the beaking of the metaphysis of both tibiae (Pelkan beak). A periosteal reaction secondary to subperiosteal bleeding is also noted.

growth plate. Such areas have been called the "white lines of scurvy" (Fig. 25.18). A ring of increased density is also seen around the secondary centers of ossification, a finding known as a Wimberger ring sign. Fractures of the metaphysis are common, producing a "corner" sign or "Pelkan beak" (see Fig. 25.18). Increased capillary fragility leads to subperiosteal and soft tissue bleeding and the formation of hematomas, which may trigger a periosteal reaction (Fig. 25.19). In adults, the bleeding may extend into the joints.

Differential Diagnosis

Scurvy should be differentiated from "battered child syndrome," congenital syphylis, and leukemia. In battered child syndrome, characteristic metaphyseal corner fractures and fractures in different healing stages are characteristic. In congenital syphylis, the epiphyseal centers are normal. In leukemia, radiolucent metaphyseal bands are common but fractures and epiphysiolysis are not part of the disorder.

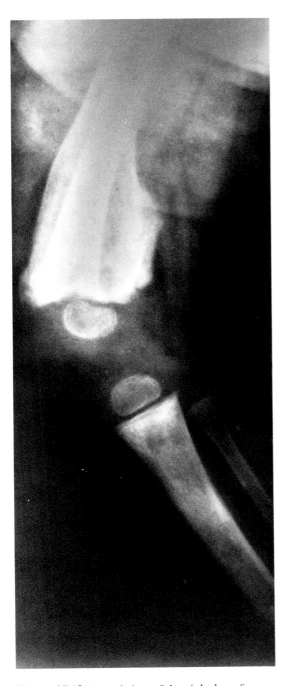

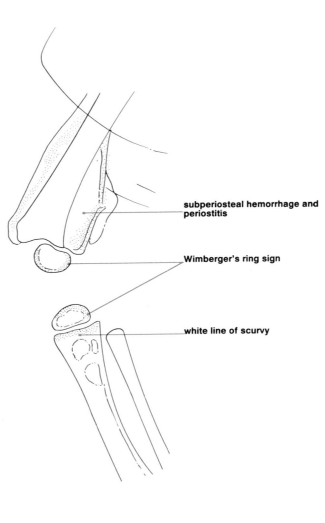

subperiosteal hemorrhage and periostitis

Wimberger's ring sign

white line of scurvy

Figure 25.19 Lateral view of the right leg of a 10-month-old infant with subperiosteal bleeding secondary to scurvy shows a marked periosteal reaction in the distal femoral diaphysis. A peripheral ring of increased density and central radiolucency, Wimberger ring sign, is evident in the posteriorly displaced ossification center of the distal femoral epiphysis.

PRACTICAL POINTS TO REMEMBER

Familial Idiopathic Hyperphosphatasia

[1] Two conditions of similar radiographic presentation are familial idiopathic hyperphosphatasia ("juvenile Paget disease") and autosomal-recessive form of hyperostosis corticalis generalisata, van Buchem disease. The radiographic features of these disorders, similar to those of Paget disease, are:
- cortical thickening and a coarse trabecular pattern to the spongiosa
- sparing of the articular ends of bones (unlike classic Paget disease).

Acromegaly

[1] In the diagnosis and evaluation of acromegaly, the following radiographic projections have specific value:
- lateral view of the skull to evaluate the thickness of the cranial vault, the size of the paranasal sinuses, and prognathism
- dorsovolar view of the hands to evaluate the sesamoid index and detect changes of the distal tufts
- lateral view of the foot to measure the heel-pad thickness
- lateral view of the spine to evaluate the intervertebral disk spaces and the posterior margins of the vertebral bodies.

[2] One of the frequent complications of acromegaly is degenerative joint disease secondary to undernourished hypertrophied articular cartilage.

Gaucher Disease

[1] Gaucher disease is a metabolic disorder characterized by the abnormal deposition of cerebrosides (glycolipids) in the reticuloendothelial system.

[2] Characteristic radiographic features of Gaucher disease include:
- Erlenmeyer-flask deformity of the distal femora
- osteonecrosis of the femoral heads
- medullary bone infarction of the long bones, frequently associated with periosteal reaction
- generalized osteopenia.

Tumoral Calcinosis

[1] Tumoral calcinosis, a condition seen predominantly in blacks, consists of multiple cystic, calcium-containing masses about the large joints (shoulders, hips, and elbows).

[2] The diagnosis of tumoral calcinosis is one of exclusion: other causes of soft tissue calcifications, such as secondary hyperparathyroidism, hypervitaminosis D, and juxtacortical myositis ossificans, must be excluded.

Hypothyroidism

[1] The fundamental radiographic feature of hypothyroidism (cretinism and juvenile myxedema) is retarded skeletal maturation, which is best demonstrated on a dorsovolar view of the hand.

[2] Other characteristic radiographic features of hypothyroidism include:
- a fragmented appearance of the ossification centers of the epiphyses
- increased density of both epiphyses and metaphyses.

[3] In the femoral heads, these features may mimic osteonecrosis (Legg-Calvé-Perthes disease) or dysplasia epiphysealis punctata (Conradi disease).

Scurvy

[1] The characteristic radiographic changes seen in scurvy (deficiency of vitamin C) include:
- generalized osteopenia
- "white lines of scurvy" adjacent to the growth plate
- Wimberger ring sign, representing increased density around ossification centers
- the "corner" sign or "Pelkan beak," representing metaphyseal fractures
- periosteal reaction secondary to subperiosteal bleeding.

[2] Conditions that should be differentiated from scurvy include:
- battered child syndrome
- congenital syphilis
- leukemia.

References

Albright F: Changes simulating Legg Perthes disease (osteochondritis deformans juvenilis) due to juvenile myxoedema. *J Bone Joint Surg* 20:764, 1938.

Amstutz HC: The hip in Gaucher's disease. *Clin Orthop* 90:83, 1973.

Bishop AF, Destovet JM, Murphy WA, Gilula LA: Tumoral calcinosis: Case report and review. *Skeletal Radiol* 8:269, 1982.

Desnick RJ: Gaucher disease (1882-1982): Centennial perspectives on the most prevalent Jewish genetic disease. *Mt Sinai J Med* 49:443, 1982.

Duncan TR: Validity of sesamoid index in diagnosis of acromegaly. *Radiology* 115:617, 1975.

Feldman RH, Lewis MM, Greenspan A, Steiner GC: Tumoral calcinosis in an infant. A case report. *Bull Hosp Jt Dis Orthop Inst* 43:78, 1983.

Goldblatt J, Sachs S, Beighton P: The orthopedic aspects of Gaucher's disease. *Clin Orthop* 137:208, 1978.

Hernandez RJ, Poznanski AK: Distinctive appearance of the distal phalanges in children with primary hypothyroidism. *Radiology* 132:83, 1979.

Hernandez RJ, Poznanski AW, Hopwood NJ: Size and skeletal maturation of the hand in children with hypothyroidism and hypopituitarism. *Am J Roentgenol* 133:405, 1979.

Hirsch M, Mogle P, Barkli Y: Neonatal Scurvy. *Pediatr Radiol* 4:251, 1976.

Inclan A, Leon P, Camejo MG: Tumoral calcinosis. *JAMA* 121:490, 1943.

Kho KM, Wright AD, Doyle FH: Heel-pad thickness in acromegaly. *Br J Radiol* 43:119, 1970.

Kleinberg DL, Young IS, Kupperman HS: The sesamoid index. An aid in the diagnosis of acromegaly. *Ann Intern Med* 64:1075, 1966.

Lafferty FW, Reynolds ES, Pearson OH: Humoral calcinosis: A metabolic disease of obscure etiology. *Am J Med* 38:105, 1965.

Lang EK, Bessler WT: The roentgenologic features of acromegaly. *Am J Roentgenol* 86:321, 1961.

Lanir A, Hadar H, Cohen I, et al: Gaucher disease: Assessment with MR imaging. *Radiology* 161:239, 1986.

Levin B: Gaucher's disease: Clinical and roentgenologic manifestations. *Am J Roentgenol* 85:685, 1961.

Lin SR, Lee KF: Relative value of some radiographic measurements of the hand in the diagnosis of acromegaly. *Invest Radiol* 6:426, 1971.

McNulty JF, Pim P: Hyperphosphatasia. Report of a case with a 30-year follow-up. *Am J Roentgenol* 115:614, 1972.

Manaster BJ, Anderson TM Jr: Tumoral calcinosis: Serial images to monitor successful dietary therapy. *Skeletal Radiol* 8:123, 1982.

Mitchell GE, Lourie H, Berne AS: The various causes of scalloped vertebrae and notes on their pathogenesis. *Radiology* 89:67, 1967.

Nerubay J, Pilderwasser D: Spontaneous bilateral distal femoral physiolysis due to scurvy. *Acta Orthop Scand* 55:18, 1984.

Palmer PES: Tumor calcinosis. *Br J Radiol* 39:518, 1966.

Smit GG, Schmaman A: Tumoral calcinosis. *J Bone Joint Surg* 49B:698, 1967.

Steinbach HL, Russell W: Measurement of the heel pad as an aid to diagnosis of acromegaly. *Radiology* 82:418, 1964.

Steinbach HL, Feldman R, Goldberg MB: Acromegaly. *Radiology* 72:535, 1959.

Stuber JL, Palacios E: Vertebral scalloping in acromegaly. *Am J Roentgenol* 112:397, 1971.

Van Buchem FSP, Hadders MN, Ubbens R: An uncommon familial systemic disease of the skeleton: Hyperostosis corticalis generalisata familiaris. *Acta Radiol* 44:109, 1955.

Van Buchem FSP, Hadders HN, Hansen JF, Woldring MG: Hyperostosis corticalis generalisata. Report of seven cases. *Am J Med* 33:38 7, 1962.

Zubrow AB, Lane JM, Parks JS: Slipped capital femoral epiphysis occurring during treatment for hypothyroidism. *J Bone Joint Surg* 60A:256, 1978.

PART VII

Congenital and Developmental Anomalies

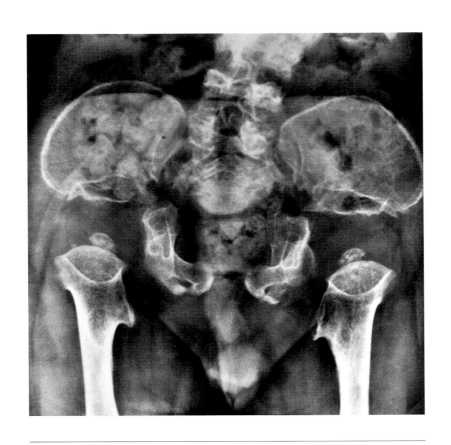

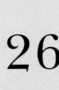

26

Radiologic Evaluation of Skeletal Anomalies

CLASSIFICATION

THE CONDITIONS DISCUSSED in this part comprise disturbances in skeletal formation, development, growth, maturation, and modeling. Some of these anomalies arise during fetal development, such as congenital absence of a whole or part of a limb, supernumerary digits in a hand or foot, or fused digits, and are obvious at the time the baby is born. Some may begin to develop during fetal life but become apparent later in childhood, such as Hurler syndrome (gargoylism) or osteogenesis imperfecta tarda. Other anomalies,

such as certain sclerosing dysplasias, develop after birth because of a genetic predisposition and become manifest later in life.

Congenital anomalies can be classified in various ways, but because of their complexity a full and detailed classification of these disorders is beyond the scope of this chapter. To simplify the variety of classifications, which are constantly changing and expanding, the congenital anomalies may be divided from the pathologic point of view into those involving disturbances of bone formation, bone growth, and bone maturation and modeling (Fig. 26.1). Anomalies of bone formation include the *complete failure of a bone to form*

Figure 26.1 Simplified Classification of Congenital Anomalies of the Skeletal System

ANOMALIES OF BONE FORMATION
Complete failure of formation (agenisis, aplasia)
Faulty formation
  Decreased number of bones
  Increased number of bones
Faulty differentiation
  Pseudoarthrosis
  Fusion (synostosis, coalition, syndactyly)

ANOMALIES OF BONE GROWTH
Aberrant size
  Undergrowth (hypoplasia, atrophy)
  Overgrowth (hypertrophy, gigantism)
Aberrant shape (deformed growth)
Aberrant fit (subluxation, dislocation)

ANOMALIES OF BONE MATURATION
    AND MODELING
Failure of endochondral bone maturation and modeling
Failure of intramembranous bone maturation and modeling
Combined failure of endochondral and intramembranmous bone
    maturation and modeling

CONSTITUTIONAL DISEASES OF BONE
Abnormalities of cartilage and/or bone growth and development
    (osteochondrodysplasias)
Malformation of individual bones, isolated or in combination
    (dysostoses)
Idiopathic osteolyses
Chromosomal aberrations and primary metabolic abnormalities

and *faulty formation* of bones, which may manifest in a decreased number of bones (agenesis and aplasia) (Fig. 26.2A) or in the number of supernumerary bones (polydactyly) (Fig. 26.2B,C). Anomalies of formation may also be encountered in aberrations involving bone *differentiation*, which include pseudoarthroses (Fig. 26.3A) and bone fusions (syndactyly and synostosis) (Fig. 26.3B,C). Disturbances in bone growth may lead to *aberrations in the size or shape* of bones. These may manifest in undergrowth (hypoplasia or atrophy)

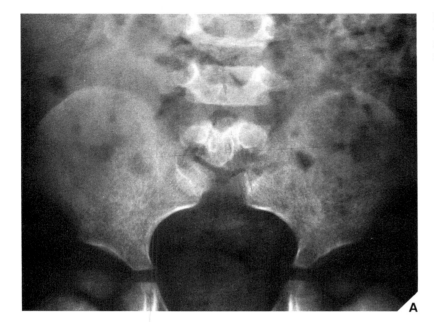

Figure 26.2 Congenital anomalies related to disturbances in bone formation may be seen in the complete failure of a bone to form, as shown on this film in a 1-year-old girl with sacral agenesis (A), or in formation of supernumerary bones, as seen in this 12-year-old boy with polydactyly in both hands (B) and in this 3-year-old girl with polydactyly in the right foot (C).

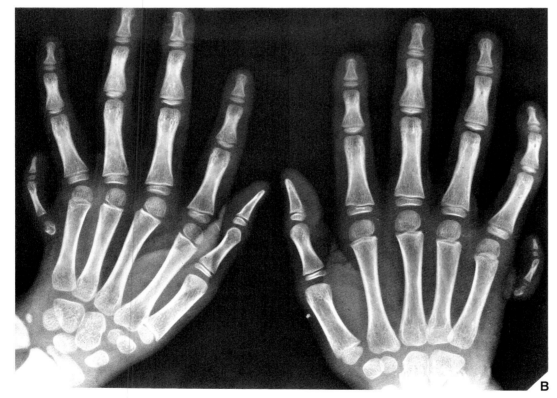

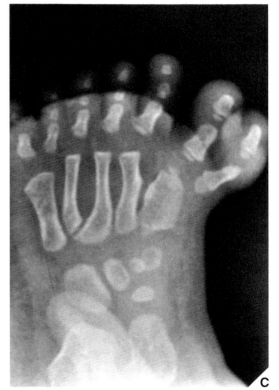

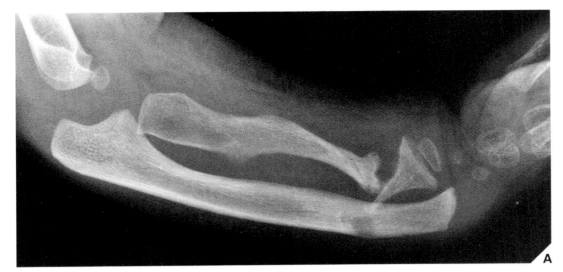

Figure 26.3 Congenital anomalies related to bone division may manifest in congenital pseudoarthrosis, seen here involving the left radius in a 4-year-old boy (A), in partial fusion (synostosis) of two bones, seen here affecting the proximal radius and ulna in a 6-year-old girl (B), or in coalition, seen in the complete fusion of the lunate and triquetrum bones in a 33-year-old man (C).

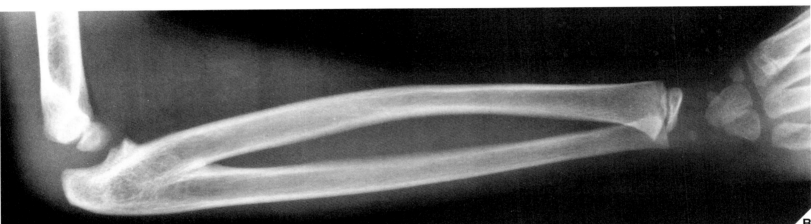

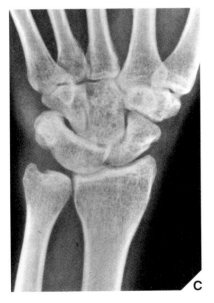

(Fig. 26.4B), in overgrowth (hypertrophy or gigantism) (Fig. 26.4), or deformed growth, such as congenital tibia vara (see Fig. 27.40). Anomalies related to bone growth may also be exhibited in abnormalities affecting the *motion in a joint*, such as contractures, subluxations, and dislocations (Fig. 26.5). Among the last group of congenital anomalies affecting the skeletal system are those exhibiting aberrations in bone *growth, maturation, and modeling*, as manifest in the various dysplasias (Fig. 26.6).

A second simple classification system is anatomic and based on the affected region of the body. This system comprises anomalies of the shoulder girdle and upper limb, pelvis and lower limb, spine, and the skeleton in general.

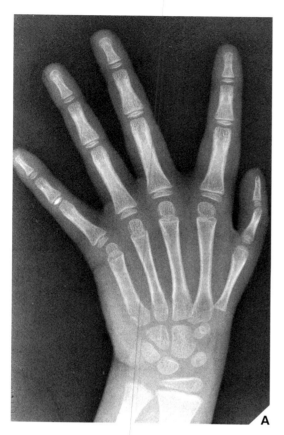

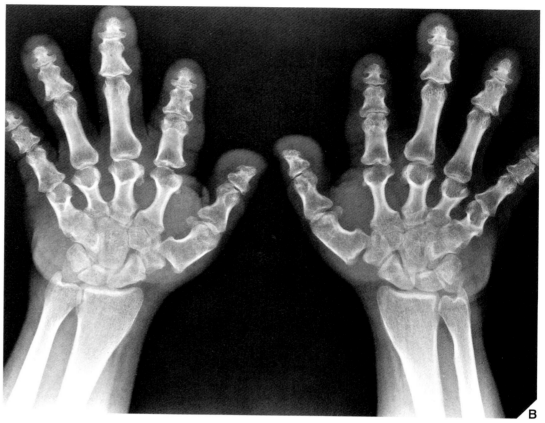

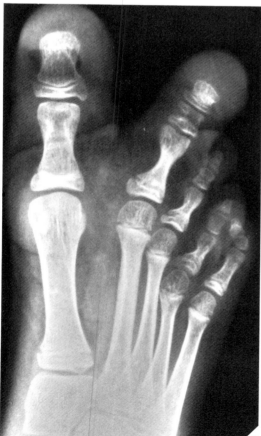

Figure 26.4 Congenital anomalies related to the size of bones may manifest in hypoplasia, as seen here in the right thumb of a 4-year-old girl (A), or in congenital brachydactyly, shown here in both hands of a 25-year-old woman (B). Overgrowth may also be encountered, as in this case of macrodactyly (megalodactyly) involving the first two digits of the left foot of a 12-year-old girl (C).

RADIOLOGIC IMAGING MODALITIES

Radiologic examination is essential for the accurate diagnosis of many congenital and developmental anomalies, which in some instances (such as osteopoikilosis or osteopathia striata) are totally asymptomatic and only revealed on radiographs obtained for other purposes. It also plays an important part in monitoring the progress of treatment. In many instances the results of therapy, whether conservative or surgical, can be assessed only on the basis of the proper radiologic examination.

The radiologic imaging modalities most frequently used in diagnosing congenital malformations of the bones and joints are the following:

1. Conventional radiography, including standard and special projections
2. Conventional tomography
3. Arthrography
4. Myelography
5. Computed tomography (CT)
6. Radionuclide imaging (scintigraphy, bone scan)
7. Sonography (ultrasound)
8. Magnetic resonance imaging (MRI)

In most instances, the diagnosis can be made on the standard radiographic projections specific for the anatomic site under investigation. As in most other orthopedic conditions, plain films should be obtained in at least two projections at 90° to one another

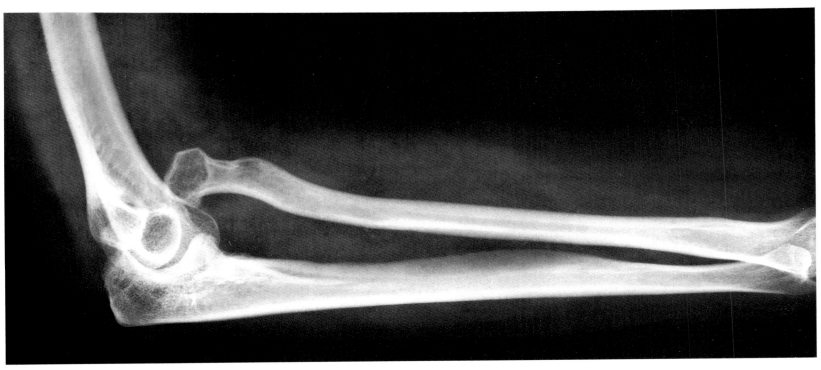

Figure 26.5 Congenital dislocation of the radial head, seen here in a 35-year-old woman, is an anomaly related to aberrant bone growth leading to a condition affecting the motion of a joint. Note the hypoplasia and abnormal shape of the radial head, an important feature differentiating this condition from traumatic dislocation.

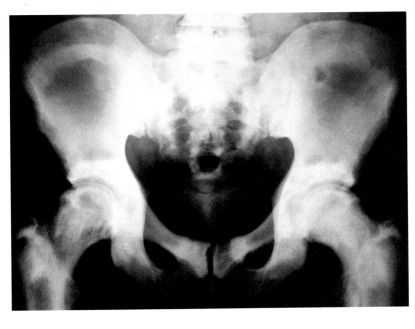

Figure 26.6 Osteopetrosis (Albers-Schönberg disease), seen here in the spine, pelvis, and both femora of a 28-year-old man, is a congenital anomaly related to the growth, development, and maturation of bone. The persistence of immature spongiosa packing the marrow cavity results in the dense marble-like appearance of the bones.

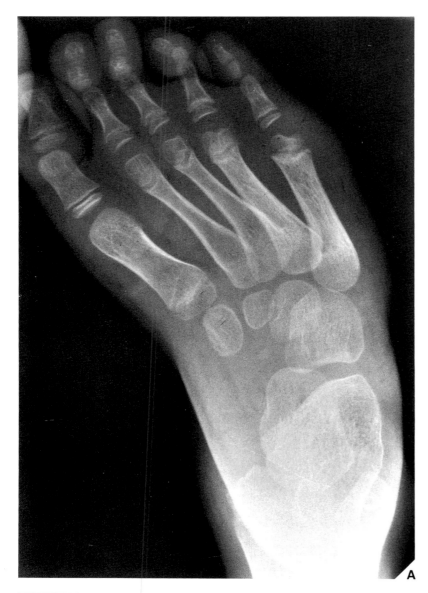

A

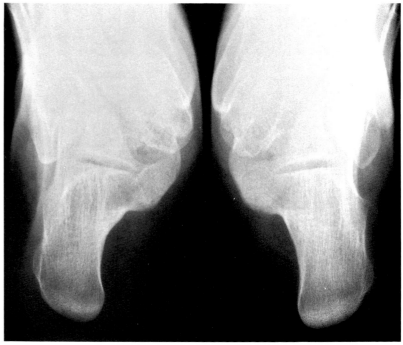

Figure 26.8 Posterior tangential (Harris-Beath) projection of both calcanei in a 23-year-old woman demonstrates bony fusion at the level of the middle facet of both subtalar joints, a diagnostic feature of a talocalcaneal coalition.

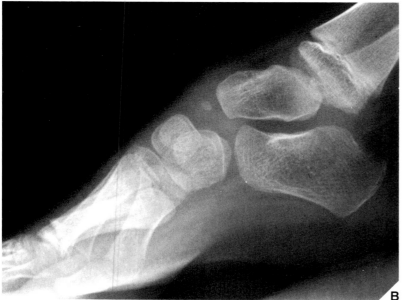

B

Figure 26.7 Dorsoplantar (A) and lateral (B) views of the foot of a 7-year-old boy are sufficient to demonstrate all the components of congenital equinovarus deformity of the foot (clubfoot), namely the equinous position of the heel, the varus position of the hindfoot, and the adduction and varus deformity of the forefoot.

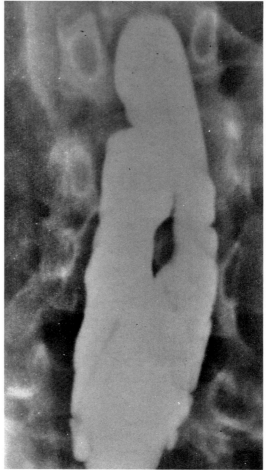

Figure 26.9 A myelogram of a 9-year-old girl demonstrates a filling defect in the center of the contrast-filled thecal sac, caused by a fibrous spur attached to the vertebral body. This finding is diagnostic of diastematomyelia, a rare congenital anomaly of the vertebrae and spinal cord. Note the associated increase in the interpedicular distances.

(Fig. 26.7; see also Fig. 4.1). Supplemental views, however, are sometimes necessary for a full evaluation of an anomaly, particularly those affecting complex structures such as the ankle and foot (Fig. 26.8). Weight-bearing views of the foot should be obtained whenever possible.

Ancillary imaging techniques play an important role in the evaluation of many congenital and developmental conditions. Myelography, for example, is valuable for detecting anomalies of the spine (Fig. 26.9). In congenital dislocations, particularly in the hip, arthrography is an essential technique (Fig. 26.10); it is also effective in demonstrating developmental anomalies affecting the articular cartilage and menisci of the knee, as in Blount disease (Fig. 26.11). CT examination is particularly valuable in the evaluation of congenital hip dislocations. Apart from providing important interpretive data about this complex anomaly, including demonstration of details of the relationship between the acetabulum and the femoral head, CT provides an accurate assessment of the degree of reduction of the head after treatment, often disclosing very subtle abnormalities not detected by plain

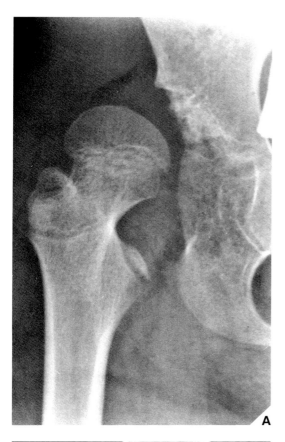

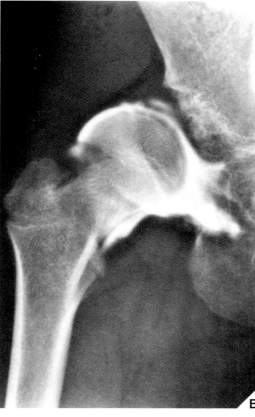

Figure 26.10 (A) Standard anteroposterior radiograph of the right hip of a 7-year-old girl who was treated conservatively for congenital hip dislocation demonstrates persistent complete dislocation. (B) Arthrography was performed to evaluate the cartilaginous structures of the joint. In addition to a deformed cartilaginous limbus, the ligamentum teres appears thickened and contrast medium has accumulated in the stretched capsule. The thickened ligamentum teres frustrated several previous attempts at closed reduction.

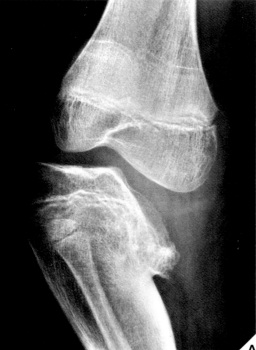

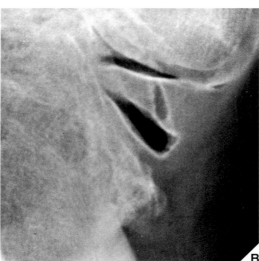

Figure 26.11 (A) Anteroposterior view of the knee of a 4-year-old boy demonstrates congenital tibia vara (Blount disease). (B) Double-contrast arthrogram of the knee shows hypertrophy of the medial meniscus and thick nonossified cartilage at the medial aspect of the proximal tibial epiphysis.

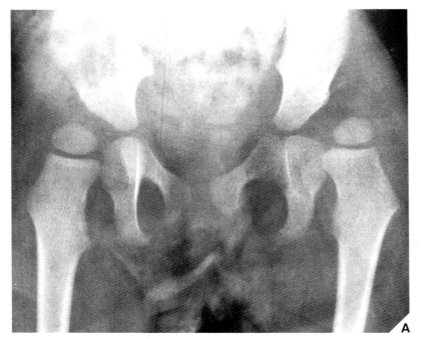

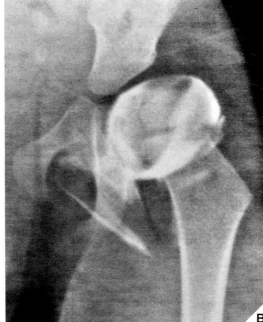

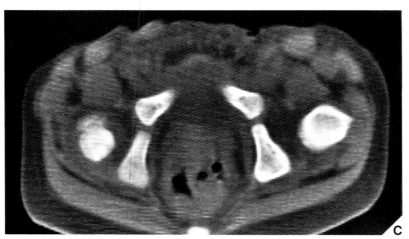

Figure 26.12 (A) Anteroposterior view of the pelvis in a 1-year-old girl demonstrates congenital dislocation of the left hip. After conservative management with a Pavlik harness, a contrast arthrogram (B) was done to evaluate the results of treatment. The femoral head appears to be well seated in the acetabulum. Note the smoothness of the Shenton-Menard line (see Fig. 27.10). (C) CT section, however, demonstrates persistence of posterolateral subluxation.

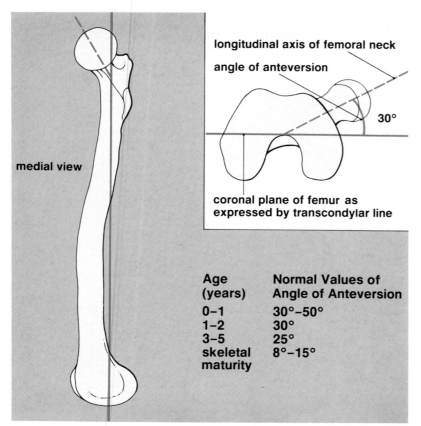

Figure 26.13 The angle of anteversion of the femoral head represents the degree of anterior torsion of the femoral head and neck from the coronal plane. It is determined by the angle formed between the longitudinal axis of the femoral neck and the coronal plane of the femur as expressed by a transcondylar line (see Fig. 26.14).

longitudinal axis of femoral neck

angle of anteversion

30°

coronal plane of femur as expressed by transcondylar line

medial view

Age (years)	Normal Values of Angle of Anteversion
0–1	30°–50°
1–2	30°
3–5	25°
skeletal maturity	8°–15°

radiography or arthrography of the hip (Fig. 26.12). A further application of CT is seen in its ability to measure the angle of anteversion of the femoral head, that is, the degree of anterior torsion of the femoral head and neck from the coronal plane (Figs. 26.13, 26.14)).

Other ancillary techniques also have important functions in the evaluation of skeletal anomalies. Radionuclide bone scan, for instance, is particularly effective in detecting silent sites of skeletal abnormality in various developmental dysplasias (Fig. 26.15).

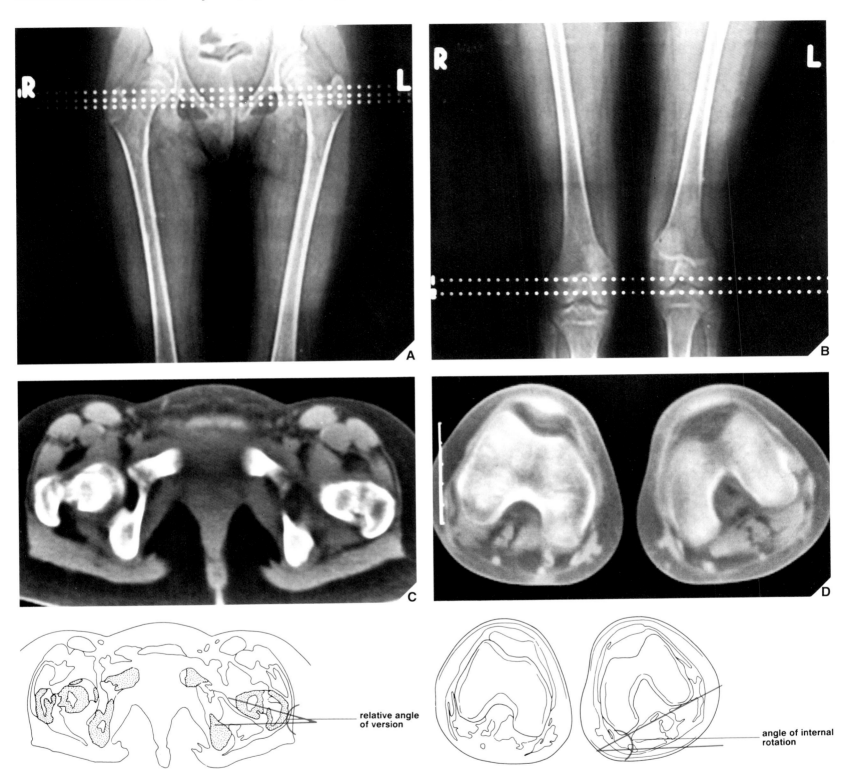

Figure 26.14 To obtain the angle of version of the femoral head on CT examination, the patient is supine, with the lower extremities in the neutral position, the feet taped together, and the knees taped to the table. Preferably, a single scanogram is obtained that includes both hips and knees on the same film; however, separate films may be obtained (A,B) if the patient is too tall. In the latter case, care should be taken not to move the patient between the two takes. On a section through the femoral neck and the upper portion of the greater trochanter (C), a line is drawn through the femoral neck, using the femoral head and greater trochanter as guides. The angle that this line forms with the horizontal line (the level of the CT table) determines the *relative* angle of anteversion (or retroversion) of the femoral head. On the CT section through the femoral condyles at the intercondylar notch (D), a line is drawn through the posterior margins of the condyles, and the angle formed by this line and the horizontal line determines the degree of internal or external rotation of the extremities. From these two measurements, a *true* angle of version (anteversion or retroversion) is calculated. If the knee is in internal rotation, as in the present case, the sum of both angles yields the degree of anteversion. If the knee is in external rotation, the angle obtained at the knee must be subtracted from the angle at the hip, yielding the degree of version.

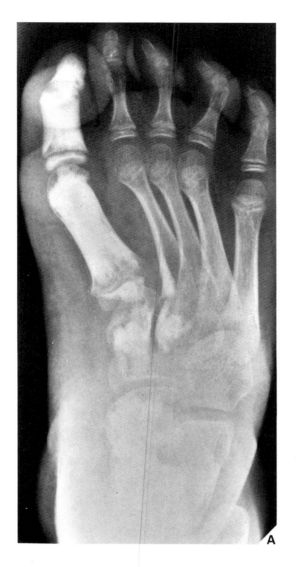

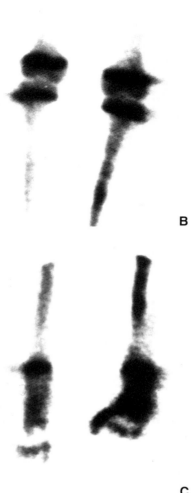

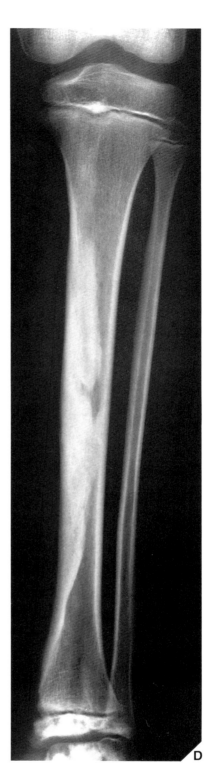

Figure 26.15
A 9-year-old boy had a deformity of the left foot since birth, which was diagnosed as a clubfoot. (A) Dorsoplantar view of the foot demonstrates the clubfoot deformity, together with sclerotic changes in the phalanges of the great toe, the first and second metatarsals, the first and second cuneiforms, the talus, and the calcaneus. Such changes are typical of melorheostosis, a form of sclerosing dysplasia. (B,C) On bone scan, the extent of skeletal involvement is indicated by increased uptake of radiopharmaceutical in not only the foot but also the left tibia, which is confirmed on a subsequent radiograph of the left leg (D).

Sonography has only recently come to be used in the diagnosis of congenital skeletal abnormalities, including hip dysplasia and dislocation. It is effective in assessing the position of the femoral head in the acetabulum, as well as the status of the cartilaginous acetabular roof and other cartilaginous structures such as the limbus that cannot be demonstrated on the standard radiographs. This technique also offers a noninvasive method of examining the infant hip, which might otherwise require arthrography. And of course, sonography also involves no exposure to ionizing radiation.

MRI is ideally suited to evaluate congenital and development anomalies of the spine since all structures, including neural components, are shown simultaneously. Since MRI evaluation is mainly an assessment of neuroanatomic development, only spin-echo T1-weighted images are usually obtained (Fig. 26.16).

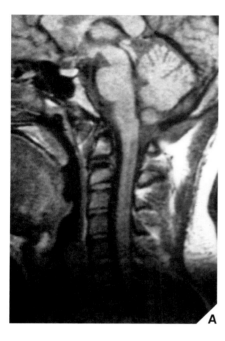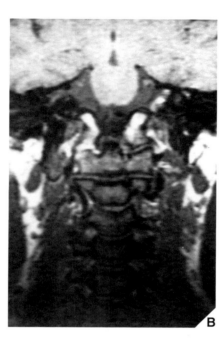

Figure 26.16 (A) Sagittal MR image (SE, TR 800/TE 20) demonstrates a hypoplastic odontoid, which arises from a normal second vertebral body. The anterior arch of the first cervical vertebra is not visualized because of fusion to the occiput. (B) Coronal MR image (SE, TR 800/TE 20) confirms that the second cervical vertebral body is normal but only a rudimentary odontoid process has formed. The atlas has fused with the occiput so that there are no occipital condyles. (From Beltran J, 1990)

PRACTICAL POINTS TO REMEMBER

[1] Congenital anomalies comprise disturbances in bone formation, bone growth, and bone maturation and modeling.

[2] Although most congenital and developmental anomalies can be diagnosed on standard radiographs, the use of ancillary techniques should be considered, such as:
- radionuclide bone scan, particularly in determining the distribution of sites of involvement in various dysplasias
- CT examination, particularly in the evaluation of congenital hip dislocation and determining the angle of version of the femoral head

- MRI, particularly in the evaluation of abnormalities of the spine.

[3] Special projections may be required for the evaluation of anomalies of complex structures such as the ankle and foot.

[4] The results and progress of treatment of various congenital disorders, especially congenital hip dislocation, can best be monitored by CT examination.

References

Bailey JA: *Disproportionate Short Stature: Diagnosis and Management.* Philadelphia, WB Saunders, 1973.

Barsky AJ: Macrodactyly. *J Bone Joint Surg,* 49A:1255, 1967.

Beighton P, Cremin B, Faure C, et al: International nomenclature of constitutional diseases of bone. *Ann Radiol* 27:275, 1984.

Beltran J: *MRI: Musculoskeletal System.* Philadelphia, Lippincott, 1990.

Berkshire SB, Maxwell EN, Sams BF: Bilateral symmetrical pseudoarthrosis in a newborn. *Radiology* 97:389, 1970.

Boal DKB, Schwenkter EP: The infant hip: Assessment with real-time US. *Radiology* 157:667, 1985.

Carlson DH: Coalition of the carpal bones. *Skeletal Radiol* 7:125, 1981.

Cleveland RH, Gilsanz V, Wilkinson RM: Congenital pseudoarthrosis of the radius. *Am J Roentgenol* 130:955, 1978.

Graf R: New possibilities for the diagnosis of congenital hip joint dislocation by ultrasonography. *J Pediatr Orthop* 3:354, 1983.

Graham CB: Assessment of bone maturation: Methods and pitfalls. *Radiol Clin North Am* 10:185, 1972.

Holston S, Carthy H: Lumbosacral agenesis: A report of three new cases and a review of the literature. *Br J Radiol* 55:629, 1982.

International nomenclature of constitutional diseases of bone. *Am J Roentgenol* 131:352, 1978.

Page LK, Post MJD: Spinal dysraphism. In: Post MJD (ed.): *Computed Tomography of the Spine.* Baltimore, Williams and Wilkins, 1984.

Rubin P: *Dynamic Classification of Bone Dysplasias.* Chicago, Year Book Med. Publ., 1972.

Smith CF: Current concepts review—tibia vara (Blount's disease). *J Bone Joint Surg* 64A:630, 1982.

Walker HS, Lufkin RB, Dietrich RB, Peacock WJ, Flannigan BD, Kangarloo H: Magnetic resonance of the pediatric spine. *RadioGraphics* 7:1129, 1987.

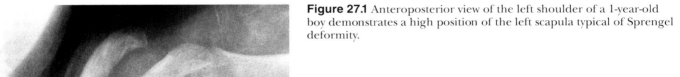

27

Anomalies of the Upper and Lower Limbs

ANOMALIES OF THE SHOULDER GIRDLE AND UPPER LIMBS
Congenital Elevation of the Scapula

SPRENGEL DEFORMITY, as congenital elevation of the scapula is also known, may be unilateral or bilateral. It is marked by the appearance of a scapula that is small, high in position, and rotated with its inferior edge pointing toward the spine—features that are easily identi-

fied on an anteroposterior view of the shoulder or chest (Fig. 27.1). The finding of a congenitally elevated scapula is important because of this condition's frequent association with other anomalies, such as scoliosis, rib anomalies, and fusion of the cervical or upper thoracic vertebrae, known as Klippel-Feil syndrome. Furthermore, there is sometimes a bony connection between the elevated scapula and one of the vertebrae (usually the C-5 or C-6 vertebra), creating what is known as the omovertebral bone (Fig. 27.2).

Figure 27.1 Anteroposterior view of the left shoulder of a 1-year-old boy demonstrates a high position of the left scapula typical of Sprengel deformity.

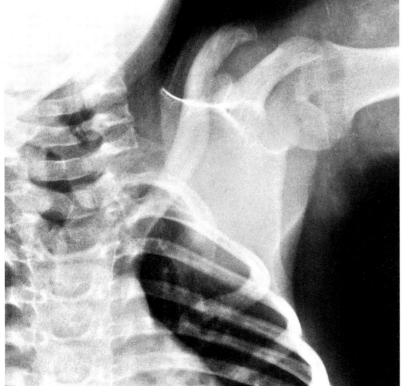

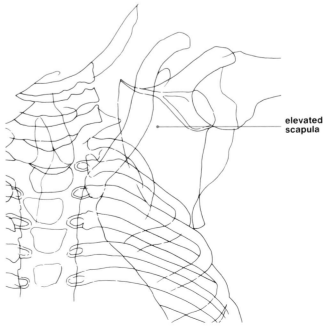

elevated scapula

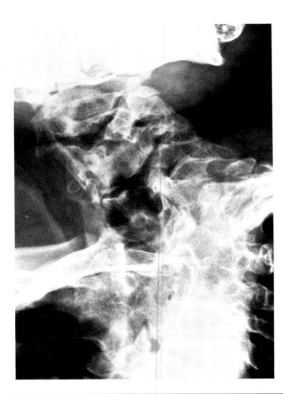
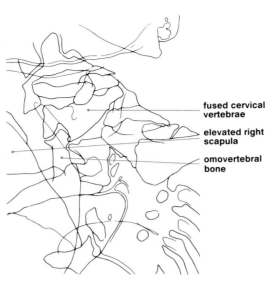

Figure 27.2 Posteroanterior view of the cervical and upper thoracic spine in a 37-year-old woman with Sprengel deformity associated with Klippel-Feil syndrome (fusion of the cervical vertebrae) shows the omovertebral bone connecting the elevated right scapula and the C-5 vertebra.

fused cervical
vertebrae

elevated right
scapula

omovertebral
bone

Figure 27.3 Radiographic Criteria for the Diagnosis of Madelung Deformity

Changes in the Radius
Double curvature (medial and dorsal)
Decrease in bone length
Triangular shape of the distal epiphysis
Premature fusion of the medial part of the distal physis, associated
    with medial and volar angulation of the articular surface
Focal radiolucent areas along the medial border of bone

Changes in the Ulna
Dorsal subluxation
Increased density (hypercondensation and distortion)
    of the ulnar head
Increase in bone length

Changes in the Carpus
Triangular configuration with the lunate at the apex
Increase in distance between the distal radius and the ulna
Decrease in carpal angle

(Modified from Dannenberg M, et al., 1939).

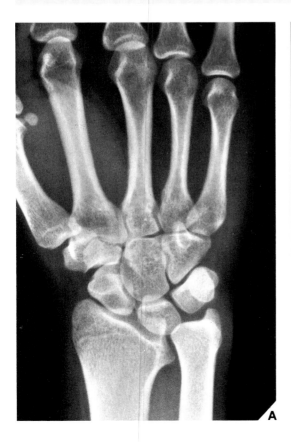
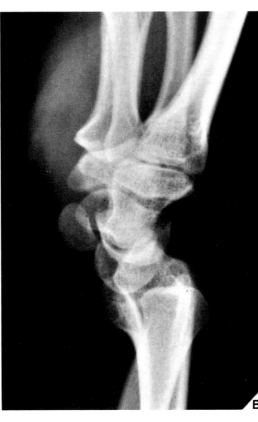

Figure 27.4 (A) Posteroanterior view of the left wrist of a 21-year-old woman with Madelung deformity shows a decrease in the length of the radius, the distal end of which has assumed a triangular shape. This is associated with a triangular configuration of the carpus, with the lunate at the apex wedged between the radius and ulna. (B) Lateral view demonstrates dorsal subluxation of the ulna.

A

B

Madelung Deformity

This developmental anomaly of the distal radius and carpus, originally described by Madelung in 1879, usually manifests in adolescent patients presenting with pain in the wrist but with no history of previous trauma or infection. Today the term *Madelung deformity* is often used to describe a variety of conditions in the wrist marked by premature fusion of the distal physis of the radius, with consequent deformity of the distal ulna and wrist. From the etiologic viewpoint, these abnormalities can be divided into posttraumatic deformities, dysplasias (such as multiple cartilaginous exostoses), and idiopathic conditions.

The radiographic criteria for the diagnosis of Madelung deformity were proposed by Dannenberg and colleagues (Fig. 27.3). The posteroanterior and lateral projections of the distal forearm and wrist are sufficient to demonstrate any of the abnormalities associated with this deformity (Fig. 27.4).

The treatment of Madelung deformity consists of arthrodesis of the radiocarpal joint by the "wedge" technique.

ANOMALIES OF THE PELVIC GIRDLE AND HIP

An overview of the most effective radiographic projections and radiologic techniques for evaluating the most common anomalies of the pelvic girdle and hip is presented in Figure 27.5.

Congenital Hip Dislocation

The hip joint is the most frequent site of congenital dislocations. The condition occurs with an incidence of 1.5 per 1000 births, and eight times more often in girls than in boys. In unilateral dislocation, the left hip is involved twice as often as the right, and bilateral dislocation occurs in more than 25% of affected children. More frequently encountered in white than in black persons, the condition is very common in Mediterranean and Scandinavian countries; it is almost unknown in China, which may be explained in part by the Chinese custom of carrying the infant on the mother's back with its hips flexed and abducted.

Figure 27.5 Most Effective Radiographic Projections and Radiologic Techniques for Evaluating Common Anomalies of the Pelvic Girdle and Hip

PROJECTION/TECHNIQUE	CRUCIAL ABNORMALITIES	PROJECTION/TECHNIQUE	CRUCIAL ABNORMALITIES
Congenital Hip Dislocation		***Legg-Calvé-Perthes Disease***	
Anteroposterior of pelvis and hips	Determination of: Hilgenreiner Y-line Acetabular index Perkins-Ombredanne line Shenton-Menard line (arc) Center-edge (C-E) angle of Wiberg Ossification center of capital femoral epiphysis Relations of femoral head and acetabulum	Anteroposterior and frog-lateral of hips	Osteonecrosis of femoral head as indicated by crescent sign and subchondral collapse Gage sign Subluxation of femoral head Horizontal orientation of growth plate Calcifications lateral to epiphysis Cystic changes in metaphysis
Anteroposterior of hips in abduction and internal rotation	Andrén-von Rosen line	Arthrography	Incongruity of hip joint Thickness of articular cartilage
Arthrography	Congruity of the joint Status of: Cartilaginous limbus (limbus thorn) Ligamentum teres Zona orbicularis	Radionuclide bone scan	Decreased uptake of isotope (earliest stage) Increased uptake of isotope (late stage)
Computed tomography (alone or with arthrography)	Relations of femoral head and acetabulum Superior, lateral, or posterior subluxation	Computed tomography and magnetic resonance imaging	Incongruity of hip joint Osteonecrosis
Sonography	Position of femoral head in acetabulum Status of: Acetabular roof Cartilaginous limbus	***Slipped Capital Femoral Epiphysis***	
Developmental Coxa Vara		Anteroposterior of hips	Loss of Capener triangle sign Periarticular osteoporosis Widening and blurring of growth plate Decreased height of femoral epiphysis Absence of intersection of epiphysis by line tangent to lateral cortex of femoral neck Herndon hump Chondrolysis (complication)
Anteroposterior of pelvis and hips	Varus angle of femoral neck and femoral shaft		
Proximal Femoral Focal Deficiency		Frog-lateral of hips	Absence of intersection of epiphysis by line tangent to lateral cortex of femoral neck Actual slippage (displacement) of femoral epiphysis
Anteroposterior of hip and proximal femur	Shortening of femur Superior, posterior, and lateral displacement of proximal femoral segment		
Arthrography	Nonossified femoral head	Radionuclide bone scan and magnetic resonance imaging	Osteonecrosis (complication)

The criteria for the diagnosis of congenital dislocation of the hip (CDH) include both physical and radiographic findings. Certain clinical signs have been identified that are helpful in the evaluation of newborns and infants for possible CDH (Fig. 27.6).

Radiographic Evaluation

Each of the stages of CDH—dysplasia of the hip, subluxation of the hip, and dislocation of the hip—has a characteristic radiographic presentation. The term *congenital hip dysplasia*, first introduced by Hilgenreiner in 1925, refers to delayed or defective development of the hip joint leading to a deranged articular relationship between an abnormal acetabulum and a deformed proximal end of the femur (Fig. 27.7). The condition is considered a precursor of subluxation and dislocation of the hip, although some authorities use the term "developmental dysplasia of the hip" (DDH) to denote all stages of CDH. In *congenital subluxation of the hip*, there is an abnormal relationship between the femoral head and the acetabulum, but the two are in contact (Fig. 27.8). *Congenital dislocation of the hip*, on the other hand, is marked by the femoral head's complete loss of contact with the acetabular cartilage; the proximal femur is displaced most often superiorly, but lateral, posterior, and posterolateral dislocation may also be seen (Fig. 27.9).

Measurements

In contrast to an adult hip, the relationship between the femoral head and the acetabulum in a newborn's hip cannot be assessed by direct visualization because the femoral head is not ossified and as a cartilaginous body it is not visible on standard films. The ossification center first appears between the ages of 3 to 6 months, and a delay in its appearance should be viewed as an indication of congenital hip dysplasia. The neck of the femur must therefore be used for ascertaining this relationship. The anteroposterior view of the pelvis serves as the basis for determining several indirect indicators of the relationship between the femoral head and acetabulum. To obtain accurate measurements, however, proper positioning of the infant is imperative; the lower extremities should be extended in the neutral position and longitudinally aligned, while the central ray should be directed toward the midline, slightly above the pubic symphysis, to assure the symmetry of both halves of the pelvis. The measurements used to evaluate the relation of the femoral head to the acetabulum are the following (Fig. 27.10):

1. The *Hilgenreiner line* or *Y-line*, which is drawn through the superior part of the triradiate cartilage, is itself a valuable indicator of femoroacetabular relations and serves as the basis for all other indicators.

Figure 27.6 Clinical Manifestations of Congenital Dislocation of the Hip

Limited abduction of the flexed hip (due to shortening and contraction of hip adductors)

Increase in depth or asymmetry of the inguinal or thigh skin folds

Shortening of one leg

Allis or Galeazzi sign*—lower position of knee of affected side when knees and hips are flexed (due to location of femoral head posterior to acetabulum in this position)

Ortolani "jerk" sign ("clunk of entry" or reduction sign)

Barlow test ("clunk of exit" or dislocation sign)

Telescoping or pistoning action of thighs* (due to lack of containment of femoral head within acetabulum)

Trendelenburg test*—dropping of normal hip when child, standing on both feet, elevates unaffected limb and bears weight on affected side (due to weakness of hip abductors)

Waddling gait*

*This finding can occur in older children.

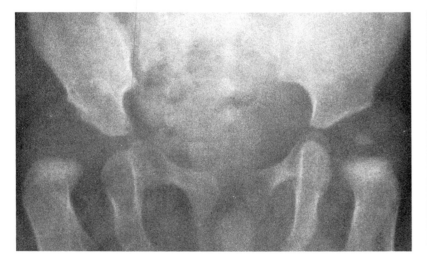

Figure 27.7 Anteroposterior view of the pelvis of a 1-year-old boy with congenital hip dysplasia shows a slightly flattened acetabulum and delayed appearance of the ossification center for the right femoral epiphysis; that of the left epiphysis is normally centered over the triradiate cartilage.

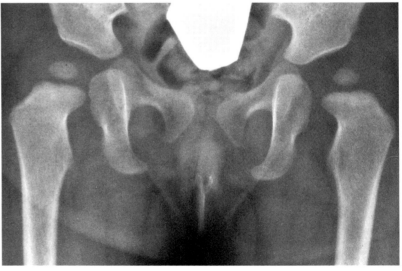

Figure 27.8 Anteroposterior view of the pelvis of a 1-year-old girl shows congenital superolateral subluxation of the left hip. Note the slightly smaller size of the left femoral epiphysis.

2. The *acetabular index*, which is an angle formed by a line tangent to the acetabular roof and the Y-line, cannot alone be diagnostic of dislocation, since it can occasionally exceed 30° in normal subjects. Generally, however, values greater than 30° are considered abnormal and indicate impending dislocation. Some investigators propose that only angles in excess of 40° are significant.

3. The *Perkins-Ombredanne line*, which is drawn perpendicular to the Y-line through the most lateral edge of the ossified acetabular cartilage, is helpful in determining subluxation and dislocation of the hip. The intersection of this line with the Y-line creates four quadrants; normally, the medial aspect of the femoral neck or the ossified capital femoral epiphysis falls in the lower medial quadrant.

4. The *Shenton-Menard line*, which forms a smooth arc through the medial aspect of the femoral neck and the superior border of the obturator foramen, may be interrupted in subluxation or dislocation of the hip. Even under normal circumstances, however, the arc may not be smooth if the radiograph is obtained with the hip in external rotation and adduction.

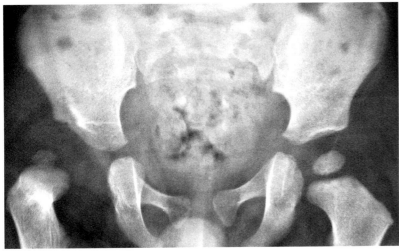

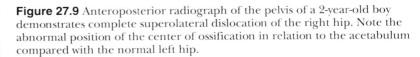

Figure 27.9 Anteroposterior radiograph of the pelvis of a 2-year-old boy demonstrates complete superolateral dislocation of the right hip. Note the abnormal position of the center of ossification in relation to the acetabulum compared with the normal left hip.

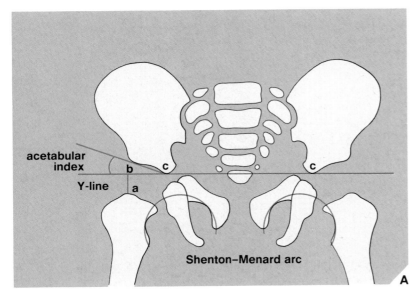

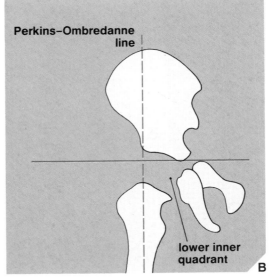

Figure 27.10 (A) The *Hilgenreiner line* or *Y-line* is drawn through the superior part of the triradiate cartilage. In normal infants, the distance represented by a line (*ab*) perpendicular to the Y-line at the most proximal point of the femoral neck should be equal on both sides of the pelvis, as should the distance represented by a line (*bc*) drawn coincident with the Y-line medially to the acetabular floor. In infants aged 6 to 7 months, the mean value for the distance (*ab*) has been determined to be 19.3 mm ± 1.5 mm; the distance for (*bc*) is 18.2 mm ± 1.4 mm. The *acetabular index* is an angle formed by a line drawn tangent to the acetabular roof from point (*c*) at the acetabular floor on the Y-line. The normal value of this angle ranges from 25° to 29°. The *Shenton-Menard line* is an arc running through the medial aspect of the femoral neck and the superior border of the obturator foramen. It should be smooth and unbroken. (B) The *Perkins-Ombredanne line* is drawn perpendicular to the Y-line through the most lateral edge of the ossified acetabular cartilage, which actually corresponds to the anteroinferior iliac spine. In normal newborns and infants, the medial aspect of the femoral neck or the ossified capital femoral epiphysis falls in the lower inner quadrant. The appearance of either of these structures in the lower outer or upper outer quadrant indicates subluxation or dislocation of the hip.

5. The *Andrén-von Rosen line*, which is drawn on a radiograph obtained with the hips abducted 45° and internally rotated, describes the relation of the longitudinal axis of the femoral shaft to the acetabulum (Fig. 27.11). In dislocation or subluxation of the hip, this line bisects or falls above the anterosuperior iliac spine.

After the capital femoral epiphysis achieves full ossification at about 4 years of age, a diagnosis of gross displacement can usually be made without difficulty. The evaluation of subtle hip dysplasias, however, can be aided by another parameter of the relation of the femoral head to the acetabulum, the *center-edge (C-E) angle of Wiberg* (Fig. 27.12). Determination of this angle is most useful after full ossifi-

cation of the femoral head, since its relationship to the acetabulum is then fully established.

Arthrography and Computed Tomography

Aside from conventional radiography, hip arthrography is the most useful technique for evaluating CDH. During the procedure, films are routinely obtained with the hip in the neutral (Fig. 27.13A) and frog-lateral positions (Fig. 27.13B), as well as in abduction, adduction, and internal rotation. In subluxation, the femoral head lies lateral to but below the margin of the acetabular cartilaginous labrum, and the joint capsule is usually loose (Fig. 27.14). In complete dislocation, the femoral head lies superior and lateral to the edge of the

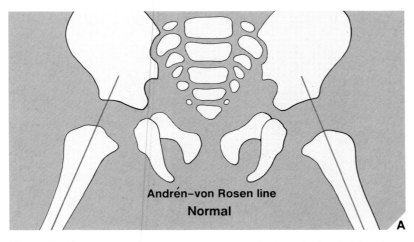

Andrén–von Rosen line
Normal

A

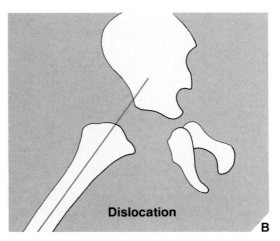

Dislocation

B

Figure 27.11 (A) The Andrén-von Rosen line, which is obtained with at least 45° of hip abduction and internal rotation, is drawn along the longitudinal axis of the femoral shaft. In normal hips, it intersects the pelvis at the upper

edge of the acetabulum. (B) In subluxation or dislocation of the hip, the line bisects or falls above the anterosuperior iliac spine.

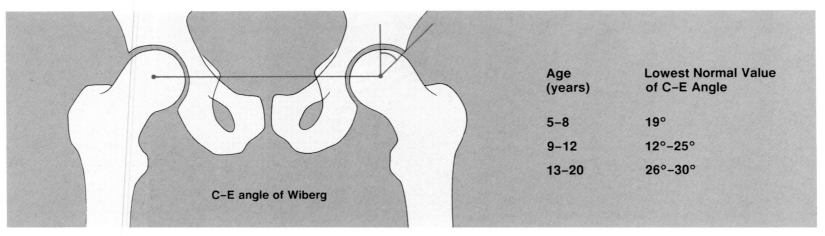

C–E angle of Wiberg

Age (years)	Lowest Normal Value of C–E Angle
5–8	19°
9–12	12°–25°
13–20	26°–30°

Figure 27.12 The center-edge (C-E) angle of Wiberg is helpful in evaluating the development of the acetabulum and its relation to the femoral head. A baseline is projected, connecting the centers of the femoral heads. The C-E angle is formed by two lines originating in the center of the femoral head,

one drawn perpendicular to the baseline into the acetabulum, and the other connecting the center of the femoral head with the superior acetabular lip. Values below the lowest normal value given for each age group indicate hip dysplasia.

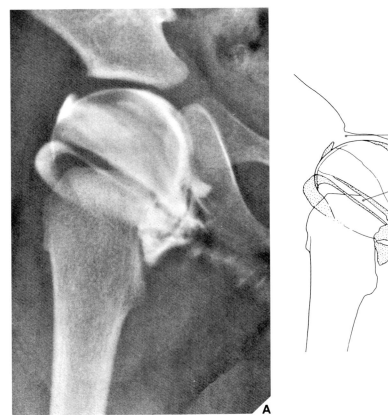
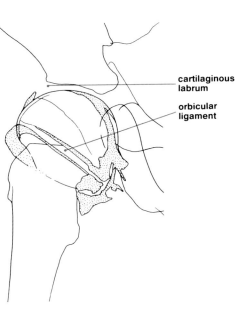
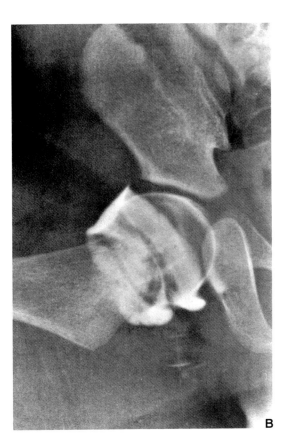

Figure 27.13 (A) Normal arthrogram of the right hip in the neutral position in a 5-month-old boy shows contrast medium accumulating in the large recesses medial and lateral to the constriction produced by the orbicular ligament. Note the smoothness and even thickness of the cartilage covering the femoral head. (B) On the normal frog-lateral view, contrast medium is seen outlining the edge of the cartilaginous labrum. The ligamentum teres can be seen medial to the femoral head, extending from the inferior portion of the acetabulum.

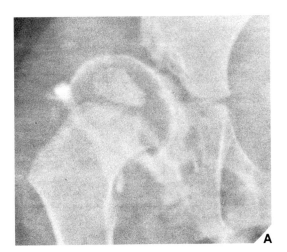
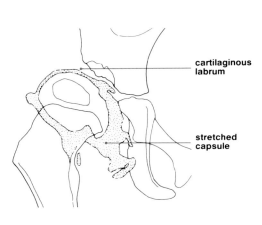
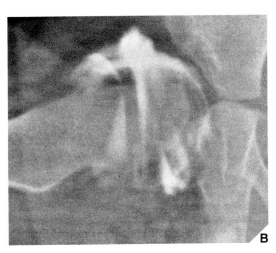

Figure 27.14 (A) Arthrogram of the right hip in the neutral position in a 1-year-old girl with congenital subluxation of the hip shows the typical displacement of the hip lateral to but below the acetabular labrum. There is accumulation of contrast agent in the stretched capsule, and the ligamentum teres is elongated. (B) In the frog-lateral position, the head moves more deeply into the acetabulum, but subluxation is still present.

labrum (Fig. 27.15). Deformities may also be encountered in the cartilaginous limbus, a structure lying between the femoral head and the acetabulum. In advanced stages it may be inverted and hypertrophied, thus making the reduction impossible. Moreover, the portion of the capsule lying medial to the femoral head is usually constricted to form an isthmus with a "figure-eight" appearance.

Computed tomography (CT), either alone (Fig. 27.16) or with arthrography, is also a frequently used modality in the evaluation of CDH. In subluxation or dislocation, the congruity of the acetabulum and the femoral head, which is normally centered over the triradiate cartilage, is disturbed (Fig. 27.17). CT has proved to be the most accurate technique for determining the degree of subluxation or dislocation. It is also an essential modality for monitoring the progress of CDH treatment.

Classification

Dunn has proposed a classification of CDH based primarily on the shape of the acetabular margins, the gross contour of the femoral head, and whether there is eversion or inversion of the limbus:

Type I   This is usually seen in neonates. The changes along the acetabular margins are mild. The femoral head, which is anteverted but spherically normal, is not completely covered by cartilage. This may lead to variable instability, particularly in extension and adduction of the hip. The labrum may also be deformed.

Type II   The hips are subluxed, and the cartilaginous labrum shows eversion. The femoral head is normally anteverted but shows a loss of sphericity. The acetabulum is shallower than in type I, and the failure of the acetabular roof to ossify laterally leads to an increased acetabular angle.

Type III There is significant deformity of the acetabulum and femoral head, which is posterosuperiorly dislocated, leading to the formation of a false acetabulum by eversion of the labrum. The limbus is hypertrophied, and the ligamentum teres is elongated and pulled, bringing with it the transverse acetabular ligament. This situation compromises the acetabular space, precluding complete reduction.

Treatment

The principle behind conservative treatment is to reduce the dislocation of the femoral head, by means of a flexion-abduction maneuver, for a period sufficient enough to permit proper growth of the head and acetabulum, which in turn insures a congruent and stable hip joint. This approach is usually taken in the very early stages of CDH and in infants under two years of age; it includes splinting, such as with the Frejka splint or Pavlik harness, as well as various traction procedures (Fig. 27.18). Colonna or Buck skin traction is usually used in children two months to 12 years of age, with a well-padded spica cast applied simultaneously to the unaffected side. Interval radiographs are obtained to monitor the progress of the traction and the descent of the femoral head. A system for this purpose, composed of various traction "stations," has been described by Gage and Winter (Fig. 27.19). It has been reported that the achievement of "station +2" by means of skeletal traction, before further treatment by open or closed reduction, is associated with a far smaller frequency of osteonecrosis of the femoral head.

When the conservative approach fails, the child is too old for conservative treatment, or the abnormalities are too extensive, surgical management is indicated. Radiologic assessment of the hip, in which CT examination plays the leading role, is mandatory prior to

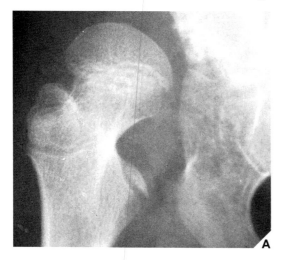
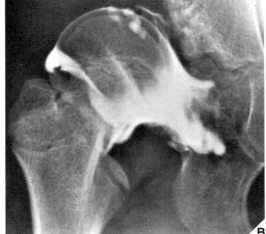

Figure 27.15 (A) Anteroposterior plain film of the right hip in an 8-year-old girl demonstrates complete superolateral dislocation of the femoral head. Note the shallow acetabulum. (B) Arthrogram of the hip shows a deformed cartilaginous limbus and stretching of the ligamentum teres. The femoral head lies superior and lateral to the edge of the cartilaginous labrum. Note the accumulation of contrast agent in the loose joint capsule.

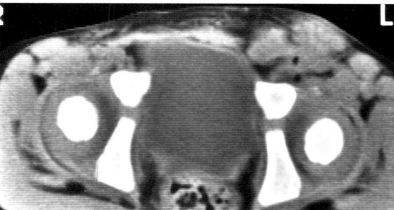

Figure 27.16 Normal CT scan of both hips in a 19-month-old infant shows good congruity of the acetabula and femoral heads, which are centered over the triradiate cartilage.

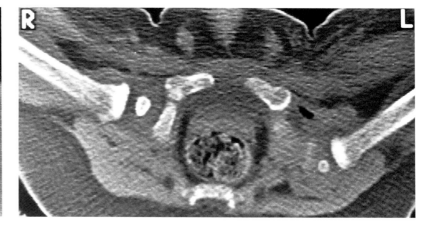

Figure 27.17 CT section through the proximal femora and hips of a 6-month-old boy shows posterolateral dislocation of the left hip. The right hip is normal.

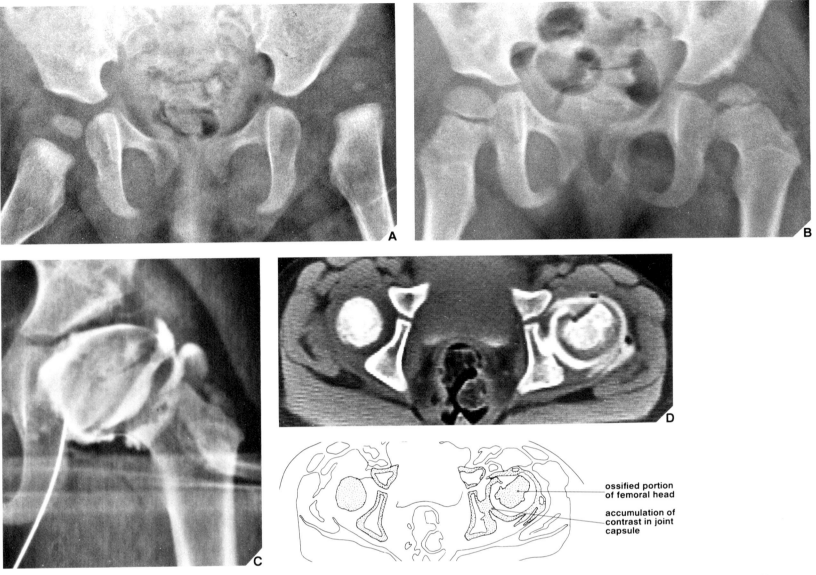

Figure 27.18 (A) Anteroposterior plain film of the pelvis in a 1-year-old boy demonstrates the typical appearance of congenital dislocation of the left hip. (B) After conservative treatment with a Pavlik harness at age 2, there is still subluxation. Note the broken Shenton-Menard arc. At age 3, after further conservative treatment by skin traction and application of a spica cast, there is almost complete reduction of subluxation, as demonstrated by contrast arthrogaphy (C). (D) CT scan, however, demonstrates some minimal residual lateral displacement of the femoral head, evident by the medial accumulation of contrast.

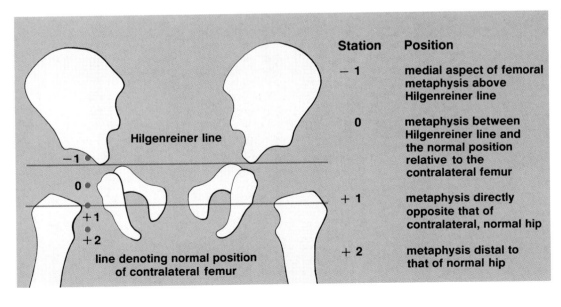

Station	Position
− 1	medial aspect of femoral metaphysis above Hilgenreiner line
0	metaphysis between Hilgenreiner line and the normal position relative to the contralateral femur
+ 1	metaphysis directly opposite that of contralateral, normal hip
+ 2	metaphysis distal to that of normal hip

Figure 27.19 The Gage and Winter system of stations for monitoring the progress of treatment by traction and the descent of the femoral head is based on the position of the proximal femoral metaphysis relative to the ipsilateral acetabulum and the contralateral normal hip.

surgical intervention since it provides the surgeon with excellent images of the anatomy of the hip, particularly the size of the femoral head, its relation to the acetabulum, and the acetabular configuration. The information regarding these structures may contraindicate the use of certain surgical procedures.

Several surgical techniques are currently used in treating CDH. The most popular procedure is the *Salter osteotomy* of the innominate bone, which may be combined with simultaneous derotational varus osteotomy of the femoral neck. It is usually performed in children aged 1 to 6 years. The principle of this technique is to redirect the abnormal orientation of the acetabulum, which in children with CDH faces more anterolaterally, thus rendering the hip stable only in abduction, flexion, and internal rotation. This redirection is accomplished by displacing the entire acetabulum anterolaterally and downward, without changing its shape or capacity, by means of a triangular bone graft (Fig. 27.20). The *Chiari pelvic osteotomy* is usually reserved for older children. This procedure displaces the femoral head medially and increases the weight-bearing surface of

the head by producing an overhanging superior acetabular ledge. This technique may also be combined with a varus derotational osteotomy of the femoral neck.

Complications
Both conservative and surgical management of CDH may be complicated by osteonecrosis of the femoral head, redislocation, infection, sciatic nerve injury, or early fusion of the growth plate due to prolonged casting. The most frequent late complication of both untreated and treated CDH is degenerative joint disease (see Chapter 12).

Proximal Femoral Focal Deficiency
Proximal femoral focal deficiency (PFFD) is a congenital anomaly characterized by dysgenesis and hypoplasia of variable segments of the proximal femur. The defect ranges in severity from femoral shortening associated with a varus deformity of the neck to the formation of only a small stub of distal femur.

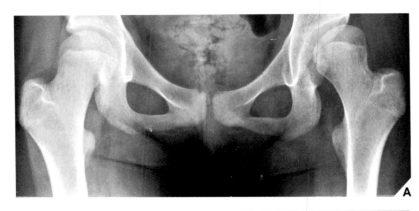
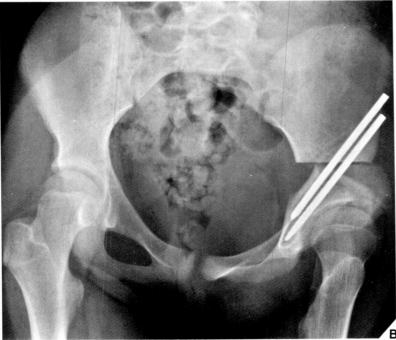
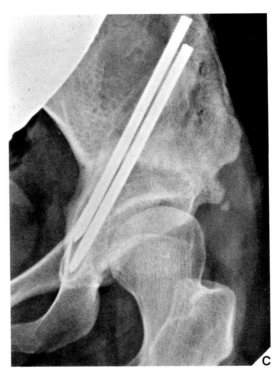

Figure 27.20 (A) Anteroposterior view of the pelvis in a 7-year-old girl with CDH shows persistent superolateral subluxation of the left hip following conservative treatment. Note the anterolateral orientation of the acetabulum in comparison with the normal right hip. (B) Postoperative film following osteotomy through the supra-acetabular portion of the iliac bone shows the acetabulum displaced anterolaterally and downward; a triangular bone graft, taken from the anterolateral aspect of the ilium, is secured by two Steinman pins at the site of the osteotomy. (C) Four years later the femoral head is completely covered by the acetabulum. Because of a valgus configuration of the femoral neck, the patient may yet require a varus derotational osteotomy.

Classification and Radiographic Evaluation

Several classifications of PFFD have been proposed. The one offered by Levinson and colleagues, which is based on the severity of the abnormalities involving the femoral head, femoral segment, and the acetabulum, is the most practical from the prognostic point of view:

Type A The femoral head is present, and the femoral segment is short. There is a varus deformity of the femoral neck. The acetabulum is normal.

Type B The femoral head is present, but there is an absence of bony connection between it and the short femoral segment. The acetabulum exhibits dysplastic changes.

Type C The femoral head is absent or represented only by an ossicle. The femoral segment is short and tapered proximally. The acetabulum is severely dysplastic.

Type D The femoral head and acetabulum are absent. The femoral segment is rudimentary, and the obturator foramen is enlarged.

Plain-film radiography is usually sufficient to make a diagnosis of proximal femoral focal deficiency. The femur is short, and the proximal segment is displaced superior, posterior, and lateral to the iliac crest; ossification of the femoral epiphysis is invariably delayed (Fig. 27.21). Arthrography is useful in the evaluation of this anomaly, particularly in its classification, since early in infancy the nonossified femoral head and acetabulum can be outlined adequately with a positive contrast agent (see Fig. 27.21C). This technique is also helpful in distinguishing proximal femoral focal deficiency from the occasionally similar presentations of congenital dislocation of the hip.

Treatment

Several surgical procedures are used to correct this anomaly, including amputation. One limb-sparing procedure involves conversion of the knee to a hip joint by flexing it 90° and fusing the femur to the pelvis. Another technique, developed by Borggreve in 1930 and called the "turn-about" procedure or "rotation-plasty" after an improvement by Van Nes, converts the foot into the knee joint; the limb is then fitted with a leg prosthesis.

Legg-Calvé-Perthes Disease

Legg-Calvé-Perthes disease, also known as coxa plana, is the name applied to osteonecrosis (ischemic necrosis) of the proximal epiphysis of the femur. It occurs five times more often in boys than in girls, usually between the ages of 4 and 8 years. Its appearance at an early age is usually associated with a better prognosis. Either hip can be affected, and bilateral involvement, which is successive rather than

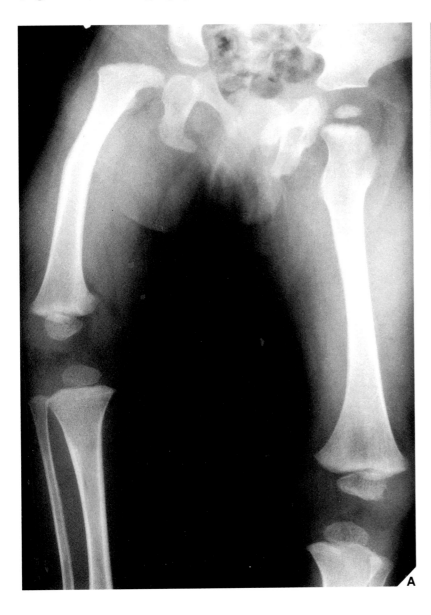

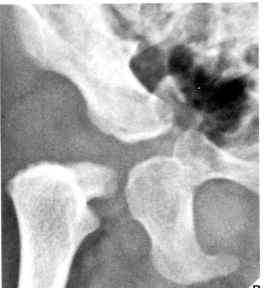

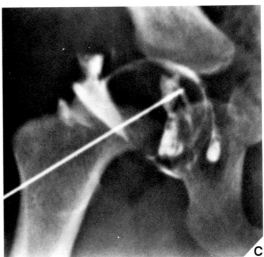

Figure 27.21 (A) Anteroposterior plain film in an 18-month-old boy who had a short right leg demonstrates a varus configuration at the right hip joint, the absence of an ossification center for the proximal femoral epiphysis, and shortening of the femur—the classic radiographic features of proximal femoral focal deficiency. (B) A coned-down view of the right hip shows superior, posterior, and lateral displacement of the proximal femoral segment in relation to the acetabulum. (C) Arthrography was performed to classify the abnormality, and the presence of the femoral head in the acetabulum and the absence of any defect in the femoral neck was found, making this a type A focal deficiency.

simultaneous, is seen in about 10% of cases (Fig. 27.22). The clinical symptoms consist of pain, limping, and limitation of motion. Not infrequently, the pain is localized not to the involved hip but to the ipsilateral knee. It is a self-limiting disorder that eventually heals, but because of the progressive deformity it produces in the shape of the femoral head and neck, it often leads to precocious osteoarthritis of the hip joint. The etiology of this anomaly has been the subject of debate. Some investigators consider it a type of idiopathic osteonecrosis, but trauma or repeated microtrauma may play a role in compromising the circulation of blood to the femoral capital epiphysis. Trueta has suggested that the blood supply to the femoral head is deficient between the ages of 4 and 8 years, and that this might be a factor in the development of the condition.

Radiologic Evaluation

Radiologic examination is essential for diagnosing Legg-Calvé-Perthes disease and for identifying its prognostic signs. Plain-film radiography is adequate for evaluating most of the features of the disease (see Fig. 27.22), while arthrography helps in the assessment of acetabular congruity, the thickness of the articular cartilage, and the degree of subluxation (Fig. 27.23). The earliest indication of Legg-Calvé-Perthes disease is demonstrated on radionuclide bone scan by a decreased uptake of tracer in the hips due to a deficient blood supply. However, with progression of the disease, an increased uptake is seen, which reflects reparative processes.

The earliest radiographic sign of Legg-Calvé-Perthes disease is periarticular osteoporosis and periarticular soft tissue swelling, with distortion of the pericapsular and iliopsoas fat planes. There may also be a discrepancy in the size of the ossification centers of the capital epiphyses. Later, lateral displacement of the affected ossification center produces widening of the medial aspect of the joint; the presence of the crescent sign (which at times may be detected only on the frog-lateral projection of the hip) (Fig. 27.24), or of radiolucent fissures in the epiphysis, indicate progression of the disease. At a more advanced stage, flattening and sclerosis of the capital epiphysis become apparent, and are associated with an increased density of the femoral head secondary to necrosis of the bone, microfractures, and reparative changes known as "creeping substitution." A vacuum phenomenon may occasionally be seen, caused by nitrogen gas released into the fissures in the capital epiphysis. Cystic changes may also be encountered in the metaphyseal segment, and later there may be broadening of the femoral neck. Throughout the course of the disease, the joint space is remarkably well preserved because the articular cartilage is not affected. Only in the end stage of Legg-Calvé-Perthes disease, when secondary osteoarthritis develops, does the joint become compromised as in primary degenerative joint disease.

The Moss technique is used to determine the degree of deformity of the femoral head. This consists of overlaying the anteroposterior radiograph of the hip with a template having concentric circles spaced 2 mm apart. If the concentricity of the femoral head

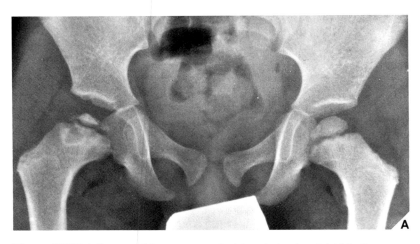
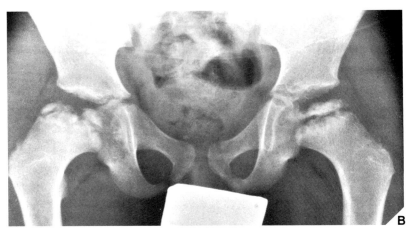

Figure 27.22 A 5-year-old boy presented with pain in the right hip for several months. (A) Anteroposterior radiograph of the pelvis and hips shows advanced Legg-Calvé-Perthes disease affecting the right hip, where osteonecrosis and collapse of the capital femoral epiphysis are apparent, as are extensive changes in the metaphysis. Note the lateral subluxation in the hip joint. The left hip is normal. (B) Three years later the left hip also became involved. Note the progression of osteonecrotic changes in the right femoral epiphysis.

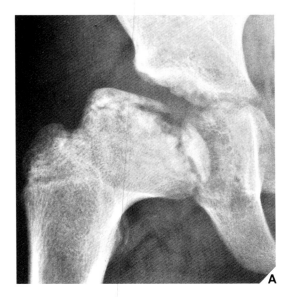
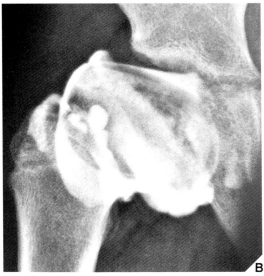

Figure 27.23 A 6-year-old boy presented with progressive pain in the right hip joint and limp for the previous eight months. (A) Anteroposterior radiograph shows a dense, flattened, and deformed femoral epiphysis, with subchondral collapse and fragmentation, diffuse metaphyseal changes, broadening of the femoral neck, and lateral subluxation—all characteristic features of Legg-Calvé-Perthes disease. (B) Contrast arthrogram demonstrates flattening of the articular cartilage at the lateral aspect of the femoral head and a relatively smooth contour of the cartilage at the anteromedial aspect. The pulling of the contrast medially indicates lateral subluxation.

deviates by more than two of the 2-mm circles, the result is rated "poor"; deviation equal to one 2-mm circle is "fair," and no deviation is rated "good." Lateral subluxation can be measured by means of the center-edge angle of Wiberg (see Fig. 27.12). It must be stressed that both measurements do not correlate well with development of secondary osteoarthritis, the main complication of Legg-Calvé-Perthes disease.

Recently some investigators have stressed the applicability of magnetic resonance imaging (MRI) in the early detection of Legg-Calvé-Perthes disease and in the evaluation of cartilaginous and synovial changes.

Classification

Several classification systems and prognostic indicators have been developed for the evaluation of Legg-Calvé-Perthes disease. Walderström proposed a three-stage system based on the progression of the osteonecrotic process. The first stage is marked by changes in the blood supply to the femoral epiphysis, with secondary alteration in the shape and density of the femoral head. In the second stage, revascularization takes place, and necrotic bone is replaced by new bone (creeping substitution). The third stage represents a healing phase of the disease in which reconstruction of the femoral epiphysis may result either in congruency of the joint or in incongruency because of deformity of the femoral head (coxa magna), with a predisposition to degenerative changes.

The Catterall classification, which has better prognostic value, divides this anomaly into four groups based on radiographic findings:

Group 1   The anterior portion of the epiphysis is involved; there is no evidence of subarticular collapse or fragmentation of the femoral head. The prognosis is good, and patients do well even without treatment, particularly those under 8 years of age.

Group 2   The anterior portion of the epiphysis is more severely affected, but the medial and lateral segments are still preserved. Small cystic changes may be seen in the metaphysis (Fig. 27.25). The prognosis is worse than that of patients in group 1, but healing may occur, particularly in children younger than 5 years.

Group 3   The entire epiphysis appears dense, yielding a "head-within-a-head" phenomenon. The changes are more generalized, and the neck becomes widened. The prognosis is poor, and more than 70% of patients require surgical intervention.

Group 4   There is marked flattening and "mushrooming" of the femoral head, eventually leading to its complete collapse; the metaphyseal changes are extensive (Fig. 27.26). The prognosis is much worse than in the previous groups.

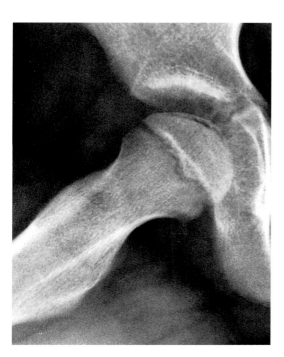

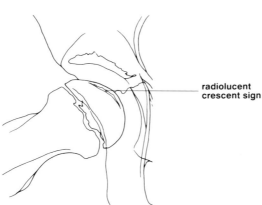

radiolucent crescent sign

Figure 27.24 Frog-lateral view of the right hip of a 7-year-old girl with Legg-Calvé-Perthes disease demonstrates the crescent sign, one of the earliest radiographic features of osteonecrosis.

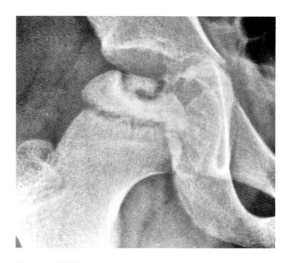

Figure 27.25 Anteroposterior view of the right hip of a 9-year-old boy demonstrates a more advanced stage of Legg-Calvé-Perthes disease (Catterall group 2). Note the central defect in the femoral head, with preservation of the lateral and medial buttresses.

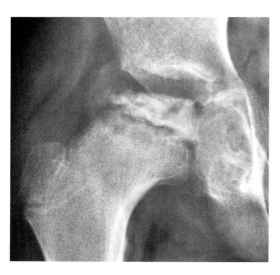

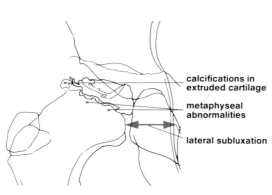

calcifications in extruded cartilage

metaphyseal abnormalities

lateral subluxation

Figure 27.26 Anteroposterior film of the right hip of an 8-year-old girl with advanced Legg-Calvé-Perthes disease (Catterall group 4) shows increased density and fragmentation of the entire femoral head. "Head-at-risk" signs are apparent in the metaphyseal changes and the lateral subluxation. Calcifications lateral to the epiphysis represent extruded cartilage and indicate pressure on the head from the lateral edge of the acetabulum.

Subsequently, Catterall improved this classification by introducing four "head-at-risk" signs that signify a poor prognosis; these features can be demonstrated on an anteroposterior projection of the hip joint:

1. Gage sign—a radiolucent, V-shaped osteoporotic segment in the lateral portion of the femoral head (Fig. 27.27)
2. Calcification lateral to the epiphysis, representing extruded cartilage and indicating pressure on the head from the lateral edge of the acetabulum (see Fig. 27.26)
3. Lateral subluxation of the femoral head (see Fig. 27.26)
4. Horizontal inclination of the growth plate, indicating physeal growth closure (see Fig. 27.22B).
5. Recently, Murphy and Marsh added a fifth sign to this group of indicators—diffuse metaphyseal changes (see Fig. 27.23A).

Patients in any of the four groups who have two or more "head-at-risk" signs have a significantly worsened prognosis. Moreover, the prognosis is poor when the disease is in a late stage at the time of diagnosis and when the patient is over 6 years of age.

Differential diagnosis

The differential diagnosis of this condition should include other causes of osteonecrosis and fragmentation of the femoral head, which may be seen, for example, in hypothyroidism, Gaucher disease, and sickle-cell anemia.

Treatment

The treatment of Legg-Calvé-Perthes disease is individualized on the basis of the clinical and radiographic findings, including the age of onset, the range of motion in the hip joint, the extent of femoral head involvement, and the presence or absence of femoral deformity and lateral subluxation. Although some authorities have suggested eliminating weight-bearing to prevent deformity of the femoral head, prevention requires measures that maintain the femoral head within the acetabulum (containment), thereby preventing extrusion and subluxation, as well as obtaining a full range of motion in the hip joint. In this respect, Salter advocates full weight-bearing together with con-

tainment methods of treatment. To minimize synovitis and its sequelae of pain and stiffness, a combination of nonweight-bearing, traction, treatment with nonsteroidal anti-inflammatory agents, and gentle range-of-motion exercises is used to enhance molding of the femoral head by the acetabulum. The surgical treatment consists of femoral (varus derotational) or pelvic (innominate bone) osteotomy, aimed at covering the femoral head with the acetabulum.

Slipped Capital Femoral Epiphysis

Slipped capital femoral epiphysis (SCFE) is a disorder of adolescence in which the femoral head gradually slips posteriorly, medially, and inferiorly with respect to the neck. Boys are affected more often than girls, and children of both sexes with this disorder are often overweight. In boys, the left hip is involved twice as often as the right, whereas in girls both hips are affected with equal frequency. Bilateral involvement occurs in 20% to 40% of patients.

Although the specific etiology of SCFE is obscure, its onset, which is usually insidious and without a history of trauma, commonly coincides with the growth spurt at puberty. Studies by Harris have suggested that an imbalance between growth hormone and sex hormones weakens the growth plate, rendering it more vulnerable to the shearing forces of weight-bearing and injury.

Regardless of its etiology, SCFE represents a Salter-Harris type I fracture (see Fig. 4.25) through the growth plate of the proximal femur. This comes about through posterior, medial, and inferior displacement of the capital epiphysis, resulting in a varus deformity in the hip joint and external rotation and adduction of the femur. Pain in the hip, or occasionally the knee, is often the presenting symptom of this condition, and physical examination may reveal shortening of the involved extremity and limitation of abduction, flexion, and internal rotation in the hip joint.

Radiographic Evaluation

The radiographic abnormalities that may be seen in SCFE depend on the degree of displacement of the capital epiphysis. The anteroposterior view of the hip, supplemented by a frog-lateral view, is usu-

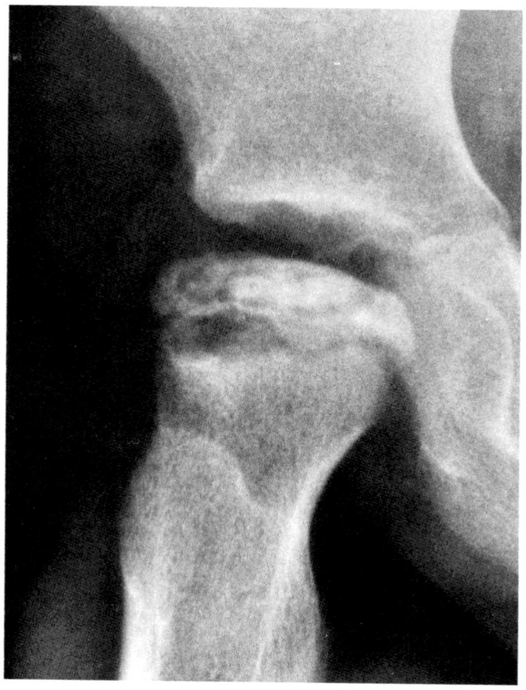

Figure 27.27 Gage sign indicating a "head-at-risk" is demonstrated in this 7-year-old girl with Legg-Calvé-Perthes disease: a V-shaped radiolucent defect in the lateral aspect of the physis.

ally sufficient to make a correct diagnosis. Several diagnostic indicators of SCFE have been identified on the anteroposterior projection of the hip (Fig. 27.28). The triangle sign of Capener may be of value in recognizing early SCFE. On a plain film of the normal adolescent hip, an intracapsular area at the medial aspect of the femoral neck is seen overlapping the posterior wall of the acetabulum, creating a dense triangular shadow; in most cases of SCFE, this triangle is lost (Fig. 27.29). In a later stage, periarticular osteoporosis becomes apparent, as well as widening and blurring of the physis and a decrease in height of the epiphysis (see Fig. 27.29). Moreover, as the disease progresses, slippage of the capital epiphysis can be identified by the absence of an intersection of the epiphysis with a line drawn

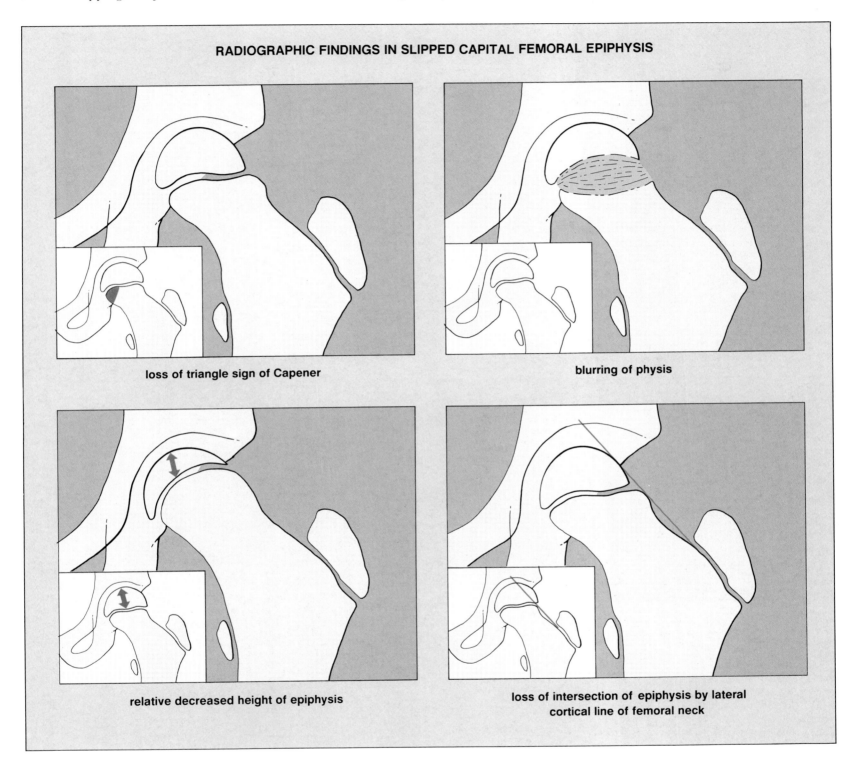

RADIOGRAPHIC FINDINGS IN SLIPPED CAPITAL FEMORAL EPIPHYSIS

loss of triangle sign of Capener

blurring of physis

relative decreased height of epiphysis

loss of intersection of epiphysis by lateral cortical line of femoral neck

Figure 27.28 Various radiographic findings have been identified as diagnostic clues to slipped capital femoral epiphysis. The insets show the normal appearance.

tangent to the lateral cortex of the femoral neck (Fig. 27.30). The frog-lateral projection of the hip reveals slippage more readily (see Fig. 27.30B), and comparison radiographs of the opposite side are helpful. Chronic stages of this disorder exhibit reactive bone formation along the superolateral aspect of the femoral neck, along with remodeling; this creates a protuberance and broadening of the femoral neck, which gives it a "pistol-grip" appearance known as a Herndon hump (Fig. 27.31). Occasionally, SCFE occurs as a result of acute trauma, in which case it is known as a transepiphyseal fracture (Fig. 27.32).

Treatment and Complications

SCFE is treated surgically by closed or open reduction of the slippage and internal fixation using various types of nails, wires, and pins to prevent further slippage and to induce closure of the physis. One of the complications of treatment is inadvertent penetration of the articular cartilage of the femoral head by a Knowles pin during placement. Lehman and colleagues have introduced a cannulated pin that prevents this complication by allowing contrast medium to be injected during surgery to determine proper placement of the pin in the femoral head on fluoroscopy. Other complications may be

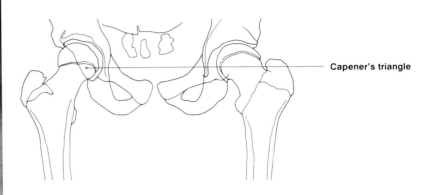

Capener's triangle

Figure 27.29 Anteroposterior view of the hips of a 12-year-old girl with slipped left capital femoral epiphysis shows the absence of a triangular density in the area of overlap of the medial segment of the femoral metaphysis

with the posterior wall of the acetabulum (Capener sign). The triangle is clearly seen in the normal right hip.

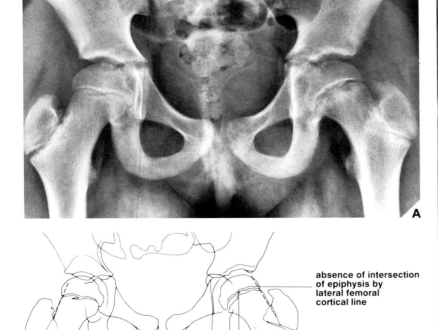

A

absence of intersection of epiphysis by lateral femoral cortical line

widening of physis

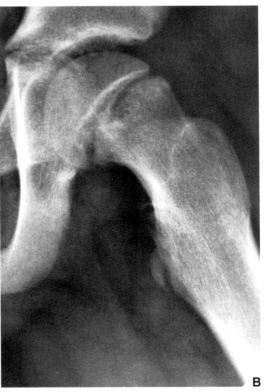

B

Figure 27.30 A 9-year-old girl presented with pain in the left hip and knee for four months. On physical examination, there was a slight limitation of abduction and internal rotation in the hip joint. (A) Anteroposterior view of the pelvis demonstrates a minimal degree of periarticular osteoporosis of the left hip, widening of the growth plate, and a slight decrease in the height of the epiphysis. Note the lack of intersection of the epiphysis by the lateral cortical line of the femoral neck. (B) Frog-lateral view of the left hip shows posteromedial slippage of the capital epiphysis.

encountered that are not necessarily related to surgical treatment. Chondrolysis is observed in about 30% to 35% of patients with SCFE and is much more common in black patients than in white. It usually occurs within one year of the slippage and may be evident by gradual narrowing of the joint space (Fig. 27.33). Osteonecrosis secondary to the precarious blood supply to the femoral head and the vulnerability of the epiphyseal vessels has been reported in about 25% of patients with SCFE (Fig. 27.34). Secondary osteoarthritis may also occur, and it can be recognized by a typical narrowing of the joint space, subchondral sclerosis, and marginal osteophyte formation (Fig. 27.35). A severe varus deformity of the femoral neck, known as coxa vara, may also be encountered.

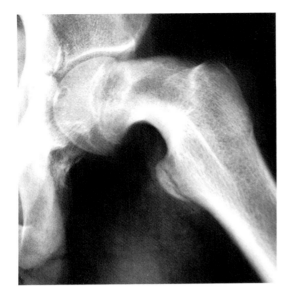

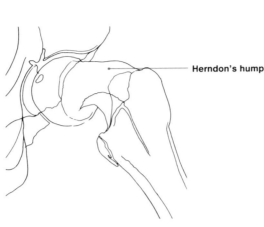

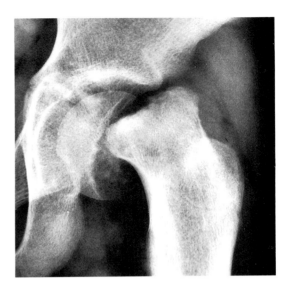

Figure 27.31 A 14-year-old boy with a 14-month history of chronic pain in the left hip was examined by a pediatrician because of significant foreshortening of the left leg and a limp. Frog-lateral view of the left hip shows changes typical of chronic slipped capital femoral epiphysis. There is a moderate degree of osteoporosis and a remodeling deformity of the femoral neck, known as a Herndon hump.

Figure 27.32 Anteroposterior view of the left hip of a 13-year-old boy who was thrown from a car in an automobile accident shows acute slippage of the femoral epiphysis. This injury represents a Salter-Harris type I fracture through the growth plate.

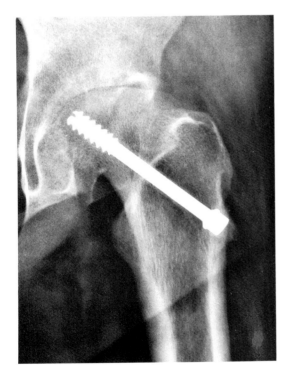

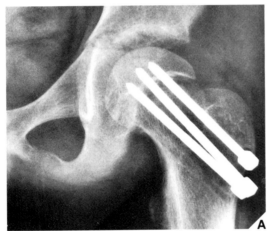

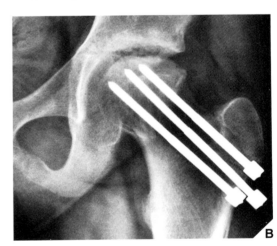

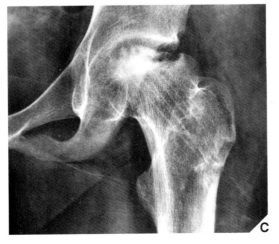

Figure 27.33 Anteroposterior view of the left hip of a 13-year-old girl who one year earlier had been treated for slipped capital femoral epiphysis shows narrowing of the joint secondary to chondrolysis, a complication of this condition.

Figure 27.34 A 12-year-old boy with a slipped left capital femoral epiphysis was treated by the insertion of three Knowles pins into the femoral head (A). Six months later, a repeat film (B) shows minimal flattening of the weight-bearing segment of the femoral epiphysis, an early sign suggesting osteonecrosis. The pins were removed. (C) On a film obtained one year later, there is an increase in density of the femoral head together with fragmentation of the epiphysis and subchondral collapse, features of advanced osteonecrosis.

ANOMALIES OF THE LOWER LIMBS

An overview of the most effective radiographic projections and radiologic techniques for evaluating common anomalies of the lower limb and foot is presented in Figure 27.36.

Congenital Tibia Vara

Blount disease, as this developmental anomaly is also known, predominantly affects the medial portion of the proximal tibial growth plate, as well as the medial segments of the tibial metaphysis and epiphysis,

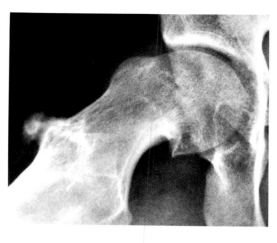

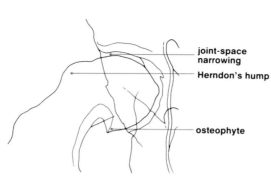

joint-space narrowing
Herndon's hump
osteophyte

Figure 27.35 Frog-lateral view of the right hip of a 14-year-old boy who developed acute slippage of the capital epiphysis at age 9 demonstrates narrowing of the joint space and osteophytosis, characteristic features of a secondary osteoarthritic process. Note the presence of a Herndon hump.

Figure 27.36 Most Effective Radiographic Projections and Radiologic Techniques for Evaluating Common Anomalies of the Lower Limb and Foot

PROJECTION/TECHNIQUE	CRUCIAL ABNORMALITIES	PROJECTION/TECHNIQUE	CRUCIAL ABNORMALITIES
Congenital Tibia Vara		**Congenital/Developmental Planovalgus Foot**	
Anteroposterior of knees	Depression of medial tibial metaphysis with beak formation	Anteroposterior of foot	Medial projection of axial line through the talus
	Varus deformity of tibia	Lateral of foot	Flattening of longitudinal arch
Conventional tomography	Premature fusion of tibial growth plate	**Congenital Vertical Talus**	
Arthrography	Hypertrophy of:	Lateral of foot	Vertical position of talus
	Nonossified portion of epiphysis		Talonavicular dislocation
			Boat-shaped or Persian-slipper appearance of foot
	Medial meniscus	With forced plantar flexion	Possibility of reduction of dislocation
Genu Valgum		Anteroposterior of foot	Flat-foot deformity
Anteroposterior of knees	Valgus deformity		Medial displacement of talus
			Abduction of forefoot
Infantile Pseudoarthrosis of the Tibia		**Calcaneonavicular Coalition**	
Anteroposterior and lateral of tibia	Bowing of tibia	Medial oblique (45°) of foot and computed tomography	Fusion of calcaneus and navicular bone
	Pseudoarthrosis		
Dysplasia Epiphysealis Hemimelica		**Talocalcaneal Coalition**	
Anteroposterior and lateral of ankle (or other affected joint)	Unilateral bulbous deformity of distal tibial (or any affected) epiphysis	Medial oblique (45°) of foot	Fusion of talus and calcaneus
		Lateral of foot	Talar beak
Talipes Equinovarus		Posterior tangential of calcaneus and computed tomography	Fusion or deformity of middle facet of subtalar joint
Anteroposterior of foot	Varus position of hindfoot	Subtalar arthrography	Cartilaginous or fibrous bridge
	Adduction and varus position of forefoot		
	Kite anteroposterior talocalcaneal angle (<20°)		
	Talus-first metatarsal (TFM) angle (>15°)		
	Metatarsal parallelism		
Lateral of foot (weight-bearing or with forced dorsiflexion)	Equinous position of the heel		
	Talocalcaneal subluxation		
	Kite lateral talocalcaneal angle (<35°)		

resulting in a varus deformity at the knee joint. The etiology of this disorder is unknown. Bateson has demonstrated convincingly that Blount disease and physiologic bowleg deformity are part of the same condition, which is influenced by both early weight-bearing and racial factors. On the basis of a study of South African black children, among whom there is an increased incidence of Blount disease (as there is in Jamaica), Bathfield and Beighton have suggested that its etiology might be related to the custom of mothers carrying children on their backs: the child's thighs are abducted and flexed, and the flexed knees gripping the mother's waist are forced to assume a varus configuration.

Two forms of Blount disease have been identified: *infantile tibia vara*, which is usually bilateral and affects children under 10 years of age, with onset most commonly between 1 and 3 years of age; and *adolescent tibia vara*, which is usually unilateral and occurs in children between the ages of 8 and 15 years. The course of the adolescent form of the disease is less severe and its incidence less frequent than in the infantile form. Regardless of its variants, Blount disease must be differentiated from other causes of tibia vara, such as those seen as sequelae to trauma.

Radiologic Evaluation and Differential Diagnosis

Radiologically, the early stages of Blount disease are marked by hypertrophy of the nonossified cartilaginous portion of the tibial epiphysis and hypertrophy of the medial meniscus, which represent compensatory changes secondary to growth arrest at the medial aspect of the physis. As the metaphysis and growth plate become depressed, the cartilage decreases in height. In advanced stages of the disease, there is premature fusion of the growth plate on the medial side, which can be demonstrated effectively by conventional tomography (Fig. 27.37). The presence of fusion is important information for surgical planning, since either resection of the bony bridge or epiphysiodesis (fusion of the physis) would be required in addition to the corrective osteotomy. Double-contrast arthrography is also a valuable technique in the radiologic evaluation of Blount disease, since it enables visualization of nonossified cartilage of the medial plateau (Fig. 27.38) and associated abnormalities of the medial meniscus (Fig. 27.39).

In most cases, it is also possible to distinguish Blount disease radiographically, particularly in its advanced stage, from developmental bowing of the legs. In Blount disease, the medial aspect of

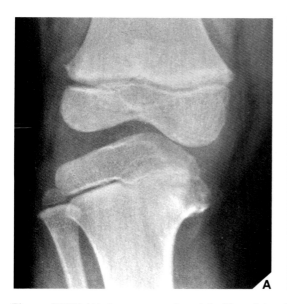
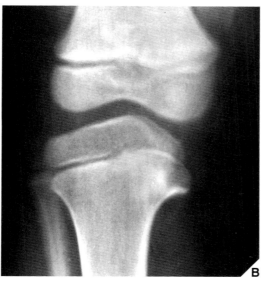
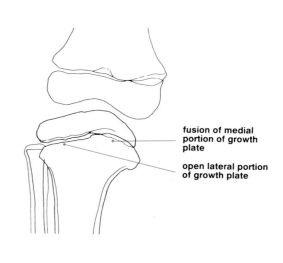

Figure 27.37 (A) Anteroposterior plain film of the right knee of an 8-year-old girl with Blount disease shows the typical changes of congenital tibia vara. There is, in addition, a possible fusion of the medial portion of the growth plate. (B) Conventional tomogram confirms the presence of a bony bridge in the medial aspect of the physis. Treatment of this condition would require either epiphysiodesis or bridge resection in addition to corrective valgus osteotomy.

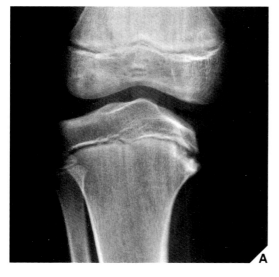
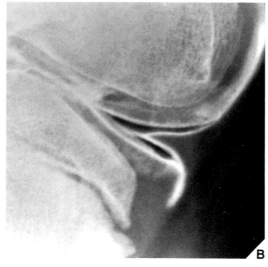
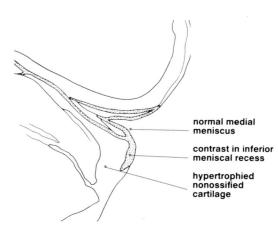

Figure 27.38 (A) Anteroposterior view of the right knee of a 10-year-old boy with Blount disease demonstrates the classic appearance of this condition, as evident in the depression of the medial metaphysis associated with a beak formation and slanting of the medial tibial epiphysis. (B) Spot film of an arthrogram shows contrast outlining the thickened nonossified cartilage of the medial tibial plateau. In this case, the medial meniscus shows no abnormalities.

the tibial metaphysis is characteristically depressed, exhibiting an abrupt angulation and formation of a beak-like prominence, which is associated with cortical thickening of the medial aspect of the tibia. Similar changes are seen in the medial aspect of the tibial epiphysis. Because of the sharp angulation of the metaphysis and adduction of the diaphysis, the tibia assumes a varus configuration (Fig. 27.40). In most instances, the lateral cortex of the tibia remains relatively straight. In developmental bowleg deformity, on the other hand, a gentle bilateral bowing is noted in both the medial and lateral femoral and tibial cortices; the growth plates appear normal, and depression of the tibial metaphysis with a beak formation is absent (Fig. 27.41). Physiologic bowing resolves to straight alignment without treatment as ambulation increases, the reversal usually beginning at about the age of 18 months. Both conditions, however, may be associated with internal tibial torsion.

Developmental bowing usually persists for about 18 to 24 months, and in most affected children, it decreases progressively, although bowing may occasionally progress with skeletal maturation. Blount disease can be differentiated from rickets on the basis of ossification of the metaphyses and the absence of widening of the growth plate (see Figs. 22.10–22.12).

Classification

Based on the progression of radiographic changes in Blount disease, Langeskjöld divided congenital tibia vara into six stages as a guideline for prognosis and treatment:

Stage I A varus deformity of the tibia, associated with irregularity of the growth plate and a small beak at the medial metaphysis; usually seen in children from 2 to 3 years of age.

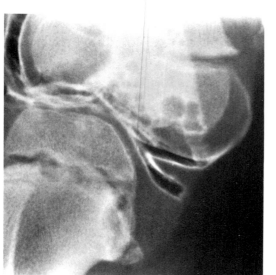

Figure 27.39
Fluoroscopic spot film of a knee arthrogram in a 4-year-old girl with advanced Blount disease affecting the right tibia shows hypertrophy of the medial aspect of the proximal tibial cartilage and an enlarged medial meniscus.

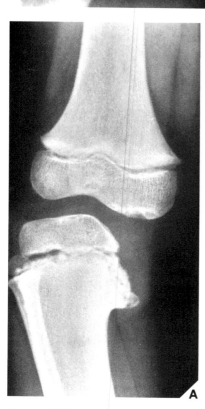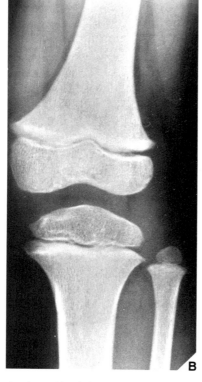

Figure 27.40 (A,B) Anteroposterior projection of both knees of a 4-year-old girl with unilateral Blount disease shows depression of the medial tibial metaphysis associated with a beak formation and medial slant of the tibial epiphysis. The left knee is normal.

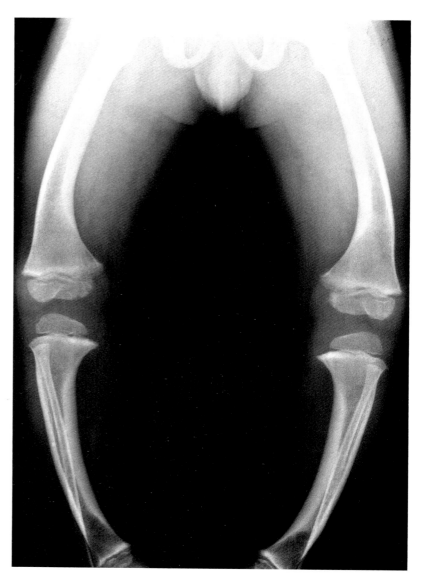

Figure 27.41 Weight-bearing (standing) anteroposterior film of the legs of a 3-year-old boy demonstrates a developmental bowleg deformity of the femora and a varus configuration of the knees. However, there are no signs of Blount disease; both proximal tibial metaphyses and growth plates are normal, although there is associated internal torsion of both tibiae and thickening of the medial femoral and tibial cortices, which is frequently seen in this condition.

Stage II   A definite depression of the medial portion of the meta-physis, associated with slanting of the medial aspect of the epiphysis; usually seen in children from 2 to 4 years of age.

Stage III   Progression of the varus deformity and a very prominent beak, with occasional fragmentation of the medial portion of the metaphysis; seen in children aged 4 to 6 years.

Stage IV   Marked narrowing of the growth plate and severe slanting of the medial aspect of the epiphysis, which shows an irregular border; usually seen in children aged 5 to 10 years.

Stage V   Marked deformity of the medial epiphysis, which is separated into two parts by a clear band, the distal part having a triangular shape; seen in children between 9 and 11 years of age.

Stage VI   A bony bridge between the epiphysis and metaphysis and possible fusion of the triangular fragment of the separated medial epiphysis to the metaphysis; seen in children between the ages of 10 and 13 years.

Stages V and VI represent phases of irreparable structural damage.

Recently, Smith introduced a simplified classification of Blount disease in an attempt to relate the grade of deformity to the need for treatment. His scheme comprises four grades: grade A, potential tibia vara; grade B, mild tibia vara; grade C, advanced tibia vara; and grade D, physeal closure.

Treatment

Blount disease is usually treated conservatively with braces. If the deformity continues to progress despite such treatment, a high tibial osteotomy may be required to achieve normal alignment of the limb; usually, correction of a rotary deformity requires an osteotomy of the proximal fibula as well. Arthrography may be required prior to surgery to determine the status of the tibial articular cartilage, information helpful in planning the degree of angular correction necessary to eliminate the deformity.

Dysplasia Epiphysealis Hemimelica

Trevor-Fairbank disease (or tarsoepiphyseal aclasis) is a developmental disorder characterized by asymmetric cartilaginous overgrowth of one or more epiphyses in the lower extremity, with a decided preference for the distal tibial epiphysis and the talus. The lesion is characteristically found on one side of the affected limb, hence the name "hemimelica." Its etiology is unknown, and there is no definite familial or hereditary predilection. Males are affected three times as often as females. Pathologically, the lesion shows similarity to an osteochondroma, and for this reason it is occasionally referred to as "epiphyseal" or "intra-articular osteochondroma." Clinically, there is deformity and restricted motion of the affected joint, and pain, particularly around the ankle, is the most frequent presenting symptom in adults.

Radiographic Evaluation and Treatment

A diagnosis of Trevor-Fairbank disease can be established through radiographic examination. It typically presents with an irregular, bulbous overgrowth of the ossification center or epiphysis on one side, resembling an osteochondroma (Fig. 26.42). Occasionally, the other ossification centers, particularly at the knee, may be similarly affected in the same individual.

Treatment for the condition is individualized according to the amount of deformity and pain; usually, surgical resection of the lesion is required. Recurrence is common.

Talipes Equinovarus

Clubfoot is a congenital deformity comprising four elements: 1) an equinous position of the heel, 2) a varus position of the hindfoot, 3) adduction and a varus deformity of the forefoot, and 4) talonavicular subluxation. Prior to the ossification of the navicular bone at 2 to 3 years of age, only the first three elements can be verified radiographically.

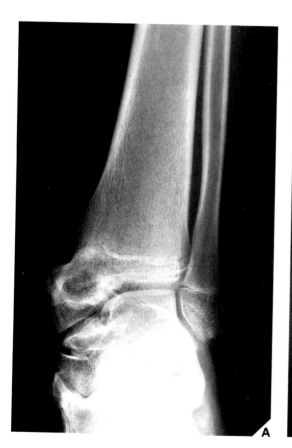
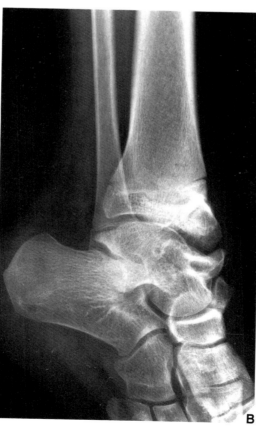

A   B

Figure 27.42 A 12-year-old girl presented with pain and limitation of motion in the ankle joint. Anteroposterior (A) and lateral (B) views of the ankle demonstrate deformity and enlargement of the medial malleolus, talus, and navicular bone, features typical of dysplasia epiphysealis hemimelica. Note that the growth disturbance is limited to the medial side of the ankle and foot. (A: reproduced with permission from Norman A, Greenspan A, 1982)

Treatment

Most cases of congenital vertical talus require surgical correction of the deformity by soft tissue release, reduction of the dislocation, and pinning of the talus to the navicular bone (Fig. 27.49). In children above 6 years of age, the navicular bone is resected. Radiographic confirmation of the correction is essential.

Tarsal Coalition

Tarsal coalition refers to the fusion of two or more tarsal bones to form a single structure. This fusion may be complete or incomplete, and the bridge may be fibrous (syndesmosis), cartilaginous (synchondrosis), or osseous (synostosis). Various bones may be affected, but most commonly the coalition occurs between the calcaneus and navic-

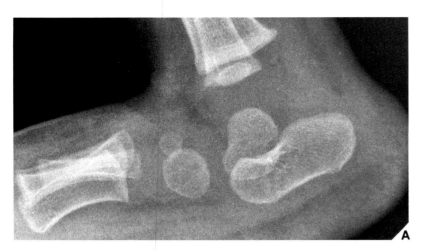

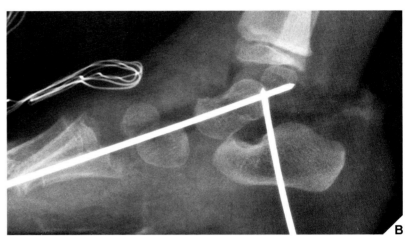

Figure 27.49 (A) Preoperative radiograph of the foot of a 2-year-old girl with congenital vertical talus shows the longitudinal axis of the talus in continuity with that of the tibia. (B) Intraoperative film demonstrates satisfactory reduction of the talonavicular dislocation.

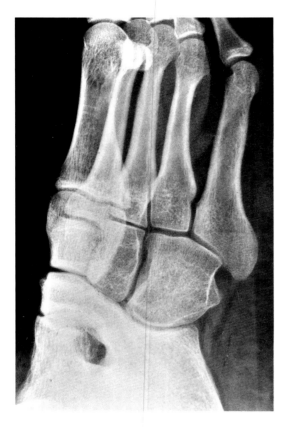

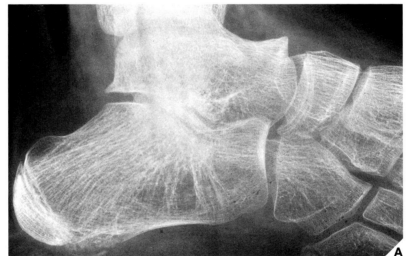

Figure 27.51
(A) Oblique projection of the hindfoot of a 12-year-old boy shows obliteration of the middle facet of the subtalar joint. Note the prominent talar beak. (B) A Harris-Beath view confirms the osseous talocalcaneal coalition.

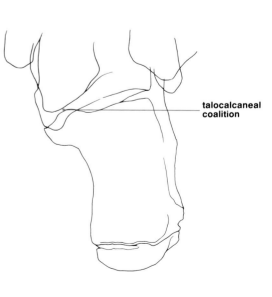

Figure 27.50 A 45° medial oblique projection of the foot of an 18-year-old boy demonstrates calcaneonavicular coalition. Note the solid osseous bridge between the two bones.

talocalcaneal coalition

ular bone, less frequently between the talus and calcaneus, and least often between the calcaneus and cuboid bone. At times, more than two bones may be affected. Despite its occurrence at birth, signs and symptoms of tarsal coalition rarely develop before the patient's second or third decade. Pain, particularly associated with prolonged walking or standing, is a typical presenting complaint, and on physical examination peroneal muscular spasm and restricted joint mobility (the so-called peroneal spastic foot) are revealed.

Although the clinical presentation usually suggests the correct diagnosis, radiographic examination is diagnostic. The primary sign of tarsal coalition is evidence of fusion. Secondary signs may also be present, representing adaptive alterations of the affected and adjacent bones and articulations.

CALCANEONAVICULAR COALITION The best projection for demonstrating this type of fusion is a 45° medial oblique view of the foot (Fig. 27.50), although conventional tomography may at times be useful. The secondary signs include hypoplasia of the talus head.

TALOCALCANEAL COALITION Since osseous fusion of the talus and calcaneus most often occurs at the level of the sustentaculum tali and the middle facet of the subtalar joint, it can effectively be demonstrated on oblique and Harris-Beath (posterior tangential) projections (Fig. 27.51); occasionally, tomography or CT examination may also be useful (Fig. 27.52). In suspected cartilaginous or fibrous union that is not readily demonstrated on plain films, secondary changes should be sought, such as close apposition of the articular surfaces of the middle facet of the subtalar joint, eburnation and sclerosis of the articular margins, and broadening or rounding of the lateral process of the talus. A common secondary sign of talocalcaneal coalition is an osseous excrescence at the dorsal aspect of the talus, forming what is called a talar beak (see Figs. 27.51A, 27.52A), which is seen in the osseous, chondrous, and fibrous types of coalition. It is important to keep in mind, however, that a similar hypertrophy of the talar ridge may be seen in other conditions as well; for example, it may be related to abnormal capsular and ligamentous traction associated with degenerative changes in the talonavicular joint (Fig. 27.53).

Demonstration of nonosseous forms of tarsal coalition may require subtalar arthrography. Similarly, when the clinical presentation is unclear and standard radiographs are equivocal, radionuclide bone scan may help localize the site of coalition by an increased uptake of radiopharmaceutical, although this is a nonspecific finding.

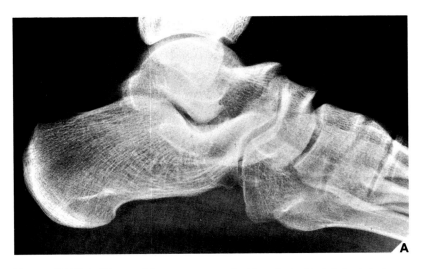

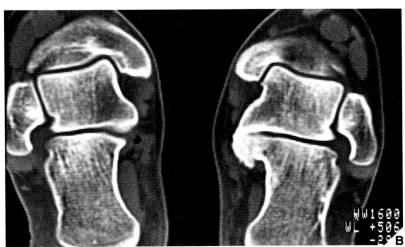

Figure 27.52 A 25-year-old man presented with pain in his left foot that was particularly pronounced after prolonged walking or standing. (A) Lateral view of the foot shows sclerotic changes in the middle facet of the subtalar joint, narrowing of the posterior talocalcaneal joint space, and a prominent talar beak—features suggesting tarsal coalition. (B) Coronal CT section clearly demonstrates narrowing of the middle facet joint space and a bony bridge. The normal right foot is shown for comparison.

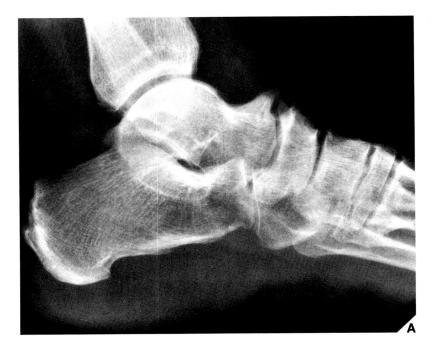

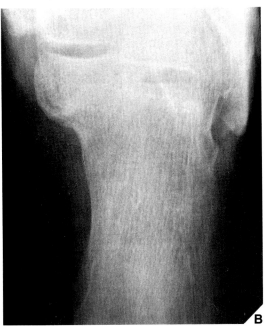

Figure 27.53 (A) Lateral view of the foot of a 61-year-old woman demonstrates a talar beak and degenerative changes in the talonavicular joint. The middle and posterior facets of the subtalar joint appear normal. (B) A Harris-Beath view shows no evidence of tarsal coalition.

PRACTICAL POINTS TO REMEMBER

Anomalies of the Shoulder Girdle and Upper Limbs

[1] Congenital elevation of the scapula (Sprengel deformity) is frequently accompanied by other anomalies, most commonly Klippel-Feil syndrome (fusion of the cervical or upper thoracic vertebrae).

[2] A Madelung deformity can be effectively evaluated on the posteroanterior and lateral projections of the distal forearm and wrist. The constant findings include:
- a decreased radial and an increased ulnar length
- medial and dorsal bowing of the radius
- a triangular configuration of the carpal bones with the lunate at the apex.

Anomalies of the Pelvic Girdle and Hip

[1] Congenital dislocation of the hip is bilateral in more than 50% of affected children; therefore, in apparently unilateral cases the unaffected hip should be carefully examined.

[2] Several lines and angles can be drawn on an anteroposterior radiograph of the pelvis and hips to help determine congenital dislocation of the hip:
- the Hilgenreiner Y-line
- the Perkins-Ombredanne line
- the Andrén-von Rosen line
- the Shenton-Menard arc
- the acetabular index
- the center-edge (C-E) angle of Wiberg.

[3] In addition to standard radiography, the radiologic evaluation of congenital dislocation of the hip requires arthrography and CT scan, which is particularly valuable in monitoring the results of treatment.

[4] Prior to conservative or surgical treatment, skin or skeletal traction is applied to bring the dislocated femoral head to "station +2" to avoid osteonecrosis of the femoral head. The Gage and Winter traction stations are determined by the position of the proximal femoral metaphysis (femoral neck) relative to the ipsilateral acetabulum and contralateral normal hip.

[5] Proximal femoral focal deficiency (PFFD) can mimic congenital hip dislocation. Arthrography is helpful in distinguishing these anomalies by demonstrating:
- presence of the femoral head in the acetabulum in type A
- a defect in the femoral neck in type B
- the absence of the femoral head in types C and D.

[6] Legg-Calvé-Perthes disease (coxa plana) represents osteonecrosis (ischemic necrosis) of the proximal epiphysis of the femur. The radiologic evaluation of this condition includes:
- a radionuclide bone scan, particularly in the early stages
- standard radiography
- contrast arthrography.

[7] The most frequently encountered radiographic findings in Legg-Calvé-Perthes disease include:
- periarticular osteoporosis
- increased density and flattening of the capital epiphysis
- a crescent sign
- fissuring and fragmentation of the epiphysis
- cystic changes in the metaphysis and broadening of the femoral neck
- lateral subluxation in the hip joint.

[8] A femoral "head-at-risk" in Legg-Calvé-Perthes disease is defined by five radiographic signs indicating a poor prognosis:
- a radiolucent, V-shaped defect in the lateral portion of the femoral head (Gage sign)
- calcifications lateral to the femoral epiphysis
- lateral subluxation of the femoral head
- a horizontal orientation of the growth plate
- diffuse metaphyseal cystic changes.

[9] A slipped capital femoral epiphysis is a Salter-Harris type I fracture through the physis, which is best demonstrated on the frog-lateral projection. Important diagnostic clues include:
- loss of the triangle sign of Capener
- decreased height of the epiphysis
- widening and blurring of the growth plate
- lack of intersection of the epiphysis by the lateral cortical line of the femoral neck.

Anomalies of the Lower Limbs

[1] Congenital tibia vara (Blount disease) can be differentiated from developmental bowing of the legs by its characteristic presentation with depression of the medial tibial metaphysis associated with abrupt angulation and the formation of a beak-like prominence on the metaphysis.

[2] Dysplasia epiphysealis hemimelica (Trevor-Fairbank disease) most often affects the ankle joint. The radiographic hallmark of this lesion, which histologically resembles osteochondroma, is an irregular bulbous overgrowth of one side of the ossification center or epiphysis.

[3] The clubfoot deformity is recognized radiographically by:
- an equinous position of the heel
- a varus position of the hindfoot
- adduction and a varus position of the forefoot
- talonavicular subluxation.

[4] In the evaluation of the clubfoot deformity, certain angles and lines drawn on the anteroposterior and lateral radiographs of the foot are helpful:
- the Kite anteroposterior and lateral talocalcaneal angles
- the talus-first metatarsal angle
- the extension of lines drawn through the longitudinal axis of the talus and the calcaneus.

[5] Proper positioning of the feet is a crucial factor in the radiographic evaluation of infants and small children. Weight-bearing films should be obtained whenever feasible; in small infants, the foot should be pressed against the radiographic cassette.

[6] Congenital vertical talus can be distinguished from developmental flat foot by the presence of dislocation in the talonavicular and talocalcaneal articulations.

[7] In tarsal coalition, the most common cause of the so-called peroneal spastic foot deformity, fusion of the affected bones (usually the talus and calcaneus or calcaneus and navicular bone) may be:
- fibrous (syndesmosis)
- cartilaginous (synchondrosis)
- osseous (synostosis).

[8] The radiologic evaluation of tarsal coalition includes:
- standard radiographs in the lateral projection (which reveals the most frequently encountered secondary sign of this condition, the formation of a talar beak), as well as in Harris-Beath and oblique projections
- conventional and computed tomography
- subtalar arthrography.

References

Bateson EM: Non-rachitic bowleg and knock-knee deformities in young Jamaican children. *Br J Radiol* 39:92, 1966.

Bateson EM: The relationship between Blount's disease and bowlegs. *Br J Radiol* 41:107, 1968.

Bathfield CA, Beighton PH: Blount's disease. A review of etiological factors in 110 patients. *Clin Orthop* 135:29, 1978.

Bloomberg TJ, Nuttall J, Stocker DJ: Radiology in early slipped femoral capital epiphysis. *Clin Radiol* 29:657, 1978.

Blount WP: Tibia vara. Osteochondrosis deformans tibiae. *J Bone Joint Surg* 19:1, 1937.

Boyer DW, Mickelson MR, Ponseti IV: Slipped capital femoral epiphysis—long-term follow-up study of 125 patients. *J Bone Joint Surg* 63A:85, 1981.

Buchanan JR, Greer RB III, Cotter JM: Management strategy for prevention of avascular necrosis during treatment of congenital dislocation of the hip. *J Bone Joint Surg* 63A:140, 1981.

Calhoun JD, Pierret G: Infantile coxa vara. *Am J Roentgenol* 115:561, 1972.

Catterall A: The natural history of Legg-Calvé-Perthes disease. *J Bone Joint Surg* 53B:37, 1971.

Catterall A: *Legg-Calvé-Perthes Disease*. Edinburgh, Churchill-Livingstone, 1982.

Chung SMK: *Hip Disorders in Infants and Children*. Philadelphia, Lea & Febiger, 1981.

Coleman SS: Diagnosis of congenital dysplasia of the hip in the newborn infant. *JAMA* 162:548, 1956.

Condon VR: Radiology of practical orthopaedic problems. *Radiol Clin North Am* 10:203, 1972.

Conway JJ, Cowell HJ: Tarsal coalition: Clinical significance and roentgenographic demonstration. *Radiology* 92:799, 1969.

Dalinka MK, Coren G, Hensinger R, Irani RN: Arthrography in Blount's disease. *Radiology* 113:161, 1974.

Dannenberg M, Anton JI, Spiegel MB: Madelung's deformity. Consideration of its roentgenological diagnostic criteria. *Am J Roentgenol* 42:671, 1939.

Deutsch AL, Resnick D, Campbell G: Computed tomography and bone scintigraphy in the evaluation of tarsal coalition. *Radiology* 144:137, 1982.

Dunn PM: The anatomy and pathology of congenital dislocation of the hip. *Clin Orthop* 119:23, 1976.

Fairbank TJ: Dysplasia epiphysealis hemimelica (tarso-epiphysial aclasis). *J Bone Joint Surg* 38B:237, 1956.

Felman AH, Kirkpatrick JA Jr: Madelung's deformity: Observations in 17 patients. *Radiology* 93:1037, 1969.

Freiberger RH, Hersh A, Harrison MO: Roentgen examination of the deformed foot. *Semin Roentgenol* 5:341, 1970.

Gage JR, Winter RB: Avascular necrosis of the capital femoral epiphysis as a complication of closed reduction of congenital dislocation of the hip. A critical review of twenty years' experience at Gillette Children's Hospital. *J Bone Joint Surg* 54A:373, 1972.

Goldman AB, Schneider R, Martel W: Acute chondrolysis complicating slipped capital femoral epiphysis: Roentgen diagnosis and differential diagnosis. *Am J Roentgenol* 130:945, 1978.

Graf R: New possibilities for the diagnosis of congenital hip joint dislocations by ultrasonography. *J Pediatr Orthop* 3:354, 1983.

Harris WR: The endocrine basis for slipping of the upper femoral epiphysis. An experimental study. *J Bone Joint Surg* 32B:5, 1950.

Haveson SB: Congenital flatfoot due to talonavicular dislocation (vertical talus). *Radiology* 72:19, 1959.

Hillmann JS, Mesgarzadeh M, Revesz G, Bonakdarpour A, Clancy M, Betz RR: Proximal femoral focal deficiency: Radiologic analysis of 49 cases. *Radiology* 165:769, 1987.

Kettelkamp DB, Campbell CJ, Bonfiglio M: Dysplasia epiphysealis hemimelica. *J Bone Joint Surg* 48A:746, 1966.

Kite NH: *The Clubfoot*. New York, Grune & Stratton, 1964.

Kleiger B, Mankin HJ: A roentgenographic study of the development of the calcaneus by means of the posterior tangential view. *J Bone Joint Surg* 43A:961, 1961.

Langeskjöld A: Tibia vara (osteochondrosis deformans tibiae). *Acta Chir Scand* 103:1, 1952.

Langeskjöld A, Riska EB: Tibia vara (osteochondrosis deformans tibiae). *J Bone Joint Surg* 46A:1405, 1964.

Lehman WB: *The Clubfoot*. Philadelphia, Lippincott, 1980.

Lehman WB: Decision-making in Legg-Calvé-Perthes disease. *Orthop Rev* 13:55, 1984.

Lehman WB, Grant AD, Nelson J, Robbins H, Milgram J: Hospital for Joint Diseases' Traction System for preliminary treatment of congenital dislocation of the hip. *J Pediatr Orthop* 3:104, 1983.

Lehman WB, Grant A, Rose D, Pugh J, Norman A: A method of evaluating possible pin penetration in slipped capital femoral epiphysis using a cannulated internal fixation device. *Clin Orthop* 186:65, 1984.

Lehman WB, Menche D, Grant A, Norman A, Pugh J: The problem of evaluating in situ pinning of slipped capital femoral epiphysis: An experimental model and a review of 63 consecutive cases. *J Pediatr Orthop* 4:297, 1984.

Lehman WB, Lubliner J, Rosen C, Grant A: Observations on the use of computerized axial tomography in the management of congenital dislocation of the hip. *Bull Hosp Jt Dis Orthop Inst* 45:21, 1985.

Levinson ED, Ozonoff MD, Royen PM: Proximal femoral focal deficiency (PFFD). *Radiology* 125:197, 1977.

Lowe HG: Necrosis of articular cartilage after slipping of capital femoral epiphysis. *J Bone Joint Surg* 52B:108, 1970.

McClure JG, Raney RB: Anomalies of the scapula. *Clin Orthop* 110:22, 1975.

McEwan DW, Dunbar JS: Radiologic study of physiologic knock knees in childhood. *J Can Assoc Radiol* 9:59, 1958.

Murphy RP, Marsh HO: Incidence and natural history of "head at risk" factor in Perthes' disease. *Clin Orthop* 132:102, 1978.

Murphy SB, Simon SR, Kijewski PK, Wilkinson RH, Griscom NT: Femoral anteversion. *J Bone Joint Surg* 69A:1169, 1987.

Norman A, Greenspan A: Bone dysplasia. In: Jahss MH (ed): *Disorders of the Foot, Vol 1*. Philadelphia, Saunders, 1982.

Ogden JA, Conlogue GJ, Phillips SB, Bronson ML: Sprengel's deformity. Radiology of the pathologic deformation. *Skeletal Radiol* 4:204, 1979.

Ogden JA, Moss HL: Pathologic anatomy of congenital hip disease. In: Weill UH (ed): *Progress in Orthopaedic Surgery, Vol 2. Acetabular Dysplasia in Childhood*. New York, Springer-Verlag, 1978.

Ramsey PL, Lasser S, MacEwen GD: Congenital dislocation of the hip. *J Bone Joint Surg* 58A:1000, 1976.

Resnick D: Talar ridges, osteophytes, and beaks: A radiologic commentary. *Radiology* 151:329, 1984.

Robbins H: Naviculectomy for congenital vertical talus. *Bull Hosp Jt Dis Orthop Inst* 37:77, 1976.

Rush BH, Bramson RT, Ogden JA: Legg-Calvé-Perthes disease: detection of cartilaginous and synovial changes with MR imaging. *Radiology* 167:473, 1988.

Salter RB: Legg-Perthes' disease. The scientific basis for methods of treatment and their indications. *Clin Orthop* 150:8, 1980.

Sartoris DJ, Resnick D: Tarsal coalition. *Arthritis Rheum* 28:331, 1985.

Scham SM: The triangular sign in the early diagnosis of slipped capital femoral epiphysis. *Clin Orthop* 103:16, 1974.

Sellers DS, Sowa DT, Moore JR, Weiland AJ: Congenital pseudoarthrosis of the forearm. *J Hand Surg* 13A:89, 1988.

Smith CF: Current concepts review—tibia vara (Blount's disease). *J Bone Joint Surg* 64A:630, 1982.

Sprengel W: Die angeborne Verschiebung des Schulterblattes nach oben. *Arch Klin Chir* 42:545, 1891.

Tachdjian MO: Reflections on complex problems of the hip in the adolescent. *Bull Hosp Jt Dis Orthop Inst* 45:1, 1985.

Tillema DA, Golding JSR: Chondrolysis following slipped capital femoral epiphysis in Jamaica. *J Bone Joint Surg* 53A:1528, 1971.

Trevor D: Tarso-epiphyseal aclasis: A congenital error of epiphyseal development. *J Bone Joint Surg* 32B:204, 1950.

Trueta J: Normal vascular anatomy of the human femoral head during growth. *J Bone Joint Surg* 39B:358, 1957.

Waldenström H: The first stages of coxa plana. *J Bone Joint Surg* 20:559, 1938.

Walters R, Simons S: Joint destruction—a sequel of unrecognized pin penetrations in patients with slipped capital femoral epiphysis. In: *The Hip Society: Proceedings of the 8th Open Scientific Meeting*. St. Louis, Mosby, 1980, p 145.

Scoliosis and Anomalies
With General Affect on the Skeleton

SCOLIOSIS

REGARDLESS OF ITS ETIOLOGY (Fig. 28.1), scoliosis is defined as a lateral curvature of the spine occurring in the coronal plane. This fact differentiates it from kyphosis, a posterior curvature of the spine in the sagittal plane; and lordosis, an anterior curvature of the spine also in the sagittal plane (Fig. 28.2). If the curve occurs in both coronal and sagittal planes, the deformity is called kyphoscoliosis. Besides a lateral curvature, scoliosis may also have a rotational component in which vertebrae rotate toward the convexity of the curve.

Idiopathic Scoliosis

Idiopathic scoliosis, which constitutes almost 70% of all scoliotic abnormalities, can be classified into three groups. The *infantile* type, of which there are two variants, occurs in children under 4 years of age; it is seen predominantly in boys, and the curvature usually occurs in the thoracic segment with its convexity to the left. In the *resolving* (benign) variant, the curve commonly does not increase beyond 30° and resolves spontaneously, requiring no treatment. The *progressive* variant carries a poor prognosis, with the potential for severe defor-

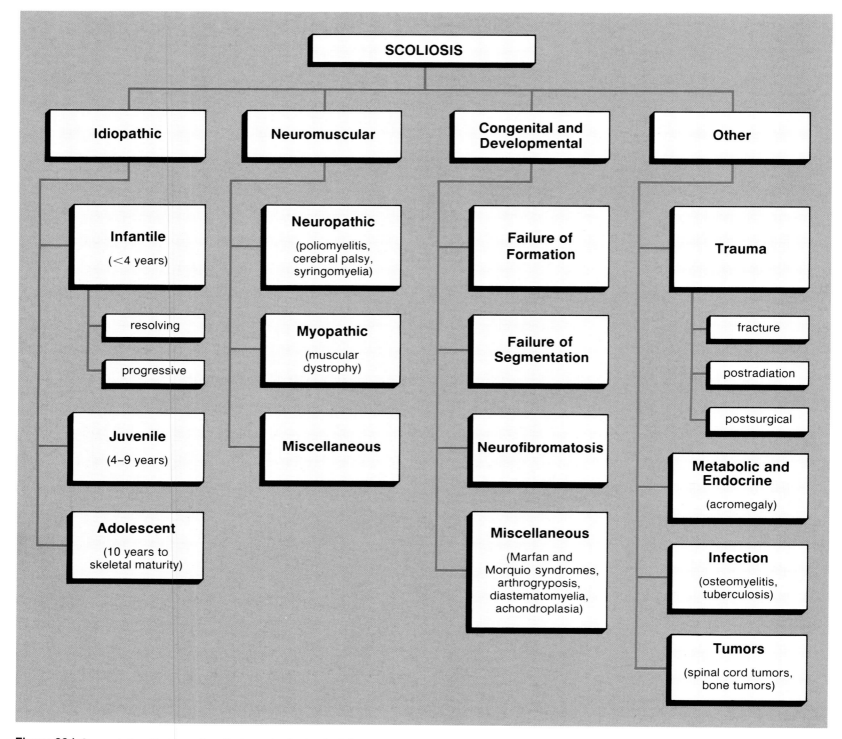

Figure 28.1 General classification of scoliosis on the basis of etiology.

mity unless aggressive treatment is initiated early in the process. *Juvenile idiopathic scoliosis* occurs equally in boys and girls from the ages of 4 to 9 years. By far the most common type of idiopathic scoliosis, comprising 85% of cases, is the *adolescent* form, seen predominantly in girls from 10 years of age to the time of skeletal maturity. The thoracic or thoracolumbar spine is most often involved, and the convexity of the curve is to the right (Fig. 28.3). Although the etiology of this type is unknown, it has been postulated that a genetic factor may be at work and that idiopathic scoliosis is a familial disorder.

Congenital Scoliosis

Congenital scoliosis is responsible for 10% of the cases of this deformity. It may generally be classified into three groups, according to MacEwen (Fig. 28.4): those resulting from a *failure in vertebral formation*, which may be partial or complete (Fig. 28.5); those caused by a *failure in vertebral segmentation*, which may be asymmetric and unilateral or symmetric and bilateral; and those resulting from a *combination* of the first two. The effects of congenital scoliosis on balance and support result in faulty biomechanics throughout the skeletal system.

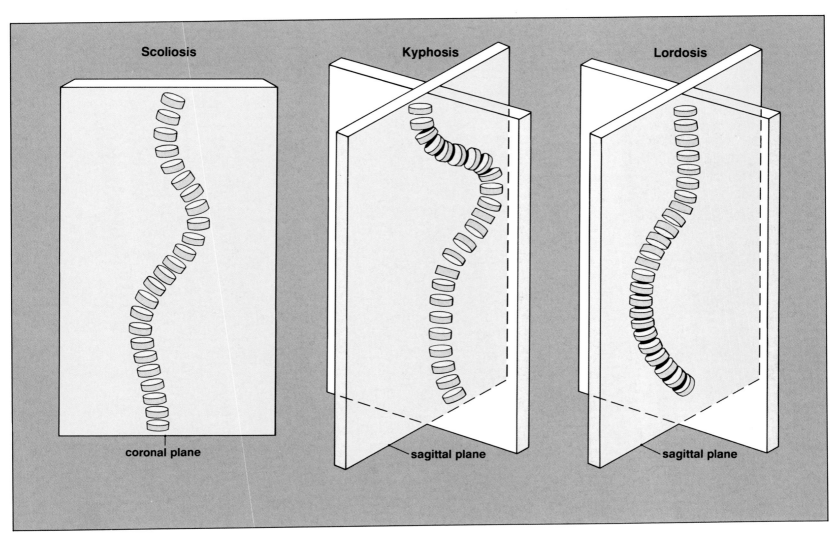

Figure 28.2 Scoliosis is a lateral curvature of the spine in the coronal (frontal) plane. Kyphosis is a posterior curvature of the spine and lordosis an anterior curvature, both occurring in the sagittal (lateral) plane.

Miscellaneous Scoliosis

Several other forms of scoliosis having specific etiology may develop, including neuromuscular, traumatic, infectious, metabolic, and secondary to tumors among others. Their discussion is beyond the scope of this text.

Radiologic Evaluation

The radiographic examination of scoliosis includes standing anteroposterior and lateral films of the entire spine; a supine anteroposterior film centered over the scoliotic curve (see Figs. 28.3, 28.5), which is used for the various measurements of spinal curvature and vertebral rotation (discussed below); and anteroposterior films obtained with the patient bending laterally to each side for evaluation of the flexible and structural components of the curve. Care should be taken to include the iliac crests in at least one of these radiographs for a determination of skeletal maturity (see Figs. 28.16, 28.17).

Ancillary techniques, such as conventional tomography and computed tomography (CT), may be required for evaluating congenital lesions such as segmentation failures. Intravenous urography (pyelography, IVP) is essential in congenital scoliosis for evaluating the presence of associated anomalies of the genitourinary tract (Fig. 28.6).

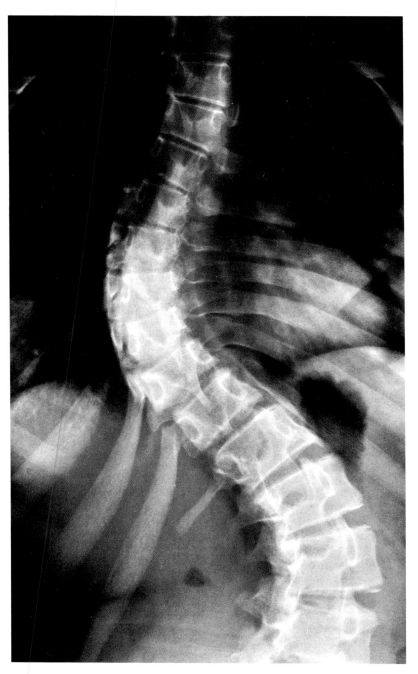

Figure 28.3 Anteroposterior view of the spine in a 15-year-old girl shows the typical features of idiopathic scoliosis involving the thoracolumbar segment. The convexity of the curve is to the right; a compensatory curve in the lumbar segment has its convexity to the left.

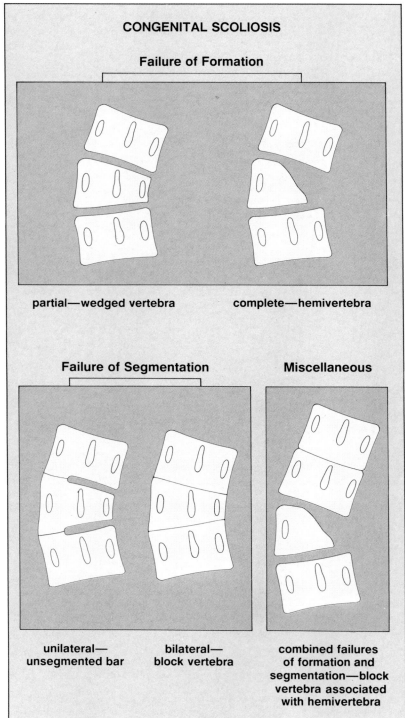

Figure 28.4 Classification of congenital scoliosis on the basis of etiology. (Adapted from MacEwen GD, et al., 1968; Winter RB, et al., 1968)

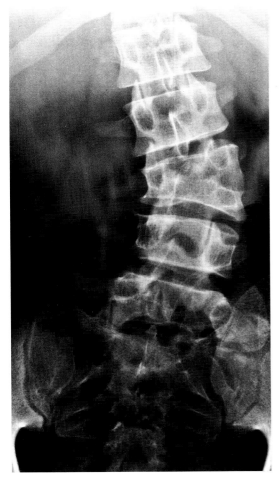

Figure 28.5 Anteroposterior view of the lumbosacral spine in a 22-year-old man demonstrates scoliosis due to hemivertebrae, a complete unilateral failure of formation. Note the deformed L-3 vertebra secondary to the faulty fusion of the hemivertebra on the left side, where two pedicles are evident. The resulting scoliosis has its convex border to the left. An associated anomaly is also apparent from the presence of the so-called transitional lumbosacral vertebra.

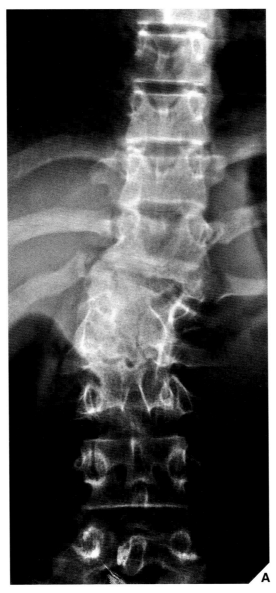

A

Figure 28.6 (A) Supine anteroposterior radiograph of the thoracolumbar spine in a 13-year-old girl shows congenital scoliosis secondary to block vertebrae consisting of a fusion of L1–3.

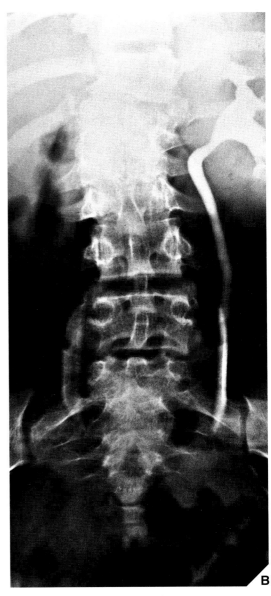

B

(B) An IVP demonstrates only the left kidney, an example of renal agenesis. Congenital scoliosis is frequently associated with urinary tract anomalies.

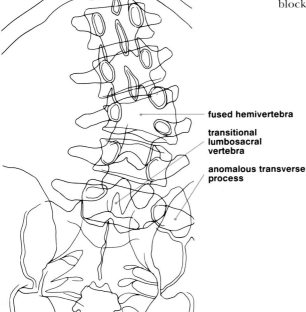

fused hemivertebra

transitional lumbosacral vertebra

anomalous transverse process

An overview of the radiographic projections and radiologic techniques used in the evaluation of scoliosis is presented in Figure 28.7.

Measurements

To evaluate the various types of scoliosis, certain terms (Fig. 28.8) and measurements must be introduced. Measurement of the severity of a scoliotic curve has practical application not only in the selection of patients for surgical treatment but also in monitoring the results of corrective therapy. Two widely accepted methods of measuring the curve are the Lippman-Cobb (Fig. 28.9) and Risser-Ferguson techniques (Fig. 28.10). The measurements obtained by these methods, however, are not comparable. The values yielded by the Lippman-Cobb method, which determines the angle of curvature only by the ends of the scoliotic curve, depending solely on the inclination of the end-vertebrae, are usually greater than those given by the Risser-Ferguson method. This also applies to the percentages of correction as determined by the two methods; the more favorable correction percentage is obtained by the Lippman-Cobb method. The latter method, which has been adopted and standardized by the Scoliosis Research Society, classifies the severity of scoliotic curvature into seven groups (Fig. 28.11).

Another technique for measuring the degree of scoliosis, introduced by Greenspan and colleagues in 1978, uses a "scoliotic index." Designed to give a more accurate and comprehensive representation of the scoliotic curve, this technique measures the deviation of each involved vertebra from the vertical spinal line as determined by points at the center of the vertebra immediately above the upper end-vertebra of the curve and at the center of the vertebra immediately below the lower end-vertebra (Fig. 28.12). Its most valuable feature is that it minimizes the influence of overcorrection of the

---

Figure 28.7 Standard Radiographic Projections and Radiologic Techniques for Evaluating Scoliosis

PROJECTION/TECHNIQUE	DEMONSTRATION	PROJECTION/TECHNIQUE	DEMONSTRATION
Anteroposterior	Lateral deviation	*Lateral*	Associated kyphosis and lordosis
	Angle of scoliosis (by Risser-Ferguson and Lippman-Cobb methods and scoliotic index)	*Conventional and Computed Tomography*	Congenital fusion of vertebrae Hemivertebrae
	Vertebral rotation (by Cobb and Moe methods)	*Myelography*	Tethering of cord
Of vertebra	Ossification of ring apophysis as determinant of skeletal maturity	*Magnetic Resonance Imaging*	Abnormalities of nerve roots Compression and displacement of thecal sac
Of pelvis	Ossification of iliac crest apophysis as determinant of skeletal maturity	*Intravenous Urography*	Associated anomalies of GU tract (in congenital scoliosis)
Lateral bending	Flexibility of curve Amount of reduction of curve		

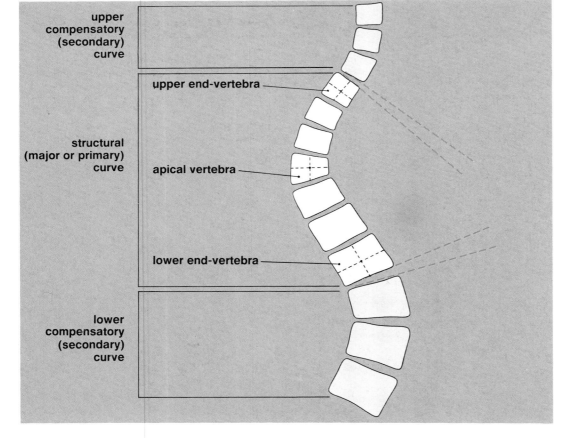

Figure 28.8 Terminology used in describing the scoliotic curve. The end-vertebrae of the curve are defined as those that tilt maximally into the concavity of the structural curve. The apical vertebra, which shows the most severe rotation and wedging, is the one whose center is most laterally displaced from the central line. The center of the apical vertebra is determined by the intersection of two lines, one drawn from the center of the upper and lower end plates and the other from the center of the lateral margins of the vertebral body. The center should not be determined by diagonal lines through the corners of the vertebral body.

end-vertebrae in the measured angle, a frequent criticism of the Lippman-Cobb technique. Furthermore, short segments or minimal curvatures, often difficult to measure with the currently accepted methods, are easily measurable with this technique.

Recently, computerized methods for measuring and analyzing the scoliotic curve have been introduced. Although more accurate than the manual methods, they require more sophisticated equipment and are more time-consuming than the methods described above.

In addition to the measurement of scoliotic curvature, the radiographic evaluation of scoliosis also requires the determination of other factors. Measurement of the degree of *rotation of the vertebrae* of the involved segment can be obtained by either of two methods currently in use. The Cobb technique for grading rotation uses the posi-

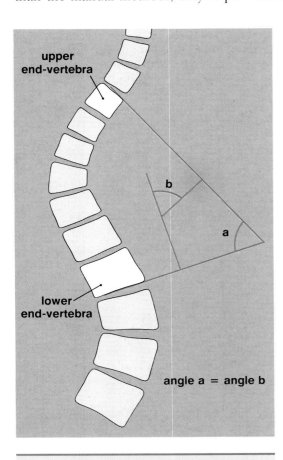

Figure 28.9 In the Lipman-Cobb method of measuring the degree of scoliotic curvature, two angles are formed by the intersection of two sets of lines. The first set of lines, one drawn tangent to the superior surface of the upper end-vertebra and the other tangent to the inferior surface of the lower end-vertebra, intersects to form angle (*a*). The intersection of the other set of lines, each drawn perpendicular to the tangential lines, forms angle (*b*). These angles are equal, and either may serve as the measurement of the degree of scoliosis.

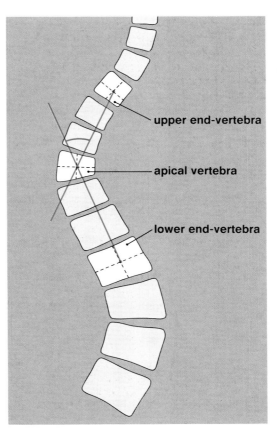

Figure 28.10 In the Risser-Ferguson method, the degree of scoliotic curvature is determined by the angle formed by the intersection of two lines at the center of the apical vertebra, the first line originating at the center of the upper end-vertebra and the other at the center of the lower end-vertebra.

Figure 28.11 Lippman-Cobb Classification of Scoliotic Curvature

GROUP	ANGLE OF CURVATURE
I	<20°
II	21°–30°
III	31°–50°
IV	51°–75°
V	76°–100°
VI	101°–125°
VII	>125°

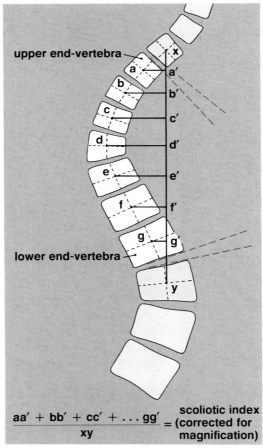

$$\frac{aa' + bb' + cc' + \ldots gg'}{xy} = \text{scoliotic index (corrected for magnification)}$$

Figure 28.12 In the measurement of scoliosis using the scoliotic index, each vertebra (*a–g*) is considered an integral part of the curve. A vertical spinal line (*xy*) is first determined whose endpoints are the centers of the vertebrae immediately above and below the upper and lower end-vertebrae of the curve. Lines are then drawn from the center of each vertebral body perpendicular to the vertical spinal line (*aa', bb', . . . gg'*). The values yielded by these lines represent the linear deviation of each vertebra; their sum, divided by the length of the vertical line (*xy*) to correct for radiographic magnification, yields the scoliotic index. A value of zero denotes a straight spine; the higher the scoliotic index the more severe the scoliosis.

tion of the spinous process as a point of reference (Fig. 28.13). On the normal anteroposterior radiograph of the spine, the spinous process appears at the center of the vertebral body if there is no rotation. As the degree of rotation increases, the spinous process migrates toward the convexity of the curve. The Moe method, also based on the measurements obtained on the anteroposterior projection of the spine, uses the symmetry of the pedicles as a point of reference, with the migration of the pedicles toward the convexity of the curve determining the degree of vertebral rotation (Fig. 28.14).

The final factor in the evaluation of scoliosis is the determination of *skeletal maturity*. This is important for both the prognosis and treatment of scoliosis, particularly the idiopathic type, since there is a potential for significant progression of the degree of curvature as long as skeletal maturity has not been reached. Skeletal age can be determined by comparison of a radiograph of a patient's hand with the standards for different ages available in radiographic atlases. It can also be assessed by radiographic observation of the ossification of the apophysis of the vertebral ring (Figs. 28.15) or, as is often done, from the ossification of the iliac apophysis (Fig. 28.16, 28.17).

Treatment

Various surgical procedures are available for the treatment of scoliosis. The main objective of surgery is to balance and fuse the spine in order to prevent the deformity from progressing; its secondary objective is to correct the scoliotic curve to the extent of its flexibility. Determining the level of fusion depends on several factors, including the etiology of the scoliosis and the age of the patient, as well as the pattern of the scoliotic curve and the extent of vertebral rotation as evaluated during the radiographic examination of the patient.

Spinal fusion is now commonly accompanied by internal fixation of the spine to provide stability. One of the most popular methods for internal fixation is the Harrington-Luque technique (Wisconsin

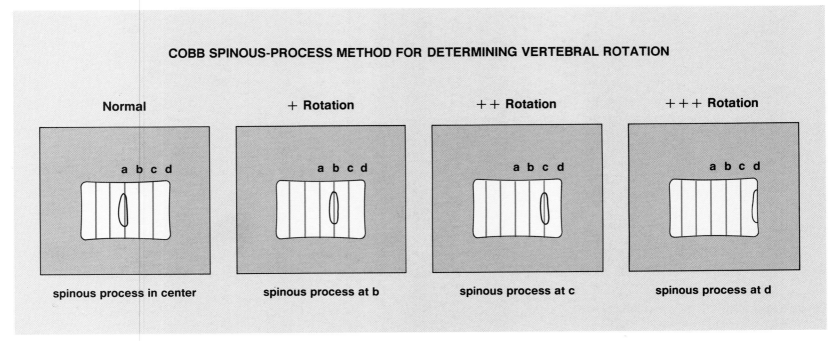

Figure 28.13 In the Cobb spinous-process method for determining rotation, the vertebra is divided into six equal parts. Normally, the spinous process appears at the center. Its migration to certain points toward the convexity of the curve marks the degree of rotation.

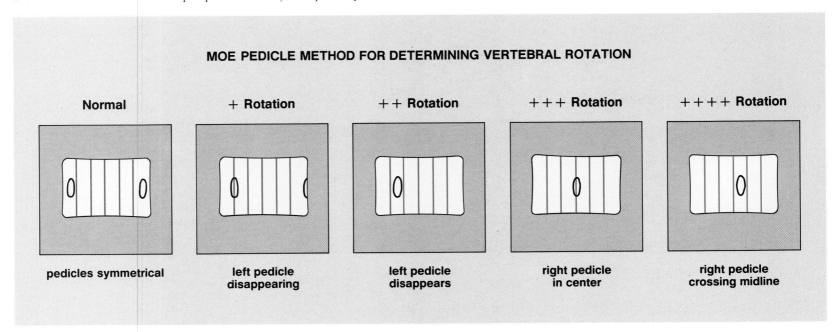

Figure 28.14 The Moe pedicle method for determining rotation divides the vertebra into six equal parts. Normally, the pedicles appear in the outer parts. Migration of a pedicle to certain points toward the convexity of the curve determines the degree of rotation.

segmental instrumentation), using square-ended distraction rods and wire loops inserted through the bases of the spinous processes and connected to two contoured paravertebral rods (Fig. 28.18). The procedure involves decortication of the laminae and spinous processes, obliteration of the posterior facet joints by removal of the cartilage, and the placement of an autogenous bone graft from the iliac crest along the concave side of the curve. The hooks of the distraction rods are inserted under the laminae at the upper and lower ends of the curve. The prebent stainless-steel paravertebral rods (Luque rods or L-rods) are anchored into the spinous process or

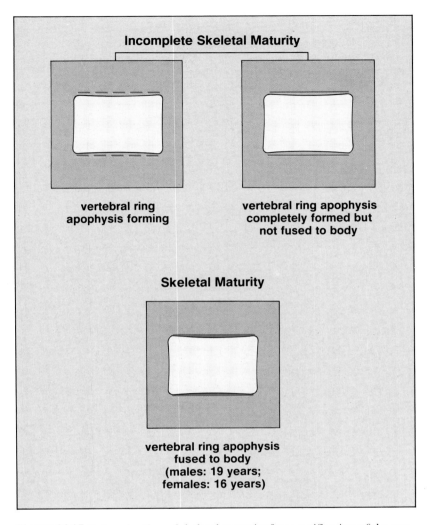

Figure 28.15 Determination of skeletal maturity from ossification of the vertebral ring apophysis.

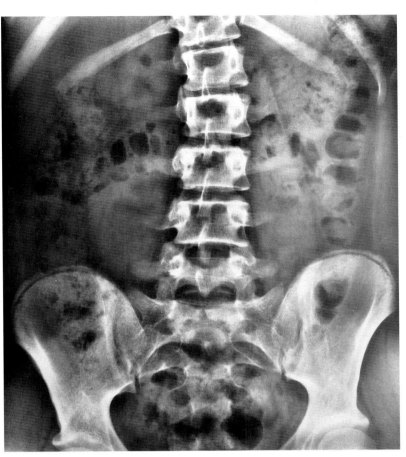

Figure 28.16 The ossification of the iliac apophysis is helpful in determining skeletal age. Progression of the apophysis in this 14-year-old girl with idiopathic scoliosis has been completed, but the lack of fusion with the iliac crest indicates continuing skeletal maturation.

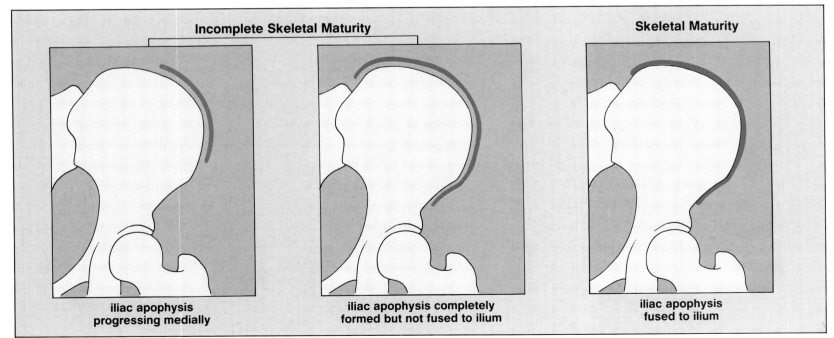

Figure 28.17 Determination of skeletal maturity from the status of ossification of the iliac apophysis.

pelvis, depending on the location of the curve; wires, passed through the base of the spinous process at each level of the spine to be fused, are then fixed to the L-rods. Variations in this technique have been employed using L-rod instrumentation alone, which involves the use of sublaminar wires fixed to the rods, or a combination of Harrington distractors and wires fixed to them. Recently, Cotrel-Dubousset spinal instrumentation using knurled rods has gained popularity. Fixation is achieved via pediculotransverse double-hook purchase at several levels. The two knurled rods are additionally stabilized by two transverse traction devices. The Dwyer technique, involving anterior fixation of the spine and obliteration of the intervertebral disks, is also used in the surgical treatment of scoliosis but more often in the paralytic types of the deformity.

The postoperative radiographic evaluation of internal fixation by the Harrington-Luque technique should focus on 1) whether the hooks of the Harrington rod are properly anchored with their brackets on the laminae of the superior and inferior vertebrae of the fused segment; 2) whether a hook has separated or been displaced; and 3) whether the rods and wires are intact. Moreover, evidence of pseu-

doarthrosis of the fused vertebrae should be sought when the postoperative loss of correction exceeds 10°; a range of 6° to 10° loss of correction is ordinarily seen. The evaluation of pseudoarthrosis may require conventional tomography in addition to the standard projections. Tomography may also be needed within six to nine months after surgery to demonstrate suspected nonunion of the bone engrafted on the concave side of the curve. Union of the graft with the spinal segment should appear solid; tomography may demonstrate radiolucent defects suggesting nonunion. Other complications involving the instrumentation may occur, such as fracture of a distraction rod or of a wire cable or screw, or excessive bending of the rods. Usually, these are easily demonstrated on standard radiographs.

ANOMALIES WITH GENERAL AFFECT ON THE SKELETON

Figure 28.19 presents an overview of radiographic projections and radiologic techniques most effective for evaluating congenital and developmental anomalies exhibiting general affect on the skeleton.

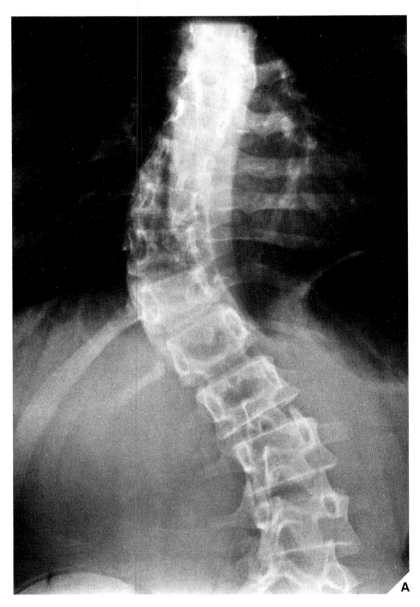

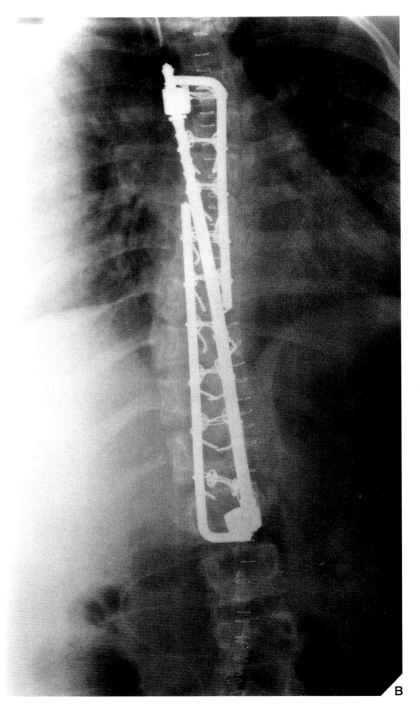

Figure 28.18 (A) Preoperative anteroposterior radiograph of the lumbar spine in a 15-year-old girl shows idiopathic dextroscoliosis. (B) Postoperative film shows the placement of the Harrington distractor and two Luque rods. Note the multiple wires fixed into the prebent L-rods.

Figure 28.19 Most Effective Radiographic Projections and Radiologic Techniques for Evaluating Common Anomalies With General Affect on the Skeleton

PROJECTION/TECHNIQUE	CRUCIAL ABNORMALITIES

Arthrogryposis

Anteroposterior, lateral, and oblique of affected joints	Multiple subluxations and dislocations
	Fat-like lucency of soft tissues
	Cubital and popliteal webbing

Down Syndrome

Anteroposterior:	
Of pelvis and hips	Hip dysplasia
Of ribs	11 pairs of ribs
Dorsovolar of both hands	Clinodactyly and hypoplasia of fifth fingers
Lateral of cervical spine	Atlantoaxial subluxation
Tomography (lateral) of cervical spine (C-1, C-2)	Hypoplastic odontoid

Neurofibromatosis

Anteroposterior, lateral, and oblique of long bones	Pit-like erosions
	Pseudoarthrosis of distal tibia and fibula
Anteroposterior:	
Of ribs	Rib notching
Of lower cervical/upper thoracic spine	Scoliosis
	Kyphoscoliosis
Oblique of cervical spine	Enlarged neural foramina
Lateral of thoracic/lumbar spine	Posterior vertebral scalloping
Myelography	Intraspinal neurofibromas
	Increased volume of enlarged subarachnoid space
	Localized dural ectasia
Computed tomography	Complications (e.g., sarcomatous degeneration)
Magnetic resonance imaging	

Osteogenesis Imperfecta

Anteroposterior, lateral, and oblique of affected bones	Osteoporosis
	Bowing deformities
	Trumpet-like metaphysis
	Fractures
Lateral of skull	Wormian bones
Anteroposterior and lateral of thoracic/lumbar spine	Kyphoscoliosis

Achondroplasia

Anteroposterior:	
Of upper and lower extremities	Shortening of tubular bones, particularly humeri and femora
Of pelvis	Rounded iliac bones
	Horizontal orientation of acetabular roofs
	Small sciatic notches
Of spine	Narrowing of interpedicular distance
Lateral of spine	Short pedicles
	Posterior scalloping of vertebral bodies
Dorsovolar of hands	Short, stubby fingers
	Separation of middle finger ("trident" appearance)
Computed tomography	Spinal stenosis
Magnetic resonance imaging	

Morquio-Brailsford Disease

Anteroposterior and lateral of spine	Oval or hook-shaped vertebrae with central beak
Anteroposterior:	
Of pelvis	Overconstriction of iliac bodies
	Wide iliac flaring
Of hips	Dysplasia of proximal femora

Hurler Syndrome

Anteroposterior and lateral:	
Of spine	Rounding and lower beaking of vertebral bodies
	Recessed hooked vertebra at apex of kyphoscoliotic curve
Of skull	Frontal bossing
	Synostosis of sagittal and lambdoidal sutures
	Thickening of calvarium
	J-shaped sella turcica
Anteroposterior of pelvis	Flaring of iliac wings
	Constriction of inferior portion of iliac body
	Shallow, obliquely oriented acetabula

Osteopetrosis

Anteroposterior and lateral:	
Of long bones	Increased density (osteosclerosis)
	Bone-in-bone appearance
Of spine	"Rugger-jersey" vertebral bodies
Anteroposterior of pelvis	Ring-like pattern of normal and abnormal bone in ilium

Pycnodysostosis

Anteroposterior and lateral of long bones	Increased density (osteosclerosis)
Dorsovolar of hands	Resorption of terminal tufts (acro-osteolysis)
Lateral of skull	Wormian bones
	Persistence of anterior and posterior fontanelles
	Obtuse (fetal) angle of mandible

Osteopoikilosis

Anteroposterior of affected bones	Dense spots at the articular ends of long bones

Osteopathia Striata

Anteroposterior of affected bones	Dense striations, particularly in metaphysis

Progressive Diaphyseal Dysplasia

Anteroposterior of long bones (particularly lower limbs)	Symmetric fusiform thickening of cortex
	Sparing of epiphyses

Melorheostosis

Anteroposterior and lateral of affected bones	Asymmetric, wavy hyperostosis (like dripping candle wax)
	Ossifications of periarticular soft tissues

Neurofibromatosis

Originally considered a disorder of neurogenic tissue (nerve-trunk tumors), neurofibromatosis (also called von Recklinghausen disease) is now believed to be a hereditary dysplasia that may involve almost every organ system of the body. It is transmitted as an autosomal-dominant trait, with more than 50% of cases reporting a family history of neurofibromatosis. Sessile or pedunculated skin lesions (mollusca fibrosa) are an almost constant finding, and café au lait spots occur in more than 90% of patients. The latter lesions have a smooth border that has been likened to the coast of California; this distinguishes them from the café au lait spots seen in fibrous dysplasia, which have rugged "coast of Maine" borders. Plexiform neurofibromatosis is a diffuse involvement of the nerves, associated with elephantoid masses of soft tissue (elephantiasis neuromatosa) and localized or generalized enlargement of a part or all of a limb. Patients with these manifestations are particularly prone to develop malignant tumors (see Fig. 18.53).

Skeletal abnormalities are often encountered in neurofibromatosis; at least 50% of patients demonstrate some bony changes, most commonly extrinsic, pit-like cortical erosions resulting from direct pressure by adjacent neurofibromas. This is commonly seen in the long bones (Fig. 28.20) and ribs. The long bones often exhibit bowing deformities, and pseudoarthroses, seen in about 10% of cases, most commonly occur in the lower tibia and fibula (Fig. 28.21).

This type of false joint formation must be differentiated from congenital pseudoarthrosis. Moreover, the long bones are the site of lesions that were once considered to represent intraosseous neurofibromas; these cyst-like radiolucencies are now regarded as lesions representing fibrous cortical defects and nonossifying fibromas, associated with neurofibromatosis. Whittling of the bones is also a typical feature of neurofibromatosis (Fig. 28.22).

The spine is the second most common site of skeletal abnormalities in neurofibromatosis. Scoliosis or kyphoscoliosis, which characteristically involves a short segment of the vertebral column with acute angulation, commonly occurs in the lower cervical or upper thoracic spine. Widening of the intervertebral foramina in the cervical segment may also occur, resulting from dumbbell-shaped neurofibromas arising in spinal nerve roots (Fig. 28.23). In the thoracic and lumbar segments, scalloping of the posterior border of verte-

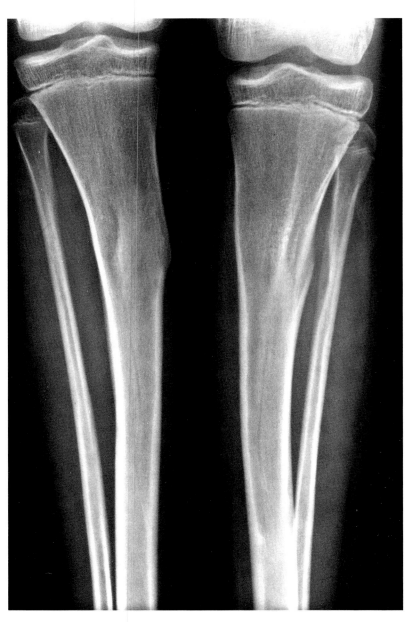

Figure 28.20 Anteroposterior view of the lower legs of an 11-year-old girl with neurofibromatosis shows pit-like erosions in the upper tibiae and fibulae, a common finding in this condition.

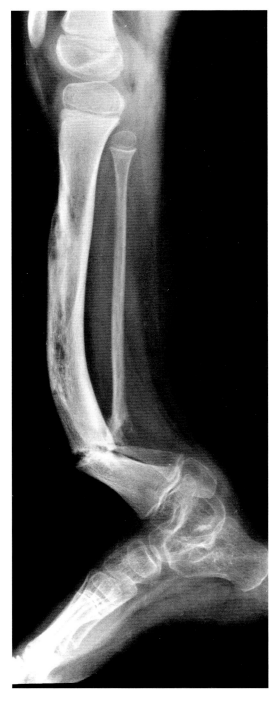

Figure 28.21 Lateral view of the right lower leg of an 11-year-old boy with generalized neurofibromatosis demonstrates anterior bowing of the distal tibia and fibula, associated with pseudoarthrosis. Note the pressure erosions in the middle third of the tibial diaphysis.

bral bodies is another characteristic feature (Fig. 28.24). Although most of these abnormalities can easily be diagnosed with conventional radiography, some ancillary techniques may be useful. Myelography is particularly valuable for demonstrating the increased volume of the enlarged subarachnoid space and the localized dural ectasia extending into the scalloped defects in the vertebral bodies; with introduction of MRI, this modality became more prevalent in investigation of the above-mentioned abnormalities.

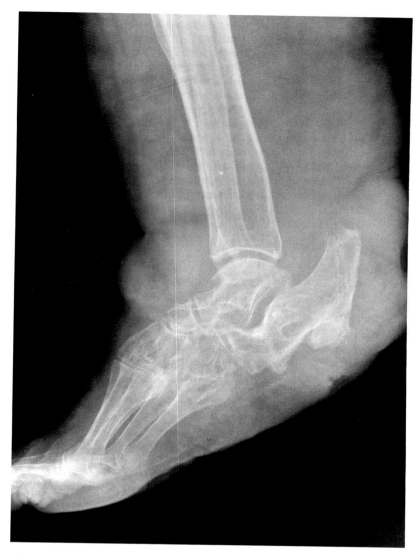

Figure 28.22 Lateral view of the lower leg and foot of a 37-year-old woman with plexiform neurofibromatosis shows whittling of the calcaneus and marked hypertrophy of the soft tissues (elephantiasis).

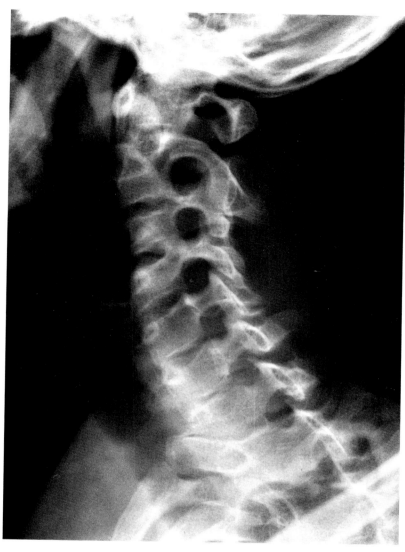

Figure 28.23 Oblique view of the cervical spine in a 26-year-old man with congenital neurofibromatosis demonstrates widening of the upper neural foramina secondary to "dumbbell" neurofibromas arising in the spinal nerve roots.

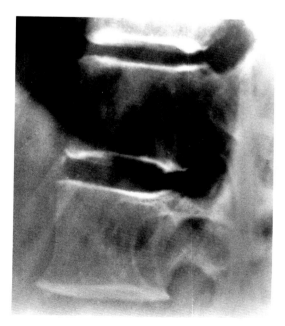

Figure 28.24 Lateral spot-film of the lower thoracic spine in a 29-year-old woman with neurofibromatosis shows scalloping of the posterior border of the T-12 vertebra, a common manifestation of this condition.

ented; and the sciatic notches are small. These features together give the hemipelvis the appearance of a ping-pong paddle. The shape of the inner contour of the pelvis has also been likened to a champagne glass (Fig. 28.30)

The most serious complication of achondroplasia is related to the spinal stenosis secondary to the typically short pedicles. Patients with the disease also occasionally develop herniation of the nucleus pulposus. CT and MRI are the procedures of choice for confirming these two complications.

It is important to note that there are two other conditions resembling achondroplasia, but they differ from it in the severity of their symptoms and in radiographic presentation. *Hypochondroplasia* is a mild form of chondrodystrophy, in which the skeletal abnormalities are less severe than in achondroplasia. The skull is unaffected. *Thanatophoric dwarfism*, on the other hand, is thought to be a severe form of achondroplasia. It is lethal either in utero or within hours to days after birth.

Mucopolysaccharidoses

The mucopolysaccharidoses constitute a group of hereditary disorders having in common an excessive accumulation of mucopolysaccharides secondary to deficiencies in specific enzymes. Although several distinctive types of mucopolysaccharidoses have been delineated (Fig. 28.31), each with distinctive clinical and radiologic features, a specific diagnosis of any of these conditions is made on the basis of the patient's age at onset, the level of neurological stunting, the amount of corneal clouding, and other clinical features. With the exception of Morquio-Brailsford disease, all of the mucopolysaccharidoses are marked by excessive urinary excretion of dermatan and heparan sulfate.

The mucopolysaccharidoses exhibit common radiographic findings. These include osteoporosis, oval or hook-shaped vertebral bodies, and an abnormal configuration of the pelvis, with overconstriction of the iliac bodies and wide flaring of the iliac wings. The tubular bones are shortened and dysplastic changes are evident in the proxi-

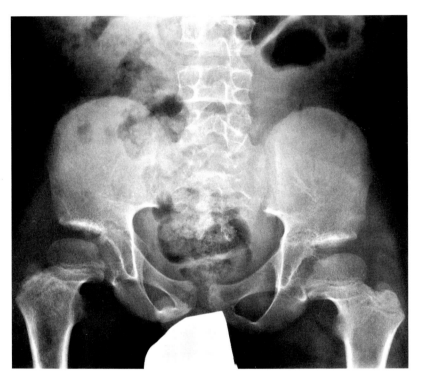

Figure 28.30 Anteroposterior view of the pelvis of a 13-year-old boy with achondroplasia shows the classic manifestations of this condition. The iliac bones are rounded, lacking their normal flaring, and the acetabular roofs are horizontal—features rendering the appearance of a ping-pong paddle. Note also the "champagne-glass" inner contour of the pelvic cavity.

Figure 28.31 Classification of the Mucopolysaccharidoses (MPS)

DESIGNATED NUMBER	EPONYM	GENETIC AND CLINICAL CHARACTERISTICS
MPS I-H	Hurler syndrome (gargoylism)	Autosomal-recessive Corneal clouding, mental retardation, hepatosplenomegaly, cardiomegaly Urinary excretion of dermatan and heparan sulfates Deficiency of α-L-iduronidase enzyme
MPS I-S	Scheie syndrome	Autosomal-recessive Corneal clouding, normal mental development, near-normal skeleton, aortic valve disease
MPS I-H/S	Hurler-Scheie compound	Urinary excretion of same product as in MPS I-H, and same enzyme deficiency
MPS II	Hunter syndrome (mild and severe variants)	Sex-chromosome-linked recessive disorder (males only) Mild mental retardation, absence of corneal clouding Urinary excretion of same product as in MPS I-H Deficiency of iduronate sulfatase
MPS III	Sanfilippo syndrome (A, B, and C variants)	Autosomal-recessive Progressive mental retardation, motor overactivity, coarse facial features Urinary excretion of heparan sulfate Deficiency of heparan-N-sulfatase
MPS IV	Morquio-Brailsford disease (type A, classic; type B, milder abnormalities)	Autosomal-recessive Short-trunk dwarfism; characteristic posture with knock knees, lumbar lordosis, and severe pectus carinatum; corneal opacities; impaired hearing; hepatosplenomegaly Urinary excretion of keratan sulfate Deficiency of galactosamine-6-sulfate sulfatase
MPS V	Redesignated MPS I-S	
MPS VI	Maroteaux-Lamy syndrome	Autosomal-recessive Normal intelligence, short stature, lumbar kyphosis, hepatosplenomegaly, joint contractures Urinary excretion of dermatan sulfate Deficiency of arylsulfatase B
MPS VII	Sly syndrome	Autosomal recessive Growth and mental retardation, hepatosplenomegaly, pulmonary infections Urinary excretion of heparan and dermatan sulfates Deficiency of β-glucuronidase
MPS VIII	DiFerrante syndrome	Probably genetic trait Short stature Urinary excretion of keratan and heparan sulfates Deficiency of glucosamine-6-sulfate sulfatase

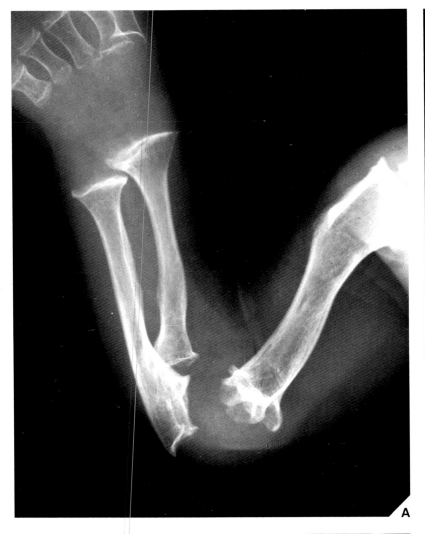

A

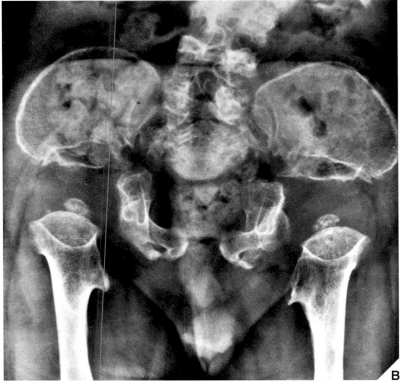

B

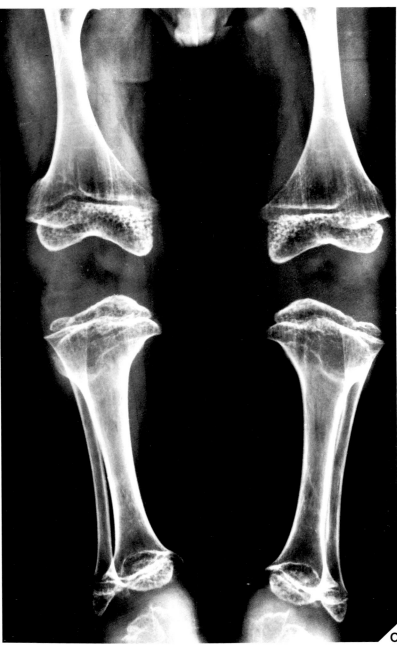

C

Figure 28.32 The classic features of Morquio-Brailsford disease are exhibited in these radiographic studies of a 3-year-old boy. (A) Plain film of the right arm shows foreshortening and deformity of the humerus, radius, and ulna, with an irregular outline of the metaphyses. (B) Anteroposterior view of the pelvis and hips shows flaring of the iliac wings and constriction of the iliac bodies. The narrowing of the pelvis at the level of the acetabula, which are distorted, produces a characteristic "wine-glass" appearance. Note the fragmentation of the ossification centers in the femoral heads and the broadening of the femoral necks, with subluxation in the hip joints and a coxa valga deformity. (C) The legs show deformities in the epiphyses of the femora and tibiae, as well as foreshortening of these bones

mal femoral epiphyses (Fig. 28.32). The mucopolysaccharidoses, however, do show variations in these radiographic abnormalities; Hurler syndrome, for example, exhibits a characteristic rounding of the vertebral end plates on the lateral projection; the vertebral bodies appear oval in shape but frequently there is a dorsolumbar gibbous with a hypoplastic hook-shaped, recessed vertebral body.

Fibrodysplasia Ossificans Progressiva (Myositis Ossificans Progressiva)

Fibrodysplasia ossificans progressiva is a rare systemic autosomal-dominant disorder with primary histopathologic abnormality in the connective tissues. Most patients are affected early in life (0–5 years), and there is no sex predominance. The earliest clinical symptom is the appearance of painful nodules and masses in the subcutaneous tissue, particularly around the head and neck, with associated stiff-ness and limitation of movement. Subsequently, excessive ossification of muscles, ligaments, and fascia occur, with the predominant sites of involvement in the head and neck, the dorsal paraspinal muscles, the shoulder girdles, and the hips. Involvement of inter-costal musculature interferes with respiration.

Clinically, the condition progresses from the shoulder girdle to the upper arms, spine, and pelvis. The natural history is one of remissions and exacerbations; death secondary to respiratory failure due to constriction of the chest wall is an almost inevitable outcome. No effective treatment is known to date.

Radiographic Evaluation

Abnormalities of the thumb and great toe are present at birth and precede the soft tissue ossification. The characteristic radiologic changes consist of agenesis, microdactyly, or congenital hallux valgus, occasionally with fusion at the metacarpophalangeal or metatarsophalangeal joints (Fig. 28.33A). Short big toes and short thumbs

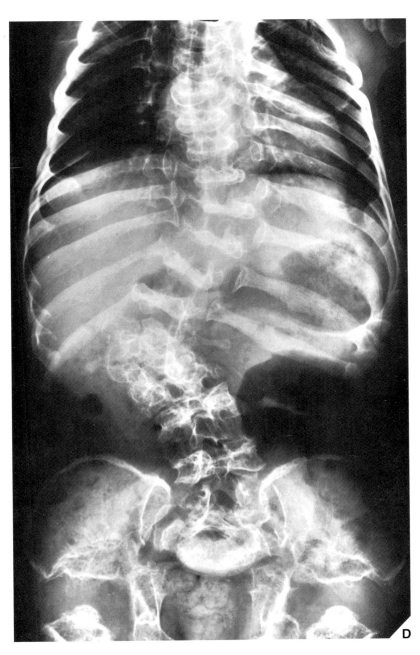

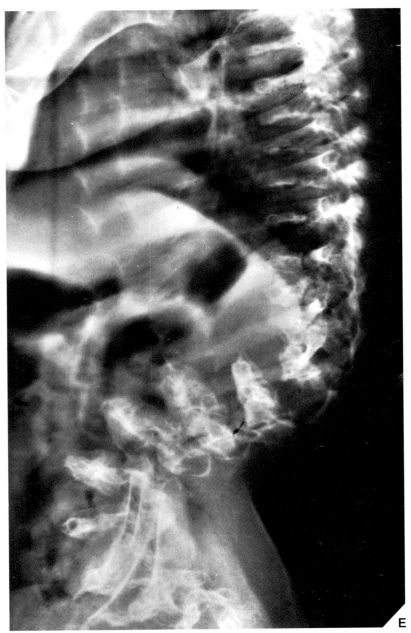

Figure 28.32 (continued) (D) Anteroposterior view of the spine shows marked kyphoscoliosis. The vertebrae are grossly deformed and flat (platyspondyly), and the ribs are wide but with narrow vertebral ends, giving them a characteristic "canoe-paddle" appearance. Note the pronounced osteoporosis. (E) Lateral view of the spine demonstrates hyperlordosis in the lumbar segment and kyphosis at the thoracolumbar junction. Note the shape of the vertebral bodies, with the characteristic irregular outline of the end plates and central, tongue-like or beak-like projections in the lumbar segment.

may be associated with clinodactyly of the fifth finger, as well as with brachydactyly. In the soft tissues, extensive ossifications are seen, along with bridging bony masses in the cervical and thoracic spine, the thorax, and the extremities (Fig. 28.33B). Involvement of the insertions of ligaments and tendons occasionally produces bony excrescences mimicking exostoses. Joint ankylosis results most often from ossification of the surrounding soft tissue, but a true intra-articular fusion may occur (Fig. 28.33C).

Histopathology

The pathologic abnormalities are similar to those of myositis ossificans circumscripta, but the zoning phenomenon of centripetal ossification is absent. The earliest histologic changes are edema and inflammatory exudate, followed by mesenchymal proliferation and formation of a large mass of collagen. This collagen is capable of accepting the deposition of calcium salts. Eventually, the lesion is transformed into irregular masses of lamellar and woven bone.

Sclerosing Dysplasias of Bone

The sclerosing bone dysplasias are a group of developmental anomalies that reflect disturbances in the formation and modeling of bone, most commonly as a result of inborn errors in metabolism. A common defect in many of these disorders is reflected in a failure of cartilage and/or bone to resorb during the process of skeletal maturation and remodeling. One defect in many cases involves the resorption capabilities of osteoclasts in the presence of normal osteoblastic activity. In other instances, the defect lies in excessive bone formation by osteoblasts, which may occur in the presence of normal or diminished osteoclastic activity. These basic errors in metabolism most commonly arise during the processes of endochondral and intramembranous ossification. All sclerosing dysplasias share the common feature of excessive bone accumulation resulting in the radiographic appear-

ance of increased bone density. Norman and Greenspan have developed a classification of these disorders based on the site of failure, whether endochondral or intramembranous, in skeletal development and maturation. Recently, Greenspan expanded and modified this classification (Fig. 28.34). The approach reflected in this classification is focused on target sites of involvement and pathomechanism of these dysplasias.

Osteopetrosis

An inherited disorder, osteopetrosis (also called Albers-Schönberg disease or marble-bone disease) involves a failure in resorption and remodeling of bone formed by endochondral ossification. The result is an excessive accumulation of primary spongiosa (calcified cartilage matrix) in the medullary portion of flat bones and both long and short tubular bones, as well as in the vertebrae. Until recently, two variants have been described. The infantile "malignant" autosomal-recessive form is recognized at birth or in early childhood, and if not treated by bone-marrow transplantation it is frequently fatal due to severe anemia secondary to substantial quantities of cartilage and immature bone packing the marrow cavity. The "benign" autosomal-dominant adult form, which is marked by sclerosis of the skeleton, is compatible with a long life span. More recent reports describe what appear to be additional variants of this developmental anomaly, which illustrate the heterogeneity of inheritance of osteopetrosis: intermediate-recessive type and autosomal-recessive type with tubular acidosis.

The radiographic hallmark of this disorder, as of all sclerosing bone dysplasias, is increased bone density. The radiographic examination also reveals a lack of differentiation between the cortex and the medullary cavity and occasionally a bone-in-bone appearance. The long and short tubular bones exhibit a club-like deformity and splaying of their ends secondary to a failure in remodeling (Figs. 28.35, 28.36). The same failure in the spine results in a charac-

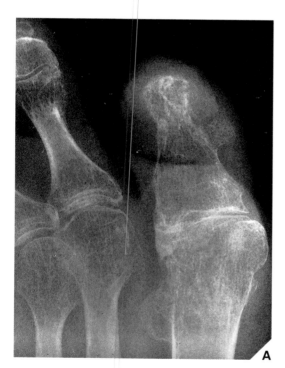
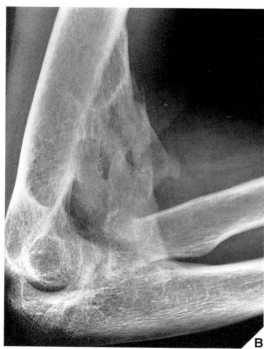
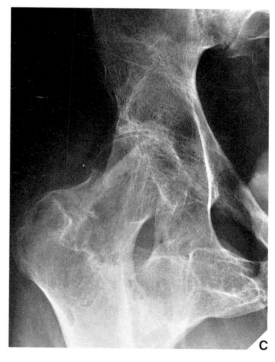

Figure 28.33 A 28-year-old man with fibrodysplasia ossificans progressiva diagnosed at age three. (A) Microdactyly of the great toe is a frequent feature of this disorder. (B) Lateral view of the elbow shows extensive ossification in the soft tissues, bridging the distal humerus to the radius and ulna. (C) Massive ossification around the hip accompanies the ankylosis of the hip joint.

Figure 28.34 Classification of Sclerosing Dysplasias of Bone

I. Dysplasias of Endochondral Bone Formation
•Affecting primary spongiosa (immature bone)
   Osteopetrosis (Albers-Schönberg disease)
     Autosomal-recessive type (lethal)
     Autosomal-dominant type
     Intermediate-recessive type
     Autosomal-recessive type with tubular acidosis (Sly disease)
   Pycnodysostosis (Maroteaux-Lamy disease)
•Affecting secondary spongiosa (mature bone)
   Enostosis (bond island)
   Osteopoikilosis (spotted bone disease)
   Osteopathia striata (Voorhoeve disease)

II. Dysplasias of Intramembranous Bone Formation
   Progressive diaphyseal dysplasia (Camurati-Engelmann disease)
   Hereditary multiple diaphyseal sclerosis (Ribbing disease)
   Endosteal hyperostosis (hyperostosis corticalis generalisata)
     Autosomal-recessive form
      van Buchem disease
      Sclerosteosis (Truswell-Hansen disease)
     Autosomal-dominant form
      Worth disease
      Nakamura disease

III. Mixed Sclerosing Dysplasias (Affecting Both Endochondral and Intramembranous Ossification)
•Affecting predominantly endochondral ossification
   Dysosteosclerosis
   Metaphyseal dysplasia (Pyle disease)
   Craniometaphyseal dysplasia
•Affecting predominantly intramembranous ossification
   Melorheostosis
   Progressive diaphyseal dysplasia with skull base involvement
     (Neuhauser variant)
   Craniodiaphyseal dysplasia
•Coexistence of two or more sclerosing bone dysplasias
     (overlap syndrome)
   Melorheostosis with osteopoikilosis and osteopathia striata
   Osteopathia striata with cranial sclerosis
     (Horan-Beighton syndrome)
   Osteopathia striata with osteopoikilosis and cranial sclerosis
   Osteopathia striata with generalized cortical hyperostosis
   Osteopathia striata with osteopetrosis
   Osteopoikilosis with progressive diaphyseal dysplasia

Reprinted with permission from Greenspan A, 1991

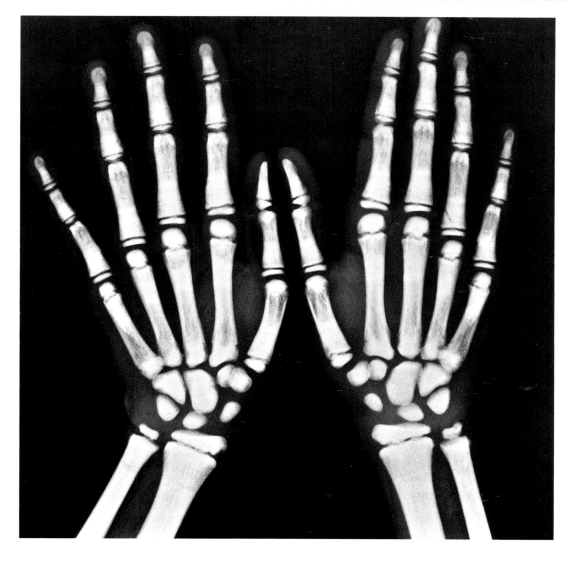

Figure 28.35 Dorsovolar film of both hands of a 7-year-old boy with osteopetrosis shows the dense sclerotic bones lacking differentiation between the cortex and medullary cavity that are characteristic of this condition. The metacarpals appear club-like due to a failure in bone remodeling.

teristic sandwich-like appearance of the vertebral bodies (Fig. 28.37). Osteopetrosis may occur in a cyclic pattern, with intervals of normal growth. This produces alternating bands of normal and abnormal bone in a ring-like pattern, which is particularly well demonstrated in the metaphysis of long bones and in flat bones such as the pelvis and scapula (Fig. 28.38).

Fractures are a frequent complication of osteopetrosis due to the brittleness of the bones.

Pycnodysostosis

Pycnodysostosis (Maroteaux-Lamy disease) is an inherited autosomal-recessive disorder whose skeletal manifestations result from a failure

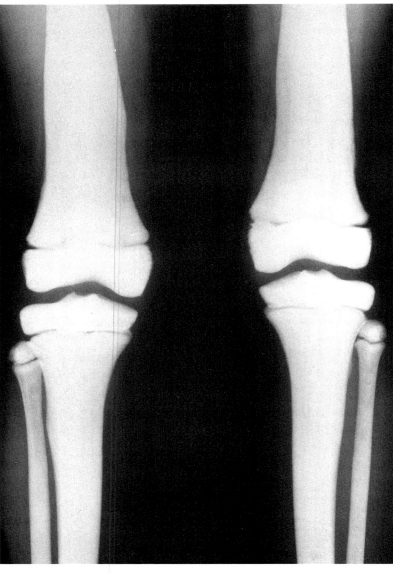

Figure 28.36 Anteroposterior view of the legs of a 10-year-old girl with osteopetrosis shows a uniform increase in bone density in the epiphyses, metaphyses, and diaphyses, with a lack of distinction between the cortical and medullary portions of the bones. The trabecular pattern is completely obliterated by the accumulation of immature bone. Note the splaying deformity of the distal femora and proximal tibiae as a result of remodeling failure.

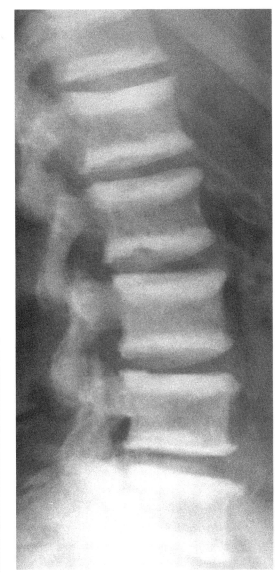

Figure 28.37 Lateral view of the thoracolumbar spine in a 14-year-old boy with osteopetrosis demonstrates the characteristic sandwich-like or "rugger-jersey" appearance seen in this disorder. Note the overall increase in bone density.

of resorption of primary spongiosa. Patients with this disease, like the artist Toulouse-Lautrec, have a disproportionately short stature, which becomes evident in early childhood. Unlike patients with osteopetrosis, however, those with pycnodysostosis are usually asymptomatic; a pathologic fracture may be the occasion of its discovery.

Radiographically, pycnodysostosis presents with the increased bone density common to all sclerosing bone dysplasias. Moreover, in the skull, there is persistence of the anterior and posterior fontanelles, wormian bones, and an obtuse angle to the ramus of the mandible (Fig. 28.39). The features distinguishing this disease from osteopetrosis are hypoplasia of the distal phalanges of the fingers and toes and resorption of the terminal tufts of the distal phalanges

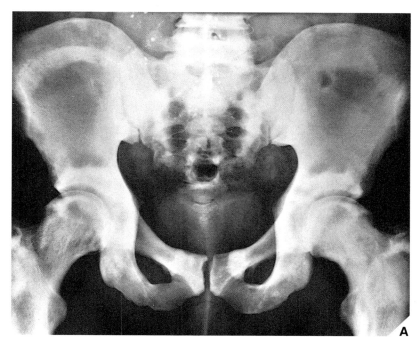

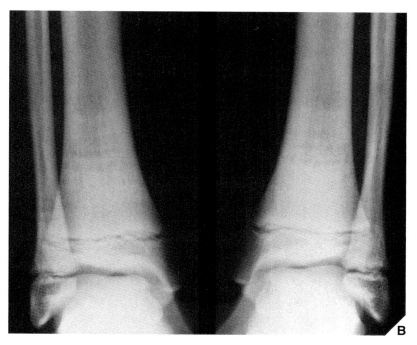

Figure 28.38 Radiographic examination of a 12-year-old girl with osteopetrosis demonstrates the cyclic pattern of this dysplasia. In the pelvis (A), alternating bands of normal (radiolucent) and abnormal (sclerotic) bone

are arranged in a ring-like pattern in both iliac wings. In both legs (B), the alternating sclerotic and radiolucent bands are seen in the distal diaphyses and metaphyses of the tibiae and fibulae.

Figure 28.39 Lateral view of the skull and facial bones of an 8-year-old pycnodysostotic patient shows persistence of the anterior and posterior fontanels and the obtuse (fetal) angle of the mandible, common manifestations of this disorder. (Courtesy of Dr. WE Berdon, New York, NY)

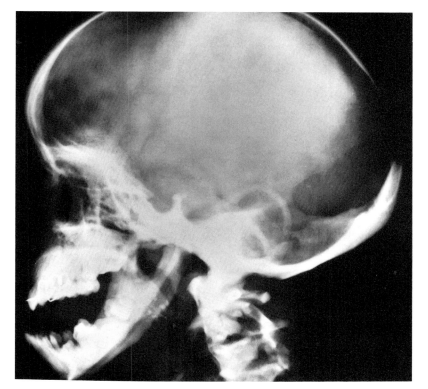

(Fig. 28.40). The latter feature, known as acro-osteolysis, may also be seen in a variety of other conditions, however.

Enostosis, Osteopoikilosis, and Osteopathia Striata

When endochondral ossification proceeds normally but mature bony trabeculae coalesce and fail to resorb and remodel, the resulting developmental anomalies are referred to as enostosis (bone island), osteopoikilosis, or osteopathia striata. The exact mode of inheritance of each is not known, but all three are probably transmitted as autosomal-dominant traits. The most common and mildest of the three is enostosis (Fig. 28.41), which is asymptomatic; it is important,

however, to differentiate this condition from an osteoid osteoma (see Figs. 15.21, 16.11) or from osteoblastic bone metastasis. Osteopoikilosis (osteopathia condensans disseminata, or "spotted-bone" disease) is also an asymptomatic disorder, and it is characterized by multiple bone islands symmetrically distributed and clustered near the articular ends of a bone (Fig. 28.42). Although plain-film radiography is usually sufficient to make a diagnosis, questionable cases may require radionuclide imaging, which is diagnostic. In osteopoikilosis a bone scan is relatively normal, unlike in metastatic disease, which invariably shows an increased uptake of radiopharmaceutical.

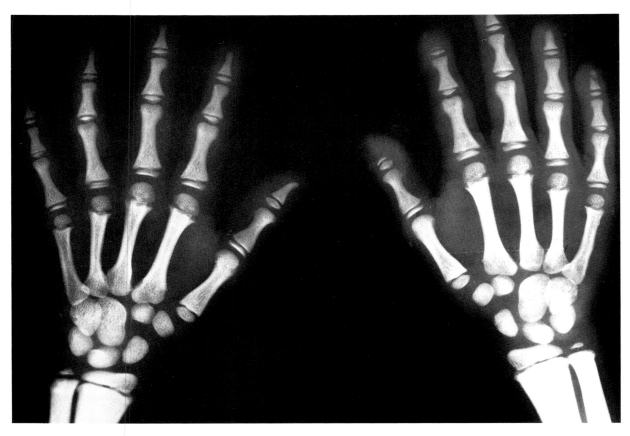

Figure 28.40 Dorsovolar projection of both hands of an 8-year-old boy with pycnodysostosis shows resorption of the terminal phalangeal tufts (acro-osteolysis), a feature differentiating this condition from osteopetrosis. (Courtesy of Dr. J Dorst, Baltimore, Md)

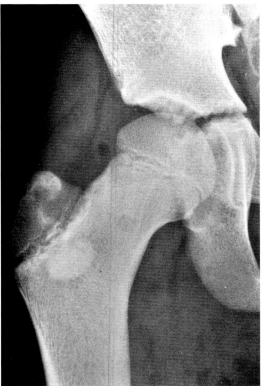

Figure 28.41 Anteroposterior view of the right hip of a 10-year-old boy who was examined for an injury to the hip reveals, as an incidental finding, a giant bone island in the femoral neck, which was completely asymptomatic.

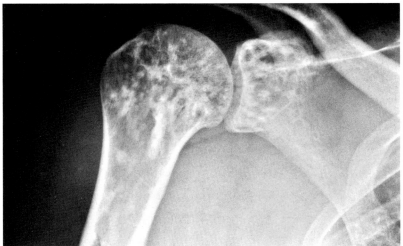

Figure 28.42 Anteroposterior radiograph of the shoulder of a 34-year-old man who had pain in his right shoulder following an automobile accident shows no fracture or dislocation. However, multiple sclerotic foci representing lesions of osteopoikilosis are apparent, scattered near the articular ends of the scapula and humerus. A subsequent bone survey showed extensive involvement of the skeleton, especially the hands, wrists, and pelvis.

Histologically, both enostoses and the lesions of osteopoikilosis are characterized by foci of compact bone scattered in the spongiosa, with prominent cement lines and occasionally a Haversian system. Clinically, osteopoikilosis must be distinguished from more severe disorders such as mastocytosis and tuberous sclerosis, as well as from osteoblastic metastatic lesions.

Osteopathia striata, the least common disorder in this group, is an asymptomatic lesion marked by fine or coarse linear striations, chiefly in the long bones and at sites of rapid growth such as the knee (Fig. 28.43) and shoulder. Several authors postulate a relationship between this disorder and osteopoikilosis; some suggest that it is in fact a variant of osteopoikilosis.

Progressive Diaphyseal Dysplasia
Failure of bone resorption and remodeling at the sites of intramembranous ossification (such as the cortex of tubular bones, the vault of the skull, the mandible, or the midsegment of the clavicle) is the abnormality typically noted in progressive diaphyseal dysplasia, also called Camurati-Engelmann disease. Like enostosis, osteopoikilosis, and osteopathia striata, this is an autosomal-dominant disorder with considerable variability of expression. Clinically, it is characterized by growth retardation, muscle wasting, pain and weakness in the extremities, and a waddling gait.

Because of its striking tendency toward symmetric involvement of the extremities, with characteristic sparing of the epiphysis and metaphysis (the sites of endochondral ossification), progressive diaphyseal dysplasia is recognized radiographically by symmetric fusiform thickening of the cortices of the long bone shafts, particularly in the lower extremities (Fig. 28.44).

A familial disorder similar to progressive diaphyseal dysplasia, described by Ribbing and later by Paul, is generally asymptomatic and exhibits limited asymmetric involvement, usually only of the long bones. Known as *hereditary multiple diaphyseal sclerosis*, this condition is generally believed to be the same disorder as Camurati-Engelmann disease.

Melorheostosis
A rare condition of unknown etiology, melorheostosis (Leri disease) shows no evidence of hereditary features. It belongs to a group of bone disorders called the mixed sclerosing dysplasias, which combine characteristics of both endochondral and intramembranous failure of ossification. The presenting symptom is pain intensified by activity. Limitation of joint motion and stiffness are common, due to contractures, soft tissue fibrosis, and periarticular bone formation in the soft tissues. It may be monostotic *(forme fruste)* or polyostotic, affecting an entire limb.

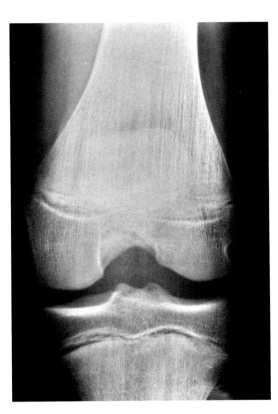

Figure 28.43 Anteroposterior view of the right knee of a 14-year-old girl who had a history of trauma reveals, as an incidental finding, fine linear striations in the diaphysis and metaphysis of the distal femur and proximal tibia, characteristic of osteopathia striata; the epiphyses, however, are spared.

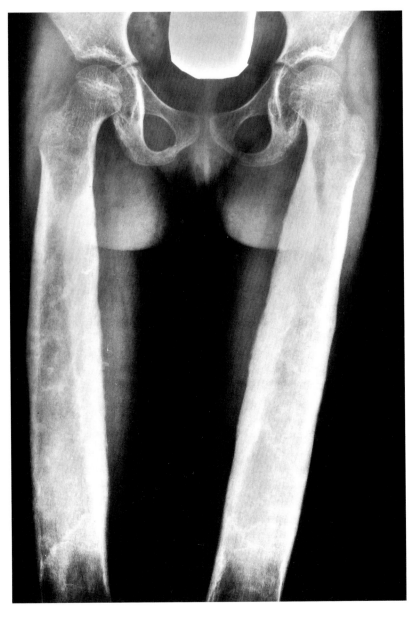

Figure 28.44
Anteroposterior view of the hips and upper femora of an 8-year-old boy with Camurati-Engelmann disease shows symmetric fusiform thickening of the cortices. Note that only the sites of intramembranous bone formation are affected, while the sites of endochondral bone formation are spared. (Courtesy of Dr. WE Berdon, New York, NY)

Standard radiography is sufficient to make a diagnosis. The lesion is characterized by a wavy hyperostosis that resembles melted wax dripping down the side of a candle, the feature from which the disease derives its name (Greek *melos*-member; *rhein*-flow); moreover, only one side of the bone is usually involved (Fig. 28.45). Associated joint abnormalities are also well delineated on standard radiographs. Radionuclide bone scan can determine other sites of skeletal involvement by demonstrating abnormal uptake of radiopharmaceutical (see Fig. 26.15).

Other Mixed Sclerosing Dysplasias

The most common of the other mixed sclerosing dysplasias is the coexistence of melorheostosis, osteopathia striata, and osteopoikilosis. The radiographic features of this "overlap syndrome" are a combination of each of these three dysplasias (Fig. 28.46), a phenomenon suggesting a common pathogenetic mechanism.

The discussion of other sclerosing dysplasias, listed in Fig. 28.34, is beyond the scope of this text.

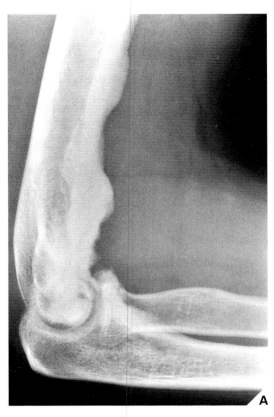

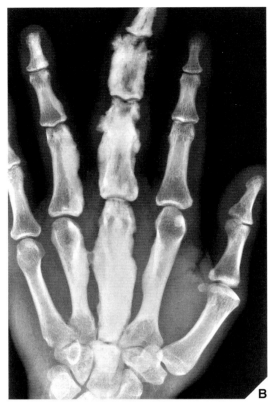

Figure 28.45 A 28-year-old man presented with pain in the right elbow and an enlargement of the middle finger of his right hand. (A) Lateral view of the elbow demonstrates a flowing hyperostosis of the anterior cortex of the distal humerus, typical of melorheostosis. Note the bridging of the joint by the lesion and the involvement of the coronoid process of the ulna. (B) Dorsovolar view of the right hand shows marked hypertrophy of the middle digit. The cortices (the sites of intramembranous ossification) are involved, as are the articular ends of the bones (the sites of endochondral ossification). This is characteristic of mixed sclerosing dysplasias.

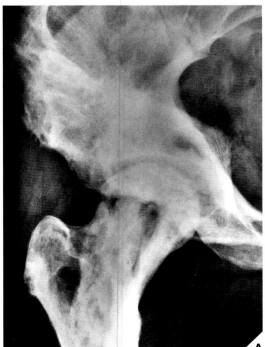

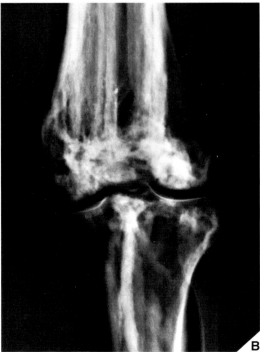

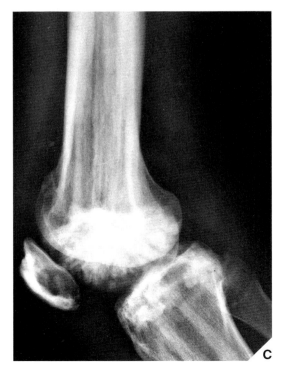

Figure 28.46 These radiographic studies in an 18-year-old male demonstrate the coexistence of melorheostosis with osteopoikilosis and osteopathia striata. (A) Anteroposterior view of the right hemipelvis and hip shows the wavy hyperostosis typical of melorheostosis affecting the iliac bone and proximal femur. Anteroposterior (B) and lateral (C) views of the knee demonstrate the linear striations characteristic of osteopathia striata in the distal femur and proximal tibia, as well as the focal densities that are the identifying feature of osteopoikilosis. (Reproduced with permission from Norman A, Greenspan A, 1986)

PRACTICAL POINTS TO REMEMBER

Scoliosis

[1] Congenital scoliosis may result from:
- a failure of vertebral formation, which may be unilateral and partial (wedged vertebra) or unilateral and complete (hemivertebra)
- a failure of segmentation, which may be unilateral (unsegmented bar) or bilateral (block vertebra)
- failures of both formation and segmentation.

[2] Idiopathic scoliosis, the most prevalent type of scoliosis (70%), can be divided into infantile (M > F), juvenile (M = F), and adolescent (M < F) categories. In the last type, the structural (major) curve is located in the thoracic or thoracolumbar segment, with its convexity to the right.

[3] In the evaluation of scoliosis, the shape of the curve usually indicates the variant, so that:
- an S-shaped curve is common in idiopathic scoliosis
- a C-shaped curve indicates the neuromuscular variant
- scoliosis marked by a sharply angled short spinal segment is most commonly congenital in origin (e.g., neurofibromatosis, hemivertebra).

[4] The scoliotic curve is described as composed of:
- a structural (major or primary) curve demarcated by upper and lower (transitional) end-vertebrae
- compensatory (secondary) curves proximal and distal to the transitional vertebrae
- an apical vertebra showing the most rotation and wedging, and whose center is most displaced from the central spinal line.

[5] Several methods for measuring the scoliotic curve are available:
- the Lippmann-Cobb method, in which the angle is determined only by the inclination of the end-vertebrae of the curve
- the Risser-Ferguson method, which utilizes three points as determinants of the curve—the centers of the upper and lower end-vertebrae and of the apical vertebra
- the scoliotic index method, which measures the deviation of each vertebra in the scoliotic curve from the central spinal line.

[6] To assure accuracy in determining the degree of correction of a scoliotic curve, the same measuring points should be used in comparing the pre- and post-treatment curvature, even if the end-vertebrae have changed their locations.

[7] The rotation of a vertebral body can be evaluated on the anteroposterior view by:
- the Cobb method, which uses the position of the spinous process as a point of reference
- the Moe method, which uses the pedicles as points of reference.

[8] The determination of skeletal maturity, an important factor in the prognosis and treatment of congenital scoliosis, may be made by:
- comparison of a radiograph of a patient's wrist and hand with standards in radiographic atlases
- evaluation of the ossification of the vertebral ring apophysis or iliac crest apophysis

Anomalies With General Affect on the Skeleton

[1] The skeletal abnormalities frequently encountered in neurofibromatosis include:
- extrinsic cortical erosions
- pseudoarthroses, particularly in the tibia and fibula
- short segment kyphoscoliosis marked by acute angulation in the lower cervical and upper thoracic spine
- enlarged neural foramina and scalloping of the posterior aspect of vertebral bodies.

[2] Malignant transformation to sarcoma is the most serious complication of the plexiform variant of neurofibromatosis.

[3] The radiographic hallmarks of osteogenesis imperfecta, a disorder characterized by excessive fragility of the bones, include:
- severe osteoporosis
- thinning of the cortices
- bone deformities, such as trumpet-shaped metaphyses
- kyphoscoliosis
- multiple fractures.

[4] Radiographically, achondroplasia is characterized by:
- rhizomelic (disproportional) dwarfism
- a configuration of the hemipelves resembling ping-pong paddles and a "champagne-glass" appearance of the inner pelvic contour
- narrowing of the interpedicular distance in the lumbar spine (spinal stenosis)
- scalloping of the posterior aspect of vertebral bodies.

[5] The various disorders constituting the mucopolysaccharidoses share common radiographic features:
- osteoporosis
- oval or hook-shaped vertebral bodies
- an abnormal configuration of the pelvis
- shortened tubular bones.

[6] Fibrodysplasia ossificans progressiva (myositis ossificans progressiva) is characterized by extensive ossifications of the muscular structures and subcutaneous tissues, leading to joint ankylosis and constriction of the chest wall. Congenital abnormalities of the thumb and great toe (agenesis, microdactyly, etc.) should alert the radiologist to the possibility of this severely crippling disorder.

[7] The sclerosing bone dysplasias share the radiographic feature of increased bone density.

[8] The radiographic hallmarks of osteopetrosis and pycnodysostosis, disorders related to the failure of endochondral ossification, are:
- a uniformly increased bone density
- the absence of remodeling
- obliteration of the boundary between the medullary cavity and cortex.

Pathologic fractures are common.

[9] The specific changes characteristic of pycnodysostosis include:
- acro-osteolysis
- obtuse angle of the mandible
- persistence of the fontanelles
- wormian bones.

[10] Enostosis, osteopoikilosis, and osteopathia striata, conditions also related to a failure of endochondral ossification, are characterized radiographically by:
- foci of sclerotic, mature bone in the medullary cavity (enostosis and osteopoikilosis)
- fine linear striations (osteopathia striata) at sites of rapid bone growth.

[11] Progressive diaphyseal dysplasia and hereditary multiple diaphyseal sclerosis, conditions related to the failure of intramembranous ossification, are recognized radiographically by thickening of the cortices of the long bones. The articular ends of the bones are, as a rule, not affected.

[12] Melorheostosis, a mixed sclerosing bone dysplasia marked by failure of both endochondral and intramembranous ossification, is recognized radiographically by a flowing hyperostosis ("wax drippings") associated with involvement of the surrounding soft tissues and joint.

References

Ablin DS, Greenspan A, Reinhart M, Grix A: Differentiation of child abuse from osteogenesis imperfecta. *Am J Roentgenol* 154:1035, 1990.

Abrahamson MN: Disseminated asymptomatic osteosclerosis with features resembling melorheostosis, osteopoikilosis and osteopathia striata. *J Bone Joint Surg* 50A:991, 1968.

Andersen PE Jr, Bollerslev J: Heterogeneity of autosomal dominant osteopetrosis. *Radiology* 164:223, 1987.

Bailey JA II: Orthopedic aspects of achondroplasia. *J Bone Joint Surg* 52A:1285, 1970.

Bauze RJ, Smith R, Francis JO: A new look at osteogenesis imperfecta. *J Bone Joint Surg* 57B:2, 1975.

Beighton P, Cremin BJ, Hamersma H: The radiology of sclerosteosis. *Br J Radiol* 49:934, 1976.

Beighton P: *Inherited Disorders of the Skeleton*. Edinburgh, Churchill-Livingstone, 1978.

Beighton P, Cremin BJ: *Sclerosing Bone Dysplasias*. Berlin-Heidelberg-New York, Springer-Verlag, 1984.

Campbell CJ, Papademetriou T, Bonfiglio M: Melorheostosis. A report of the clinical, roentgenographic and pathological findings in fourteen cases. *J Bone Joint Surg* 50A:1281, 1968.

Carlsen DH: Osteopathic striata revisited. *Can Assoc Radiol J* 28:190, 1977.

Cobb JR: Outline for the study of scoliosis. Instructional Course Lectures. *Am Acad Orthop Surgeons* 5:261, 1948.

Connor J, Evans DA: Genetic aspects of fibrodysplasia ossificans progressiva. *J Med Genet* 19:35, 1982.

Connor J, Evans DA: Fibrodysplasia ossificans progressiva. *J Bone Joint Surg* 64B:76, 1982.

Cremin B, Connor J, Beighton P: The radiological spectrum of fibrodysplasia ossificans progressiva. *Clin Radiol* 33:499, 1982.

D'Agostino A, Soule E, Miller R: Sarcomas of the peripheral nerves and somatic tissue associated with multiple neurofibromatosis (von Recklinghausen's disease). *Cancer* 16:1015, 1963.

Eggli KD: The mucopolysaccharidoses. In: Taveras JM, Ferrucci JT (eds): *Radiology—Diagnosis, Imaging, Intervention*. Philadelphia, Lippincott, 1986.

Elmore SM: Pycnodysostosis. A review. *J Bone Joint Surg* 49A:153, 1967.

Fairbank, HAT: *An Atlas of General Affections of the Skeleton*. Edinburgh, Livingstone, 1951.

Falvo KA, Root L, Bullough PG: Osteogenesis imperfecta: Clinical evaluation and management. *J Bone Joint Surg* 56A:783, 1974.

Felson B: Dwarfs and other little people. *Semin Roentgenol* 8:133, 1973.

Gehweiler JA, Bland WR, Carden TS Jr, Daffner RH: Osteopathia striata—Voorhoeve's disease: Review of the roentgen manifestations. *Am J Roentgenol* 118:450, 1973.

George K, Rippstein JA: A comparative study of the two popular methods of measuring scoliotic deformity of the spine. *J Bone Joint Surg* 43A:809, 1961.

Gertner JM, Root L: Osteogenesis imperfecta. *Orthop Clin North Am* 21:151, 1990.

Goldstein LA, Waugh TR: Classification and terminology of scoliosis. *Clin Orthop* 93:10, 1973.

Greenspan A, Pugh JW, Norman A, Norman RS: Scoliotic index: A comparative evaluation of methods for the measurement of scoliosis. *Bull Hosp Jt Dis Orthop Inst* 39:117, 1978.

Greenspan A, Steiner G, Knutzon R: Bone island (enostosis): Clinical significance and radiologic and pathologic correlations. *Skeletal Radiol* 20:85, 1990.

Greenspan A: Sclerosing bone dysplasias—a target sites approach. *Skeletal Radiol* 1991 (in press).

Harrington PR, Dickson JM: An eleven-year clinical investigation of Harrington instrumentation: A preliminary report on 578 cases. *Clin Orthop* 93:113, 1973.

Hoppenfeld S, *Scoliosis: A Manual of Concept and Treatment*. Philadelphia, Lippincott, 1967.

Hundley JD, Wilson FC: Progressive diaphyseal dysplasia. Review of the literature and report of seven cases in one family. *J Bone Joint Surg* 55A:461, 1973.

Jacobson HG: Dense bone—too much bone: Radiological considerations and differential diagnosis. Part I. *Skeletal Radiol* 13:1, 1985.

Kaftori JK, Kleinhaus U, Naveh Y: Progressive diaphyseal dysplasia (Camurati-Engelmann): Radiographic follow-up and CT findings. *Radiology* 164:777, 1987.

Klatte EC, Franken EA, Smith JA: The radiographic spectrum in neurofibromatosis. *Semin Roentgenol* 11:17, 1976.

Kleinman PK: Differentiation of child abuse and osteogenesis imperfecta: Medical and legal implications. *Am J Roentgenol* 154:1047, 1990.

Lagier R, Mbakop A, Bigler A: Osteopoikilosis: A radiological and pathological study. *Skeletal Radiol* 11:161, 1984.

Langer LO Jr, Baumann PA, Gorlin RJ: Achondroplasia. *Am J Roentgenol* 100:12, 1967.

MacEven GD, Conway JJ, Miller WT: Congenital scoliosis with a unilateral bar. *Radiology* 90:711, 1968.

McKusick V: *Hereditary Disorders of Connective Tissue*, ed 4. St. Louis, Mosby, 1972.

Norman A: Myositis ossifcans and fibrodysplasia ossificans progressiva. In: Taveras JM, Ferrucci JT (eds): *Radiology—Diagnosis, Imaging, Intervention, vol 5*. Philadelphia, Lippincott, 1986, chapter 132.

Norman A, Greenspan A: Bone dysplasias. In: Jahss MH (ed): *Disorders of the Foot, vol. 1*. Philadelphia, Saunders, 1982.

Norman A, Greenspan A: Sclerosing dysplasias of bone. In: Taveras JM, Ferrucci JT (eds): *Radiology—Diagnosis, Imaging, Intervention, vol 5*. Philadelphia, Lippincott, 1986.

Norman A, Greenspan A: Bone dysplasias. In: Jahss MH (ed): *Disorders of the Foot and Ankle. Medical and Surgical Management, vol I*. Philadelphia, Saunders, 1991.

Ozonoff M: *Pediatric Orthopaedic Radiology*. Philadelphia, Saunders, 1979.

Palmer PES, Thomas JEP: Case reports. Osteopetrosis with unusual changes in the skull and digits. *Br J Radiol* 31:705, 1958.

Paul LW: Hereditary, multiple, diphyseal sclerosis (Ribbing). *Radiology* 60:412, 1953.

Resnick D, Nemcek AA Jr, Haghighi P: Spinal enostoses (bone islands). *Radiology* 147:373, 1983.

Ribbing S: Hereditary, multiple, diaphyseal sclerosis. *Acta Radiol* 31:522, 1949.

Riccardi VM: von Recklinghausen's neurofibromatosis. *N Engl J Med* 305:1617, 1981.

Rubin P: *Dynamic Classification of Bone Dysplasias.* Chicago, Year Book Medical Publishers, 1964.

Schwartz A, Ramos R: Neurofibromatosis and multiple nonossifying fibromas. *Am J Roentgenol* 135:617, 1980.

Sillence DO: Osteogenesis imperfecta: An expanding panorama of variants. *Clin Orthop* 159:11, 1981.

Sillence DO, Senn A, Danks DM: Genetic heterogeneity in osteogenesis imperfecta. *J Med Genet* 16:101, 1979.

Silverman BJ, Greenbarg PE: Internal fixation of the spine for idiopathic scoliosis using square-ended distraction rods and lamina wiring (Harrington-Luque technique). *Bull Hosp Jt Dis Orthop Inst* 44:41, 1984.

Spranger JW, Langer LO Jr, Wiederman HR: *Bone Dysplasias. An Atlas of Constitutional Disorders of Skeletal Development.* Philadelphia, Saunders, 1974.

Stevenson R, Howell R, McKusick V, et al: The iduronidase deficient mucopolysaccharidoses: Clinical and roentgenographic features. *Pediatrics* 57:111, 1976.

Taitz LS: Child abuse and osteogenesis imperfecta. *Br Med J* 295:1082, 1987.

Walker GF: Mixed sclerosing bone dystrophies. *J Bone Joint Surg* 46B:546, 1964.

Whyte MP, Murphy WA, Siegel BA: ^{99m}Tc-pyrophosphate bone imaging in osteopoikilosis, osteopathic striata and melorheostosis. *Radiology* 127:439, 1978.

Whyte MP, Murphy WA, Fallon MD, Hahn TJ: Mixed-sclerosing-bone-dystrophy: Report of a case and review of the literature. *Skeletal Radiol* 6:95, 1981.

Winter RB, Moe JH, Eilers VE: Congenital scoliosis. A study of 234 patients treated and untreated. *J Bone Joint Surg* 50A: 1, 1968.

Wynne-Davies R, Fairbank TJ: *Fairbank's Atlas of General Affections of the Skeleton,* ed 2. New York, Churchill-Livingstone, 1976.

Yaghmai I: Spine changes in neurofibromatosis. *Radiology* 6:261, 1986.

Index

Note: The numbers in **boldface** type refer to Figure numbers.

A

Achondroplasia, 28.17–28.18, **28.19, 28.28–28.30**
Acquired immune deficiency syndrome (AIDS), 14.14
Acromegaly, **12.15**, 14.13, 25.1–25.6, **25.3**
    practical points to remember, 25.14
    radiographic evaluation, 25.4–25.6, **25.4–25.8**
Acromioclavicular separation, 5.21–5.22, **5.37–5.40**
Adamantinoma, 17.11, 18.25, **18.46, 18.47**
Adhesive capsulitis, 5.21, **5.36**
AIDS. *See* Acquired immune deficiency syndrome
Albers-Schönberg disease. *See* Osteopetrosis
Albright-McCune syndrome, **17.19**
ALD. *See* Serum creatine phosphokinase
Alkaptonuria (ochronosis), 14.12, **14.17**
Amyloidosis, 14.13–14.14, **14.18**
Aneurysmal bone cyst, 17.15–17.17, **17.30–17.33**
    treatment, 17.17, **17.34**
Angiography, 2.6, **4.10, 15.13–15.15**
Ankle and foot
    ancillary imaging techniques for evaluating
        injury to, **9.26**
    anatomic-radiologic considerations, 9.1–9.14, **9.1–9.27**
    complications, 9.38
    injury to the ankle, 9.16–9.31, **9.28, 9.29**
        fractures about the ankle joint, 9.16–9.25, **9.30**
            classification, 9.18
                bimalleolar, **9.32**
                complex fractures, **9.34**
                trimalleolar, **9.33**
                unimalleolar, **9.31**
            fracture of the distal tibia, 9.18–9.23
                pylon fracture, 9.18–9.20, **9.35**
                Tillaux fracture, 9.20–9.22, **9.36–9.38**
                triplanar (Marmor-Lynn) fracture, 9.22–9.23,
                    9.40–9.42
            fractures of the fibula, 9.23–9.25, **9.43**
                Dupuytren fracture, 9.23, **9.44**
                Maisonneuve fracture, 9.25, **9.45, 9.46**
                Pott fracture, 9.23
             triplanar (Marmor-Lynn) fracture, 9.22–9.23
            Wagstaffe-LeFort fracture, 9.22, **9.39**
        injury to the soft tissues about the ankle joint and
            foot, 9.25–9.31, **9.28, 9.29, 9.47–9.50**
            tear of the distal anterior tibiofibular ligament,
                9.29–9.31, **9.56, 9.57**
            tear of the lateral collateral ligament, 9.27–9.29,
                9.28, 9.52–9.55
            tear of the medial collateral ligament, 9.26–9.27,
                9.29, 9.51
            tendon ruptures, 9.29–9.31, **9.58–9.60**
        Lauge-Hansen classification of ankle injuries, **9.47**
    injury to the foot, 9.31–9.38
        dislocations in the foot, 9.36–9.38
            in the subtalar joint, 9.37

peritalar, 9.37, **9.70**
        total talar, 9.37
        tarsometatarsal, 9.37–9.38, **9.71, 9.72**
    fractures of the foot, 9.31–9.36
        fractures of the calcaneus, 9.31–9.32, **9.61–9.65**
        fractures of the talus, 9.35, **9.66, 9.67**
        Jones fracture, 9.35–9.36, **9.68, 9.69**
  practical points to remember, 9.39
  standard and special radiographic projections for
    evaluating injury to the ankle and foot, **9.25**
Arthritides
  clinical and radiographic hallmarks of metabolic,
    endocrine, and miscellaneous, **14.9**
  connective tissue, 14.1–14.9
    clinical and radiographic hallmarks of, **14.1**
    mixed (MCTD), 14.6–14.8
    polymyositis and dermatomyositis, 14.6
    scleroderma, 14.5–14.6, **14.6–14.8**
    systemic lupus erythematosus (SLE), 14.1–14.5,
      14.2–14.5
    vasculitis, 14.8–14.9
  infectious, **11.21, 11.23**, 19.2, **19.3**, 20.7–20.11
    nonpyogenic joint infections, 20.9–20.11
        other infectious arthritides, 20.9–20.11, **20.20**
        tuberculous arthritis, 20.9, **20.17–20.19**
    practical points to remember, 20.18
    pyogenic joint infections, 20.7–20.9, **20.15, 20.16**
        complications, **19.16**, 20.9
  inflammatory. *See* Inflammatory arthritides
  metabolic and endocrine, 14.9–14.13, **14.9**
    acromegaly, **12.15**, 14.13
    alkaptonuria (ochronosis), 14.12, **14.17**
    CHA crystal deposition disease, 14.10–14.11, **14.15**
    CPPD crystal deposition disease, 14.10
        clinical features, 14.10
        radiographic features, 14.10, **14.14**
    gout, 14.9–14.10
        examination of synovial fluid, 14.9
        hyperuricemia, 14.9
        radiographic features, 14.9–14.10, **14.10–14.13**
    hemochromotosis, **12.16**, 14.11–14.12, **14.16**
    hyperparathyroidism, 14.12–14.13
  miscellaneous arthropathies, 14.13–14.14
    and acquired immune deficiency syndrome
      (AIDS), 14.14
    amyloidosis, 14.13–14.14, **14.18**
    hemophilia, **11.16**, 14.14, **14.19**
    infectious, 14.14
    Jaccoud arthritis, 14.14
    multicentric reticulohistiocytosis, 14.14
  posttraumatic, 4.28, **4.58, 4.59**
  practical points to remember, 14.16
  radiologic evaluation of, 11.1–11.31, **11.1**
    diagnosis, 11.12–11.25
        clinical information, 11.12–11.13
        radiographic features, 11.13–11.25, **11.17–11.22**
            distribution of the articular lesion,
              11.24–11.25, **11.38**

Q

R

S

U

V

W

Y